18th Edition

HARRISON'S®

Principles of
INTERNAL
MEDICINE

SELF-ASSESSMENT
AND BOARD REVIEW

Editorial Board

18th Edition

HARRISON'S®
Principles of INTERNAL MEDICINE

SELF-ASSESSMENT AND BOARD REVIEW

For use with the 18th edition of HARRISON'S PRINCIPLES OF INTERNAL MEDICINE

EDITED BY

CHARLES M. WIENER, MD

Dean/CEO
Perdana University Graduate School of Medicine
Selangor, Malaysia
Professor of Medicine and Physiology
Johns Hopkins University School of Medicine
Baltimore, Maryland

CYNTHIA D. BROWN, MD

Assistant Professor of Medicine
Division of Pulmonary and Critical Care Medicine
University of Virginia
Charlottesville, Virginia

ANNA R. HEMNES, MD

Assistant Professor, Division of Allergy, Pulmonary,
 and Critical Care Medicine
Vanderbilt University Medical Center
Nashville, Tennessee

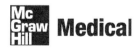

New York   Chicago   San Francisco   Lisbon   London   Madrid   Mexico City
Milan   New Delhi   San Juan   Seoul   Singapore   Sydney   Toronto

Harrison's®
PRINCIPLES OF INTERNAL MEDICINE, 18th Edition

1 2 3 4 5 6 7 8 9 0   QDB/QDB   17 16 15 14 13 12

ISBN 978-0-07-177195-5
MHID 0-07-177195-6
ISSN 2167-7808

Notice

Medicine is an ever-changing science. As new research and clinical experience broaden our knowledge, changes in treatment and drug therapy are required. The authors and the publisher of this work have checked with sources believed to be reliable in their efforts to provide information that is complete and generally in accord with the standards accepted at the time of publication. However, in view of the possibility of human error or changes in medical sciences, neither the authors nor the publisher nor any other party who has been involved in the preparation or publication of this work warrants that the information contained herein is in every respect accurate or complete, and they disclaim all responsibility for any errors or omissions or for the results obtained from use of the information contained in this work. Readers are encouraged to confirm the information contained herein with other sources. For example and in particular, readers are advised to check the product information sheet included in the package of each drug they plan to administer to be certain that the information contained in this work is accurate and that changes have not been made in the recommended dose or in the contraindications for administration. This recommendation is of particular importance in connection with new or infrequently used drugs.

This book was set in Minion Pro by Cenveo Publisher Services.
The editors were James F. Shanahan and Kim J. Davis.
The production supervisor was Catherine H. Saggese.
Project management was provided by Manisha Singh of Cenveo Publisher Services.
Quad/Graphics was the printer and binder.

This book is printed on acid-free paper.

International Edition ISBN 978-0-07-178847-2; MHID 0-07-178847-6. Copyright © 2012. Exclusive rights by The McGraw-Hill Companies, Inc., for manufacture and export. This book cannot be re-exported from the country to which it is consigned by McGraw-Hill. The International Edition is not available in North America.

McGraw-Hill books are available at special quantity discounts to use as premiums and sales promotions, or for use in corporate training programs. To contact a representative please e-mail us at bulksales@mcgraw-hill.com.

CONTENTS

PREFACE

This is the third edition of *Harrison's Self-Assessment and Board Review* that we have had the honor of working on. We thank the editors of the 18th edition of *Harrison's Principles of Internal Medicine* for their continued confidence in our ability to produce a worthwhile companion to their exceptional textbook. It is truly inspirational to remind ourselves why we love medicine broadly, and internal medicine specifically.

The care of patients is a privilege. As physicians, we owe it to our patients to be intelligent, contemporary, and curious. Continuing education takes many forms; many of us enjoy the intellectual stimulation and active learning challenge of the question-answer format. It is in that spirit that we offer the 18th edition of the *Self-Assessment and Board Review* to students, housestaff, and practitioners. We hope that from it you will learn, read, investigate, and question. The questions and answers are particularly conducive to collaboration and discussion with colleagues. This edition contains over 1100 questions that, whenever possible, utilize realistic patient scenarios including radiographic or pathologic images. Similarly, our answers attempt to explain the correct or best choice, often supported with figures from the 18th edition of *Harrison's Principles of Internal Medicine* to stimulate learning.

All of the authors have physically left the Osler Medical Service at Johns Hopkins Hospital. However, our experiences with colleagues and patients at Hopkins have defined our professional lives. In the words of William Osler, *"We are here to add what we can to life, not to get what we can from life."* We hope this addition to your life stimulates your mind, challenges your thinking, and translates to your patients.

Of course, none of this would be possible without the loving support of our families, for which we are truly thankful. They were patient and encouraging as we transformed (often not quietly) a mountain of page proofs into this book.

SECTION I

Introduction to Clinical Medicine

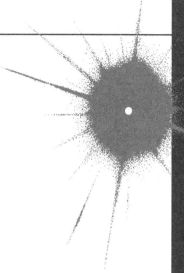

QUESTIONS

DIRECTIONS: Choose the **one best** response to each question.

I-1. Which of the following is the best definition of evidence-based medicine?

   A. A summary of existing data from existing clinical trials with a critical methodological review and statistical analysis of summative data

   B. A type of research that compares the results of one approach to treating a disease with another approach to treating the same disease

   C. Clinical decision making support tools developed by professional organizations that include expert opinions and data from clinical trials

   D. Clinical decision making supported by data, preferably from randomized controlled clinical trials

   E. One physician's clinical experience in caring for multiple patients with a specific disorder over many years

I-2. All of the following are part of the informed consent process EXCEPT:

   A. Alternatives and likely consequences of the alternatives to the procedure

   B. Ascertainment of understanding by the patient

   C. Discussion of the details of the procedure

   D. Outlining the patient's wishes if he or she becomes unable to make decisions

   E. Risks and benefits of the procedure

I-3. Which of the following is the standard measure for determining the impact of a health condition on a population?

   A. Disability-adjusted life years

   B. Infant mortality

   C. Life expectancy

   D. Standardized mortality ratio

   E. Years of life lost

I-4. In high-income countries, what category of disease accounts for the greatest percentage of disability-adjusted life years lost?

   A. Alcohol abuse

   B. Chronic obstructive pulmonary disease

   C. Diabetes mellitus

   D. Ischemic heart disease

   E. Unipolar depressive disorders

I-5. What is the leading cause of death in low-income countries?

   A. Diarrheal diseases

   B. Human immunodeficiency virus

   D. Ischemic heart disease

   D. Lower respiratory disease

   E. Malaria

I-6. You are working with the public health minister of Malawi in a project to decrease malarial deaths in children younger than 5 years of age. All of the following strategies are part of the World Health Organization Roll Back Malaria plan EXCEPT:

   A. Artemisinin-based combination therapy

   B. Early treatment with chloroquine alone

   C. Indoor residual spraying

   D. Insecticide-treated bed nets

   E. Intermittent preventive treatment during pregnancy

I-7. A 38-year-old woman is evaluated for chest pain. She has no risk factors for coronary artery disease, but a stress test is ordered by a physician in the emergency department. You are called for a cardiology consult when an exercise ECG stress test result is positive. You estimate that the pretest probability of coronary artery disease is 10% and determine that this is most likely a false-positive stress test with a low posttest probability of coronary artery disease. This is an example of which of the following principles used in medical decision making?

A. Bayes' theorem
B. High positive predictive value
C. High specificity
D. Low negative predictive value
E. Low sensitivity

I-8. A new diagnostic test for predicting latent tuberculosis is introduced into clinical practice. In clinical trials, it was determined to have a sensitivity of 90% and a specificity of 80%. A specific clinical population of 1000 individuals has a prevalence of tuberculosis of 10%. How many individuals with latent tuberculosis would be correctly identified in this population?

A. 10
B. 80
C. 90
D. 100
E. 180

I-9. In the above scenario, how many individuals would be erroneously told they have latent tuberculosis?

A. 10
B. 90
C. 180
D. 720
E. 900

I-10. A receiver operating characteristic (ROC) curve is constructed for a new test for disease X. All of the following statements regarding the ROC curve are true EXCEPT:

A. One criticism of the ROC curve is that it is developed for testing only one test or clinical parameter with exclusion of other potentially relevant data.
B. The ROC curve allows the selection of a threshold value for a test that yields the best sensitivity with the fewest false-positive test results.
C. The axes of the ROC curve are sensitivity versus 1 − specificity.
D. The ideal ROC curve would have a value of 0.5.
E. The value of the ROC curve is calculated as the area under the curve generated from the true-positive rate versus the false-positive rate.

I-11. Which of the following values is affected by the disease prevalence in a population?

A. Number needed to treat
B. Positive likelihood ratio
C. Positive predictive value
D. Sensitivity
E. Specificity

I-12. Drug X is investigated in a meta-analysis for its effect on mortality after a myocardial infarction. It is found that mortality drops from 10 to 2% when this drug is administered. What is the absolute risk reduction conferred by drug X?

A. 2%
B. 8%
C. 20%
D. 200%
E. None of the above

I-13. How many patients will have to be treated with drug X to prevent one death?

A. 2
B. 8
C. 12.5
D. 50
E. 93

I-14. When considering a potential screening test, what endpoints should be considered to assess the potential gain from a proposed intervention?

A. Absolute and relative impact of screening on the disease outcome
B. Cost per life year saved
C. Increase in the average life expectancy for the entire population
D. Number of subjects screened to alter the outcome in one individual
E. All of the above

I-15. A 55-year-old man who smokes cigarettes is enrolled in a lung cancer screening trial based on performance of yearly CT scans over a period of 5 years. At year 2, he is found to have a 2-cm right lower lobe lung nodule that is a non–small cell lung cancer upon surgical removal. At that time, there were no positive lymph nodes. The cancer recurs, and the patient subsequently dies from lung cancer 6 years after his initial diagnosis. A person with a similar smoking history who is not participating in the trial is discovered to have a 3-cm lung nodule that is also non–small cell lung cancer. Upon surgical resection, one lymph node is positive. This person also dies from lung cancer after a period of 3 years. What conclusion can be made about the use of the CT screening for lung cancer in these patients?

A. CT screening for lung cancer improves mortality in smokers.
B. It is unable to be determined if CT screening for lung cancer led to any difference in survival because one cannot determine if lag time bias is present.
C. It is unable to be determined if CT screening for lung cancer led to any difference in survival because one cannot determine if lead time bias is present.
D. Selection bias may cause apparent differences in survival in this trial, and one should be cautious in making conclusions with regards to CT screening for lung cancer.
E. The radiation received as part of the CT scan screening led to lung cancer in the initial patient and contributed to the first patient's overall mortality.

I-16. According to the U.S. Preventive Services Task Force, what is the recommended screening interval for thyroid disease in women older than the age of 30 years?

A. Every 5 years beginning at age 30 years
B. Once at age 30 years
C. Once at age 30 years and again in 10 years if the test result is normal
D. Periodically
E. There is no recommended screening for thyroid disease recommended by the U.S. Preventive Services Task Force

I-17. Which preventative intervention leads to the largest average increase in life expectancy for a target population?

A. A regular exercise program for a 40-year-old man
B. Getting a 35-year-old smoker to quit smoking
C. Mammography in women age 50–70 years
D. Pap smears in women age 18–65 years
E. Prostate-specific antigen (PSA) and digital rectal examination for a man older than 50 years old

I-18. All of the following patients should receive a lipid screening profile EXCEPT:

A. A 16-year-old boy with type 1 diabetes
B. A 17-year-old female teen who recently began smoking
C. A 23-year-old healthy man who is starting his first job
D. A 48-year-old woman beginning menopause
E. A 62-year-old man with no past medical history

I-19. A 43-year-old woman is diagnosed with pulmonary blastomycosis and is initiated on therapy with oral itraconazole therapy. All of the following could affect the bioavailability of this drug EXCEPT:

A. Coadministration with a cola beverage
B. Coadministration with oral contraceptive pills
C. Formulation of the drug (liquid vs. capsule)
D. pH of the stomach
E. Presence of food in the stomach

I-20. A 24-year-old woman with cystic fibrosis is admitted to the hospital with an exacerbation. She is known to be colonized with *Pseudomonas aeruginosa* and is started on intravenous therapy with cefepime 1 g IV every 8 hours and tobramycin 10 mg/kg IV once daily. You want to ensure that the risk of nephrotoxicity is low. When should the tobramycin level be checked?

A. 30 minutes after the first dose
B. 2 hours after the first dose
C. 2 hours before second dose
D. Immediately before the fourth dose
E. There is no need to check drug levels if the patient has normal renal function

I-21. A 68-year-old man with ischemic cardiomyopathy has been treated with digoxin 250 μg daily for the past year. He has chronic kidney disease with a stable baseline creatinine of 2.1 mg/dL. He is initiated on an oral amiodarone load for new-onset atrial fibrillation with rapid ventricular response. Over 1 week, he develops increasing nausea, vomiting, and fatigue. On presentation to the emergency department, he is lethargic and difficult to arouse with a heart rate of 45 beats/min and a blood pressure of 88/50 mmHg. His laboratory values demonstrate a potassium of 5.2 meq/L, creatinine of 3.0 mg/dL, and a digoxin level of 13 ng/mL. His ECG shows complete heart block. What is the most appropriate treatment for this patient?

A. Digitalis-specific antibody (Fab) fragments alone
B. Digitalis-specific antibody fragments plus hemodialysis
C. Digitalis-specific antibody fragments plus hemoperfusion
D. Plasmapheresis alone
E. Volume resuscitation and observation

I-22. A 48-year-old woman with a generalized seizure disorder has been taking phenytoin for the past 10 years with good control of her disease. She also has a history of hepatitis C virus infection acquired via a blood transfusion received after an automobile accident in her teens. She currently takes phenytoin 100 mg tid, lactulose 30 g tid, and spironolactone 25 mg daily. She is brought to the emergency department by her husband, who reports that she has had increasing lethargy for the past week. On examination, her blood pressure is 100/60 mmHg, heart rate is 88 beats/min, respiratory rate is 20 breaths/min, and oxygen saturation is 98% on room air. She is afebrile. She is minimally responsive to voice and follows no commands. There is no nuchal rigidity. Her abdomen is distended with a positive fluid wave but without tenderness. She has spider angiomata, caput medusa, and palmar erythema. She does not appear to have asterixis. She does have horizontal nystagmus on examination. Her laboratory values include Na, 134 meq/L; potassium, 3.9 meq/L; chloride, 104 meq/L; and bicarbonate, 20 meq/L. Creatinine is 1.0 mg/dL. The white blood cell count is 10,000/μL with a normal differential. Her liver function tests are unchanged from baseline with the exception of an albumin that is now 2.1 g/dL compared with 3 months ago when her level was 2.9 g/dL. Ammonia level is 15 μmol/L, and her phenytoin level is 17 mg/L. A paracentesis shows a white blood cell count of 100/μL that is 80% neutrophils. What test would be most likely to demonstrate the cause of the patient's change in mental status?

A. CT scan of the head
B. Electroencephalogram (EEG)
C. Free phenytoin level
D. Gram stain of ascites fluid
E. Gram stain of cerebrospinal fluid (CSF)

I-23. A 55-year-old Japanese woman is found to have a 3-cm mass in the right lower lobe of the lung. She is a lifelong nonsmoker. The mass is positive on positron emission tomography scan as are contralateral and ipsilateral lymph nodes in the mediastinum. A biopsy demonstrates the mass to be a moderately differentiated adenocarcinoma, and a left hilar lymph node also demonstrates adenocarcinoma. Clinically, this places the patient as a stage IIIB non–small cell lung cancer, and the patient and her oncologist decide to treat with chemotherapy. Molecular testing demonstrates an exon 19 deletion in the tyrosine kinase domain of the epidermal growth factor receptor and no mutation in k-ras. What is the best choice for initial chemotherapy in this patient?

A. Carboplatin plus paclitaxel
B. Carboplatin and paclitaxel plus erlotinib
C. Docetaxel alone
D. Erlotinib alone
E. Gemcitabine plus docetaxel

I-24. A 26-year-old woman received an allogeneic bone marrow transplant 9 months ago for acute myelogenous leukemia. Her transplant course is complicated by graft-versus-host disease with diarrhea, weight loss, and skin rash. She is immunosuppressed with tacrolimus 1 mg bid and prednisone 7.5 mg daily. She recently was admitted to the hospital with shortness of breath and fevers to 101.5°F. She has a chest CT showing nodular pneumonia, and fungal organisms are seen on a transbronchial lung biopsy. The culture demonstrates *Aspergillus fumigatus*, and a serum galactomannan level is elevated. She is initiated on therapy with voriconazole 6 mg/kg IV every 12 hours for 1 day, decreasing to 4 mg/kg IV every 12 hours beginning on day 2. Two days after starting voriconazole, she is no longer febrile but is complaining of headaches and tremors. Her blood pressure is 150/92 mmHg, up from 108/60 mmHg on admission. On examination, she has developed 1+ pitting edema in the lower extremities. Her creatinine has risen to 1.7 mg/dL from 0.8 mg/dL on admission. What is the most likely cause of the patient's current clinical picture?

A. *Aspergillus* meningitis
B. Congestive heart failure
C. Recurrent graft-versus-host disease
D. Tacrolimus toxicity
E. Thrombotic thrombocytopenic purpura caused by voriconazole

I-25. A 45-year-old man is diagnosed with primary syphilis after development of a penile ulcer. Results of a rapid plasma reagin and fluorescent treponemal antibody absorption tests are both positive. He is treated with benzathine penicillin G 2.4 million units intramuscularly as a one-time dose. Ten days after the injection, the patient presents to the emergency department complaining of fevers, rash, and diffuse joint pains with muscle aches. On physical examination, the patient has a temperature of 38.3°F, heart rate of 110 beats/min, and blood pressure of 112/76 mmHg. His HEENT, chest, cardiovascular, and abdominal examination findings are normal. He has an urticarial rash on trunk, back, and extremities. There is swelling and warmth of the knees, wrists, and metacarpophalangeal joints bilaterally. In addition, there is pain with palpation of the tendinous insertions of the Achilles tendons and patellar tendons bilaterally. The penile ulcer has a dry base and has decreased in size compared with previously. Laboratory studies show a white cell count of 10,100/μL (80% neutrophils, 15% lymphocytes, 3% monocytes, and 2% eosinophils). The erythrocyte sedimentation rate is 55 seconds. Antinuclear antibodies and rheumatoid factor results are negative. A urethral swab is negative for *Chlamydia trachomatis* and *Neisseria gonorrhea*. What is the most likely diagnosis?

A. Disseminated gonococcal infection
B. Inadequate treatment of secondary syphilis
C. Jarisch-Herxheimer reaction
D. Seronegative rheumatoid arthritis
E. Serum sickness caused by benzathine penicillin

I-26. Which of the following classes of medicines has been linked to the occurrence of hip fractures in elderly adults?

A. Benzodiazepines
B. Opiates
C. Angiotensin-converting enzyme inhibitors
D. Beta-blockers
E. Atypical antipsychotics

I-27. Patients taking which of the following drugs should be advised to avoid drinking grapefruit juice?

A. Amoxicillin
B. Aspirin
C. Atorvastatin
D. Prevacid
E. Sildenafil

I-28. Which of the following diseases is responsible for a greater percentage of deaths in women compared with men?

A. Alzheimer's disease
B. Cerebrovascular disease
C. Chronic obstructive pulmonary disease
D. Sepsis
E. All of the above

I-29. Which of the following statements regarding coronary heart disease (CHD) in women when compared with men is TRUE?

A. Angina is a rare symptom in women with CHD.
B. At the time of diagnosis of CHD, women typically have fewer comorbidities compared with men.
C. Physicians are less likely to consider CHD in women and are also less likely to recommend both diagnostic and therapeutic procedures in women.
D. Women and men present with CHD at similar ages.
E. Women are more likely to present with ventricular tachycardia, but men more commonly have cardiac arrest or cardiogenic shock.

I-30. Which of the following is an independent risk factor for coronary heart disease in women but not men?

A. Elevated total triglyceride levels
B. Hypertension
C. Low high-density lipoprotein cholesterol
D. Obesity
E. Smoking

I-31. All of the following diseases are more common in women than men EXCEPT:

A. Depression
B. Hypertension
C. Obesity
D. Rheumatoid arthritis
E. Type 1 diabetes mellitus

I-32. Which of the following statements regarding Alzheimer's disease and gender are true?

A. Alzheimer's disease affects men and women at equal rates.
B. Alzheimer's disease affects men two times more commonly than women.
C. In a recent placebo-controlled trial, postmenopausal hormone therapy did not show improvement in disease progression in women with Alzheimer's disease.
D. The difference in deaths from Alzheimer's disease between men and women can be entirely accounted for by the difference in life expectancy between men and women.
E. Women with Alzheimer's disease have higher levels of circulating estrogen than women without Alzheimer's disease.

I-33. All of the following are changes in the cardiovascular system seen in pregnancy EXCEPT:

A. Decreased blood pressure
B. Increased cardiac output
C. Increased heart rate
D. Increased plasma volume
E. Increased systemic vascular resistance

I-34. A 36-year-old woman has a history of hypertension and is planning on starting a family. She is currently taking lisinopril 10 mg daily for control of her blood pressure. She wants to stop taking her oral contraceptive medications. Her current blood pressure is 128/83 mmHg. What do you advise her about ongoing treatment with antihypertensive medications?

A. Because the cardiovascular changes that occur during pregnancy lead to a fall in blood pressure, she can safely discontinue her lisinopril when she stops her oral contraceptives.
B. She should continue lisinopril and start hydrochlorothiazide.
C. She should discontinue lisinopril and start irbesartan.
D. She should discontinue lisinopril and start labetalol.
E. She should not get pregnant because she is high risk of complications.

I-35. Which of the following cardiovascular conditions is a contraindication to pregnancy?

A. Atrial septal defect without Eisenmenger syndrome
B. Idiopathic pulmonary arterial hypertension
C. Marfan syndrome
D. Mitral regurgitation
E. Prior peripartum cardiomyopathy with a current ejection fraction of 65%

I-36. A 33-year-old woman with diabetes mellitus and hypertension presents to the hospital with seizures during week 37 of her pregnancy. Her blood pressure is 156/92 mmHg. She has 4+ proteinuria. Management should include all of the following EXCEPT:

A. Emergent delivery
B. Intravenous labetalol
C. Intravenous magnesium sulfate
D. Intravenous phenytoin

I-37. A 27-year-old woman develops left leg swelling during week 20 of her pregnancy. Left lower extremity ultrasonogram reveals a left iliac vein deep venous thrombosis (DVT). Proper management includes:

A. Bedrest
B. Catheter-directed thrombolysis
C. Enoxaparin
D. Inferior vena cava filter placement
E. Warfarin

I-38. In which of the following categories should women undergo routine screening for gestational diabetes?

A. Age greater than 25 years
B. Body mass index greater than 25 kg/m^2
C. Family history of diabetes mellitus in a first-degree relative
D. African American
E. All of the above

I-39. Which of the following surgeries would be considered at the greatest risk for postsurgical complications?

A. Carotid endarterectomy
B. Non-emergent repair of a thoracic aortic aneurysm
C. Resection of a 5-cm lung cancer
D. Total colectomy for colon cancer
E. Total hip replacement

I-40. A 64-year-old man is contemplating undergoing elective cholecystectomy for biliary colic and cholelithiasis. He has a history of coronary artery disease with coronary artery bypass surgery performed at the age of 51 after an anterior wall myocardial infarction. His most recent ejection fraction 2 years previously was 35%. He also has a 45 pack-year history of tobacco, quitting after his surgery 13 years previously. Since his bypass surgery, he reports failure to return to full functional capacity. You ask him about his current exercise capacity. Which of the following would be considered poor exercise tolerance and increase his risk of perioperative complications?

A. Inability to achieve 4 metabolic equivalents during an exercise test
B. Inability to carry 15–20 lb
C. Inability to climb two flights of stairs at a normal pace
D. Inability to walk four blocks at a normal pace
E. All of the above

I-41. A 74-year-old man is scheduled to undergo total colectomy for recurrent life-threatening diverticular bleeding. He denies any chest pain with exertion but is limited in his physical activity because of degenerative arthritis of his knees. He has no history of coronary artery disease or congestive heart failure but does have diabetes mellitus and hypertension. His current medications include aspirin 81 mg daily, atorvastatin 10 mg daily, enalapril 20 mg daily, and insulin glargine 25 units daily in combination with insulin lispro on a sliding scale. His blood pressure is 128/86 mmHg. His physical examination findings are normal. His most recent hemoglobin A1C is 6.3%, and his creatinine is 1.5 mg/dL. You elect to perform an electrocardiogram preoperatively, and it demonstrates Q waves in leads II, III, and aVF. Based on this information, what is his expected his postoperative risk of a major cardiac event?

A. 0.5%
B. 1%
C. 5%
D. 10%
E. 20%

I-42. All of the following are risk factors for postoperative pulmonary complications EXCEPT:

A. Age greater than 60 years
B. Asthma with a peak expiratory flow rate of 220 L/min
C. Chronic obstructive pulmonary disease
D. Congestive heart failure
E. Forced expiratory volume in 1 second of 1.5 L

I-43. You are caring for a 56-year-old woman who was admitted to the hospital with a change in mental status. She underwent a right-sided mastectomy and axillary lymph node dissection 3 years previously for stage IIIB ductal carcinoma. Serum calcium is elevated at 15.3 mg/dL. A chest radiograph demonstrates innumerable pulmonary nodules, and a head CT shows a brain mass in the right frontal lobe with surrounding edema. Despite correcting her calcium and treating cerebral edema, the patient remains confused. You approach the family to discuss the diagnosis of widely metastatic disease and the patient's poor prognosis. Which

of the following is NOT a component of the seven elements for communicating bad news (P-SPIKES approach)?

A. Assess the family's perception of her current illness and the status of her underlying cancer diagnosis.
B. Empathize with the family's feelings and provide emotional support.
C. Prepare mentally for the discussion.
D. Provide an appropriate setting for discussion.
E. Schedule a follow-up meeting in 1 day to reassess whether there are additional informational and emotional needs.

I-44. Which of the following is not a component of a living will?

A. Delineation of specific interventions that would be acceptable to the patient under certain conditions
B. Description of values that should guide discussions regarding terminal care
C. Designation of a health care proxy
D. General statements regarding whether the patient desires receipt of life-sustaining interventions such as mechanical ventilation

I-45. A 72-year-old woman has stage IV ovarian cancer with diffuse peritoneal studding. She is developing increasing pain in her abdomen and is admitted to the hospital for pain control. She previously was treated with oxycodone 10 mg orally every 6 hours as needed. Upon admission, she is initiated on morphine intravenously via patient-controlled analgesia. During the first 48 hours of her hospitalization, she received an average daily dose of morphine 90 mg and reports adequate pain control unless she is walking. What is the most appropriate opioid regimen for transitioning this patient to oral pain medication?

	Sustained-Release Morphine	Immediate-Release Morphine
A.	None	15 mg every 4 hours as needed
B.	45 mg twice daily	5 mg every 4 hours as needed
C.	45 mg twice daily	15 mg every 4 hours as needed
D.	90 mg twice daily	15 mg every 4 hours as needed
E.	90 mg three time daily	15 mg every 4 hours as needed

I-46. You are asked to consult on 62-year-old man who was recently found to have newly metastatic disease. He was originally diagnosed with cancer of the prostate 5 years previously and presented to the hospital with back pain and weakness. Magnetic resonance imaging (MRI) demonstrated bony metastases to his L2 and L5 vertebrae with spinal cord compression at the L2 level only. On bone scan images, there was evidence of widespread bony metastases. He has been started on radiation and hormonal therapy, and his disease has shown some response. However, he has become quite depressed since the metastatic disease was found. His family reports that he is sleeping for 18 or more hours daily and has stopped eating. His weight is down 12 lb over 4 weeks. He expresses profound fatigue, hopelessness, and a feeling of sadness. He claims to have no interest in his usual activities and no longer interacts with his grandchildren. What is the best approach to treating this patient's depression?

A. Do not initiate pharmacologic therapy because the patient is experiencing an appropriate reaction to his newly diagnosed metastatic disease.

B. Initiate therapy with doxepin 75 mg nightly.

C. Initiate therapy with fluoxetine 10 mg daily.

D. Initiate therapy with fluoxetine 10 mg daily and methylphenidate 2.5 mg twice daily in the morning and at noon.

E. Initiate therapy with methylphenidate 2.5 mg twice daily in the morning and at noon.

I-47. You are treating a 76-year-old woman with Alzheimer's disease admitted to the intensive care unit for aspiration pneumonia. After 7 days of mechanical ventilation, her family requests that care be withdrawn. The patient is palliated with fentanyl intravenously at a rate of 25 μg/hr and midazolam intravenously at 2 mg/hr. You are urgently called to the bedside 15 minutes after the patient is extubated because the patient's daughter is distraught. She states that you are "drowning" her mother and is upset because her mother appears to be struggling to breathe. When you enter the room, you hear a gurgling noise that is coming from accumulated secretions in the oropharynx. You suction the patient for liberal amounts of thin salivary secretions and reassure the daughter that you will make her mother as comfortable as possible. Which of the following interventions may help with the treatment of the patient's oral secretions?

A. Increased infusion rate of fentanyl

B. *N*-acetylcysteine nebulized

C. Pilocarpine drops

D. Placement of a nasal trumpet and oral airway to allow easier access for aggressive suctioning

E. Scopolamine patches

I-48. Which of the following is the most common type of preventable adverse event in hospitalized patients?

A. Adverse drug events

B. Diagnostic failures

C. Falls

D. Technical complications of procedures

E. Wound infections

I-49. All of the following statements regarding the use of complementary and alternative medicine (CAM) in the US are true EXCEPT:

A. Acupuncture is the most frequently used CAM approach in the US

B. CAM approaches represent approximately 10% of out-of-pocket medical expenses in the US

C. Control of back or musculoskeletal pain is a common reason for US patients to utilize CAM approaches

D. Recent estimates suggest 30-40% of Americans use CAM approaches

E. The most common reasons US patients seek CAM approaches is for management of symptoms poorly controlled by conventional approaches

I-50. Independent of insurance status, income, age, and comorbid conditions, African American patients are less likely to receive equivalent levels of care compared with white patients for the following scenarios:

A. Prescription of analgesic for pain control

B. Referral to renal transplantation

C. Surgical treatment for lung cancer

D. Utilization of cardiac diagnostic and therapeutic procedures

E. All of the above

I-51. All of the following statements regarding the difference between breast cancer in pregnant versus nonpregnant women are true EXCEPT:

A. Estrogen-positive tumors are more common in pregnant women.

B. Her-2 positivity is more common in pregnant women.

C. A higher stage is more common in pregnant women.

D. Positive lymph nodes are more common in pregnant women.

E. Tumor size at diagnosis is larger in pregnant women.

I-52. A 32-year-old woman seeks evaluation for cough that has been present for 4 months. She reports that the cough is present day and night. It does awaken her from sleep and is worse in the early morning hours. She also notes the cough to be worse in cold weather and after exercise. She describes the cough as dry and has no associated shortness of breath or wheezing. She gives no antecedent history of an upper respiratory tract infection that preceded the onset of cough. She has a medical history of pulmonary embolus occurring in the postpartum period 6 years previously. Her only medication is norgestimate/ethinyl estradiol. She works as an elementary school teacher. On review of systems, she reports intermittent itchy eyes and runny nose that is worse in the spring and fall. She denies postnasal drip and heartburn. Her physical examination findings are normal with the exception of coughing when breathing through an open mouth. A chest radiograph is also normal. Spirometry demonstrates a forced expiratory volume in 1 second (FEV_1) of 3.0 L (85% predicted), forced vital capacity (FVC) of 3.75 L (88% predicted), and FEV_1/FVC ratio of 80%. After administration of a bronchodilator, the FEV_1 increases to 3.3 L (10% change). What would you recommend next in the evaluation and treatment of this patient?

A. Initiate a nasal corticosteroid.

B. Initiate a proton pump inhibitor.

C. Perform a methacholine challenge test.

D. Perform a nasopharyngeal culture for *Bordetella pertussis.*

E. Reassure the patient that there are no pulmonary abnormalities and continue supportive care.

I-53. A 56-year-old man presents to his primary care physician complaining of coughing up blood. He has felt ill for the past 4 days with a low-grade fever and cough. The cough was initially productive of yellow-green sputum, but it now is sputum mixed with red blood. He estimates that he has produced about 1–2 tsp (5–10 mL) of blood in the past day. He smokes 1 pack of cigarettes daily and has done so since the 15 years of age. He is known to have moderate chronic obstructive pulmonary disease and coronary artery disease. He takes aspirin, metoprolol, lisinopril, tiotropium, and albuterol as needed. His physical examination is notable for a temperature of 37.8°C (100.0°F). Bilateral expiratory wheezing and coarse rhonchi are heard on examination. Chest radiograph is normal. What is the most likely cause of hemoptysis in this individual?

A. Acute bronchitis
B. Infection with tuberculosis
C. Lung abscess
D. Lung cancer
E. Medications

I-54. A 65-year-old man with a known squamous cell carcinoma near the right upper lobe bronchus is admitted to intensive care after coughing up more than 100 mL of bright red blood. He appears in significant respiratory distress with an oxygen saturation of 78% on room air. He continues to have violent coughing with ongoing hemoptysis. He had a prior pulmonary embolus and is being treated with warfarin. His last INR was therapeutic at 2.5 three days previously. All of the following would be useful in the immediate management of this patient EXCEPT:

A. Consultation with anesthesia for placement of a dual-lumen endotracheal tube.
B. Consultation with interventional radiology for embolization.
C. Consultation with thoracic surgery for urgent surgical intervention if conservative management fails.
D. Correction of the patient's coagulopathy.
E. Positioning of the patient in the left lateral decubitus position.

I-55. Microbial agents have been used as bioweapons since ancient times. All of the following are key features of microbial agents that are used as bioweapons EXCEPT:

A. Environmental stability
B. High morbidity and mortality rates
C. Lack of rapid diagnostic capability
D. Lack of readily available antibiotic treatment
E. Lack of universally available and effective vaccine

I-56. Ten individuals in Arizona are hospitalized over a 4-week period with fever and rapidly enlarging and painful lymph nodes. Seven of these individuals experience severe sepsis, and three die. While reviewing the epidemiologic characteristics of these individuals, you note that they are all illegal immigrants and have recently stayed in the same immigrant camp. Blood cultures are growing gram-negative rods that are identified as

Yersinia pestis. You notify local public health officials and the Centers for Disease Control and Prevention. Which of the following factors indicate that this is NOT likely to be an act of bioterrorism?

A. The area affected was limited to a small immigrant camp.
B. The individuals presented with symptoms of bubonic plague rather than pneumonic plague.
C. The individuals were in close contact with one another, suggesting possible person-to-person transmission.
D. The mortality rate was less than 50%.
E. *Yersinia pestis* is not environmentally stable for longer than 1 hour.

I-57. Which of the following routes of dispersal are likely for botulinum toxin used as a bioweapon?

A. Aerosol
B. Contamination of the food supply
C. Contamination of the water supply
D. A and B
E. All of the above

I-58. Anthrax spores can remain dormant in the respiratory tract for how long?

A. 1 week
B. 6 weeks
C. 6 months
D. 1 year
E. 3 years

I-59. Twenty recent attendees at a National Football League game arrive at the emergency department complaining of shortness of breath, fever, and malaise. Chest radiographs show mediastinal widening on several of these patients, prompting a concern for inhalational anthrax as a result of a bioterror attack. Antibiotics are initiated, and the Centers for Disease Control and Prevention is notified. What form of isolation should be instituted for these patients in the hospital?

A. Airborne
B. Contact
C. Droplet
D. None

I-60. The Centers for Disease Control and Prevention (CDC) has designated several biologic agents as category A in their ability to be used as bioweapons. Category A agents include agents that can be easily disseminated or transmitted, result in high mortality, can cause public panic, and require special action for public health preparedness. All of the following agents are considered category A EXCEPT:

A. *Bacillus anthracis*
B. *Francisella tularensis*
C. Ricin toxin from *Ricinus communis*
D. Smallpox
E. *Yersinia pestis*

I-61. All of the following chemical agents of bioterrorism are correctly identified by their mechanism of injury EXCEPT:

A. Arsine—asphyxiant
B. Chlorine gas—pulmonary damage
C. Cyanogen chloride—nerve agent
D. Mustard gas—vesicant
E. Sarin—nerve agent

I-62. Over the course of 12 hours, 24 individuals present to a single emergency department complaining of a sunburn-like reaction with development of large blisters. Most of these individuals are also experiencing irritation of the eyes, nose, and pharynx. Two individuals developed progressive dyspnea, severe cough, and stridor requiring endotracheal intubation. On physical examination, all of the patients exhibited conjunctivitis and nasal congestion. Erythema of the skin was greatest in the axillae, neck, and antecubital fossae. Many of the affected had large, thin-walled bullae on the extremities that were filled with a clear or straw-colored fluid. On further questioning, all of the affected individuals had been shopping at a local mall within the past 24 hours and ate at the food court. Many commented on a strong odor of burning garlic in the food court at that time. You suspect a bioterrorism act. Which of the following is TRUE with regard to the likely agent causing the patients' symptoms?

A. 2-Pralidoxime should be administered to all affected individuals.
B. The associated mortality rate of this agent is more than 50%.
C. The cause of respiratory distress in affected individuals is related to direct alveolar injury and adult respiratory distress syndrome.
D. The erythema that occurs can be delayed as long as 2 days after exposure and depends on several factors, including ambient temperature and humidity.
E. The fluid within the bullae should be treated as a hazardous substance that can lead to local reactions and blistering with exposure.

I-63. A 24-year-old man is evaluated immediately after exposure to chlorine gas as an act of chemical terrorism. He currently denies dyspnea. His respiratory rate is 16 breaths/min and oxygen saturation is 97% on room air. All of the following should be included in the immediate treatment of this individual EXCEPT:

A. Aggressive bathing of all exposed skin areas
B. Flushing of the eyes with water or normal saline
C. Forced rest and fresh air
D. Immediate removal of clothing if no frostbite
E. Maintenance of a semiupright position

I-64. You are a physician working in an urban emergency department when several patients are brought in after the release of an unknown gas at the performance of a symphony. You are evaluating a 52-year-old woman who is not able to talk clearly because of excessive salivation and rhinorrhea, although she is able to tell you that she feels as if she lost her sight immediately upon exposure. At present, she also has nausea, vomiting, diarrhea, and muscle twitching. On physical examination, the patient has a blood pressure of 156/92 mmHg, a heart rate of 92, a respiratory rate of 30 breaths/min, and a temperature of 37.4°C (99.3°F). She has pinpoint pupils with profuse rhinorrhea and salivation. She also is coughing profusely, with production of copious amounts of clear secretions. A lung examination reveals wheezing on expiration in bilateral lung fields. The patient has a regular rate and rhythm with normal heart sounds. Bowel sounds are hyperactive, but the abdomen is not tender. She is having diffuse fasciculations. At the end of your examination, the patient abruptly develops tonic-clonic seizures. Which of the following agents is most likely to cause this patient's symptoms?

A. Arsine
B. Cyanogen chloride
C. Nitrogen mustard
D. Sarin
E. VX

I-65. All the following should be used in the treatment of this patient EXCEPT:

A. Atropine
B. Decontamination
C. Diazepam
D. Phenytoin
E. 2-Pralidoxime chloride

I-66. All of the following statements are true regarding the results of detonation of a low-yield nuclear device by a terror group EXCEPT:

A. After recovery of initial exposure symptoms, the patient remains at risk of systemic illness for up to 6 weeks.
B. Appropriate medical therapy can change the LD50 from approximately 4–8 gray (Gy).
C. Initial mortality is mostly caused by shock blast and thermal damage.
D. Most of the total mortality is related to release of alpha and beta particles.
E. The hematopoietic, gastrointestinal, and neurologic systems are most likely involved in acute radiation syndrome.

I-67. A "dirty" bomb is detonated in downtown Boston. The bomb was composed of cesium-137 with trinitrotoluene. In the immediate aftermath, an estimated 30 people were killed because of the power of the blast. The fallout area was about 0.5 mile, with radiation exposure of about 1.8 Gy. An estimated 5000 people have been potentially exposed to beta and gamma radiation. Most of these individuals show no sign of any injury, but about 60 people have evidence of thermal injury. What is the most appropriate approach to treating the injured victims?

A. All individuals who have been exposed should be treated with potassium iodide.

B. All individuals who have been exposed should be treated with Prussian blue.

C. All individuals should be decontaminated before transportation to the nearest medical center for emergency care to prevent exposure of health care workers.

D. Severely injured individuals should be transported to the hospital for emergency care after removing the victims' clothes because the risk of exposure to health care workers is low.

E. With this degree of radiation exposure, no further testing and treatment are needed.

I-68. A 37-year-old woman is brought to the ICU after her elective laparoscopic cholecystectomy is complicated by a temperature of 105°F, tachycardia, and systemic hypotension. Examination is notable for diffuse muscular rigidity. Which of the following drugs should be administered immediately?

A. Acetaminophen
B. Dantrolene
C. Haloperidol
D. Hydrocortisone
E. Ibuprofen

I-69. Hyperthermia is defined as:

A. A core temperature greater than 40.0°C
B. A core temperature greater than 41.5°C
C. An uncontrolled increase in body temperature despite a normal hypothalamic temperature setting
D. An elevated temperature that normalizes with antipyretic therapy
E. Temperature greater than 40.0°C, rigidity, and autonomic dysregulation

I-70. Which of the following conditions is associated with increased susceptibility to heat stroke in elderly adults?

A. A heat wave
B. Antiparkinsonian therapy
C. Bedridden status
D. Diuretic therapy
E. All of the above

I-71. A recent 18-year-old immigrant from Kenya presents to a university clinic with fever, nasal congestion, severe fatigue, and a rash. The rash started with discrete lesions at the hairline that coalesced as the rash spread caudally. There is sparing of the palms and soles. Small white spots with a surrounding red halo are noted on examination of the palate. The patient is at risk for developing which of the following in the future?

A. Encephalitis
B. Epiglottitis
C. Opportunistic infections
D. Postherpetic neuralgia
E. Splenic rupture

I-72. A 23-year-old woman with a chronic lower extremity ulcer related to prior trauma presents with rash, hypotension, and fever. She has had no recent travel or outdoor exposure and is up to date on all of her vaccinations. She does not use IV drugs. On examination, the ulcer looks clean with a well-granulated base and no erythema, warmth, or pustular discharge. However, the patient does have diffuse erythema that is most prominent on her palms, conjunctiva, and oral mucosa. Other than profound hypotension and tachycardia, the remainder of the examination is nonfocal. Laboratory results are notable for a creatinine of 2.8 mg/dL, aspartate aminotransferase of 250 U/L, alanine aminotransferase of 328 U/L, total bilirubin of 3.2 mg/dL, direct bilirubin of 0.5 mg/dL, INR of 1.5, activated partial thromboplastin time of 1.6 × control, and platelets at 94,000/μL. Ferritin is 1300 μg/mL. The patient is started on broad-spectrum antibiotics after appropriate blood cultures are drawn and is resuscitated with IV fluid and vasopressors. Her blood cultures are negative at 72 hours; at this point, her fingertips start to desquamate. What is the most likely diagnosis?

A. Juvenile rheumatoid arthritis (JRA)
B. Leptospirosis
C. Staphylococcal toxic shock syndrome
D. Streptococcal toxic shock syndrome
E. Typhoid fever

I-73. A 75-year-old man with chronic systolic heart failure requiring high-dose diuretics and lisinopril is seen by his primary care physician for acute onset of right great toe pain with redness and swelling. He is unable to bear weight on this foot. On examination, he is afebrile and has normal vital signs. His complaints in his right great toe are verified. No other joints are involved, and he appears otherwise to be in well-compensated heart failure. Prednisone and allopurinol are prescribed. Five days later, the patient is seen in the emergency department with a temperature of 101°F and a rash throughout his body and mouth. On examination, he has diffuse erythema, areas of skin exfoliation, and oral and orbital edema. Mucous membranes are not involved. Laboratory studies show mild transaminitis and peripheral eosinophilia. Which of the following syndromes describes this condition?

A. Acute bacterial endocarditis
B. Angioedema caused by lisinopril
C. Drug-induced hypersensitivity syndrome caused by allopurinol
D. MRSA cellulitis
E. Staphylococcal toxic shock syndrome caused by septic arthritis

I-74. A 50-year-old man is evaluated for fevers and weight loss of uncertain etiology. He first developed symptoms 3 months previously. He reports daily fevers to as high as 39.4°C (103°F) with night sweats and fatigue. Over this same period, his appetite has been decreased, and he has lost 50 lb compared with his weight at his last annual examination. Fevers have been documented in his primary care physician's office to as high as 38.7°C (101.7°F). He has no exposures or ill contacts. His medical history is significant for diabetes mellitus, obesity, and obstructive sleep apnea. He is taking insulin glargine 50 U daily. He works in a warehouse driving a forklift. He has not traveled outside of his home area in a rural part of Virginia. He has never received a blood transfusion and is married with one female sexual partner for the past 25 years. On examination, no focal findings are identified. Multiple laboratory studies have been performed that have shown nonspecific findings only with exception of an elevated calcium at 11.2 g/dL. A complete blood count showed a white blood cell count of 15,700/μL with 80% polymorphonuclear cells, 15% lymphocytes, 3% eosinophils, and 2% monocytes. The peripheral smear is normal. The hematocrit is 34.7%. His erythrocyte sedimentation rate (ESR) is elevated at 57 mm/hr. A rheumatologic panel is normal, and the ferritin is 521 ng/mL. Liver and kidney function are normal. The serum protein electrophoresis demonstrated polyclonal gammopathy. HIV, Epstein-Barr virus (EBV), and cytomegalovirus (CMV) testing are negative. The urine Histoplasma antigen result is negative. Routine blood cultures for bacteria, chest radiograph, and purified protein derivative (PPD) testing results are negative. A CT scan of the chest, abdomen, and pelvis has borderline enlargement of lymph nodes in the abdomen and retroperitoneum to 1.2 cm. What would be the next best step in determining the etiology of fever in this patient?

A. Empiric treatment with corticosteroids
B. Empiric treatment for *Mycobacterium tuberculosis*
C. Needle biopsy of enlarged lymph nodes
D. PET-CT imaging
E. Serum angiotensin-converting enzyme levels

I-75. A 48-year-old man is brought to the emergency department (ED) in January after being found unresponsive in a city park. He has alcoholism and was last seen by his daughter about 12 hours before being brought to the ED. At that time, he left their home intoxicated and agitated. He left seeking additional alcohol because his daughter had poured out his last bottle of vodka hoping that he would seek treatment. On presentation, he has a core body temperature of 88.5°F (31.4°C), heart rate of 48 beats/min, respiratory rate of 28 breaths/min, and blood pressure of 88/44 mmHg; oxygen saturation is unable to be obtained. The arterial blood gas demonstrates a pH of 7.05, $PaCO_2$ of 32 mmHg, and PaO_2 of 56 mmHg. Initial blood chemistries demonstrate a sodium of 132 meq/L, potassium of 5.2 meq/L, chloride of 94 meq/L, bicarbonate of 10 meq/L, blood urea nitrogen of 56 mg/dL, and creatinine of 1.8 mg/dL. Serum glucose is 63 mg/dL. The serum ethanol level is 65 mg/dL. The measured osmolality is 328 mOsm/kg. ECG demonstrates sinus bradycardia with a long first-degree atrioventricular block and J waves. In addition to initiating a rewarming protocol, what additional tests should be performed in this patient?

A. Endotracheal intubation with hyperventilation to a goal $PaCO_2$ of less than 20 mmHg
B. Intravenous hydration with a 1–2 L bolus of warmed lactated Ringer's solution
C. No other measures are necessary because interpretation of the acid–base status is unreliable with this degree of hypothermia.
D. Measure levels of ethylene glycol and methanol
E. Placement of a transvenous cardiac pacemaker

I-76. A homeless man is evaluated in the emergency department. He has noted that after he slept outside during a particularly cold night his left foot has become clumsy and feels "dead." On examination, the foot has hemorrhagic vesicles distributed throughout the foot distal to the ankle. The foot is cool and has no sensation to pain or temperature. The right foot is hyperemic but does not have vesicles and has normal sensation. The remainder of the physical examination findings are normal. Which of the following statements regarding the management of this disorder is true?

A. Active foot rewarming should not be attempted.
B. During the period of rewarming, intense pain can be anticipated.
C. Heparin has been shown to improve outcomes in this disorder.
D. Immediate amputation is indicated.
E. Normal sensation is likely to return with rewarming.

I-77. A 25-year-old woman becomes lightheaded and experiences a syncopal event while having her blood drawn during a cholesterol screening. She has no medical history and takes no medications. She experiences a brief loss of consciousness for about 20 seconds. She has no seizure-like activity and immediately returns to her usual level of functioning. She is diagnosed with vasovagal syncope, and no follow-up testing is recommended. Which of the following statements regarding neurally mediated syncope is TRUE?

A. Neurally mediated syncope occurs when there are abnormalities of the autonomic nervous system.
B. Proximal and distal myoclonus do not occur during neurally mediated syncope and should increase the likelihood of a seizure.
C. The final pathway of neurally mediated syncope results in a surge of the sympathetic nervous system with inhibition of the parasympathetic nervous system.
D. The primary therapy for neurally mediated syncope is reassurance, avoidance of triggers, and plasma volume expansion.
E. The usual finding with cardiovascular monitoring is hypotension and tachycardia.

I-78. A 76-year-old woman is brought to the emergency department after a syncopal event that occurred while she was singing in her church choir. She has a history of hypertension, diabetes mellitus, and chronic kidney disease (stage III). She does recall at least two prior episodes of syncope similar to this one. Her medications include insulin glargine 40 units daily, lispro insulin sliding scale, lisinopril 20 mg daily, and hydrochlorothiazide 25 mg daily. By the time she arrived in the emergency department, she reports feeling back to her usual self. She does recall feeling somewhat lightheaded before the syncopal events but does not recall the event itself. Witnesses report some jerking of her upper extremities. She regained full consciousness in less than 2 minutes. Her current vital signs include blood pressure of 110/62 mmHg, heart rate of 84 beats/min, respiratory rate of 16 breaths/min, and oxygen saturation of 95% on room air. She is afebrile. Her physical examination is unremarkable and includes a normal neurologic examination. Which of the following would be least helpful in determining the etiology of the patient's syncope?

A. CT scan of the head
B. Electrocardiogram
C. Fingerstick glucose measurement
D. Orthostatic blood pressure measurement
E. Tilt table testing

I-79. A 48-year-old man presents to the emergency department complaining of dizziness. He describes it as a sensation that the room is spinning. All of the following would be consistent with a central cause of vertigo EXCEPT:

A. Absence of tinnitus
B. Gaze-evoked nystagmus
C. Hiccups
D. Inhibition of nystagmus by visual fixation
E. Purely vertical nystagmus

I-80. A 62-year-old woman presents complaining of severe dizziness. She notes it especially when she turns over in bed and immediately upon standing. Her initial physical examination findings are normal. Upon further testing, you ask the patient to sit with her head turned 45 degrees to the right. You lower the patient to the supine position and extend the head backward 20 degrees. This maneuver immediately reproduces the patient's symptoms, and you note torsional nystagmus. What is the most appropriate next step in evaluation and treatment of this patient?

A. MRI of the brainstem
B. Methylprednisolone taper beginning at 100 mg daily
C. Repositioning (Epley) maneuvers
D. Rizatriptan 10 mg orally once
E. Valacyclovir 1000 mg three times daily for 7 days

I-81. A 42-year-old man presents complaining of progressive weakness over a period of several months. He reports tripping over his toes while walking and has dropped a cup of hot coffee on one occasion because he felt too weak to continue to hold it. A disorder affecting lower motor neurons is suspected. All of the following findings would be found in an individual with a disease primarily affecting lower motor neurons EXCEPT:

A. Decreased muscle tone
B. Distal greater than proximal weakness
C. Fasciculations
D. Hyperactive tendon reflexes
E. Severe muscle atrophy

I-82. A 78-year-old man is seen in clinic because of recent falls. He reports gait difficulties with a sensation of being off balance at times. One recent fall caused a shoulder injury requiring surgery to repair a torn rotation cuff. In epidemiologic case series, what is the most common cause of gait disorders?

A. Cerebellar degeneration
B. Cerebrovascular disease with multiple infarcts
C. Cervical myelopathy
D. Parkinson's disease
E. Sensory deficits

I-83. A 65-year-old man presents complaining of frequent falls and gait abnormalities. He first noticed the difficulty about 6 months ago. He has a history of hypertension and hypothyroidism and hyperlipidemia. His current medications include amlodipine 10 mg daily, simvastatin 20 mg daily, and levothyroxine 75 μg daily. On neurologic examination, you observe his gait to be wide based with short, shuffling steps. He has difficulty rising from his chair and initiating his gait. Upon turning, he takes multiple steps and appears unsteady. However, cerebellar testing results are normal, including heel-to-shin and Romberg testing. He has no evidence of sensory deficits in the lower extremities, and strength is 5/5 throughout all tested muscle groups. He shows no evidence of muscle spasticity on passive movement. His neurologic examination is consistent with which of the following causes?

A. Alcoholic cerebellar degeneration
B. Communicating hydrocephalus
C. Neurosyphilis
D. Multiple system atrophy
E. Lumbar myelopathy

I-84. A 74-year-old woman is admitted to the medical intensive care unit with confusion and sepsis from a urinary origin. Her initial blood pressure was 70/40 mmHg with a heart rate of 130 beats/min. She is volume resuscitated but requires dopamine to maintain an adequate blood pressure. Her mental status improved initially, but now she is agitated and pulling at her IV catheters. She is screaming that she is trapped, and she is not oriented to place or year. All of the following statements regarding the patient's condition are true EXCEPT:

A. An episode of delirium is associated with an in-hospital mortality rate of 25% to 33%.
B. A patient who has an episode of delirium in the hospital is more likely to be discharged to a nursing home.
C. Delirium is associated with an increased risk of all-cause mortality for at least 1 year after hospital discharge.
D. Delirium is typically short-lived and does not persist longer than several days.
E. Individuals who experience delirium have longer lengths of stay in the hospital.

I-85. You are covering the night shift at a local hospital and are called acutely to the bedside of a 62-year-old man to evaluate a change in his mental status. He was admitted 36 hours previously for treatment of community-acquired pneumonia. He received treatment with levofloxacin 500 mg daily and required oxygen 2 L/min. He has a medical history of tobacco abuse, diabetes mellitus, and hypertension. He reports alcohol intake of 2–4 beers daily. His vital signs at 10 PM were blood pressure of 138/85 mmHg, heart rate of 92 beats/min, respiratory rate of 20 breaths/min, temperature of 37.4°C (99.3°F), and SaO$_2$ of 92% on oxygen 2 L/min. Currently, the patient is agitated and pacing his room. He is reporting that he needs to leave the "meeting" immediately and go home. He states that if he does not do this, someone is going to take his house and car away. He has removed his IV and oxygen tubing from his nose. His last vital signs taken 30 minutes previously were blood pressure of 156/92 mmHg, heart rate of 118 beats/min, respiratory rate of 26 breaths/min, temperature of 38.3°C (100.9°F), and oxygen saturation of 87% on room air. He is noted to be somewhat tremulous and diaphoretic. All of the following should be considered as part of the patient's diagnostic workup EXCEPT:

A. Arterial blood gas testing
B. Brain imaging with MRI or head CT
C. Fingerstick glucose testing
D. More thorough review of the patient's alcohol intake with his wife
E. Review of the recent medications received by the patient

I-86. Delirium, an acute confusional state, is a common disorder that remains a major cause of morbidity and mortality in the United States. Which of the following patients is at the highest risk for developing delirium?

A. A 36-year-old man admitted to the medical ward with a deep venous thrombosis
B. A 55-year-old man postoperative day 2 from a total colectomy
C. A 68-year-old woman admitted to the intensive care unit (ICU) with esophageal rupture
D. A 74-year-old woman in the preoperative clinic before hip surgery
E. An 84-year-old man living in an assisted living facility

I-87. Which of the following is the most common finding in aphasic patients?

A. Alexia
B. Anomia
C. Comprehension
D. Fluency
E. Repetition

I-88. A 65-year-old man experiences an ischemic cerebrovascular accident affecting the territory of the right anterior cerebral artery. After the stroke, an assessment reveals the findings shown in Figure I-88. What diagnosis does this figure suggest?

A. Construction apraxia
B. Hemianopia
C. Hemineglect
D. Object agnosia
E. Simultanagnosia

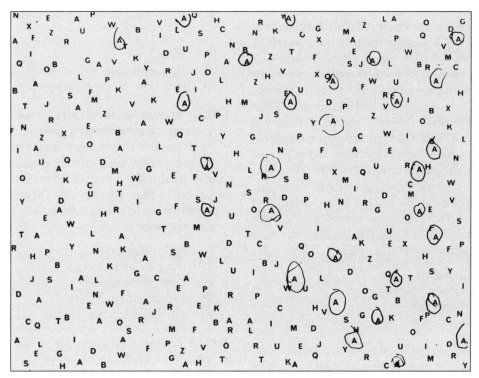

FIGURE I-88

I-89. A 42-year-old man is evaluated for excessive sleepiness that is interfering with his ability to work. He works at a glass factory that requires him to work rotating shifts. He typically cycles across day (7 AM–3 PM), evening (3 PM–11 PM), and night (11 PM–7 AM) shifts over the course of 4 weeks. He notes the problem to be most severe when he is on the night shift. Twice he has fallen asleep on the job. Although no accidents have occurred, he has been threatened with loss of his job if he falls asleep again. His preferred sleep schedule is 10 PM until 6 AM, but even when he is working day shifts, he typically only sleeps from about 10:30 PM until 5:30 AM. However, he feels fully functional at work on day and evening shifts. After his night shifts, he states that he finds it difficult to sleep when he first gets home, frequently not falling asleep until 10 AM or later. He is up by about 3 PM when his children arrive home from school. He drinks about 2 cups of coffee daily but tries to avoid drinking more than this. He does not snore and has a body mass index of 21.3 kg/m². All of the following are reasonable approaches to treatment in this man EXCEPT:

A. Avoidance of bright light in the morning after his shifts
B. Exercise in the early evening before going to work
C. Melatonin 3 mg taken at bedtime on the morning after a night shift
D. Modafinil 200 mg taken 30–60 minutes before starting a shift
E. Strategic napping of no more than 20 minutes during breaks at work

I-90. A 45-year-old woman presents for evaluation of abnormal sensations in her legs that keep her from sleeping at night. She first notices the symptoms around 8 PM when she is sitting quietly watching television. She describes the symptoms as "ants crawling in my veins." Although the symptoms are not painful, they are very uncomfortable and worsen when she lies down at night. They interfere with her ability to fall asleep about four times weekly. If she gets out of bed to walk or rubs her legs, the symptoms disappear almost immediately only to recur as soon as she is still. She also sometimes takes a very hot bath to alleviate the symptoms. During sleep, her husband complains that she kicks him throughout the night. She has no history of neurologic or renal disease. She currently is perimenopausal and has been experiencing very heavy and prolonged menstrual cycles over the past several months. The physical examination findings, including thorough neurologic examination, are normal. Her hemoglobin is 9.8 g/dL and hematocrit is 30.1%. The mean corpuscular volume is 68 fL. Serum ferritin is 12 ng/mL. Which is the most appropriate initial therapy for this patient?

A. Carbidopa/levodopa
B. Hormone replacement therapy
C. Iron supplementation
D. Oxycodone
E. Pramipexole

I-91. A 20-year-old man presents for evaluation of excessive daytime somnolence. He is finding it increasingly difficult to stay awake during his classes. Recently, his grades have fallen because whenever he tries to read, he finds himself drifting off. He finds that his alertness is best after exercising or brief naps of 10–30 minutes. Because of this, he states that he takes 5 or 10 "catnaps" daily. The sleepiness persists despite averaging 9 hours of sleep nightly. In addition to excessive somnolence, he reports occasional hallucinations that occur as he is falling asleep. He describes these occurrences as a voice calling his name as he drifts off. Perhaps once weekly, he awakens from sleep but is unable to move for a period of about 30 seconds. He has never had apparent loss of consciousness but states that whenever he is laughing, he feels heaviness in his neck and arms. Once he had to lean against a wall to keep from falling down. He undergoes an overnight sleep study and multiple sleep latency test. There is no sleep apnea. His mean sleep latency on five naps is 2.3 minutes. In three of the five naps, rapid eye movement sleep is present. Which of the following findings of this patient is most specific for the diagnosis of narcolepsy?

A. Cataplexy
B. Excessive daytime somnolence
C. Hypnagogic hallucinations
D. Rapid eye movement sleep in more than two naps on a multiple sleep latency test
E. Sleep paralysis

I-92. Which of the following is the most common sleep disorder in the U.S. population?

A. Delayed sleep phase syndrome
B. Insomnia
C. Obstructive sleep apnea
D. Narcolepsy
E. Restless legs syndrome

I-93. In which stage of sleep are the parasomnias somnambulism and night terrors most likely to occur?

A. Stage 1
B. Stage 2
C. Slow-wave sleep
D. Rapid eye movement sleep

I-94. A 44-year-old man is seen in the emergency department after a motor vehicle accident. The patient says, "I never saw that car coming from the right side." On physical examination, his pupils are equal and reactive to light. His visual acuity is normal; however, there are visual field defects in both eyes laterally (bitemporal hemianopia). Which of the following is most likely to be found on further evaluation?

A. Retinal detachment
B. Occipital lobe glioma
C. Optic nerve injury
D. Parietal lobe infarction
E. Pituitary adenoma

I-95. A 42-year-old construction worker complains of waking up with a red, painful left eye. She often works without goggles at her construction site. Her history is notable for hypertension, inflammatory bowel disease, diabetes, and prior IV drug use. Her only current medication is lisinopril. On examination, the left eye is diffusely red and sensitive to light. The eyelids are normal. In dim light, visual acuity is normal in both eyes. All of the following diagnoses will explain her findings EXCEPT:

A. Acute angle-closure glaucoma
B. Anterior uveitis
C. Corneal abrasion
D. Posterior uveitis
E. Transient ischemic attack

I-96. A 75-year-old triathlete complains of gradually worsening vision over the past year. It seems to be involving near and far vision. The patient has never required corrective lenses and has no significant medical history other than diet-controlled hypertension. He takes no regular medications. Physical examination is normal except for bilateral visual acuity of 20/100. There are no focal visual field defects and no redness of the eyes or eyelids. Which of the following is the most likely diagnosis?

A. Age-related macular degeneration
B. Blepharitis
C. Diabetic retinopathy
D. Episcleritis
E. Retinal detachment

I-97. All of the following statements regarding olfaction are true EXCEPT:

A. Decrements in olfaction may lead to nutritional deficiency.
B. More than 40% of patients with traumatic anosmia will regain normal function over time.
C. Significant decrements in olfaction are present in more than 50% of the population 80 years and older.
D. The most common identifiable cause of long-lasting or permanent loss of olfaction in outpatients is severe respiratory infection.
E. Women identify odorants better than men at all ages.

I-98. A 64-year-old man is evaluated for hearing loss that he thinks is worse in his left ear. His wife and children have told him for years that he does not listen to them. Recently, he has failed to hear the chime of the alarm on his digital watch, and he admits to focusing on the lips of individuals speaking to him because he sometimes has difficulties in word recognition. In addition, he reports a continuous buzzing that is louder in his left ear. He denies any sensation of vertigo, headaches, or balance difficulties. He has worked in a factory for many years that makes parts for airplanes, and the machinery that he works with sits to his left primarily. He has no family history of deafness, although his father had hearing loss as he aged. He has a medical history of hypertension, hyperlipidemia, and coronary artery disease. You suspect sensorineural hearing loss related to exposure to the intense noise in the factory for many decades. Which of the following findings would you expect on physical examination?

A. A deep tympanic retraction pocket seen above the pars flaccida on the tympanic membrane.
B. Cerumen impaction in the external auditory canal.
C. Hearing loss that is greater at lower frequencies on pure tone audiometry.
D. Increased intensity of sound when a tuning fork is placed on the mastoid process when compared with placement near the auditory canal.
E. Increased intensity of sound in the right ear when a tuning fork is placed in the midline of the forehead.

I-99. A 32-year-old woman presents to her primary care physician complaining of nasal congestion and drainage and headache. Her symptoms originally began about 7 days ago with rhinorrhea and sore throat. For the past 5 days, she has been having increasing feelings of fullness and pressure in the maxillary area that is causing her headaches. The pressure is worse when she bends over, and she also notices it while lying in bed at night. She is otherwise healthy and has not had fevers. On physical examination, there is purulent nasal drainage and pain with palpation over bilateral maxillary sinuses. What is the best approach to ongoing management of this patient?

A. Initiate therapy with amoxicillin 500 mg three times daily for 10 days.
B. Initiate therapy with levofloxacin 500 mg daily for 10 days.
C. Perform a sinus aspirate for culture and sensitivities.
D. Perform a sinus CT.
E. Treat with oral decongestants and nasal saline lavage.

I-100. A 28-year-old man seeks evaluation for sore throat for 2 days. He has not had a cough or rhinorrhea. He has no other medical conditions and works as a daycare provider. On examination, tonsillar hypertrophy with membranous exudate is present. What is the next step in the management of this patient?

A. Empiric treatment with amoxicillin 500 mg twice daily for 10 days
B. Rapid antigen detection test for *Streptococcus pyogenes* only
C. Rapid antigen detection test for *Streptococcus pyogenes* plus throat culture if the rapid test result is negative
D. Rapid antigen detection test for *Streptococcus pyogenes* plus a throat culture regardless of result
E. Throat culture only

I-101. A 62-year-old man presents to his physician complaining of shortness of breath. All of the following findings are consistent with left ventricular dysfunction as a cause of the patient's dyspnea EXCEPT:

A. Feeling of chest tightness
B. Nocturnal dyspnea
C. Orthopnea
D. Pulsus paradoxus greater than 10 mmHg
E. Sensation of air hunger

I-102. A 42-year-old woman seeks evaluation for a cough that has been present for almost 3 months. The cough is mostly dry and non-productive, but occasionally productive of yellow phlegm. She reports that the cough is worse at night and often wakes her from sleep. She denies any recent upper respiratory tract infection, allergic rhinitis, fever, chills or cough. She recalls her mother told her that she had asthma as a child but she has never felt symptomatic wheezing as an adult. She exercises regularly but continues to smoke 1 pack per day of cigarettes; she'd like to quit. The patient takes no medications. Her physical examination is unremarkable. Which of the following is indicated at this point?

A. Chest PET-CT
B. Chest radiograph
C. Measurement of serum angiotensin-converting enzyme (ACE)
D. Measurement of serum IgE
E. Sinus CT

I-103. In the patient described above, her chest radiograph is normal and further history reveals a long history of symptoms suggestive of GERD. She also admits that her cough is worse on nights after a large or late meal. She often has a bad taste in her mouth as she starts coughing. Based on this information, which of the following would be a reasonable empiric therapeutic trial?

A. Inhaled corticosteroid
B. Inhaled long acting beta agonist
C. Nasal corticosteroid
D. Oral proton pump inhibitor
E. Oral triple antibiotic therapy for *H. pylori*

I-104. A 48-year-old man is evaluated for hypoxia of unknown etiology. He recently has noticed shortness of breath that is worse with exertion and in the upright position. It is relieved with lying down. On physical examination, he is visibly dyspneic with minimal exertion. He is noted to have a resting oxygen saturation of 89% on room air. When lying down, his oxygen saturation increases to 93%. His pulmonary examination shows no wheezes or crackles. His cardiac examination findings are normal without murmur. His chest radiograph reports a possible 1-cm lung nodule in the right lower lobe. On 100% oxygen and in the upright position, the patient has an oxygen saturation of 90%. What is the most likely cause of the patient's hypoxia?

A. Circulatory hypoxia
B. Hypoventilation
C. Intracardiac right-to-left shunting
D. Intrapulmonary right-to-left shunting
E. Ventilation–perfusion mismatch

I-105. A patient is evaluated in the emergency department for peripheral cyanosis. All of the following are potential etiologies EXCEPT:

A. Cold exposure
B. Deep venous thrombosis
C. Methemoglobinemia
D. Peripheral vascular disease
E. Raynaud's phenomenon

I-106. An 18-year-old college freshman is being evaluated for a heart murmur heard at health screening. She reports an active lifestyle, no past medical history, and no cardiac symptoms. She has a midsystolic murmur that follows a nonejection sound and crescendos with S2. The murmur duration is greater when going from supine to standing and decreases when squatting. The murmur is heard best along the lower left sternal border and apex. Her electrocardiogram is normal. Which of the following is the most likely condition causing the murmur?

A. Aortic stenosis
B. Hypertrophic obstructive cardiomyopathy
C. Mitral valve prolapse
D. Pulmonic stenosis
E. Tricuspid regurgitation

I-107. Which of the following characteristics makes a heart murmur more likely to be caused by tricuspid regurgitation than mitral regurgitation?

A. Decreased intensity with amyl nitrate
B. Inaudible A2 at the apex
C. Prominent c-v wave in jugular pulse
D. Onset signaled by a midsystolic click
E. Wide splitting of S2

I-108. You are examining a 25-year-old patient in clinic who came in for a routine examination. Cardiac auscultation reveals a second heart sound that is split and does not vary with respiration. There is also a grade 2–3 midsystolic murmur at the midsternal border. Which of the following is most likely?

A. Atrial septal defect
B. Hypertrophic obstructive cardiomyopathy
C. Left bundle branch block
D. Normal physiology
E. Pulmonary hypertension

I-109. A 32-year-old woman presents to her physician complaining of hair loss. She is currently 10 weeks postpartum after delivery of a normal healthy baby girl. She admits to having increased stress and sleep loss because her child has colic. She also has not been able to nurse because of poor milk production. On examination, the patient's hair does not appear to have decreased density. With a gentle tug, more than 10 hairs come out but are not broken and all appear normal. There are no scalp lesions. What do you recommend for this patient?

A. Careful evaluation of the patient's hair care products for a potential cause
B. Reassurance only
C. Referral for counseling for trichotillomania
D. Treatment with minoxidil
E. Treatment with topical steroids

I-110. A 26-year-old man develops diffuse itching, wheezing, and laryngeal edema within minutes of receiving intravenous radiocontrast media for an intravenous pyelogram. He has not previously received contrast dye per his recollection. He is treated with supportive care and recovers without further complications. Which of the following best describes the mechanism of the patient's reaction to the contrast media?

A. Cross-linking of IgE molecules fixed to sensitized cells in the presence of a specific drug-protein conjugate
B. Deposition of circulating immune complexes
C. Development of drug-specific T-cell immunogenicity
D. Direct mast cell degranulation
E. Hepatic metabolism into toxic intermediate

I-111. A 44-year-old woman is prescribed phenytoin for the development of complex partial seizures. One month after initiating the medication, she is evaluated for a diffuse erythematous eruption with associated fever to 101.3°F. She is noted to have facial edema with diffusely enlarged lymph nodes along the cervical, axillary, and inguinal areas. Her white cell count is 14,500/μL (75% neutrophils, 12% lymphocytes, 5% atypical lymphocytes, and 8% eosinophils). A basic metabolic panel is normal, but elevations in the liver functions tests are noted with an AST of 124 U/L, ALT of 148 U/L, alkaline phosphatase of 114 U/L, and total bilirubin of 2.2 mg/dL. All of the following are indicated in the management of this patient EXCEPT:

A. Administration of carbamazepine 200 mg twice daily
B. Administration of prednisone 1.5–2 mg/kg daily
C. Administration of topical glucocorticoids
D. Discontinuation of phenytoin
E. Evaluation for development of thyroiditis for up to 6 months

I-112. Which of the following drugs is associated with development of both phototoxicity and photoallergy?

A. Amiodarone
B. Diclofenac
C. Doxycycline
D. Hydrochlorothiazide
E. Levofloxacin

I-113. You are seeing a patient in follow-up in whom you have begun an evaluation for an elevated hematocrit. You suspect polycythemia vera based on a history of aquagenic pruritus and splenomegaly. Which set of laboratory tests is consistent with the diagnosis of polycythemia vera?

A. Elevated red blood cell mass, high serum erythropoietin levels, and normal oxygen saturation
B. Elevated red blood cell mass, low serum erythropoietin levels, and normal oxygen saturation
C. Normal red blood cell mass, high serum erythropoietin levels, and low arterial oxygen saturation
D. Normal red blood cell mass, low serum erythropoietin levels, and low arterial oxygen saturation

I-114. All of the following are common manifestations of bleeding caused by von Willebrand disease EXCEPT:

A. Angiodysplasia of the small bowel
B. Epistaxis
C. Menorrhagia
D. Postpartum hemorrhage
E. Spontaneous hemarthrosis

I-115. A 68-year-old man is admitted to the intensive care unit with spontaneous retroperitoneal bleeding and hypotension. He has a medical history of hypertension, diabetes mellitus, and chronic kidney disease stage III. His medications include lisinopril, amlodipine, sitagliptin, and glimepiride. On initial presentation, he is in pain and has a blood pressure of 70/40 mmHg with a heart rate of 132 beats/min. His hemoglobin on admission is 5.3 g/dL and hematocrit is 16.0%. His coagulation studies demonstrate an aPTT of 64 seconds and a PT of 12.1 seconds (INR 1.0). Mixing studies (1:1) are performed. Immediately, the aPTT decreases to 42 seconds. At 1 hour, the aPTT is 56 seconds, and at 2 hours, it is 68 seconds. Thrombin time and reptilase time are normal. Fibrinogen is also normal. What is the most likely cause of the patient's coagulopathy?

A. Acquired factor VIII deficiency
B. Acquired factor VIII inhibitor
C. Heparin
D. Lupus anticoagulant
E. Vitamin K deficiency

I-116. A 54-year-old man is seen in the clinic complaining of painless enlargement of lymph nodes in his neck. He has not otherwise been ill and denies fevers, chills, weight loss, and fatigue. His past medical history is remarkable for pulmonary tuberculosis that was treated 10 years previously under directly observed therapy. He currently takes no medications. He is a heterosexual man in a monogamous relationship for 25 years. He denies illicit drug use. He has smoked 1½ packs of cigarettes daily since 16 years of age. He works as a logger. On physical examination, the patient is thin, but not ill-appearing. He is not febrile and has normal vital signs. He has dental caries noted with gingivitis. In the right supraclavicular area, there is a hard and fixed lymph node measuring 2.5 × 2.0 cm in size. Lymph nodes less than 1 cm in size are noted in the anterior cervical chain. There is no axillary or inguinal lymphadenopathy. His liver and spleen are not enlarged. Which of the following factors in history or physical examination increases the likelihood that the lymph node enlargement is caused by malignancy?

A. Age greater than 50 years
B. Location in the supraclavicular area
C. Presence of a lymph node that is hard and fixed
D. Size greater than 2.25 cm^2 (1.5 × 1.5 cm)
E. All of the above

I-117. A 24-year-old woman presents for a routine checkup and complains only of small masses in her groin. She states that they have been present for at least 3 years. She denies fever, malaise, weight loss, and anorexia. She works as a sailing instructor and competes in triathlons. On physical examination, she is noted to have several palpable 1-cm inguinal lymph nodes that are mobile, nontender, and discrete. There is no other lymphadenopathy or focal findings on examination. What should be the next step in management?

A. Bone marrow biopsy
B. CT scan of the chest, abdomen, and pelvis
C. Excisional biopsy
D. Fine-needle aspiration for culture and cytopathology
E. Pelvic ultrasonography
F. Reassurance

I-118. All of the following diseases are associated with massive splenomegaly (spleen extends 8 cm below the costal margin or weighs >1000 g) EXCEPT:

A. Autoimmune hemolytic anemia
B. Chronic lymphocytic leukemia
C. Cirrhosis with portal hypertension
D. Marginal zone lymphoma
E. Myelofibrosis with myeloid metaplasia

I-119. The presence of Howell-Jolly bodies, Heinz bodies, basophilic stippling, and nucleated red blood cells in a patient with hairy cell leukemia before any treatment intervention implies which of the following?

A. Diffuse splenic infiltration by tumor
B. Disseminated intravascular coagulation (DIC)
C. Hemolytic anemia
D. Pancytopenia
E. Transformation to acute leukemia

I-120. Which of the following is true regarding infection risk after elective splenectomy?

A. Patients are at no increased risk of viral infection after splenectomy.
B. Patients should be vaccinated 2 weeks after splenectomy.
C. Splenectomy patients over the age of 50 are at greatest risk for postsplenectomy sepsis.
D. *Staphylococcus aureus* is the most commonly implicated organism in postsplenectomy sepsis.
E. The risk of infection after splenectomy increases with time.

I-121. An 18-year-old man is seen in consultation for a pulmonary abscess caused by infection with *Staphylococcus aureus*. He had been in his usual state of health until 1 week ago when he developed fevers and a cough. He has no ill contacts and presents in the summer. His medical history is significant for episodes of axillary and perianal abscesses requiring incision and drainage. He cannot specifically recall how often this has occurred, but he does know it has been more than five times that he can recall. In one instance, he recalls a lymph node became enlarged to the point that it "popped" and drained spontaneously. He also reports frequent aphthous ulcers and is treated for eczema. On physical examination, his height is 5'3". He appears ill with a temperature of 39.6°C. Eczematous dermatitis is present in the scalp and periorbital area. There are crackles at the left lung base. Axillary lymphadenopathy is present bilaterally and is tender. The spleen in enlarged. His laboratory studies show a white blood cell count of 12,500/μL (94% neutrophils), hemoglobin of 11.3 g/dL, hematocrit of 34.2%, and platelets of 320,000/μL. Granulomatous inflammation is seen on lymph node biopsy. Which of the following tests are most likely found in this patient?

A. Elevated angiotensin-converting enzyme level
B. Eosinophilia
C. Giant primary granules in neutrophils
D. Mutations of the tumor necrosis factor-alpha receptor
E. Positive nitroblue tetrazolium dye test

I-122. A 72-year-old man with chronic obstructive pulmonary disease and stable coronary disease presents to the emergency department with several days of worsening productive cough, fevers, malaise, and diffuse muscle aches. A chest radiograph demonstrates a new lobar infiltrate. Laboratory measurements reveal a total white blood cell count of 12,100 cells/μL with a neutrophilic predominance of 86% and 8% band forms. He is diagnosed with community-acquired pneumonia, and antibiotic treatment is initiated. Under normal, or "nonstress," conditions, what percentage of the total body neutrophils are present in the circulation?

A. 2%
B. 10%
C. 25%
D. 40%
E. 90%

I-123. A patient with longstanding HIV infection, alcoholism, and asthma is seen in the emergency department for 1–2 days of severe wheezing. He has not been taking any medicines for months. He is admitted to the hospital and treated with nebulized therapy and systemic glucocorticoids. His CD4 count is 8 and viral load is greater than 750,000. His total white blood cell (WBC) count is 3200 cells/μL with 90% neutrophils. He is accepted into an inpatient substance abuse rehabilitation program and before discharge is started on opportunistic infection prophylaxis, bronchodilators, a prednisone taper over 2 weeks, ranitidine, and highly active antiretroviral therapy. The rehabilitation center pages you 2 weeks later; a routine laboratory check reveals a total WBC count of 900 cells/μL with 5% neutrophils. Which of the following new drugs would most likely explain this patient's neutropenia?

A. Darunavir
B. Efavirenz
C. Ranitidine
D. Prednisone
E. Trimethoprim–sulfamethoxazole

I-124. All of the following statements regarding mercury exposure or poisoning are true EXCEPT:

A. Chronic mercury poisoning is best assessed using hair samples.
B. Ethyl mercury preservative in multiuse vaccines has not been implicated in causing autism.
C. Exposure to as little as a few drops of dimethylmercury may be lethal.
D. Offspring of mothers who ingested mercury-contaminated fish are at higher risk of neurobehavioral abnormalities.
E. Pregnant women should avoid consumption of sardines and mackerel.

I-125. A 39-year-old man comes to clinic reporting a 4-day illness that began while he was in the Caribbean on vacation. A few hours after attending a large seafood buffet, he developed abdominal pain, chills, nausea, and diarrhea. Soon thereafter, he noticed diffused paresthesias, throat numbness, and fatigue. The symptoms slowly improved over 2 days, and he returned home yesterday. Today he noticed while washing that cold water felt hot and warm water felt cold. He is concerned about this new symptom. All of the following are true regarding his illness EXCEPT:

A. His symptoms should improve over weeks to months.
B. It is likely caused by ingestion of contaminated snapper or grouper.
C. It is likely caused by ingestion of undercooked oysters or clams.
D. Subsequent episodes may be more severe.
E. No diagnostic laboratory test is available.

I-126. Which of the following is the most common cause of death from poisoning?

A. Acetaminophen
B. Carbon monoxide
C. Chlorine gas
D. Insecticide
E. Tricyclic antidepressants

I-127. Which of the following is a distinguishing feature of amphetamine overdose versus other causes of sympathetic overstimulation caused by drug overdose or withdrawal?

A. Hallucination
B. Hot, dry, flushed skin and urinary retention
C. History of benzodiazepine abuse
D. Markedly increased blood pressure, heart rate, and end-organ damage in the absence of hallucination
E. Nystagmus

I-128. A patient with metabolic acidosis, reduced anion gap, and increased osmolal gap is most likely to have which of the following toxic ingestions?

A. Lithium
B. Methanol
C. Oxycodone
D. Propylene glycol
E. Salicylate

I-129. Which of the following is true regarding drug effects after an overdose compared with a reference dose?

A. Drug effects begin earlier, peak earlier, and last longer.
B. Drug effects begin earlier, peak later, and last longer.
C. Drug effects begin earlier, peak later, and last shorter.
D. Drug effects begin later, peak earlier, and last shorter.
E. Drug effects begin later, peak later, and last longer.

I-130. Which of the following statements regarding gastric decontamination for toxin ingestion is true?

A. Activated charcoal's most common side effect is aspiration.
B. Gastric lavage via nasogastric tube is preferred over the use of activated charcoal when therapeutic endoscopy may also be warranted.
C. Syrup of ipecac has no role in the hospital setting.
D. There are insufficient data to support or exclude a benefit when gastric decontamination is used more than 1 hour after a toxic ingestion.
E. All of the above are true.

I-131. One of your patients is contemplating a trekking trip to Nepal at elevations between 2500 and 3000 m. Five years ago, while skiing at Telluride (altitude, 2650 m), she recalls having headache, nausea, and fatigue within 1 day of arriving that lasted about 2–3 days. All of the following are true regarding the development of acute mountain sickness in this patient EXCEPT:

A. Acetazolamide starting 1 day before ascent is effective in decreasing the risk.
B. Gingko biloba is not effective in decreasing the risk.
C. Gradual ascent is protective.
D. Her prior episode increases her risk for this trip.
E. Improved physical conditioning before the trip decreases the risk.

I-132. A 36-year-old man develops shortness of breath, dyspnea, and dry cough 3 days after arriving for helicopter snowboarding in the Bugaboo mountain range in British Columbia (elevation, 3000 m). Over the next 12 hours, he becomes more short of breath and produces pink, frothy sputum. An EMT-trained guide hears crackles on chest examination. All of the following are true regarding his illness EXCEPT:

A. Descent and oxygen are most therapeutic.
B. Exercise increased his risk.
C. Fever and leukocytosis may occur.
D. He should never risk return to high altitude after recovery.
E. Pretreatment with nifedipine or tadalafil would have lowered his risk.

I-133. Which of the following is considered an absolute contraindication to hyperbaric oxygen therapy?

A. Carbon monoxide poisoning
B. History of COPD
C. History of high altitude pulmonary edema
D. Radiation proctitis
E. Untreated pneumothorax

I-134. A 35-year-old woman is scuba diving while vacationing in Malaysia. During her last dive of the day, her regulator malfunctions, requiring her to ascend from 20 m to the surface rapidly. Upon returning to the boat, she feels well. However, about 6 hours after returning to shore, she develops diffuse itching and muscle aches, leg pain, blurred vision, slurred speech, and nausea. Which of the following statements regarding her condition is true?

A. Decompression illness is unlikely at 20-m water depth.
B. Inhalation of 100% oxygen is contraindicated.
C. She can never again scuba dive to a depth greater than 6 m.
D. She should receive recompression and hyperbaric oxygen therapy.
E. She should remain upright as much as possible.

I-135. Which of the following statements regarding the distinction between acute lung injury (ALI) and acute respiratory distress syndrome (ARDS) is true?

A. ALI and ARDS can be distinguished by radiographic testing.
B. ALI and ARDS can be distinguished by the magnitude of the PaO_2/FIO_2 ratio.
C. ALI can be diagnosed in the presence of elevated left atrial pressure, but ARDS can not.
D. ALI is caused by direct lung injury, but ARDS is the result of secondary lung injury.
E. The risk of ALI but not ARDS increases with multiple predisposing conditions.

I-136. Which of the following has been demonstrated to reduce mortality in patients with ARDS?

A. High-dose glucocorticoids within 48 hours of presentation
B. High-frequency mechanical ventilation
C. Inhaled nitric oxide
D. Low tidal volume mechanical ventilation
E. Surfactant replacement

I-137. A 38-year-old man is hospitalized in the ICU with ARDS after a motor vehicle accident with multiple long bone fractures, substantial blood loss, and hypotension. By day 2 of hospitalization, he is off vasopressors but is requiring a high FIO_2 and positive end-expiratory pressure (PEEP) to maintain adequate oxygenation. His family is asking about the short- and long-term prognosis for recovery. All of the following statements about his prognosis are true EXCEPT:

A. He has a greater chance of survival than a patient with similar physiology who is older than 70 years old.
B. His overall mortality from ARDS is approximately 25–45%.
C. If he survives, he is likely to have some degree of depression or posttraumatic stress disorder.
D. If he survives, he likely will have normal or near normal lung function.
E. The most likely cause of mortality is hypoxemic respiratory failure.

I-138. Clinical trials support the use of noninvasive ventilation in which of the following patients?

A. A 33-year-old man who was rescued from a motor vehicle accident. He is unarousable with possible internal injuries. Room air blood gas is 7.30 (pH), PCO_2 50 mmHg, PO_2 60 mmHg.
B. A 49-year-old woman with end-stage renal disease admitted with presumed staphylococcal sepsis from her hemodialysis catheter. She is somnolent, blood pressure is 80/50 mmHg, heart rate is 105 beats/min, and room air oxygen saturation is 95%.
C. A 58-year-old woman with a history of cirrhotic liver disease admitted with a presumed esophageal variceal bleed. Her blood pressure is 75/55 mmHg, and she has a heart rate of 110 beats/min. She is awake and alert.
D. A 62-year-old man with a long history of COPD admitted with an exacerbation related to an upper respiratory tract infection. He is in marked respiratory distress but is awake and alert. Chest radiograph only shows hyperinflation. His room air arterial blood gas is pH, 7.28; PCO_2, 75 mmHg; and PO_2, 46 mmHg.
E. A 74-year-old man with cardiogenic shock and an acute ST-segment elevation myocardial infarction. His blood pressure is 84/65 mmHg, heart rate is 110 beats/min, respiratory rate is 24 breaths/min, and room air oxygen saturation is 85%.

I-139. You are caring for a patient on mechanical ventilation in the intensive care unit. Whenever the patient initiates a breath, no matter her spontaneous respiratory rate, she gets a fixed volume breath from the machine that does not change from breath to breath. After receiving a dose of sedation, she does not initiate any breaths, but the machine delivers the same volume breath at periodic fixed intervals during this time. Which of the following modes of mechanical ventilation is this patient receiving?

A. Assist control
B. Continuous positive airway pressure
C. Pressure control
D. Pressure support
E. Synchronized intermittent mandatory ventilation (SIMV)

I-140. A 68-year-old woman has been receiving mechanical ventilation for 10 days for community-acquired pneumonia. You are attempting to decide whether the patient is appropriate for a spontaneous breathing trial. All of the following factors would indicate that the patient is likely to be successfully extubated EXCEPT:

A. Alert mental status
B. PEEP of 5 cmH_2O
C. pH greater than 7.35
D. Rapid shallow breathing index (respiratory rate/tidal volume) greater than 105
E. SaO_2 greater than 90% and FIO_2 less than 0.5

I-141. A 45-year-old woman with HIV is admitted to the intensive care unit with pneumonia and pneumothorax secondary to infection with *Pneumocystis jiroveci*. She requires mechanical ventilatory support, chest tube placement, and central venous access. The ventilator settings are PC mode; inspiratory pressure, 30 cmH_2O, 1.0; and PEEP, 10 cmH_2O. An arterial blood gas measured on these settings shows: pH 7.32, 46 mmHg, and 62 mmHg. All of the following are important supportive measures for this patient EXCEPT:

A. Analgesia to maintain patient comfort
B. Daily change of ventilator circuit
C. Gastric acid suppression
D. Nutritional support
E. Prophylaxis against deep venous thrombosis

I-142. All of the following statements about the physiology of mechanical ventilation are true EXCEPT:

A. Application of PEEP decreases left ventricular preload and afterload.
B. High inspired tidal volumes contribute to the development of acute lung injury caused by overdistention of alveoli with resultant alveolar damage.
C. Increasing the inspiratory flow rate will decrease the ratio of inspiration to expiration (I:E) and allow more time for expiration.
D. Mechanical ventilation provides assistance with inspiration and expiration.
E. PEEP helps prevent alveolar collapse at end-expiration.

I-143. A 64-year-old man requires endotracheal intubation and mechanical ventilation for chronic obstructive pulmonary disease. He was paralyzed with rocuronium for intubation. His initial ventilator settings were AC mode; respiratory rate 10 breaths/minute; FIO_2 1.0; Vt (tidal volume) 550 mL; and positive end-expiratory pressure 0 cm H_2O. On admission to the intensive care unit the patient remains paralzyed; arterial blood gas is pH 7.22, PCO_2 78 mmHg, PO_2 394 mmHg. The FIO_2 is decreased to 0.6. Thirty minutes later you are called to the bedside to evaluate the patient for hypotension. Current vital signs are blood pressure 80/40 mmHg, heart rate, 133 beats/min; respiratory rate, 24/minute; and oxygen saturation 92%. Physical examination shows the patient is agitated and moving all extremities, a prolonged expiration with wheezing continuing until the initiation of the next breath. Breath sounds are heard in both lung fields. The high-pressure alarm on the ventilator is triggering. What should be done first in treating this patient's hypotension?

A. Administer a fluid bolus of 500 mL.
B. Disconnect the patient from the ventilator.
C. Initiate a continuous IV infusion of midazolam.
D. Initiate a continuous IV infusion of norepinephrine.
E. Perform tube thoracostomy on the right side.

I-144. All of the following are relative contraindications for the use of succinylcholine as a paralytic for endotracheal intubation EXCEPT:

A. Acetaminophen overdose
B. Acute renal failure
C. Crush injuries
D. Muscular dystrophy
E. Tumor lysis syndrome

I-145. Match the following vasopressors with the statement that best describes their action on the cardiovascular system.

1. Dobutamine
2. Low-dose dopamine (2–4 μg/kg/min)
3. Norepinephrine
4. Phenylephrine
A. Acts solely at α-adrenergic receptors to cause vasoconstriction
B. Acts at $β_1$-adrenergic receptors and dopaminergic receptors to increase cardiac contractility and heart rate; also causes vasodilatation and increased splanchnic and renal blood flow
C. Acts at $β_1$- and, to a lesser extent, $β_2$-adrenergic receptors to increase cardiac contractility, heart rate, and vasodilatation
D. Acts at α- and $β_1$-adrenergic receptors to increase heart rate, cardiac contractility, and vasoconstriction

I-146. An 86-year-old nursing home resident is brought by ambulance to the local emergency department. He was found unresponsive in his bed immersed in black stool. Apparently, he had not been feeling well for 1–2 days, had complained of vague abdominal pain, and had decreased oral intake; no further history is available from the nursing home staff. His past medical history is remarkable for Alzheimer's dementia and treated prostate cancer. The emergency responders were able to appreciate a faint pulse and obtained a blood pressure of 91/49 mmHg and a heart rate of 120 beats/min. In the emergency department, his pressure is 88/51 mmHg and heart rate is 131 beats/min. He is moaning and obtunded, localizes to pain, and has flat neck veins. Skin tenting is noted. A central venous catheter is placed that reveals CVP less than 5 mmHg, specimens for initial laboratory testing are sent off, and electrocardiogram and chest x-ray are obtained. Catheterization of the bladder yields no urine. Anesthesiology has been called to the bedside and is assessing the patient's airway. What is the best immediate step in management?

A. Infuse hypertonic saline to increase the rate of vascular filling.
B. Infuse isotonic crystalloid solution via IV wide open.
C. Infuse a colloidal solution rapidly.
D. Initiate inotropic support with dobutamine.
E. Initiate IV pressors starting with Levophed.

I-147. In the patient described above, which of the following is true regarding his clinical condition?

A. Loss of 20–40% of the blood volume leads to shock physiology.

B. Loss of less than 20% of the blood volume will manifest as orthostasis.

C. Oliguria is a crucial prognostic sign of impending vascular collapse.

D. Symptoms of hypovolemic shock differ from those of hemorrhagic shock.

E. The first sign of hypovolemic shock is mental obtundation.

I-148. A 52-year-old man presents with crushing substernal chest pain. He has a history of coronary artery disease and has had two non–ST-segment elevation myocardial inf-arctions in the past 5 years, both requiring percutaneous intervention and intracoronary stent placement. His electro-cardiogram shows ST elevations across the precordial leads, and he is taken emergently to the catheterization laboratory. After angioplasty and stent placement, he is transferred to the coronary care unit. His vital signs are stable on transfer; how-ever, 20 minutes after arrival, he is found to be unresponsive. His radial pulse is thready, extremities are cool, and blood pressure is difficult to obtain; with a manual cuff, it is 65/40 mmHg. The nurse turns to you and asks what you would like to do next. Which of the following accurately represents the physiologic characteristics of this patient's condition?

	Central Venous Pressure	Cardiac Output	Systemic Vascular Resistance
A.	Decreased	Decreased	Decreased
B.	Decreased	Increased	Decreased
C.	Increased	Increased	Decreased
D.	Increased	Decreased	Increased
E.	Decreased	Decreased	Increased

I-149. All of the following are factors that are related to the increased incidence of sepsis in the United States EXCEPT:

A. Aging of the population

B. Increased longevity of individuals with chronic disease

C. Increased risk of sepsis in individuals without comorbidities

D. Increased risk of sepsis in individuals with AIDS

E. Increased use of immunosuppressive drugs

I-150. A 68-year-old woman is brought to the emergency department for fever and lethargy. She first felt ill yester-day and experienced generalized body aches. Overnight, she developed a fever of 39.6°C and had shaking chills. By this morning, she was feeling very fatigued. Her son feels that she has had periods of waxing and waning mental status. She denies cough, nausea, vomiting, diarrhea, and abdominal pain. She has a medical history of rheumatoid arthritis. She takes prednisone, 10 mg daily, and meth-otrexate, 15 mg weekly. On examination, she is lethargic but appropriate. Her vital signs are blood pressure of 85/50

mmHg, heart rate of 122 beats/min, temperature of 39.1°C, respiratory rate of 24 breaths/min, and oxygen saturation of 97% on room air. Physical examination shows clear lung fields and a regular tachycardia without murmur. There is no abdominal tenderness or masses. Stool is negative for occult blood. There are no rashes. Hematologic studies show a white blood cell count of 24,200/μL with a differ-ential of 82% PMNs, 8% band forms, 6% lymphocytes, and 3% monocytes. Hemoglobin is 8.2 g/dL. A urinalysis has numerous white blood cells with gram-negative bacteria on Gram stain. Chemistries reveal the following: bicarbonate of 16 meq/L, BUN of 60 mg/dL, and creatinine of 2.4 mg/dL. After fluid administration of 2 L, the patient has a blood pressure of 88/54 mmHg and a heart rate of 112 beats/min with a central venous pressure of 18 cmH₂O. There is 25 mL of urine output in the first hour. The patient has been ini-tiated on antibiotics with cefepime. What should be done next for the treatment of this patient's hypotension?

A. Dopamine, 3 μg/kg/min IV

B. Hydrocortisone, 50 mg IV every 6 hours

C. Norepinephrine, 2 μg/min IV

D. Ongoing colloid administration at 500–1000 mL/h

E. Transfusion of 2 units of packed red blood cells

I-151. All of the following statements about the pathogenesis of sepsis and septic shock are true EXCEPT:

A. Blood cultures are positive in only 20–40% of cases of severe sepsis.

B. Microbial invasion of the bloodstream is not neces-sary for the development of severe sepsis.

C. Serum levels of TNF-alpha are typically reduced in patients with severe sepsis or septic shock.

D. The hallmark of septic shock is a marked decrease in peripheral vascular resistance that occurs despite increased plasma levels of catecholamines.

E. Widespread vascular endothelial injury is present in severe sepsis and is mediated by cytokines and proco-agulant factors that stimulate intravascular thrombosis.

I-152. Which of the following treatments is recommended to improve mortality in septic shock?

A. Activated protein C (drotrecogin alpha)

B. Administration of antibiotics within 1 hour of presentation

C. Bicarbonate therapy for severe acidosis

D. Erythropoietin

E. Vasopressin infusion

I-153. All of the following statements regarding cardiogenic shock are true EXCEPT:

A. Approximately 80% of cases of cardiogenic shock complicating acute myocardial infarction are attributable to acute severe mitral regurgitation.
B. Cardiogenic shock is more common in ST-segment elevation than non–ST-segment elevation myocardial infarction.
C. Cardiogenic shock is uncommon in inferior wall myocardial infarction.
D. Cardiogenic shock may occur in the absence of significant coronary stenosis.
E. Pulmonary capillary wedge pressure is elevated in cardiogenic shock.

I-154. Aortic counterpulsation with an intra-aortic balloon pump has which of the following as an advantage over therapy with infused vasopressors or inotropes in a patient with acute ST-segment elevation myocardial infarction and cardiogenic shock?

A. Increased heart rate
B. Increased left ventricular afterload
C. Lower diastolic blood pressure
D. Not contraindicated in acute aortic regurgitation
E. Reduced myocardial oxygen consumption

I-155. Which of the following is the most common electrical mechanism to explain sudden cardiac death?

A. Asystole
B. Bradycardia
C. Pulseless electrical activity (PEA)
D. Pulseless ventricular tachycardia (PVT)
E. Ventricular fibrillation

I-156. All of the following statements regarding successful resuscitation from sudden cardiac death are true EXCEPT:

A. Advanced age does not affect the likelihood of immediate resuscitation, only the probability of hospital discharge.
B. After cardiac out of hospital cardiac arrest, survival rates are approximately 25% if defibrillation is administered after 5 minutes.
C. If the initial rhythm in an out-of-hospital cardiac arrest is pulseless ventricular tachycardia, the patient has a higher probability of survival than asystole.
D. Prompt CPR followed by prompt defibrillation improves outcomes in all settings.
E. The probability of survival from cardiac arrest is higher if the event takes place in a public setting than at home.

I-157. A 28-year-old woman has severe head trauma after a motor vehicle accident. One year after the accident, she is noted to have spontaneous eye opening and is able to track an object visually at times. She does not speak or follow any commands. She breathes independently but is fed through a gastrostomy tube. She can move all extremities spontaneously but without purposeful movement. What term best describes this patient's condition?

A. Coma
B. Locked-in
C. Minimally conscious state
D. Persistent vegetative state
E. Vegetative state

I-158. A 52-year-old man is evaluated after a large subarachnoid hemorrhage (SAH) from a ruptured cerebral aneurysm. There is concern that the patient has brain death. What test is most commonly used to diagnose brain death in this situation?

A. Apnea testing
B. Cerebral angiography
C. Demonstration of absent cranial nerve reflexes
D. Demonstration of fixed and dilated pupils
E. Performance of transcranial Doppler ultrasonography

I-159. Which of the following neurologic phenomena is classically associated with herniation of the brain through the foramen magnum?

A. Third-nerve compression and ipsilateral papillary dilation
B. Catatonia
C. "Locked-in" state
D. Miotic pupils
E. Respiratory arrest

I-160. A 72-year-old woman is admitted to the intensive care unit after a cardiac arrest at home. She had a witnessed collapse, and her family immediately began to perform cardiopulmonary resuscitation. Emergency medical service arrived within 10 minutes, and the initial cardiac rhythm demonstrated ventricular fibrillation. Spontaneous circulation returned after defibrillation, and the estimated time the patient was without a pulse was 15–20 minutes. The patient is brought to hospital and remains intubated, paralyzed, and sedated in the coronary care unit. She is being treated with medically induced hypothermia and is completely unresponsive to all stimuli 12 hours after the initial event. Her pupils are 3 mm and respond sluggishly to light. She has no cough or gag reflex. Intermittent myoclonic jerks are seen. The family has concerns about her neurologic prognosis after her prolonged cardiac arrest. What advice do you give the family regarding prognosis in this situation?

A. An MRI scan of the brain should be performed before determining neurologic outcome.
B. Apnea testing will be performed at the first opportunity to determine if the patient has suffered brain death.
C. Given the immediate actions of the family to initiate cardiopulmonary resuscitation, the patient has a greater than 50% chance to have good neurologic outcomes.
D. It is impossible to predict the patient's likelihood of neurologic recovery as her examination is unreliable in the face of sedation and hypothermia.
E. No information regarding prognosis can be determined until 72 hours have passed.

I-161. A 52-year-old man presents to the emergency department complaining of the worst headache of his life that is unresolving. It began abruptly 3 days before presentation and is worse with bending over. It rapidly increased in intensity over 30 minutes, but he did not seek medical care at that time. Over the ensuing 72 hours, the headache has persisted although lessened in intensity. He has not lost consciousness and has no other neurologic symptoms. His vision is normal, but he does report that light is painful to his eyes. His past medical history is notable for hypertension, but he takes his medications irregularly. Upon arrival to the emergency department, his initial blood pressure is 232/128 mmHg with a heart rate of 112 beats/min. No nuchal rigidity is present. A head CT shows no acute bleeding and no mass effect. What is the next best step in the management of this patient?

A. Cerebral angiography
B. CT angiography
C. Lumbar puncture
D. Magnetic resonance angiography
E. Treat with sumatriptan

I-162. A 56-year-old man is admitted to intensive care with a subarachnoid hemorrhage. Upon admission, he is unresponsive, and his head CT shows evidence of blood in the third ventricle with midline shift. He undergoes successful coiling of an aneurysm of the anterior cerebral artery. All of the following would be indicated in the management of this patient EXCEPT:

A. Glucocorticoids
B. Hypernatremia
C. Nimodipine
D. Ventriculostomy
E. Volume expansion

I-163. A 56-year-old man is admitted to the intensive care unit with a hypertensive crisis after cocaine use. Initial blood pressure is 245/132 mmHg. On physical examination, the patient is unresponsive except to painful stimuli. He has been intubated for airway protection and is being mechanically ventilated, with a respiratory rate of 14 breaths/min. His pupils are reactive to light, and he has normal corneal, cough, and gag reflexes. The patient has a dense left hemiparesis. When presented with painful stimuli, the patient responds with flexure posturing on the right side. Computed tomography (CT) reveals a large area of intracranial bleeding in the right frontoparietal area. Over the next several hours, the patient deteriorates. The most recent examination reveals a blood pressure of 189/100 mmHg. The patient now has a dilated pupil on the right side. The patient continues to have corneal reflexes. You suspect rising intracranial pressure related to the intracranial bleed. All but which of the following can be done to decrease the patient's intracranial pressure?

A. Administer intravenous mannitol at a dose of 1 g/kg body weight.
B. Administer hypertonic fluids to achieve a goal sodium level of 155–160 meq/L.
C. Consult neurosurgery for an urgent ventriculostomy.
D. Initiate intravenous nitroprusside to decrease the mean arterial pressure (MAP) to a goal of 100 mmHg.
E. Increase the respiratory rate to 30 breaths/min.

I-164. A 64-year-old man presents to the emergency department complaining of shortness of breath and facial swelling. He smokes 1 pack of cigarettes daily and has done so since the age of 16 years. On physical examination, he has dyspnea at an angle of 45 degrees or less. His vital signs are heart rate of 124 beats/min, blood pressure of 164/98 mmHg, respiratory rate of 28 breaths/min, temperature of 37.6°C (99.6°F), and oxygen saturation of 89% on room air. Pulsus paradoxus is not present. His neck veins are dilated and do not collapse with inspiration. Collateral venous dilation is noted on the upper chest wall. There is facial edema and 1+ edema of the upper extremities bilaterally. Cyanosis is present. There is dullness to percussion and decreased breath sounds over the lower half of the right lung field. Given this clinical scenario, what would be the most likely finding on CT examination of the chest?

A. A central mass lesion obstructing the right mainstem bronchus
B. A large apical mass invading the chest wall and brachial plexus
C. A large pericardial effusion
D. A massive pleural effusion leading to opacification of the right hemithorax
E. Enlarged mediastinal lymph nodes causing obstruction of the superior vena cava

I-165. In the scenario in question I-165, the initial therapy of this patient includes all of the following EXCEPT:

A. Administration of furosemide as needed to achieve diuresis
B. Elevation of the head of the bed to 45 degrees
C. Emergent radiation
D. Low-sodium diet
E. Oxygen

I-166. A 58-year-old woman with known stage IV breast cancer presents to the emergency department with an inability to move her legs. She has had lower back pain for the past 4 days and has found it difficult to lie down. There is no radiating pain. Earlier today, the patient lost the ability to move either of her legs. In addition, she has been incontinent of urine recently. She has been diagnosed previously with metastatic disease to the lung and pleura from her breast cancer but was not known to have spinal or brain metastases. Her physical examination confirms absence of movement in the bilateral lower extremities associated with decreased to absent sensation below the umbilicus. There is increased tone and 3+ deep tendon reflexes in the lower extremities with crossed adduction. Anal sphincter tone is decreased, and the anal wink reflex is absent. What is the most important first step to take in the management of this patient?

A. Administer dexamethasone 10 mg intravenously.
B. Consult neurosurgery for emergent spinal decompression.
C. Consult radiation oncology for emergent spinal radiation.
D. Perform MRI of the brain.
E. Perform MRI of the entire spinal cord.

I-167. A 21-year-old man is treated with induction chemotherapy for acute lymphoblastic leukemia. His initial white blood cell count before treatment was 156,000/μL. All of the following are expected complications during his treatment EXCEPT:

A. Acute kidney injury
B. Hypercalcemia
C. Hyperkalemia
D. Hyperphosphatemia
E. Hyperuricemia

I-168. All of the following would be important for prevention of these complications EXCEPT:

A. Administration of allopurinol 300 mg/m^2 daily
B. Administration of intravenous fluids at a minimum of 3000 mL/m^2 daily
C. Alkalinization of the urine to a pH of greater than 7.0 by administration of sodium bicarbonate
D. Frequent monitoring of serum chemistries every 4 hours
E. Prophylactic hemodialysis before initiating chemotherapy

ANSWERS

I-1. **The answer is D.** *(Chap. 1)* Evidence-based medicine (EBM) is an important cornerstone to the effective and efficient practice of internal medicine. EBM refers to the concept that clinical decisions should be supported by data with the strongest evidence gleaned from randomized controlled clinical trials. Clearly, in some situations, it is impossible or unethical to perform randomized controlled trials, and data from observational studies such as cohort or case-control studies supply important information regarding disease associations. Professional organizations and government agencies use EBM to develop clinical practice guidelines. These guidelines combine the best available evidence from clinical and observational studies with expert opinion to develop clinical-decision support tools (option C). The purpose of clinical guidelines is to provide a framework for diagnosis and treatment of a specific clinical problem in a cost-effective and efficient manner. When multiple clinical trials have been published, accumulated data can be summarized in a systematic review (option A). In a systematic review, the researchers carefully scrutinize the methods of published trials for inclusion into the review and use statistical analysis to attempt to provide additional strength to clinical findings. A new branch of research called comparative effectiveness research (option B) attempts to compare different approaches to treating disease to determine effectiveness from both a clinical and cost-effectiveness standpoint. A variety of methods can be used, and systematic reviews are an important tool in comparative effectiveness research. The weakest type of evidence is anecdotal evidence (option E), which is one individual's clinical experience in treating a disease and can be biased by prior experiences.

I-2. **The answer is D.** *(Chap. 1)* Before performing any procedure, a physician has the ethical duty to discuss the details of the procedure with the patient and ensuring that he or she understands before proceeding. This process includes ensuring that the patient has the mental capacity to provide consent, outlining the risks and benefits of the procedure, and discussing alternatives and potential consequences of these alternatives. Informed consent does not require that a patient outline his or her wishes if he or she becomes incompetent to make decisions. This is accomplished in an advanced directive, which can outline the goals of care and also appoint someone to make medical decisions.

I-3. **The answer is A.** *(Chap. 2)* Disability-adjusted life years (DALYs) is the standard measure for determining global burden of disease by the World Health Organization. This measure takes into account both absolute years of life lost because of disease (premature death) as well as productive years lost because of disability. DALYs is believed to more accurately reflect the true effects of disease within a population because individuals who become disabled cannot contribute fully to society. Life expectancy, years of life lost because of disease, standardized mortality ratios, and infant mortality do provide important information about the general health of a population but do not capture the true burden of disease.

I-4.   **The answer is E.** *(Chap. 2)* The causes of morbidity and burden of disease in a population differ from the absolute causes of mortality in a population. Unipolar depressive disorder accounts for 10.0 million disability-adjusted life years lost (DALYs) in high-income countries. Depression is quite common in the general population of developed countries. However, the death rate from depression is low and is mainly reflected in suicides. Thus, depression creates disability and lost productivity without a significant impact on years of life lost. Depression often presents at young ages and persists or recurs throughout a lifetime, leading to significant morbidity over time. After unipolar depressive disorder, the leading causes of DALYs lost in high-income countries are ischemic heart disease, cerebrovascular disease, Alzheimer's disease and other dementia, and alcohol use disorders. However, worldwide, the leading cause of DALYs is lower respiratory infections caused by the high burden of disease in low-income countries with an estimated 76.9 million DALYs lost because of lower respiratory infections in low-income countries. Additionally, in low-income countries, the top five causes of DALYs are related to infectious diseases (diarrheal diseases, HIV, malaria) and prematurity.

I-5.   **The answer is D.** *(Chap. 2)* Although ischemic heart disease is the leading cause of death worldwide, low-income countries have a disproportionate number of deaths caused by lower respiratory tract infections. This primarily reflects the large numbers of individuals in low-income countries who die of tuberculosis and other infectious pneumonias. Ischemic heart disease is the second leading cause of death in low-income countries.

I-6.   **The answer is B.** *(Chap. 2)* Global health experts have developed priorities for improving global health in conjunction with the World Health Organization (WHO). Many of these efforts are focused on the prevention, early recognition, and treatment of infectious diseases in developing countries and the developing world. Among infectious causes of disease, malaria ranks as the third most deadly. In 2001, the WHO Roll Back Malaria campaign was endorsed by heads of state in Africa in an effort to develop a coordinated plan for malaria prevention and treatment. A major goal of the Roll Back Malaria campaign was to prevent gains in disease prevention in one country from being lost because of lack of a coordinated effort in neighboring countries. This effort involves a multifaceted approach that includes vector control, prevention of transmission, and early recognition and treatment. Insecticide-treated bed nets are a simple and cost-effective method of reducing malaria transmission with a 50% decreased incidence of malaria in individuals who sleep under these bed nets. Indoor residual spraying is also an important factor in decreasing malaria transmission as outdoor vector control alone is ineffective in controlling transmission. It has been found that 80% of structures in a community must be treated to decrease disease transmission. Another important part of decreasing disease transmission is to give at least two doses of effective antimalarial drugs during pregnancy to decrease placental transmission of disease. If disease is unable to be prevented, it is important to recognize and treat the disease early. Chloroquine resistance has emerged in many areas around the world, particularly in sub-Saharan Africa, the Middle East, India, Southeast Asia, and parts of South America. Given the widespread chloroquine resistance, the WHO now recommends only artemisinin-based combination therapy for falciparum malaria infection.

I-7.   **The answer is A.** *(Chap. 3)* Bayes' theorem is a statistical model based on conditional probabilities that is useful in medical decision making. The three components of Bayes' theorem as it relates to medical decision making are the pretest probability of disease, the sensitivity of the test, and the specificity of the test. These factors are combined into the following formula:

$$\text{Posttest probability} = \frac{\text{Pretest probability} \times \text{Test sensitivity}}{\begin{array}{c}(\text{Pretest probability} \times \text{Test sensitivity}) + \\ [(1 - \text{Pretest probability}) \times \text{False-positive rate}]\end{array}}$$

In most occasions, the pretest probability is an estimate based on the prevalence of disease in the population and the clinical situation. The false-positive rate is $1 -$ specificity. In this clinical scenario, the pretest probability of disease was estimated at 10%, and the treadmill ECG stress test has an average sensitivity of 66% and a specificity of 84%. Based on the formula above, the posttest probability would be low at only 31%.

$$\text{Posttest probability} = (0.10)(0.66)/[(0.10)(0.66) + (0.90)(0.16)] = 0.31$$

I-8 and I-9. The answers are C and C, respectively. *(Chap. 3)* In evaluating the usefulness of a test, it is imperative to understand the clinical implications of the sensitivity and specificity of that test. Simply, the sensitivity is the proportion of people with disease that are correctly identified by the test—the true-positive rate. Alternatively, the specificity can be viewed as the true-negative rate and is the proportion of individuals without disease who would have a negative test result. The perfect test would have a sensitivity of 100% and a specificity of 100%, but this is unachievable in clinical practice. Sensitivity and specificity are inherent properties of the test and are not affected by the disease prevalence. However, by obtaining information about the prevalence of the disease in the population, one can generate a two-by-two table, as shown below. This table is used to generate the total number of patients in each group of the population. The sensitivity of the test is $TP/(TP + FN)$. The specificity is $TN/(TN + FP)$. In this case, the disease prevalence is 10%. In a population of 1000 individuals, 100 would truly have latent tuberculosis, and the table is filled in as follows:

		Latent Tuberculosis	
		+	−
Test	+	90	180
	−	10	720

I-10. The answer is D. *(Chap. 3)* A receiver operating characteristic (ROC) curve plots sensitivity (or true-positive rate) on the y-axis and $1 -$ specificity (or false-positive rate) on the x-axis. Each point on the curve represents a cutoff point of sensitivity and $1 -$ specificity, and these cutoff points are used to select the threshold value for a diagnostic test that yields the best trade-off between true-positive and false-positive tests. The area under the curve can be used as a quantitative measure of the information content of a test. Values range from 0.5 (a 45-degree line) representing no diagnostic information to 1.0 for an ideal test. In the medical literature, ROC curves are often used to compare alternative diagnostic tests, but the interpretation of a specific test and ROC curve is not as simple in clinical practice. One criticism of the ROC curve is that it only evaluates only one test parameter with exclusion of other potentially relevant clinical data. Also, one must consider the underlying population in which the ROC curve was validated and how generalizable this is the entire population with disease.

I-11. The answer is C. *(Chap. 3)* The positive and negative predictive values of a test are strongly influenced by the prevalence of disease in a population. The positive predictive value is calculated as the number of true-positive test results divided by the number of all positive test values. Alternatively, the negative predictive value is calculated as the number of true-negative test results divided by the number of all negative test results. For example, in a population of 1000 with a disease prevalence of 5%, a specific test has a sensitivity of 95% and a specificity of 80%. In this setting, the two-by-two table would be completed as follows:

		Disease	
		+	–
Test	+	48	190
	–	2	760

Thus, the positive predictive value of the test would be [48/(48 + 190)] × 100 = 20.2%, and the negative predictive value would be [760/(760 + 2)] ×100 = 99.7%.

The sensitivity and specificity of the test, however, are properties of the test and are not affected by disease prevalence. Positive and negative likelihood ratios are calculated from the sensitivity and specificity and are defined as the ratio of the probability of a given test result (positive or negative) in an individual with disease to the probability of that test result in a patient without disease. For a positive likelihood ratio, a higher ratio indicates that a test performs better at identifying a patient with disease. For the negative likelihood ratio, a smaller ratio performs better at ruling out disease. The number needed to treat is a measure of the effectiveness of an intervention. It is simply calculated as 1 divided by the absolute reduction in risk related to the intervention.

I-12 and I-13. The answers are B and C, respectively. *(Chap. 3)* The goal of a meta-analysis is to summarize the treatment benefit conferred by an intervention by combining and summarizing data available from multiple clinical trials. Meta-analyses often focus on summary measures of relative risk reductions expressed by the relative risk or odds ratios; however, clinicians should also understand the absolute risk reduction (ARR) related to an intervention. This is the difference in mortality (or another endpoint) between the treatment and the placebo arms. In this case, the absolute risk reduction is 10% − 2% = 8%. From this number, one can calculate the number needed to treat (NNT), which is 1/ ARR. The NNT is the number of patients who must receive the intervention to prevent one death (or another outcome assessed in the study). In this case, the NNT is 1/8% = 12.5 patients.

I-14. **The answer is E.** *(Chap. 4)* Within a population, it is certainly impractical to perform all possible screening procedures for the variety of diseases that exist in that population. This approach would be overwhelming to the medical community and would not be cost effective. Indeed, the amount of monetary and psychological stress that would occur from pursuing false-positive test results would add an additional burden on the population. When determining which procedures should be considered as screening tests, a variety of endpoints can be used. One of these is to determine how many individuals would need to be screened in the population to prevent or alter the outcome in one individual with disease. Although this can be statistically determined, there are no recommendations for what the threshold value should be and may change based on the invasiveness or cost of the test and the potential outcome avoided. Additionally, one should consider both the absolute and relative impact of screening on disease outcome. Another measure used in considering the utility of screening tests is the cost per life year saved. Most measures are considered cost effective if they cost less than $30,000 to $50,000 per year of life saved. This measure is also sometimes adjusted for the quality of life as well and presented as quality-adjusted life years saved. A final measure that is used in determining the effectiveness of a screening test is the effect of the screening test on life expectancy of the entire population. When applying the test across the entire population, this number is surprisingly small, and a goal of about 1 month is desirable for a population-based screening strategy.

I-15. **The answer is C.** *(Chap. 4)* Evaluating the utility of screening tests requires also understanding the potential biases that can exist when interpreting data from screening trials. One of the most difficult to ascertain but potentially the most confounding is lead time bias. Simply, lead time bias refers to the bias that occurs when one finds a tumor at an earlier clinical stage than would be expected from usual care but ultimately does not lead to an overall change in the outcome. In this case, the apparent difference in time to diagnosis and death likely represents lead time bias. To fully determine this, one would need to know outcome data for the entire trial. In the case of lead time bias, one would find that although the number of tumors diagnosed at early stages was increased, the overall mortality would be the same. The recently published Lung Cancer Screening Trial (*N Engl J Med,* August 4, 2011) showed that low-dose helical CT scan in high-risk patients was associated 20% reduction in risk of dying from lung cancer compared with chest x-ray. Although this was the first clinical trial to show a radiologic intervention reducing mortality from lung cancer, how these results will translate into clinical practice and cost effectiveness is still uncertain.

I-16. **The answer is E.** *(Chap. 4)* The U.S. Preventive Services Task Force (USPSTF) is an independent panel of experts selected by the federal government to provide evidence-based guidelines for prevention and screening for disease. The panel typically consists of primary care providers from internal medicine, family medicine, pediatrics, and obstetrics and gynecology. The USPSTF provides guidelines on a variety of measures, including blood pressure, height, weight, cholesterol, Pap smears, mammography, colorectal cancer screening, and adult immunizations. However, the most recent review of the evidence by the USPSTF concluded that there was insufficient evidence to recommend screening for thyroid disease in adults. Notably, the USPSTF also recommends against screening for prostate cancer in men older than 75 years and states that there is insufficient evidence for screening among younger men.

I-17. **The answer is B.** *(Chap. 4)* Predicted increases in life expectancy are average numbers that apply to populations, not individuals. Because we often do not understand the true nature of risk of disease, screening and lifestyle interventions usually benefit a small proportion of the total population. For screening tests, false-positive test results may also increase the risk of diagnostic tests. Although Pap smears increase life expectancy overall by only 2–3 months, for an individual at risk of cervical cancer, Pap smear screening may add many years to life. The average life expectancy increases resulting from mammography (1 month), PSA (2 weeks), and exercise (1–2 years) are less than from quitting smoking (3–5 years).

I-18. **The answer is B.** *(Chaps. 4 and 235)* Current guidelines from the National Cholesterol Education Project Adult Treatment Panel III recommend screening in all adults older than 20 years old. The testing should include fasting total cholesterol, triglycerides, low-density lipoprotein cholesterol, and high-density lipoprotein cholesterol. The screening should be repeated every 5 years. All patients with type 1 diabetes should have lipids followed closely to decrease cardiovascular risk by combining the results of lipid screening with other risk factors to determine risk category and intensity of recommended treatment.

I-19. **The answer is B.** *(Chap. 5)* Bioavailability is the amount of the drug that is available to the systemic circulation when administered by routes other than the intravenous route. In this setting, bioavailability may be much less than 100%. The primary factors affecting bioavailability are the amount of drug that is absorbed and metabolism of the drug before entering the systemic circulation (the first-pass effect). Oral itraconazole is the recommended treatment for mild blastomycosis, but a problem with use of this drug is its bioavailability, which is estimated at about 55%. Although oral itraconazole does not experience a significant first-pass effect, its absorption from the stomach can be quite variable under different conditions. A first important consideration is the drug preparation. Whereas the liquid formulation should be taken on an empty stomach, the capsule should be taken after a meal. Furthermore, having an acid pH improves bioavailability, and use of gastric acid suppressors such as H2 blockers or proton pump inhibitors should be avoided with itraconazole use. When acid suppressors cannot be withheld, it is recommended to coadminister itraconazole with a cola beverage, which has been shown to enhance absorption in some clinical trials. Oral contraceptive pills will not affect the bioavailability of itraconazole; however, azole antifungals (including itraconazole) inhibit CYP450 3A4 and may increase the serum levels of estrogens and progestins.

I-20. **The answer is D.** *(Chap. 5)* Aminoglycoside antibiotics (tobramycin, gentamicin, amikacin) are active against *Pseudomonas aeruginosa* and are recommended for treatment of exacerbations of cystic fibrosis in combination with a beta-lactam antibiotic. The volume of distribution is increased in cystic fibrosis, altering drug metabolism and often necessitating higher doses than are normally given. To ensure therapeutic concentrations of tobramycin, a peak level should be check about 30 minutes after completion of an infusion. To reduce the risk of nephrotoxicity, a trough level should be checked immediately before the administration of a dose to ensure that the drug has been adequately metabolized. To ensure that steady-state concentration has been achieved, it is recommended that these levels be checked after three to five doses.

I-21. **The answer is A.** *(Chap. 5)* Digitalis is a cardiac glycoside that exerts its effect via reversible inhibition of the sodium–potassium–ATPase pump. The cellular effect of this inhibition is to increase intracellular sodium and decrease extracellular potassium. The increase in intracellular sodium leads to a change in the membrane potential of the cell and an influx of calcium. This influx of calcium improves inotropy of the heart and leads to increased vagal tone with resultant decrease in heart rate through action at the sinoatrial and atrioventricular nodes. Digoxin is a drug with a narrow therapeutic window, meaning that the effective dose and the toxic dose are close to one another. Digoxin is a substrate for P-glycoprotein, which is an efflux pump that excretes drugs into the proximal tubule of the kidney. Caution must be taken when introducing a new medication that is an inhibitor of P-glycoprotein because these drugs can increase the serum concentration of digoxin. Examples of inhibitors of P-glycoprotein include amiodarone, clarithromycin, verapamil, and diltiazem. In this patient, initiation of an oral amiodarone load in the face of the patient's known renal insufficiency was sufficient to cause digoxin toxicity. The typical manifestations of digoxin toxicity in this patient with a subacute onset include lethargy, generalized weakness, and delirium. Gastrointestinal manifestations may be seen but are less pronounced that in acute overdoses. The cardiac manifestations of digoxin toxicity are of the greatest concern, and the electrocardiogram can demonstrate a wide range of abnormalities, including bradycardia, atrial tachyarrhythmias, atrioventricular block, and ventricular tachycardia or fibrillation. The ECG can evolve over time, so continuous cardiac monitoring is warranted. Electrolyte abnormalities are common, especially hyperkalemia caused by the effects on the sodium–potassium–ATPase pump. However, in chronic toxicity, hypokalemia can also be seen. Worsening renal function is also a frequent manifestation and is often the cause for the rise in digoxin levels. The therapeutic range of digoxin is between 0.8 and 2 ng/mL. However, the level may not correlate well with the development of toxicity. Levels greater than 10 ng/mL often require treatment with digoxin-specific antibody fragments (Fab). This patient has other indications for use of Fab fragments as well given the complete heart block on ECG. Thus, observation alone is not an appropriate choice in this patient. Fab fragments are highly effective in the management of cardiac arrhythmias and are given as a single intravenous dose. Given the large molecular weight of digoxin and large volume of distribution, neither hemodialysis nor hemoperfusion is effective in elimination of digoxin. There are case reports of combined use of Fab fragments and plasmapheresis in individuals with profound renal failure, but this is not a standard option.

I-22. **The answer is C.** *(Chap. 5)* Some medications circulate in the plasma partially bound to plasma proteins. In this setting, only unbound (or free) drug can distribute to the sites of action to exert pharmacologic effects. Examples of medications that are bound to plasma proteins include phenytoin, warfarin, valproic acid, and amiodarone. Hypoalbuminemia can lead to increased free levels of drugs that are more highly protein bound and can lead to drug toxicity at total drug levels that are not typically considered toxic. In this case, the patient has evidence of worsening liver disease with a low albumin level that has lead to signs and symptoms of phenytoin toxicity. A free drug level should be checked to confirm this. Although phenytoin can be used safely in those with mild liver disease, it should be discontinued in individuals with evidence of cirrhosis, which this patient clearly exhibits. Signs and symptoms of phenytoin toxicity include slurred speech, horizontal nystagmus, and altered mental status that can progress to obtundation and coma. Typically, severe phenytoin toxicity is not encountered unless the total phenytoin level is greater than 30 μg/mL. However, in the case of hypoalbuminemia, the total level can substantially misrepresent the free level of drug. When the free phenytoin level was checked in this case, it was elevated at 5 μg/mL (therapeutic range, 1.0–2.5 μg/mL). Other less likely possibilities in the differential diagnosis of this patient include nonconvulsive status epilepticus and hepatic encephalopathy, but the presence of horizontal nystagmus is more suggestive of phenytoin toxicity. Infection is also a common cause of altered mental status in individuals with cirrhosis. However, the ascitic fluid does not support a diagnosis of spontaneous bacterial peritonitis that may be associated with a positive Gram stain of the ascites fluid. The history and physical examination are not consistent with a diagnosis of bacterial meningitis, and a head CT is not likely to provide additional information in this clinical setting.

I-23. **The answer is D.** (*Chap. 5; VD Cataldo et al:* N Engl J Med *364:947, 2011.*) In the past decades, increasing interest and research has occurred in the area of genetic variability with respect to drug effects, particularly in the area of cancer chemotherapy. Each individual tumor contains multiple mutations that exhibit different biologic advantages that promote proliferation of tumor cells and escape from immune attack by the host. As investigators have learned more about the function of these mutations, drug development has concurrently allowed specific therapies directed against a particular mutation. Some specific examples of chemotherapeutic successes with targeted chemotherapy include use of imatinib in chronic myelogenous leukemia and gastrointestinal stroma tumors. In non–small cell lung cancer (NSCLC; adenocarcinoma and squamous cell carcinoma), targeted chemotherapeutic agents have included small molecule epidermal growth factor receptor (EGFR) tyrosine kinase inhibitors, a monoclonal antibody against vascular endothelial growth factor, and a monoclonal antibody that binds to EGFR. Current research is continuing to define the most appropriate role of these agents in the treatment of NSCLC. Recently, the National Comprehensive Cancer Network recognized the EGFR tyrosine kinase inhibitor erlotinib as second- and third-line therapy in individuals who have advanced stage NSCLC with good performance status. However, in individuals with activating mutations of the EGFR, erlotinib monotherapy is recommended. The two most common mutations are deletions of exon 19 and an arginine for leucine substitution at position 858 in exon 21. In clinical trials, individuals with these mutations, treatment with erlotinib or gefitinib is associated with an initial response rate of 55–90%. Moreover, those with activating mutations of EGFR have improved progression-free survival when treated with erlotinib or gefitinib. On the other hand, those without these mutations have been shown to do worse with these medications. Therefore, it is important to perform testing for mutations of EGFR before using either of these medications. Other clinical predictors of response to the EGFR tyrosine kinase inhibitors are female sex, lack of tobacco use, adenocarcinoma by pathology, and individuals of East Asian descent.

I-24. **The answer is D.** (*Chap. 5*) Calcineurin inhibitors such as tacrolimus and cyclosporine are immunosuppressive agents that are used after solid organ transplants as well as for treatment of graft-versus-host disease (GVHD) in bone marrow transplant patients. These drugs are primarily metabolized via the cytochrome P450 pathway and excreted into bile. Many drugs and foods can be inhibitors or inducers of this pathway, and thoughtful consideration of possible drug interactions must be considered when starting any patient on a new medication while on tacrolimus or cyclosporine. In this case, voriconazole inhibits metabolism of tacrolimus, leading to increased serum concentrations of the drug. The clinical signs and symptoms of tacrolimus toxicity include hypertension, edema, headaches, insomnia, and tremor. In addition, elevated levels of tacrolimus can lead to worsening renal function and electrolyte abnormalities, including hyperkalemia, hypomagnesemia, hypophosphatemia, and hyperglycemia. It is recommended that the tacrolimus dose be decreased to one-third of the original dose when it is necessary to co-administer tacrolimus and voriconazole. *Aspergillus* meningitis is a rare infection that typically results from direct invasion from a rhinosinusitis. Congestive heart failure is unlikely in the clinical scenario because this is a young woman with no known heart disease and the neurologic symptoms are not consistent with that diagnosis. GVHD occurs when transplanted immune cells recognizes the host cells as foreign and initiates an immune response. GVHD occurs after allogeneic hematopoietic stem cell transplants, and there is increased risk of GVHD in those with a greater disparity of human leukocyte antigens between the graft and the host. GVHD presents acutely with a diffuse maculopapular rash, fever, elevations in bilirubin and alkaline phosphatase, and diarrhea with abdominal cramping. There are case reports of nephritic syndrome related to GVHD, but renal involvement is not common. Also unlikely are neurologic symptoms, headache, hypertension, and tremor. Thrombotic thrombocytopenic purpura (TTP) could be considered in an individual with renal disease, altered mental status, and hypertension if there was concurrent evidence of an intravascular hemolytic process. However, TTP has not been associated with administration of voriconazole.

I-25.   **The answer is E.** *(Chap. 5)* Adverse drug reactions create significant morbidity in the treatment of disease. The most common classes of drugs that cause adverse events are antimicrobials, nonsteroidal anti-inflammatory drugs and aspirin, analgesics, anticoagulants, glucocorticoids, antineoplastics, diuretics, digoxin, and hypoglycemic agents. These drugs account for about 90% of all adverse drug events. Adverse drug events can be broadly classified as related or unrelated to the intended pharmacologic action. In this case, the patient has developed serum sickness (option E) after administration of benzathine penicillin. Serum sickness is an immunologic reaction to penicillin that is not a part of the intended pharmacologic action of the drug. Serum sickness is a type III immune complex mediated reaction that occurs when complex of drug and the appropriate antibody are deposited on endothelial cells. After the first exposure to the drug, it takes about 1–2 weeks for the immune reaction to occur, although with subsequent exposures, this would occur more quickly. Deposition of the immune complexes leads to complement activation with neutrophilic inflammation. Clinically, serum sickness presents as fever, urticarial rash, lymphadenopathy, inflammatory arthritis, and glomerulonephritis. Clinical recovery typically occurs in 7–28 days. Common pharmacologic causes of serum sickness are antibiotics and foreign proteins, including streptokinase, vaccines, and therapeutic antibodies. Secondary syphilis typically does not present until 4–10 weeks after primary infection. The rash typically is an erythematous maculopapular eruption that affects the palms and soles. Secondary syphilis should be adequately treated by the patient's single dose of benzathine penicillin as long as the primary infection occurred with the past year. A Jarisch-Herxheimer reaction occurs when there is a systemic reaction to the killing of syphilis organisms. It begins in the first 24 hours after treatment and is associated with fevers, myalgias, headaches, and tachycardia. Disseminated gonococcal infection presents as an asymmetric migratory polyarthritis with fever and a papular or pustular rash. Septic arthritis may occur. A negative urethral swab result does not rule out this possibility, but the clinical presentation is not consistent with disseminated gonococcal infection. Approximately 10–20% of patients with rheumatoid arthritis have a negative rheumatoid factor. Although the disease most often presents with a symmetric inflammatory arthritis of the larger joints, the acute presentation of this patient makes this diagnosis less likely.

I-26.   **The answer is A.** *(Chap. 5)* In population surveys of noninstitutionalized elderly adults, up to 10% had at least one adverse drug reaction in the prior year. Adverse drug reactions are common in elderly adults and are related to altered drug sensitivity, impaired renal or hepatic clearance, impaired homeostatic mechanisms, and drug interactions. Long half-life benzodiazepines are linked to the increased occurrence of hip fractures in elderly adults. The association may be caused by the increased risk of falling (related to sedation) in a population with a high prevalence of osteoporosis. This association may also be true for other drugs with sedative properties such as opioids or antipsychotics. Exaggerated responses to cardiovascular drugs such as angiotensin-converting enzyme inhibitors may occur because of a blunted vasoconstrictor or chronotropic response to reduced blood pressure. Conversely, elderly patients often display decreased sensitivity to beta-blockers.

I-27.   **The answer is C.** *(Chap. 5)* Grapefruit juice inhibits CYP3A4 in the liver, particularly at high doses. This can cause decreased drug elimination via hepatic metabolism and increase potential drug toxicities. Atorvastatin is metabolized via this pathway. Drugs that may enhance atorvastatin toxicity via this mechanism include phenytoin, ritonavir, clarithro-mycin, and azole antifungals. Aspirin is cleared via renal mechanisms. Prevacid can cause impaired absorption of other drugs via its effect on gastric pH. Sildenafil is a phosphodieste-rase inhibitor that may enhance the effect of nitrate medications and cause hypotension.

I-28.   **The answer is E.** *(Chap. 6)* The top two causes of death for men and women are the same—heart disease and cancer. These two broad categories of disease account for more than 50% of all deaths in men and 47% of deaths in women. Likewise, the number one cause of cancer death (lung cancer) is the same in men and women. After this, there are significant differences in the major causes of death between the sexes. Cerebrovascu-lar disease is the third most common cause of death in women responsible for 6.7% of death, but in men, it is only the fifth most common cause of death with only 4.5% of all deaths. Although chronic lower respiratory disease is the fourth most common cause of death in both men and women, the percentage of deaths from chronic lower respi-ratory disease in women is 5.3% compared with 4.9% in men. Other diseases that are responsible for a greater percentage of deaths in women are Alzheimer's disease, sepsis, pneumonia, and hypertension.

I-29.   **The answer is C.** *(Chap. 6)* Coronary heart disease (CHD) is the most common cause of death in men and women, but important sex differences exist in the presentation and treatment of CHD. At the time of presentation of CHD, women are about 10–15 years older than men with CHD. In addition, women have a greater number of medical comorbidities at the time of diagnosis, including hypertension, heart failure, and diabetes mellitus. Angina is the most common presenting symptom of CHD in women and may have atypical features, including nausea, indigestion, and upper back pain. Women who present with a myocardial infarction (MI) more often present with cardiogenic shock or cardiac arrest, but men have a greater risk of ventricular tachycardia on presentation with MI. In the past, women had a greater risk of death from MI when presenting at younger ages, but this gap has decreased in recent years. However, women are still referred less often by physicians for diagnostic and therapeutic cardiovascular procedures, and there are more false-positive and false-negative diagnostic test results in women. Women are also less likely to receive angioplasty, thrombolysis, coronary artery bypass grafting, aspi-rin, and beta-blockers. Despite this, the 5- and 10-year survival rates after coronary artery bypass grafting are the same for men and women.

I-30.   **The answer is A.** *(Chap. 6)* In general, the risk factors for coronary heart disease (CHD) are similar in men and women. However, an elevated total triglyceride level has been demonstrated to be an independent risk factor in women but not men. Low high-density lipoprotein and diabetes mellitus are also stronger risk factors in women, but they also influence CHD in men. Other shared risk factors include elevated total cholesterol, hyper-tension, obesity, smoking, and lack of physical activity.

I-31.   **The answer is E.** *(Chap. 6)* Sex differences exist in the prevalence of many common dis-eases. Hypertension is more common in women, particularly in those older than 60 years. In addition, most autoimmune diseases are more common in women, including rheu-matoid arthritis, systemic lupus erythematosus, and autoimmune thyroid disease. Major depression is twice as common in women than men, and this is true even in developing countries. Other psychological disorders that are more common in women are eating dis-orders and anxiety. Endocrine disorders, including obesity and osteoporosis, are more common in women, and 80% of patients referred for bariatric surgery are women. How-ever, the prevalence of both type 1 and type 2 diabetes mellitus is the same between men and women.

I-32.   **The answer is C.** *(Chap. 6)* Alzheimer's disease (AD) affects women twice as commonly as men. This sex difference cannot fully be explained by the difference in life expectancy between men and women. The brains of women differ from men in terms of size, struc-ture, and functional organization. In addition, it is thought that estrogen may play a role in the development of AD. Women with AD have lower levels of circulating estrogen than age-controlled women without disease. Although observational studies suggested a protective effect of estrogen replacement therapy on the development of AD, this was not borne out in randomized and blinded placebo-controlled trials. Indeed, the largest trial to date demonstrated an increase in dementia and mild cognitive impairment in individuals receiving either estrogen or combined hormone replacement therapy.

I-33.　**The answer is E.** *(Chap. 7)* The cardiovascular system undergoes many changes in a pregnant woman to accommodate the needs of the developing fetus. Plasma volume begins to expand early in pregnancy and ultimately is increased by about 40–50% at term. Coincident with the increased plasma volume, cardiac output increases as well by about 40%. Although this is primarily attributable to increases in stroke volume, heart rate also increases in pregnancy by about 10 beats/min. In the second trimester, systemic vascular resistance falls, and subsequently blood pressure decreases as well. Thus, a blood pressure greater than 140/90 mmHg is considered abnormal and is associated with increased maternal and fetal morbidity and mortality.

I-34.　**The answer is D.** *(Chap. 7)* Chronic essential hypertension occurs in up to 5% of all pregnancies. Although hypertension is not a contraindication to pregnancy, the condition is associated with an increased risk of intrauterine growth restriction, preeclampsia, placental abruption, and perinatal mortality. The cardiovascular changes of pregnancy typically do lead to a fall in systemic vascular resistance and a fall in blood pressure in the second trimester, but it is not safe to discontinue medications in those with a prior diagnosis of hypertension if the blood pressure in the first trimester is greater than 120/80 mmHg. When choosing an antihypertensive medication in pregnancy, angiotensin-converting enzyme inhibitors and angiotensin receptor blockers should be strictly avoided because they are known to cause birth defects, including congenital malformations and intrauterine death, particularly in the second and third trimesters. The most common medications used in pregnancy are α-methyldopa, labetalol, and nifedipine. Although these medications have limited data from randomized controlled trials, there is a long history of safety with use of these medications. Diuretics such as hydrochlorothiazide appear also to be safe in pregnancy, although there are concerns that use of diuretics would impair the volume expansion that occurs during pregnancy.

I-35.　**The answer is B.** *(Chaps. 7 and 150)* Most cardiovascular conditions can be managed safely in pregnancy, although these pregnancies are often considered high risk. The conditions that are considered to be contraindications to pregnancy are idiopathic pulmonary arterial hypertension and Eisenmenger syndrome (congenital heart disease resulting in pulmonary hypertension with right-to-left shunting). In these cases, it is typically recommended to terminate the pregnancy because there is a high risk of maternal and fetal death. Peripartum cardiomyopathy can recur in subsequent pregnancies, and it is recommended that individuals with an abnormal ejection fraction avoid further pregnancies. Approximately 15% of individuals with Marfan syndrome will have a major cardiovascular complication in pregnancy, although the condition is not considered a contraindication to pregnancy. An aortic root diameter of less than 40 mm is generally associated with the best outcomes in pregnancy. The valvular heart disease with the greatest risk in pregnancy is mitral stenosis. There is an increased risk of pulmonary edema, and pulmonary hypertension is a common long-term consequence of mitral stenosis. However, aortic stenosis, aortic regurgitation, and mitral regurgitation are typically well tolerated. Congenital heart disease in the mother is associated with an increased risk of congenital heart disease in the offspring, but atrial and ventricular septal defects are usually well tolerated in pregnancy as long as there is no evidence of Eisenmenger syndrome.

I-36.　**The answer is D.** *(Chap. 7)* This patient has severe eclampsia, and delivery should be performed as rapidly as possible. Mild eclampsia is the presence of new-onset hypertension and proteinuria in a pregnant woman after 20 weeks' gestation. Severe eclampsia is eclampsia complicated by central nervous system symptoms (including seizure), marked hypertension, severe proteinuria, renal failure, pulmonary edema, thrombocytopenia, or disseminated intravascular coagulation. Delivery in a mother with severe eclampsia before 37 weeks' gestation decreases maternal morbidity but increases fetal risks of complications of prematurity. Aggressive management of blood pressure, usually with labetalol or hydralazine intravenously, decreases the maternal risk of stroke. However, similar to any hypertensive crisis, the decrease in blood pressure should be achieved slowly to avoid hypotension and risk of decreased blood flow to the fetus. Eclamptic seizures should be controlled with magnesium sulfate; it has been shown to be superior to phenytoin and diazepam in large randomized clinical trials.

I-37.   **The answer is C.** *(Chap. 7)* Pregnancy causes a hypercoagulable state, and deep venous thrombosis (DVT) occurs in about 1 in 2000 pregnancies. DVT occurs more commonly in the left leg than the right leg during pregnancy because of compression of the left iliac vein by the gravid uterus. In addition, pregnancy represents a procoagulant states with increases in factors V and VII and decreases in proteins C and S. Approximately 25% of pregnant women with DVT have a factor V Leiden mutation, which also predisposes to preeclampsia. Warfarin is strictly contraindicated because of a risk of fetal abnormality. Low-molecular-weight heparin (LMWH) is appropriate therapy at this point in pregnancy but is typically switched to unfractionated heparin 4 weeks before anticipated delivery because LMWH may be associated with an increased risk of epidural hematoma. Ambulation, rather than bedrest, should be encouraged as with all DVTs. There is no proven role for local thrombolytics or an inferior vena cava filter in pregnancy. The latter would be considered only when anticoagulation is not possible.

I-38.   **The answer is E.** *(Chap. 7)* Pregnancy complicated by diabetes is associated with greater maternal and perinatal morbidity and mortality rates and occurs in 4% of all pregnancies. Women with gestational diabetes are at increased risk of preeclampsia, delivering infants large for gestational age, and birth lacerations. Their infants are at risk of hypoglycemia and birth injury. Appropriate therapy can reduce these risks. All women should be screened for gestational diabetes unless they fall into a low-risk group. Low-risk groups include age younger than 25 years, body mass index less than 25 kg/m², no maternal history of macrosomia or gestational diabetes, no diabetes in any first-degree relative, and those who are not members of a high-risk ethnic group (African American, Hispanic, or Native American).

I-39.   **The answer is B.** *(Chap. 8)* Medical providers are often asked to provide guidance regarding the postoperative risk of complications after a variety of noncardiac surgical procedures. When evaluating risk of complications, it is useful to categorize the surgical procedures into a low, intermediate, or higher risk category. Individuals who are at the highest risk of complications include those undergoing an emergent major operation, especially in elderly adults. Other higher risk procedures include aortic and other noncarotid major vascular surgery and surgeries with a prolonged operative time and large anticipated blood loss or fluid shifts (e.g., pancreaticoduodenectomy or Whipple procedure). Surgeries that are believed to be an intermediate risk include major thoracic surgery, major abdominal surgery, carotid endarterectomy, head and neck surgery, orthopedic surgery, and prostate surgery. Lower risk procedures include eye, skin, and superficial surgery as well as endoscopy.

I-40.   **The answer is E.** *(Chap. 8)* Poor exercise tolerance is an important predictor of postoperative complications. To standardize the determination of functional status, general guidelines are available that attempt to categorize the risk of complications according to functional status (Table I-40). The risk of postoperative complications increases when an individual cannot meet a metabolic equivalent (MET) level of 4. General activities that require a MET level of 4 include carrying 15–20 lb, playing golf, and playing doubles tennis. In addition, individuals experience increased risk of postoperative complications if they are unable to walk four blocks or climb two flights of stairs when walking at a normal pace. Individuals at highest risk of postoperative complications in relation to exercise capacity are those who have difficulty performing activities of daily living because of dyspnea, angina, or excessive fatigue.

TABLE I-40 Functional Status

Higher Risk↕	• Difficulty with adult activities of daily living
	• Cannot walk four blocks or up two flights of stairs or unable to meet a MET level of 4
	• Inactive but no limitation
	• Active: easily does vigorous tasks
Lower	• Performs regular vigorous exercises

Abbreviation: MET, metabolic equivalents.

Source: From Fleisher LA et al: ACC/AHA guideline for perioperative cardiovascular evaluation for noncardiac surgery: A report of the American College of Cardiology/American Heart Association Task Force on Practice Guidelines (Writing Committee to Revise the 2002 Guidelines on Perioperative Cardiovascular Evaluation for Noncardiac Surgery). *Circulation* 116:1971, 2007.

I-41.   **The answer is D.** *(Chap. 8)* Cardiovascular events continue to be a major source of morbidity and mortality after surgical interventions, and preoperative prediction of those individuals at the highest risk of cardiovascular events has been an area of much research. Over the years, a variety of risk stratification tools have been developed to assist clinicians in determining which patients may benefit from preoperative noninvasive cardiac testing or initiation of preoperative preventive medical management. One of the simplest and most widely used is the revised cardiac risk index (RCRI), which scores patients on a scale from 0–6. The six factors that comprise the RCRI (Table I-41) are high-risk surgical procedures, known ischemic heart disease, congestive heart failure, cerebrovascular disease, diabetes mellitus requiring insulin, and chronic kidney disease with a creatinine greater than 2 mg/dL. An individual would be considered as

TABLE I-41 Revised Cardiac Risk Index Clinical Markers

High-Risk Surgical Procedures

Vascular surgery

Major intraperitoneal or intrathoracic procedures

Ischemic Heart Disease

History of myocardial infarction

Current angina considered to be ischemic

Requiring sublingual nitroglycerin

Positive exercise test

Pathological Q waves on ECG

History of PTCA or CABG with current angina considered to be ischemic

Congestive Heart Failure

Left ventricular failure by physical examination

History of paroxysmal nocturnal dyspnea

History of pulmonary edema

S3 gallop on cardiac auscultation

Bilateral rales on pulmonary auscultation

Pulmonary edema on chest radiograph

Cerebrovascular Disease

History of transient ischemic attack

History of cerebrovascular accident

Diabetes Mellitus

Treatment with insulin

Chronic Renal Insufficiency

Serum creatinine >2 mg/dL

Abbreviations: CABG, coronary artery bypass grafting; ECG, electrocardiogram; PTCA, percutaneous transluminal coronary angioplasty.

Source: Adapted from Lee TH et al: Derivation and prospective validation of a simple index for prediction of cardiac risk of major noncardiac surgery. *Circulation* 100:1043, 1999, with permission.

having ischemic heart disease if he or she had a history of angina, myocardial infarction, or prior angioplasty or bypass surgery. In addition, ischemic heart disease would be considered present if a patient was requiring sublingual nitroglycerin, had a positive exercise test result, or had pathologic Q waves on the electrocardiogram (ECG). Therefore, the patient has a RCRI score of 3 (high-risk surgery, ischemic heart disease by ECG, and diabetes mellitus requiring insulin).

Individuals with scores of 3 or higher fall in the highest risk category of the RCRI. These individuals have an estimated postoperative risk of major cardiovascular events between 9 and 11%. If an individual has a risk score of 2, the risk of postoperative cardiovascular events is 4–6.6%. There is a 1% risk of postoperative events with a risk score of 1 and a 0.5% risk with a risk score of 0. No group has a risk score as high as 20% using this methodology.

I-42.   **The answer is B.** *(Chap. 8)* Pulmonary and cardiovascular complications are a major source of morbidity and mortality after surgery. Primary care physicians are often asked to determine a patient's postoperative risk of pulmonary complications. Factors identified by the American College of Physicians as conferring an increased risk of pulmonary complications are shown in Table I-42. Although many of these factors are directly related to pulmonary function, some of these are not. Notably, the presence of congestive heart failure and a serum albumin level of less than 3.5 g/dL predict postoperative pulmonary complications. Asthma is not a predictor of pulmonary complications as long as the disease is under sufficient control. Factors listed in the table that are useful determinants of asthma control include peak expiratory flow rate greater than 100 L or 50% predicted and forced expiratory volume in 1 second of less than 2 L.

TABLE I-42   **Predisposing Risk Factors for Pulmonary Complications**

1. Upper respiratory tract infection: cough, dyspnea
2. Age greater than 60 years
3. COPD
4. American Society of Anesthesiologists Class ≥2
5. Functionally dependent
6. Congestive heart failure
7. Serum albumin <3.5 g/dL
8. FEV_1 <2 L
9. MVV <50% of predicted
10. PEF <100 L or 50% predicted value
11. PCO_2 ≥45 mmHg
12. PO_2 ≤50 mmHg

Abbreviations: COPD, chronic obstructive pulmonary disease; FEV_1, forced expiratory volume in 1 second; MVV, maximum voluntary ventilation; PEF, peak expiratory flow rate; PCO_2, partial pressure of carbon dioxide; PO_2, partial pressure of oxygen.
Source: Modified from Smetana GW et al: Preoperative pulmonary risk stratification for noncardiothoracic surgery: Systematic review for the American College of Physicians. *Ann Intern Med* 144:581, 2006 and Mohr DN et al: *Postgrad Med* 100:247, 1996, with permission.

I-43.   **The answer is E.** *(Chap. 9)* Communication of bad news is an inherent component of the physician–patient relationship, and these conversations often occur in a hospital setting where the treating provider is not the primary care provider for the patient. Many physicians struggle with providing clear and effective communication to patients who are seriously ill and their family members. In the scenario presented in this case, it is necessary to have a discussion about the patient's poor prognosis and determine the goals of care without the input of the patient because her mental status remains altered. Failure to provide clear communication in the appropriate environment can lead to tension in the relationship between the physician and patient and may lead to overly aggressive treatment. The P-SPIKES approach (Table I-43) has been advocated as a simple framework to assist physicians in effectively communicating bad news to patients. The components of this communication tool are:

- Preparation—Review what information needs to be communicated and plan how emotional support will be provided.
- Setting of interaction—This step is often the most neglected. Ensure a quiet and private environment and attempt to minimize any interruptions.
- Patient (or family) perceptions and preparation—Assess what the patient and family know about the current condition. Use open-ended questions.
- Invitation and information needs—Ask the patient or family what they would like to know and also what limits they want regarding bad information
- Knowledge of the condition—Provide the patient and family with the bad news and assess understanding.
- Empathy and exploration—Empathize with the patient and family's feelings and offer emotional support. Allow plenty of time for questions and exploration of their feelings.
- Summary and planning—Outline the next steps for the patient and family. Recommend a timeline to achieve the goals of care.

TABLE I-43 Elements of Communicating Bad News—The P-SPIKES Approach

Acronym	Step	Aim of the Interaction	Preparations, Questions, or Phrases
P	Preparation	Mentally prepare for the interaction with the patient or family (or both).	Review what information needs to be communicated. Plan how you will provide emotional support. Rehearse key steps and phrases in the interaction.
S	Setting of the interaction	Ensure the appropriate setting for a serious and potentially emotionally charged discussion.	Ensure that patient, family, and appropriate social supports are present. Devote sufficient time. Ensure privacy and prevent interruptions by people, beeper, or phone. Bring a box of tissues.
P	Patient's perception and preparation	Begin the discussion by establishing the baseline and whether the patient and family can grasp the information. Ease tension by having the patient and family contribute.	Start with open-ended questions to encourage participation. Possible phrases to use: *What do you understand about your illness? When you first had symptom X, what did you think it might be? What did Dr. X tell you when he or she sent you here? What do you think is going to happen?*
I	Invitation and information needs	Discover what information needs the patient and family have and what limits they want regarding the bad information.	Possible phrases to use: *If this condition turns out to be something serious, do you want to know? Would you like me to tell you all the details of your condition? If not, who would you like me to talk to?*
K	Knowledge of the condition	Provide the bad news or other information to the patient and family sensitively.	Do not just dump the information on the patient and family. Check for patient and family understanding. Possible phrases to use: *I feel bad to have to tell you this, but … Unfortunately, the tests showed … I'm afraid the news is not good …*
E	Empathy and exploration	Identify the cause of the emotions (e.g., poor prognosis). Empathize with the patient and family's feelings. Explore by asking open-ended questions.	Strong feelings in reaction to bad news are normal. Acknowledge what the patient and family are feeling. Remind them such feelings are normal, even if frightening. Give them time to respond. Remind patient and family you will not abandon them. Possible phrases to use: *I imagine this is very hard for you to hear. You look very upset. Tell me how you are feeling. I wish the news were different. We'll do whatever we can to help you.*
S	Summary and planning	Delineate for the patient and the family the next steps, including additional tests or interventions.	It is the unknown and uncertain that can increase anxiety. Recommend a schedule with goals and landmarks. Provide your rationale for the patient and family to accept (or reject). If the patient and family are not ready to discuss the next steps, schedule a follow-up visit.

Source: Adapted from Buckman R: *How to Break Bad News: A Guide for Health Care Professionals.* Baltimore, Johns Hopkins University Press, 1992.

Setting a follow-up meeting is not a primary component of the P-SPIKES framework but may be necessary when a family or patient is not emotionally ready to discuss the next steps in the care plan.

I-44.   **The answer is C.** *(Chap. 9)* Advance care planning documentation is an increasing component of medical practice. As of 2006, 48 states and the District of Columbia had enacted legislation regarding advance care planning. The two broad types of advance care planning documentation are living wills and designation of a health care proxy (option C). Although these two documents are often combined into a single document, designation of a health care proxy is not one of the primary components of a living will. The living will (or instructional directive) delineates the patient's preferences (option A) regarding treatment under different scenarios (e.g., whether condition is perceived as terminal). These documents can be very specific to a condition such as cancer but may also be very broad in the case of elderly individuals who do not currently have a terminal condition but want to outline their wishes for care in the event of an unexpected health crisis. Examples of what this might include general statements regarding the receipt of life-sustaining therapies (option D) and the values that should guide the decisions regarding terminal care (option B).

I-45.   **The answer is D.** *(Chap. 9)* Depression is difficult to diagnose in individuals with terminal illness and is often an overlooked symptom by physicians because many individual believe it a normal component of terminal illness. Furthermore, symptoms commonly associated with depression such as insomnia and anorexia are also frequently seen in serious illness or occur as a side effect of treatment. Although about 75% of terminally ill patients express some depressive symptoms, only 25% or less have major depression. When assessing depression in terminally ill individuals, one should focus on symptoms pertaining to the dysphoric mood, including helplessness, hopelessness, and anhedonia. It is inappropriate to do nothing in when one believes major depression is occurring (option A). The approach to treatment should include nonpharmacologic and pharmacologic therapies. The pharmacologic approach to depression should be the same in terminally ill individuals as in non–terminally ill individuals. If an individual has a prognosis of several months or longer, selective serotonin reuptake inhibitors (fluoxetine, paroxetine) or serotonin–noradrenaline reuptake inhibitors (venlafaxine) are the preferred treatment because of their efficacy and side effect profile. However, these medications take several weeks to become effective. Thus, starting fluoxetine alone (option C) is not preferred. In patients with major depression and fatigue or opioid-induced somnolence, combining a traditional antidepressant with a psychostimulant is appropriate (option D). Psychostimulants are also indicated in individuals with a poor prognosis who are not expected to live long enough to experience the benefits of treatment with a traditional antidepressant. A variety of psychostimulant medications are available, including methylphenidate, modafinil, dextroamphetamine, and pemoline. Because this patient has a prognosis of several months or longer, methylphenidate alone is not recommended (option E). Because of their side effect profile, tricyclic antidepressants (option A) are not used in the treatment of depression in terminally ill patients unless they are used as adjunctive treatment for chronic pain.

I-46.   **The answer is C.** *(Chap. 9)* A primary goal of palliative care medicine is to control pain in patients who are terminally ill. Surveys have found that 36–90% of individuals with advanced cancer have substantial pain, and an individualized treatment plan is necessary for each patient. For individuals with continuous pain, opioid analgesics should be administered on a scheduled basis around the clock at an interval based on the half-life of the medication chosen. Extended-release preparations are frequently used because of their longer half-lives. However, it is inappropriate to start immediately with an extended-release preparation. In this scenario, the patient was treated with a continuous intravenous infusion via patient-controlled analgesia for 48 hours to determine her baseline opioid needs. The average daily dose of morphine required was 90 mg. This total dose should be administered in divided doses two or three times daily (either 45 mg twice daily or 30 mg three times daily). In addition, an immediate-release preparation should be available for administration for breakthrough pain. The recommended dose of the immediate-release preparation is 20% of the baseline dose. In this case, the dose would be 18 mg and could be given as either 15 or 20 mg four times daily as needed.

I-47. **The answer is E.** *(Chap. 9)* Withdrawal of care is a common occurrence in intensive care units. More than 90% of Americans die without performance of cardiopulmonary resuscitation. When a family decides to withdraw care, the treating care team of doctors, nurses, and respiratory therapists must work together to ensure that the dying process will be comfortable for both the patient and the family. Commonly, patients receive a combination of anxiolytics and opioid analgesics. These medications also provide relief of dyspnea in the dying patient. However, they have little effect on oropharyngeal secretions (option A). The accumulation of secretions in the oropharynx can produce agitation, labored breathing, and noisy breathing that has been labeled the "death rattle." This can be quite distressing to the family. Treatments for excessive oropharyngeal secretions are primarily anticholinergic medications, including scopolamine delivered transdermally (option E) or intravenously, atropine, and glycopyrrolate. Although placement of a nasal trumpet or oral airway (option D) may allow better access for suctioning of secretions, these can be uncomfortable or even painful interventions that are typically discouraged in a palliative care situation. *N*-acetylcysteine (option B) can be used as a mucolytic agent to thin lower respiratory secretions. Pilocarpine (option C) is a cholinergic stimulant and increases salivary production.

I-48. **The answer is A.** *(Chap. 10)* In recent years, there has been increasing focus on both the safety and quality of health care provided throughout the world. An Institute of Medicine report identified safety as an essential component of quality in health care. Improving safety and quality in health care relies on understanding the frequency and type of adverse events that occur in the health care system. An adverse event is defined as an injury caused by medical management rather than the underlying disease of the patient. One of the largest studies that has attempted to quantify adverse events in hospitalized patients was the Harvard Medical Practice Study. In this study, the most common adverse event was an adverse drug event, which occurred in 19% of hospitalizations. Other common adverse events included wound infections (14%), technical complications of a procedure (13%), diagnostic mishaps (15%), and falls (5%).

I-49. **The answer is A.** *(Chap. e2)* Since 1993, numerous population studies have shown that 30–40% of American adults seek and or use at least one complementary and alternative medicine (CAM) approach. The most prevalent are nonmineral nonvitamin dietary supplements, relaxation, medication, massage, and chiropractic care. Approximately 1% of Americans use acupuncture. The most common reasons are for back or musculoskeletal pain and control of symptoms not adequately addressed by conventional therapy. CAM expenses are estimated to be $34 billion per year, representing 1.5% of total health care expenditures and 11% of out-of-pocket expenses.

I-50. **The answer is E.** *(Chap. e4)* Minority patients have poorer health outcomes from many preventable and treatable conditions such as cardiovascular disease, asthma, diabetes, cancer, and others. The causes of these differences are multifactorial and include social determinants (education, socioeconomic status, environment) and access to care (which often leads to more serious illness before seeking care). However, there are also clearly described racial differences in quality of care when patients enter the health care system. These differences have been found in cardiovascular, oncologic, renal, diabetic, and palliative care. Eliminating these differences will require systematic changes in health system factors, provider-level factors, and patient-level factors.

I-51. **The answer is A.** *(Chap. e6)* Breast cancer in pregnant women is defined as cancer diagnosed during pregnancy or up to 1 year after delivery. Only about 5% of all breast cancers occur in women younger than 40 years of age, and of those, approximately 25% are pregnancy-associated cancer. Needle biopsy of breast masses in pregnant women is often nondiagnostic, and false-positive test results may occur. Breast cancers diagnosed during pregnancy have a worse outcome than other breast cancers. The cancers tend to be diagnosed at a later stage (often the signs are thought to be related to pregnancy) and tend to have a more aggressive behavior. Approximately 30% of breast cancers found in pregnancy are estrogen receptor positive in contrast to 60–70% being estrogen receptor positive overall. Larger tumor size, positive axillary nodes, Her-2 positivity, and higher stage are all more common in pregnant women.

I-52.   **The answer is C.** *(Chap. 34)* Chronic cough is one of the most common causes of referral to pulmonary, allergy, and otolaryngology practices and is frequently encountered in primary care. A cough is classified as chronic when it persists for longer than 8 weeks and has a wide range of differential diagnoses, including cardiac, pulmonary, upper airway, and gastrointestinal diseases. The initial history and physical examination is important in providing clues to the potential etiology, particularly in the setting of a normal chest radiograph and examination. The most common causes of chronic cough in an otherwise normal individual are cough-variant asthma, gastroesophageal reflux disease, postnasal drip, and medications. In this patient, there are clues that should lead one to suspect cough-variant asthma as a potential cause. Asthma can present only with cough. Although this presentation is more common in children, it can present this way in adults as well. This patient does have triggers that include cold air and exercise, both of which can lead to increased bronchoconstriction. In addition, the parasympathetic–sympathetic balance favors bronchoconstriction that is worse in the early morning hours with cough late at night. Although spirometry demonstrating reversible airflow obstruction is typically seen in asthma, asthma has significant clinical variability, and lung function varies over time. In this patient, the spirometry results are normal, and the bronchodilator response is insufficient to diagnose reversibility, which requires a response of at least 12% and an increase of at least 200 mL in either the forced expiratory volume in 1 second (FEV_1) or forced vital capacity (FVC). To establish the diagnosis more definitively, demonstration of a fall in FEV_1 of at least 20% during a bronchoprovocation test with methacholine would be sufficient in this clinical scenario to diagnose asthma and would be safe to perform in this patient with normal pulmonary function at baseline. An alternative approach would be to treat empirically with low-dose inhaled corticosteroids given the clinical history.

   In many cases, the cause of chronic cough is multifactorial. This patient has minor symptoms of allergic rhinitis, which may be a contributing factor. Nasal corticosteroids may also be required, but given the reported triggers, would not be sole treatment. The patient gives no history to suggest GERD, which may be clinically silent. If the cough failed to improve with treatment for asthma, antacid medications may be indicated. Finally, increasing numbers of adults are becoming infected with *Bordetella pertussis* because individual immunity wanes in adulthood, and more parents are electing to forego childhood immunizations. In this scenario, the patient typically gives a history of an upper respiratory infection with a strong cough at the onset of the illness. When the illness has progresses to the recovery phase, diagnosis is typically made by serology, and culture is not useful.

I-53.   **The answer is A.** *(Chap. 34)* Hemoptysis is a relatively common symptom that causes a significant degree of distress in the patient. In most individuals, the hemoptysis is mild and self-limited despite the anxiety that it causes. Worldwide, tuberculosis remains the most common cause of hemoptysis. However, in the United States, the most common cause of hemoptysis is acute bronchitis of viral or bacterial etiology. Given the acute nature of the illness and mild degree of hemoptysis, this patient's presentation would be most consistent with the diagnosis of acute bronchitis. Antiplatelet or anticoagulant agents may increase the risk of bleeding but are not sufficient in the absence of an underlying cause to initiate hemoptysis. Moreover, these agents are typically associated with underlying alveolar rather than airway damage. Most patients who experience hemoptysis fear lung cancer, which can present with acute hemoptysis, but this patient's report of primarily blood-streaked sputum would make this less likely, especially in the face of a normal chest radiograph. Lung abscesses rarely present with hemoptysis, and the typical presentation is one of a prolonged illness.

I-54. **The answer is E.** *(Chap. 34)* Life-threatening hemoptysis is a medical emergency. Defining *massive hemoptysis* can be difficult but generally should be viewed as any amount of hemoptysis that can lead to airway obstruction because most patients who die of hemoptysis die from asphyxiation and airway obstruction. The immediate management of hemoptysis is to establish a patent airway and establish the site of bleeding. The initial step is to place the patient with the bleeding side in a dependent position. In this patient with a known lesion of the right upper lobe, he should be placed with the right side (not left) in a dependent position. The patient should be intubated with the largest possible endotracheal tube to allow for adequate suctioning. When immediately available, placement of a dual-lumen endotracheal tube can allow selective ventilation of the nonbleeding lung while providing access to continue suctioning from the affected side. Certainly, correction of any underlying coagulopathy would be important in the management of this patient. If conservative measures fail to stop the bleeding, the first step is to attempt embolization of the bleeding artery, but in rare instances, urgent surgical intervention may be required.

I-55. **The answer is D.** *(Chap. 221)* Microbial agents have been used as bioweapons as far back as the sixth century BC when water supplies were poisoned with *Claviceps purpurea* by the Assyrians. In modern times, science that has been often sponsored by governmental agencies has lead to new ways to enhance and spread microbial bioweapons. Bioterrorism should be delineated from biowarfare. Although bioterrorism has the potential to lead to thousands of deaths if used in a large-scale manner, the primary impact is the fear and terror generated by the attack. However, biowarfare specifically targets mass casualties and seeks to weaken the enemy. The Working Group for Civilian Biodefense has outlined key features that characterize agents that are the most effective bioweapons. These 10 features are:

1. High morbidity and mortality rates
2. Potential for person-to-person spread
3. Low infective dose and highly infectious by the aerosol route
4. Lack of rapid diagnostic capability
5. Lack of a universally available effective vaccine
6. Potential to cause anxiety
7. Availability of pathogen and feasibility of production
8. Environmental stability
9. Database of prior research and development
10. Potential to be weaponized

A lack of effective and available treatment is not one of the characteristics of an effective bioweapon. *Bacillus anthracis* is the causative organism of anthrax, one of the most prototypical microbial bioweapons, but many antibiotics have efficacy against anthrax and can be lifesaving if initiated early.

I-56. **The answer is B.** *(Chap. 221)* *Yersinia pestis* is a gram-negative rod that causes the plague and has been one of the most widely used bioweapons over the centuries. Although *Y. pestis* lacks environmental stability, it is highly contagious and has a high mortality rate, making it an effective agent of bioterrorism. There are two major syndromes caused by *Y. pestis* that reflect the mode of infection. These patients presented with symptoms typical of bubonic plague, which still exists widely in nature. In the United States, the area with the greatest number of naturally occurring cases of bubonic plague is in the Southwest with transmission occurring via contact with infected animals or fleas. In this case, infected animals or fleas were present in the concentrated population of an immigrant camp that had poor sanitation. After an individual is bitten by an infected vector, the bacteria travel through the lymphatics to regional lymph nodes, where they are phagocytized but not destroyed. The organisms can then multiply with the cells, leading to inflammation, painful and markedly enlarged lymph nodes, and fever. The affected lymph nodes can develop necrosis and are characteristically called buboes. Infection can progress to severe sepsis and death. The mortality rate for treated bubonic plague is 1–15% and 40–60% in untreated cases. When *Y. pestis* is used as an agent of bioterrorism, it is aerosolized to a large area, and the affected cases present primarily with pneumonic plague. Pneumonic plague presents with fever, cough, hemoptysis, and gastrointestinal symptoms that occur 1–6 days after exposure. Without treatment, pneumonic plague has an 85% morality rate with death occurring rapidly within 2–6 days. The treatment for *Y. pestis* could include aminoglycosides or doxycycline.

I-57.   **The answer is D.** *(Chap. 221)* In the event of a bioterrorism attack, botulinum toxin would be most likely delivered by either aerosol or contamination of the food supply. Contamination of the water supply is possible, but it is not an optimal route for bioterrorism. Botulinum toxin is inactivated by chlorine, which is used in many water supplies for purification. In addition, heating any food or water to greater than 85°C for longer than 5 minutes will inactivate the toxin. Finally, there is an environmental decay rate of 1% per minute. So the time interval between release and ingestion would need to be very short, which would be difficult with an entire city water supply.

I-58.   **The answer is B.** *(Chap. 221)* Anthrax is caused by the gram-positive spore-forming rod *Bacillus* anthrax. Anthrax spores may be the prototypical disease of bioterrorism. Although not spread person to person, inhalational anthrax has a high mortality and a low infective dose (five spores) and may be spread widely with aerosols after bioengineering. It is well documented that anthrax spores were produced and stored as potential bioweapons. In 2001, the United States was exposed to anthrax spores delivered as a powder in letters. Of 11 patients with inhalation anthrax, five died. All 11 patients with cutaneous anthrax survived. Because anthrax spores can remain dormant in the respiratory tract for 6 weeks, the incubation period can be quite long, and postexposure antibiotics are recommended for 60 days. Trials of a recombinant vaccine are underway.

I-59.   **The answer is D.** *(Chap. 221)* The three major clinical forms of anthrax are gastrointestinal (GI), cutaneous, and inhalational. GI anthrax results from eating contaminated meat and is an unlikely bioweapon. Cutaneous anthrax results from contact with the spores and results in a black eschar lesion. Cutaneous anthrax had a 20% mortality before antibiotics became available. Inhalational anthrax typically presents with the most deadly form and is the most likely bioweapon. The spores are phagocytosed by alveolar macrophages and transported to the mediastinum. Subsequent germination, toxin elaboration, and hematogenous spread cause septic shock. A characteristic radiographic finding is mediastinal widening and pleural effusion. Prompt initiation of antibiotics is essential because the mortality rate is likely 100% without specific treatment. Inhalational anthrax is not known to be contagious. Provided that there is no concern for release of another highly infectious agent such as smallpox, only routine precautions are warranted.

I-60.   **The answer is C.** *(Chap. 221)* Using the characteristics listed in the question, the Centers for Disease Control and Prevention developed classifications of biologic agents that are based on their potential to be used as bioweapons. Six types of agents have been designated as category A: *Bacillus anthracis*, botulinum toxin, *Yersinia pestis*, smallpox, tularemia, and the many viruses that cause viral hemorrhagic fever. Those viruses include Lassa virus, Rift Valley fever virus, Ebola virus, and yellow fever virus.

I-61.   **The answer is C.** *(Chap. 222)* Chemical agents were first used in modern warfare during World War I when 1.3 million died as a result of chemical agents. Since then, chemical agents have been used during warfare and bioterrorism, but most agents have a fairly low associated mortality rate. The chemical agents generally fall into one of five categories: nerve agents, asphyxiants, pulmonary damaging, vesicants, and behavior altering or incapacitating. Nerve agents include cyclohexyl sarin, sarin, soman, tabun, and VX and largely exert their effects through acetylcholinesterase inhibition. The most common asphyxiant is cyanide, which is liberated through cyanogen chloride or hydrogen cyanide. Chlorine gas, hydrogen chloride, nitrogen oxide, and phosgene are common agents that primarily cause pulmonary damage and adult respiratory distress syndrome. Vesicants include mustard gas and phosgene oxime, and agent 15/BZ is the primary chemical causing alterations in behavior or incapacitation.

I-62.   **The answer is D.** *(Chap. 222)* Sulfur mustard was first used as a chemical warfare agent in World War I. This agent is considered a vesicant and has a characteristic odor of burning garlic or horseradish. It is a threat to all exposed epithelial surfaces, and the most commonly affected organs are the eyes, skin, and airways. Large exposures can lead to bone marrow suppression. Erythema resembling a sunburn is one of the earliest manifestations of sulfur mustard exposure and begins within 2 hours to 2 days of exposure. The timing of exposure can be delayed as long as 2 days depending on the severity of exposure, ambient temperature, and humidity. The most sensitive body areas are warm, moist locations, including the axillae, perineum, external genitalia, neck, and antecubital fossae. Blistering of the skin is frequent and may be anything from small vesicles to large bullae. The bullae are dome shaped and flaccid. Filled with clear or straw-colored fluid, these bullae are not hazardous because the fluid does not contain any vesicant substances. The respiratory passages are also affected. With mild exposure, the only manifestation may be a complaint of irritation and congestion. Laryngospasm may occur. In severe cases, there is necrosis of the airways with pseudomembrane formation. The damage that occurs after sulfur mustard exposure is airway predominant, and alveolar damage is very rare. The eyes are particularly sensitive to sulfur mustard and have a shorter latency period than the skin injury. Almost all exposed individuals develop redness of the eyes. With higher exposure, there is a greater severity of conjunctivitis and corneal damage. The cause of death after mustard gas exposure is sepsis or respiratory failure, but the mortality rate is typically low. Even during World War I, when antibiotics and endotracheal intubation were not available, the mortality rate was only 1.9%. There is no antidote to sulfur mustard. Complete decontamination in 2 minutes stops clinical injury, and decontamination within 5 minutes can decrease skin injury by half. Treatment is largely supportive.

I-63.   **The answer is A.** *(Chap. 222)* Chlorine gas exposure primarily causes pulmonary damage and edema with respiratory distress syndrome. The initial decontamination of a victim exposed to chlorine gas should include removal of all clothing if no frostbite is present. The victim should gently wash the skin with soap and water with care to avoid aggressive bathing that may lead to serious abrasion of the skin. The eyes are flushed with water or normal saline. Supportive care should include forced rest, fresh air, and maintenance of a semiupright position. Oxygen is not required because the patient is not hypoxemic or in any respiratory distress. Delayed pulmonary edema can occur even if the patient is initially asymptomatic. Thus, observation for a period of time after exposure is required.

I-64 and I-65.   **The answers are D and D, respectively.** *(Chap. 222)* This patient has symptoms of an acute cholinergic crisis as seen in cases of organophosphate poisoning. Organophosphates are the "classic" nerve agents, and several different compounds may act in this manner, including sarin, tabun, soman, and cyclosarin. Except for agent VX, all of the organophosphates are liquid at standard room temperature and pressure and are highly volatile, with the onset of symptoms occurring within minutes to hours after exposure. VX is an oily liquid with a low vapor pressure; therefore, it does not acutely cause symptoms. However, it is an environmental hazard because it can persist in the environment for a longer period. Organophosphates act by inhibiting tissue synaptic acetylcholinesterase. Symptoms differ between vapor exposure and liquid exposure because the organophosphate acts in the tissue upon contact. The first organ exposed with vapor exposure is the eyes, causing rapid and persistent pupillary constriction. After the sarin gas attacks in the Tokyo subway in 1994 and 1995, survivors frequently complained that their "world went black" as the first symptom of exposure. This is rapidly followed by rhinorrhea, excessive salivation, and lacrimation. In the airways, organophosphates cause bronchorrhea and bronchospasm. It is in the alveoli that organophosphates gain the greatest extent of entry into the blood. As organophosphates circulate, other symptoms appear, including nausea, vomiting, diarrhea, and muscle fasciculations. Death occurs with central nervous system penetration causing central apnea and status epilepticus. The effects on the heart rate and blood pressure are unpredictable.

Treatment requires a multifocal approach. Initially, decontamination of clothing and wounds is important for both the patient and the caregiver. Clothing should be removed before contact with the health care provider. In Tokyo, 10% of emergency personnel developed miosis related to contact with patients' clothing. Three classes of medication are important in treating organophosphate poisoning, anticholinergics, oximes, and anticonvulsant agents. Initially, atropine at doses of 2–6 mg should be given intravenously or intramuscularly to reverse the effects of organophosphates at muscarinic receptors; it has no effect on nicotinic receptors. Thus, atropine rapidly treats life-threatening respiratory depression but does not affect neuromuscular or sympathetic effects. This should be followed by the administration of an oxime, which is a nucleophile compound that reactivates the cholinesterase whose active site has been bound to a nerve agent. Depending on the nerve agent used, oxime may not be helpful because it is unable to bind to "aged" complexes that have undergone degradation of a side chain of the nerve agent, making it negatively charged. Soman undergoes aging within 2 minutes, thus rendering oxime therapy useless. The currently approved oxime in the United States is 2-pralidoxime. Finally, the only anticonvulsant class of drugs that is effective in seizures caused by organophosphate poisoning is the benzodiazepines. The dose required is frequently higher than that used for epileptic seizures, requiring the equivalent of 40 mg of diazepam given in frequent doses. All other classes of anticonvulsant medications, including phenytoin, barbiturates, carbamazepine, and valproic acid, will not improve seizures related to organophosphate poisoning.

I-66. **The answer is D.** *(Chap. 223)* Detonation of a nuclear device is the most likely scenario of radiation bioterror. The initial blast will cause acute mortality caused by the shock wave and thermal damage. Subsequent mortality would be caused by acute radiation exposure and fallout to more distant populations that largely depend on weather patterns. The initial detonation releases mostly highly damaging gamma particles and neutrons. Alpha and beta particles are not highly toxic in this situation. Alpha particles are large, have limiting penetrating power, and are stopped by cloth and human skin. Beta particles, although small, travel only a short distance (a few millimeters) in tissue and cause mostly burn-type injuries. Radioactive iodine is a beta particle emitter. Acute radiation syndrome causes death by hematopoietic bone marrow suppression and aplasia; gastrointestinal tract damage with malabsorption and translocation of bacteria; and in severe cases, neurologic damage. Appropriate medical supportive therapy can reduce mortality and allow patient with more severe exposure to survive. Radiation causes dose-dependent bone marrow suppression that is irreversible at high doses. Bone marrow transplantation is controversial in cases of non-recovery of bone marrow. The acute exposure symptoms, predominantly thermal injury, respiratory distress, and GI symptoms, make resolve within days. However, subsequent bone marrow dysfunction typically develops within 2 weeks but may take as long as 6 weeks to manifest.

I-67. **The answer is D.** *(Chap. 223)* Much of the initial damage related to a "dirty" bomb is related to the power of the blast rather than the radiation. After a terrorist attack, it is important to identify all individuals who might have been exposed to radiation. The initial treatment of these individuals should be to stabilize and treat the most severely injured ones. Those with severe injuries should have contaminated clothing removed before transportation to the emergency department, but further care should not be withheld for additional decontamination because the risk of exposure to health care workers is low. Individuals with minor injuries who can be safely decontaminated without increasing the risk of medical complications should be transported to a centralized area for decontamination. A further consideration regarding treatment after radiation exposure is the total dose of radiation that an individual was exposed to. At a dose less than 2 Gy, there are usually no significant adverse outcomes, and no specific treatment is recommended unless symptoms develop. Many individuals will develop flulike symptoms. However, a complete blood count should be obtained every 6 hours for the first 24 hours because bone marrow suppression can develop with radiation exposure as low as 0.7 Gy. The earliest sign of this is a fall in the lymphocyte count of greater than 50%. Potential treatments of radiation exposure include use of colony-stimulating factors and supportive transfusions. Stem cell transfusion and bone marrow transplantation can be considered in the case of severe pancytopenia that does not recover. However, this is controversial, given the lack of experience with the procedure for this indication. After the Chernobyl nuclear reactor accident, none of the bone marrow transplants were successful.

I-68. **The answer is B.** *(Chap. 16)* The patient has a classic presentation of malignant hyperthermia likely caused by succinylcholine or inhalational anesthetic administration as part of her anesthetic regimen. This syndrome occurs in individuals with inherited abnormality of skeletal muscle sarcoplasmic reticulum that causes a rise in intracellular calcium content after inhalational anesthetic or succinylcholine administration. The syndrome presents with hyperthermia, or an uncontrolled increase in body temperature that exceeds the ability of the body to lose heat; muscular rigidity; and acidosis, cardiovascular instability, and rhabdomyolysis. Because the temperature dysregulation is not attributable to alteration in hypothalamic set point, antipyretics such as acetaminophen, ibuprofen, and corticosteroids are ineffective at treating the condition. Haloperidol is associated with neuroleptic malignant syndrome and should not be used to treat this condition. Physical cooling in addition to dantrolene are the treatments of choice. Dantrolene disrupts excitation–contraction coupling in skeletal muscle, thereby diminishing thermogenesis. Dantrolene may also be used in neuroleptic malignant syndrome and occasionally the serotonin syndrome.

I-69. **The answer is C.** *(Chap. 16)* Hyperthermia occurs when exogenous heat exposure or an endogenous heat-producing process, such as neuroleptic malignant syndrome or malignant hyperthermia, leads to high internal temperatures despite a normal hypothalamic temperature set point. Fever occurs when a pyrogen such as a microbial toxin, microbe particle, or cytokine resets the hypothalamus to a higher temperature. A particular temperature cutoff point does not define hyperthermia. Rigidity and autonomic dysregulation are characteristic of malignant hyperthermia, a subset of hyperthermia. Fever, not hyperthermia, responds to antipyretics.

I-70. **The answer is E.** *(Chap. 17)* Elderly adults and young children are at highest risk of nonexertional heat stroke. Environmental stress (heat wave) is the most common precipitating factor, particularly in bedridden individuals and individuals living in poorly ventilated or non–air-conditioned conditions. Medications such as antiparkinson treatment, diuretics, and anticholinergics increase the risk of heat stroke.

I-71. **The answer is A.** *(Chap. 17)* Based on the characteristic rash and Koplik's spots, this patient has measles. A rare but feared complication of measles is subacute sclerosing panencephalitis. His examination does not support epiglottitis because he has no drooling or dysphagia. His rash is not characteristic of acute HIV infection, and he lacks the pharyngitis and arthralgias commonly seen with this diagnosis. The rash is not consistent with herpes zoster, and he is quite young to have this condition. Splenic rupture occasionally occurs with infectious mononucleosis, but this patient has no pharyngitis, lymphadenopathy, or splenomegaly to suggest this diagnosis. Because of mandatory vaccination, measles is very uncommon in the United States (as well as central and south America); almost all cases are imported. However, countries with lower rates of vaccination still have endemic measles.

I-72. **The answer is C.** *(Chap. 17)* This case is likely toxic shock syndrome, given the clinical appearance of septic shock with no positive blood cultures. The characteristic diffuse rash, as well as the lack of a primary infected site, make *Staphylococcus* the most likely inciting agent. Streptococcal toxic shock usually has a prominent primary site of infection, but the diffuse rash is usually much more subtle than in this case. Staphylococcal toxic shock can be associated with immunosuppression, surgical wounds, or retained tampons. Mere *Staphylococcus aureus* colonization (with an appropriate toxigenic strain) can incite toxic shock. Centers for Disease Control and Prevention guidelines state that measles, Rocky Mountain spotted fever, and leptospirosis need to be ruled out serologically to confirm the diagnosis. However, this patient is at very low risk for these diagnoses based on vaccination and travel history. Juvenile rheumatoid arthritis would become a consideration only if the fevers were more prolonged and there was documented evidence of organomegaly and enlarged lymph nodes.

I-73. **The answer is C.** *(Chap. 17)* Although he never underwent joint fluid sampling, the presentation of monoarticular arthritis of the great toe in the context of a patient taking diuretics makes gout very likely. Allopurinol, although effective at controlling hyperuricemia, is a frequent culprit in drug-induced hypersensitivity syndromes. This syndrome generally presents with evidence of systemic hypersensitivity, including rash, eosinophilia, and often renal or hepatic dysfunction. Desquamative erythroderma and toxic epidermal necrolysis have been described additionally with allopurinol, but the absence of mucous membrane involvement makes TEN less likely. The absence of preexisting septic arthritis makes toxic shock less likely. Angioedema is not known to be associated with diffuse erythroderma. Diffuse erythema is not a feature of bacterial endocarditis, which frequently has associated focal skin lesions such as Osler lesions or Janeway nodes. Finally, in the absence of a focal area of infection, MRSA cellulitis would not explain the findings.

I-74.   **The answer is C.** *(Chap. 18)* Fever of unknown origin (FUO) is defined as the presence of fevers to greater than 38.3°C (101.0°F) on several occasions occurring for more than 3 weeks without a defined cause after appropriate investigation into potential causes have failed to yield a diagnosis. Initial laboratory investigation into an FUO should include a complete blood count with differential, peripheral blood smear, ESR, C-reactive protein, electrolytes, creatinine, calcium, liver function tests, urinalysis, and muscle enzymes. In addition, specific testing for a variety of infections should be performed, including VDRL for syphilis, HIV, CMV, EBV, PPD testing, and blood, sputum, and urine cultures if appropriate. Finally, the workup should include evaluation for inflammatory disorders. These tests include antinuclear antibodies, rheumatoid factor, ferritin, iron, and transferrin. This patient has had a significant workup that has demonstrated primarily nonspecific findings, including elevation in the erythrocyte sedimentation rate and ferritin as well as borderline enlargement of multiple lymph nodes. The only finding that may help define further workup is the elevation in calcium levels. When combined with the clinical symptoms and prominent lymph nodes, this could suggest granulomatous diseases, including disseminated tuberculosis, fungal infections, or sarcoidosis. The next step in the work up of this patient would be to obtain a sample from an enlarged lymph node for cultures and pathology to confirm granulomatous inflammation and provide additional samples for microbiology. In recent studies, up to 30% of individuals will not have an identified cause of FUO, and infectious etiologies continue to comprise 25% of all FUO. The most common infection causing FUO is extrapulmonary tuberculosis, which may be difficult to diagnose because PPD is often negative in these individuals. However, one would not consider empirical therapy if the possibility to obtain definitive diagnosis exists through a procedure such as a needle biopsy because it is prudent to have not only the diagnosis but also the sensitivity profile of the organism to ensure appropriate therapy. Even in the presence of granulomatous infection, sarcoidosis would be considered a diagnosis of exclusion and would require definitive negative mycobacterial cultures before considering therapy with corticosteroids. Serum angiotensin-converting enzyme levels are neither appropriately sensitive nor specific for diagnosis of sarcoidosis and should not be used to determine if therapy is needed. PET-CT imaging would be unlikely to be helpful in this situation because the presence of granulomatous inflammation can lead to false-positive results or will confirm the presence of already characterized abnormal lymph nodes.

I-75.   **The answer is D.** *(Chap. 19)* When evaluating a patient with hypothermia, it is important to consider all the possible factors that could contribute to hypothermia because treatment of hypothermia alone without treating the underlying cause could lead to delayed diagnosis and poor outcomes. In some instances, it is clear that the cause of hypothermia is simply prolonged exposure to cold without proper clothing. However, in patients such as this one, the clinician will need to look for findings that would be unexpected in a patient with hypothermia. This patient has a moderate degree of hypothermia (between 28.0°C and 32.2°C). At this range of hypothermia, the expected clinical presentation would be one of a global slowing of metabolism. Clinically, this would include a depressed level of consciousness with papillary dilatation. Often, these individuals experience a paradoxical instinct to take off their clothes. In addition, the heart rate, blood pressure, and respiratory rate would be expected to decrease. Carbon dioxide production by tissues typically decreases by 50% for each 8°C drop in body temperature. A common error in the treatment of individuals with hypothermia is overly aggressive hyperventilation in the face of this known decrease in carbon dioxide production.

In this patient, despite the hypothermia there is an increased respiratory rate in the setting of a metabolic acidosis. This finding suggests a lesion in the central nervous system or ingestion of an alcohol that would lead to a metabolic acidosis. Ingestion is confirmed by the presence of a very high anion gap (28) as well as an osmolar gap. The osmolar gap can be calculated as (Sodium × 2) + (BUN/2.8) + (Glucose/18) + (Ethanol/4.6). In this patient, the calculated osmolarity would be 301.6. Thus, the osmolar gap is 26, indicating the presence of some other osmotically active compound. In this case, it is prudent to measure toxic alcohol levels such as methanol and ethylene glycol.

In the management of the patient's hypothermia, warmed intravenous fluids may be indicated. However, lactated Ringer's solution should be avoided because the liver may be unable to metabolize lactate and lead to worsening metabolic acidosis. The cardiac complications of hypothermia may lead to bradyarrhythmias, but cardiac pacing is rarely indicated. If required, the transthoracic route is preferred because placement of any leads into the heart may lead to refractory ventricular arrhythmias.

I-76.   **The answer is B.** *(Chap. 19)* This patient presents with frostbite of the left foot. The most common presenting symptom of this disorder is sensory changes that affect pain and temperature. Physical examination can have a multitude of findings, depending on the degree of tissue damage. Mild frostbite will show erythema and anesthesia. With more extensive damage, bullae and vesicles will develop. Hemorrhagic vesicles are caused by injury to the microvasculature. The prognosis is most favorable when the presenting area is warm and has a normal color. Treatment is with rapid rewarming, which usually is accomplished with a 37–40°C (98.6–104°F) water bath. The period of rewarming can be intensely painful for the patient, and often narcotic analgesia is warranted. If the pain is intolerable, the temperature of the water bath can be dropped slightly. Compartment syndrome can develop with rewarming and should be investigated if cyanosis persists after rewarming. No medications have been shown to improve outcomes, including heparin, steroids, calcium channel blockers, and hyperbaric oxygen. In the absence of wet gangrene or another emergent surgical indication, decisions about the need for amputation or debridement should be deferred until the boundaries of the tissue injury are well demarcated. After recovery from the initial insult, these patients often have neuronal injury with abnormal sympathetic tone in the extremity. Other remote complications include cutaneous carcinomas; nail deformities; and, in children, epiphyseal damage.

I-77.   **The answer is D.** *(Chap. 20)* Syncope is a common medical complaint that occurs when there is global cerebral hypoperfusion. Syncope accounts for 3% of all emergency department visits and 1% of all hospitalizations. Additionally, it is estimated that 35% of all individuals will experience at least one syncopal event in their lifetimes. The most common cause of syncope in young adults is neurally mediated syncope. The incidence of neurally mediated syncope is higher in females and has a familial predisposition. Neurally mediated syncope represents a complex reflex arc of the autonomic nervous system and inherently requires an intact autonomic nervous system to occur. The final pathway of neurally mediated syncope is a surge of parasympathetic activity with inhibition of the sympathetic nervous system. This results in hypotension with accompanying bradycardia. Syncope occurs when blood flow to the brain drops abruptly. Triggers of the reflex pathway are varied. Vasovagal syncope is one category without a clearly defined trigger but can occur with intense emotions, strong odors, or orthostatic stress. Individuals who faint at the sight of blood experience vasovagal syncope. Neurally mediated syncope can also be brought about by specific situations such as cough, micturition, swallowing, or carotid sensitivity. The primary symptoms of neurally mediated syncope include premonitory symptoms such as lightheadedness and dizziness as well as parasympathetic symptoms such as diaphoresis, pallor, hyperventilation, pallor, and palpitation. Myoclonic jerks of the extremities can occur and be difficult to distinguish from seizure activity. On rare occasions, an individual may experience urinary incontinence, but fecal incontinence does not occur. Individuals usually recover very quickly from neurally mediated syncope with a rapid return to consciousness and previous level of alertness. Reassurance and avoidance of triggers are the primary treatments. Liberal intake of fluids and salt expand plasma volume and are protective against syncopal events. In randomized controlled trials, isometric counterpressure maneuvers (leg crossing or handgrip) are also protective. In patients with refractory syncope, fludrocortisone, beta-blockers, or vasoconstricting agents have been used with clinical success, although there are no clinical trial data to support their use.

I-78. **The answer is A.** *(Chap. 20)* The cornerstone of the evaluation of syncope is to perform an thorough history and examination. Clues to the cause of syncope include the presence of prodromal symptoms, presence of injury, and eyewitness accounts of the event. Neurally mediated syncope is one of the most common causes of syncope and often has preceding lightheadedness or dizziness. Orthostatic hypotension is also frequently preceded by symptoms of lightheadedness and is more common in older individuals. Likewise, older individuals are at greater risk of cardiac syncope. Cardiac syncope needs to be considered as cardiac syncope caused by structural heart disease or primary arrhythmia is associated with an increased risk of sudden cardiac death. Cardiac syncope is more likely to occur without warning symptoms and is more likely to have associated serious injury. Hypoglycemia can present with syncope as well and needs to be considered in this case. Neurologic causes of syncope include seizures and vertebrobasilar insufficiency. A cerebrovascular accident does not commonly cause syncope because bihemispheric disruption of cerebral blood flow is necessary to cause loss of consciousness.

In this individual, evaluation should include fingerstick glucose measurement, orthostatic blood pressures, and an electrocardiogram. Tilt table testing can be considered, particularly because the patient has had recurrent episodes of syncope in the past. A head CT scan, however, should not be a routine part of the evaluation of syncope unless there is concern about a head injury that occurred as a result of the syncope.

I-79. **The answer is D.** *(Chap. 21)* Dizziness is a common complaint affecting approximately 20% of the population over the course of the year. Most dizziness is benign, self-limited, and must be distinguished from vertigo. Although dizziness is often described as a sensation of lightheadedness, vertigo is more often described as a sensation that the room is spinning. Vertigo is most commonly from peripheral causes affecting labyrinths of the inner ear or the vestibular nerve. However, central lesions of the brainstem and cerebellum can also lead to vertigo. Features of the history and physical examination can be useful in determining central versus peripheral causes of vertigo. By history, deafness or tinnitus is typically absent with central lesions. On physical examination, spontaneous nystagmus is most often a sign of central vertigo, although it can be seen with acute vestibular neuritis. Specific patterns of vertigo that are characteristic of lesions in the cerebellar pathways are vertical nystagmus with a downward fast phase (downbeat nystagmus) and horizontal nystagmus that changes direction with gaze (gaze-evoked nystagmus). Alternatively, in peripheral vertigo, nystagmus typically is provoked by positional maneuvers and can be inhibited by visual fixation. Visual fixation does not, however, inhibit nystagmus in central lesions. Finally, central causes of nystagmus are more likely to be associated with other symptoms that would lead one to suspect a central cause. These include hiccups, diplopia, cranial neuropathies, and dysarthria.

I-80. **The answer is C.** *(Chap. 21)* The symptoms and physical examination of this patient are typical of benign paroxysmal positional vertigo (BPPV). Episodes of BPPV are typically quite brief, lasting no more than 1 minute, and are brought about by changes in position relative to gravity. Typical movements that elicit the vertigo are lying down, rolling over in bed, rising from the supine position, and tilting the head to look upward. The labyrinth of the inner ear is responsible for process information with regards to position and movement. It consists of three semicircular canals: the superior canal, the posterior canal, and the horizontal canal. BPPV results when calcium carbonate crystals called otoconia migrate from the utricle of the inner ear into the semicircular canals. By far, the most commonly affected canal is the posterior one. When this occurs, vertigo is accompanied by nystagmus that beats upward and torsionally toward the affected ear. This can be brought about by the Dix-Hallpike maneuver, which is described in the clinical scenario. Less commonly, the horizontal canal is affected, leading to horizontal nystagmus. The primary treatment of BPPV is repositioning therapy that uses gravity to remove the otoconia from the affected canal. The Epley maneuver is the most common repositioning procedure.

The history and physical examination are not consistent with a central cause of vertigo; therefore, a brain MRI is not indicated. Methylprednisolone is the primary treatment of acute vestibular neuritis if used within the first 3 days of symptoms. Acute vestibular neuritis often presents with more prolonged symptoms that persist even when there is no movement of the head. Most patients recover spontaneously, but when used early, methylprednisolone will decrease the duration of symptoms. There is no indication for the use of antiviral therapy unless there is obvious herpes zoster infection. Likewise, the symptoms are not consistent with migrainous vertigo, which would be persistent for hours and not be affected by positional changes. Thus, the use of rizatriptan would not be helpful.

I-81. **The answer is D.** *(Chap. 22)* Complaints of weakness in a patient have a multitude of causes, and it is important to perform a thorough history and physical examination to help localize the site of weakness. Lower motor neuron diseases occur when there is destruction of the cell bodies of the lower motor neurons in the brainstem or the anterior horn of the spinal cord. Lower motor neuron diseases can also occur because of direct axonal dysfunction and demyelination. The primary presenting symptoms are those of distal muscle weakness such as tripping or decreased hand grip strength. When a motor neuron becomes diseased, it may discharge spontaneously, leading to muscle fasciculations that are not seen in disease of the upper motor neurons or myopathies. Additionally, on physical examination, lower motor neuron disease leads to decreases in muscle tone and decreased or absent deep tendon reflexes. Over time, severe muscle atrophy can occur. A Babinski sign should not be present. If there is evidence of a Babinski sign in the presence of lower motor neuron disease, this should raise the suspicion of a disorder affecting both upper and lower motor neurons such as amyotrophic lateral sclerosis.

I-82. **The answer is E.** *(Chap. 24)* Approximately 15% of individuals older than 65 years have an identifiable gait disorder. By age 80 years, 25% of individuals require a mechanical aid to assist ambulation. Proper maintenance of gait requires a complex interaction between central nervous system centers to integrate postural control and locomotion. The cerebellum, brainstem, and motor cortex simultaneously process information regarding the environment and purpose of the motion to allow for proper gait and avoidance of falls. Any disorder affecting either sensory input regarding the environment or central nervous system output has the potential to affect gait. In most case series, the most common cause of gait disorders is a sensory deficit. The causes of sensory deficits can quite broad and include peripheral sensory neuropathy from a variety of causes, including diabetes mellitus, peripheral vascular disease, and vitamin B_{12} deficiency, among many others. Other common causes of gait disorders include myelopathy and multiple cerebrovascular infarcts. Although Parkinson's disease is almost inevitably marked by gait abnormalities, it occurs less commonly in the general population than the previously discussed disorders. Likewise, cerebellar degeneration is frequently associated with gait disturbance but is a less common disorder in the general population.

I-83. **The answer is B.** *(Chap. 24)* Characteristics found during the neurologic examination can assist with the localization of disease in gait disorders. In this case, the patient presents with signs of a frontal gait disorder or parkinsonism. The specific characteristics that would be seen with a frontal gait disorder are a wide-based stance with slow and short shuffling steps. The patient may have difficulty rising from a chair and has a slow, hesitating start. Likewise, there is great difficult with turning with multiple steps required to complete a turn. The patient has very significant postural instability. However, cerebellar signs are typically absent. Romberg sign may or may not be positive, and seated cerebellar testing results are normal, including heel-to-shin testing and rapid alternating movements. Additionally, there should otherwise be normal muscle bulk and tone without sensory or strength deficits. The most common cause of frontal gait disorders (sometimes known as gait apraxia) is cerebrovascular disease, especially small vessel subcortical disease. Communicating hydrocephalus also presents with a gait disorder of this type. In some individuals, the gait disorder precedes other typical symptoms such as incontinence or mental status change.

Alcoholic cerebellar degeneration and multiple system atrophy present with signs of cerebellar ataxia. Characteristics of cerebellar ataxia include a wide-based gait with variable velocity. Gait initiation is normal, but the patient is hesitant during turns. The stride is lurching and irregular. Falls are a late event. The heel-to-shin test is abnormal, and the Romberg test is variably positive.

Neurosyphilis and lumbar myelopathy are examples of sensory ataxia. Sensory ataxia presents with frequent falls. The gait with sensory ataxia, however, is narrow based. Often the patient is noted to be looking down while walking. The patient tends to walk slowly but have path deviation. Gait is initiated normal, but the patient may have some difficulty with turning. The Romberg test is typically unsteady and may result in falls.

I-84. **The answer is D.** *(Chap. 25)* Delirium is an acute confusional state that most frequently occurs in the context of an acute medical illness. Fluctuating levels of cognitive function with a particular deficit of attention are the primary clinical features of delirium. All levels of cognitive function, however, are invariably involved, including memory, language, and executive functioning. Other common associated symptoms are sleep–wake disturbances, hallucinations or delusions, affect changes, and changes in heart rate or blood pressure. Delirium remains a clinical diagnosis and is believed to affect as much as 50% of hospitalized patients. For elderly patients in intensive care, the incidence rises to between 70 and 87%. However, it has been estimated the diagnosis is missed in one-third of individuals with delirium. Once thought of as an acute but benign condition, increasing research is demonstrating delirium to have persisting effects on cognition and functioning. Delirium typically is short lived, but some episodes of delirium can last for weeks, months, or even years. When delirium persists for longer periods of time, it is thought to represent inadequate treatment of the cause of delirium or permanent neuronal damage from the episode. Delirium also has significant associated morbidity and mortality. A single episode of delirium in hospitalized patients has been associated with an in-hospital mortality rate as high as 25–33%. However, the increased mortality is not simply limited to the hospital stay. Individuals experiencing delirium in the hospital have increased mortality for the next several months to years. In addition, these individuals experience a longer hospital length of stay and are less likely to return to functional independence. Individuals who experience delirium are more likely to be discharged to nursing home care and are at increased risk of rehospitalization.

I-85. **The answer is B.** *(Chap. 25)* This patient has features of acute delirium, which can be precipitated by many causes in hospitalized patients. Broad categories of causes of delirium include toxins, medication reactions, metabolic disorders, infections, endocrine disorders, cerebrovascular disorders (especially hypertensive encephalopathy), autoimmune disorders, seizures, neoplastic disorders, and hospitalization. Although the list of causes is broad, the initial history and physical examination are important to establish potential etiologies of delirium and guide further workup. In most patients with delirium, it is difficult to obtain an accurate history; therefore, it is important to seek out a spouse of family member to outline the history further. In this case, there are features that could suggest alcohol withdrawal (hypertension, tachycardia, fevers, tremors), and one should clarify his alcohol intake with his wife. Another primary consideration in determining the etiology of a delirium episode is the time course over which it evolves and the current medications. Particularly in older hospitalized individuals, common medications used as sleep aids, such as diphenhydramine, can have a paradoxical effect with delirium and agitation. It is estimated that as many as one-third of episodes of delirium in hospitalized patients are the result of medications. Worsening infection also needs to be considered because the change in the patient's vital signs could be indicative of an infectious source, although the elevated blood pressure is not consistent with this. Because the patient has required oxygen during his hospitalization, it is important to check an oxygen saturation or arterial blood gas because acute hypoxemia or hypercarbia can precipitate delirium. Likewise, given the patient's history of diabetes mellitus, a fingerstick glucose is necessary because hypoglycemia could also lead to alterations in mental status with evidence of tachycardia, tremor, and diaphoresis. Other initial tests to consider in an individual with delirium are electrolytes and basic liver and kidney function. Although commonly ordered, brain imaging is most often not helpful in the evaluation of delirium.

I-86. **The answer is C.** *(Chap. 25)* *Confusion* is defined as a mental and behavioral state of reduced comprehension, coherence, and capacity to reason. *Delirium* is used to describe an acute confusional state. Delirium often goes unrecognized despite clear evidence that it is often a cognitive manifestation of many medical and neurologic illnesses. Delirium is a clinical diagnosis that may be hyperactive (e.g., alcohol withdrawal) or hypoactive (e.g., opiate intoxication). There is often dramatic fluctuation between states. Delirium is associated with a substantial mortality rate with in-hospital mortality estimates ranging from 25–33%. Overall estimates of delirium in hospitalized patients range from 15–55% with higher rates in elderly adults. Patients in the intensive care unit have especially high rates of delirium, ranging from 70–87%. The clinic setting represents the lowest risk. Postoperative patients, especially after hip surgery, have an incidence of delirium that is somewhat higher than patients admitted to the medical wards.

I-87.   **The answer is B.** (*Chap. 26*) When evaluating someone who reports difficulty with language, it is important to assess speech in several different domains, which are spontaneous speech, comprehension, repetition, naming, reading, and writing. *Anomia* refers to the inability to name common objects and is the most common finding in patients with aphasia. Indeed, anomia is present in all types of aphasia except pure word deafness or pure alexia. Anomia can present in many fashions, including complete an inability to name, provision of a related word ("pen" for "pencil"), a description of the word ("a thing for writing"), or the wrong word. Fluency is assessed by listening to spontaneous speech. Fluency is decreased in Broca's or global aphasia but is relatively preserved in other forms of aphasia. Comprehension is assessed by asking patients to follow conversation and provide simple answers (yes/no, pointing to appropriate objects). The most common aphasia presenting with deficits of comprehension is Wernicke's aphasia in which fluent but nonsensical spontaneous speech (word salad) is present. Repetition asks patients to repeat a string of words, sentences, or a single word and is impaired in many types of aphasia. In addition, repetition of tongue twisters can be useful in the evaluation of dysarthria or palilalia as well. Alexia refers to the inability to read aloud or comprehend written language.

I-88.   **The answer is C.** (*Chap. 26*) The parietofrontal area of the brain is responsible for spatial orientation. The major components of the network include the cingulate cortex, posterior parietal cortex, and the frontal eye fields. In addition, subcortical areas in the striatum and thalamus are also important. Together, these systems integrate information to maintain spatial cognition, and a lesion in any of these areas can lead to hemispatial neglect. In neglect syndromes, three behavioral manifestations are seen: Sensory events in the neglected hemisphere have less overall impact; there is a paucity of conscious acts directed toward the neglected hemisphere; and the patient behaves as if the neglected hemisphere is devalued. In Figure I-88, almost all of the As (the target) represented on the left half of the figure are missed. This is an example of a target detection task. Hemianopia alone is not sufficient to cause this finding because the individual can turn his or her head left and right to identify the targets.

Bilateral disorders of the parietofrontal area of the brain can lead to severe spatial disorientation known as Balint's syndrome. In Balint's syndrome, there is inability to orderly scan the environment (oculomotor apraxia) and inaccurate manual reaching for objects (optic apraxia). A third finding in Balint's syndrome is simultanagnosia. Simultanagnosia is the inability to integrate information in the center of the gaze with peripheral information. An example is a target detection test in which only the A's present in the outer portion of the figure would be indicated. Individuals with this finding also tend to miss the larger objects in a figure and would not be able to accurately identify the target when it was made much larger than the surrounding letters. Construction apraxia refers to the inability to copy a simple line drawing such as a house or star and occurs most commonly in association with parietal lesions. Object agnosia is the inability to name a generic object or describe its use in contrast to anomia when an individual should be able to describe the use of the object even if it cannot be named. The defect in the object agnosia is usually in the territory of the bilateral posterior cerebral arteries.

I-89.   **The answer is C.** (*Chap. 27*) Shift work sleep disorder is a disorder of the circadian rhythm that is common in any individual who has to commonly work at night. At present, an estimated 7 million individuals in the United States work permanently at night or on rotating shifts. Increasing research devoted to sleep disorders in night shift workers has demonstrated that the circadian rhythm never fully shifts to allow one to perform at full alertness at night. The reason for this is likely multifactorial and includes the fact that most individuals who work at night try to abruptly shift their sleep schedules to a more normal pattern on days when they are not working. Consequently, night shift workers often have chronic sleep deprivation, increased length of time awake before starting work, and misalignment of their circadian phase with the intrinsic circadian phase. The results of this lead to decreased alertness and increased errors during night shifts. In an estimated 5–10% of individuals working night shifts, the excessive sleepiness during the night and insomnia during the day are deemed to be clinically significant. Strategies for treating shift work sleep disorder use a combination of behavioral and pharmacologic strategies. Caffeine does promote wakefulness, but the effects are not long lasting, and tolerance develops over time. Brief periods of exercise frequently boost alertness and can be used before starting a night shift or during the shift at times of increased sleepiness. Many sleep experts support strategic napping during shifts for no more than 20 minutes at times of circadian nadirs. Naps longer than 20 minutes can lead to sleep inertia during which an individual may feel very disoriented and groggy and experience a decline in motor skills upon abrupt awakening from sleep. Bright lights before and during night shift work may improve alertness, but one must be careful to avoid bright lights in the morning after a night shift because light entrainment is a powerful stimulus of the internal circadian clock. If an individual is exposed to bright light in the morning, it will interfere with the ability to fall asleep during the day. Night shift workers should be encouraged to wear dark sunglasses in the morning on the way home. Sleep during the day is frequently disrupted in night shift workers. Creating a quiet, dark, and comfortable environment is important, and sleep should be a priority for the individual during the day. The only pharmacologic therapy approved by the Food and Drug Administration for treatment of shift work sleep disorder is modafinil 200 mg taken 20–30 minutes before the start of a night shift. Modafinil has been demonstrated to increase sleep latency and decrease attentional failures during night shifts but does not alleviate the feelings of excessive sleepiness. Melatonin is not one of the recommended therapies for shift work sleep disorder. If used, it should be taken 2–3 hours before bedtime rather than right before bedtime to simulate the normal peaks and troughs of melatonin secretion.

I-90. **The answer is C.** *(Chap. 27)* This patient complains of symptoms that are consistent with restless legs syndrome (RLS). This disorder affects 1–5% of young to middle-aged individuals and many as 20% of older individuals. The symptom of RLS is a nonspecific uncomfortable sensation in the legs that begins during periods of quiescence and is associated with the irresistible urge to move. Patients frequently find it difficult to describe their symptoms but usually describe the sensation as deep within the affected limb. Rarely is the sensation described as distinctly painful unless an underlying neuropathy is also present. The severity of the disorder tends to wax and wane over time and tends to worsen with sleep deprivation, caffeine intake, pregnancy, and alcohol. Renal disease, neuropathy, and iron deficiency are known secondary causes of RLS symptoms. In this patient, correcting the iron deficiency is the best choice for initial therapy because this may entirely relieve the symptoms of RLS. For individuals with primary RLS (not related to another medical condition), the dopaminergic agents are the treatment of choice. Pramipexole or ropinirole is recommended as first-line treatment. Although carbidopa/levodopa is highly effective, individuals have a high risk of developing augmented symptoms over time with increasingly higher doses needed to control the symptoms. Other options for treating RLS include narcotics, benzodiazepines, and gabapentin. Hormone replacement therapy has no role in the treatment of RLS.

I-91. **The answer is A.** *(Chap. 27)* Narcolepsy is a sleep disorder characterized by excessive sleepiness with intrusion of rapid eye movement (REM) sleep into wakefulness. Narcolepsy affects about one in 4000 individuals in the United States with a genetic predisposition. Recent research has demonstrated that narcolepsy with cataplexy is associated with low or undetectable levels of the neurotransmitter hypocretin (orexin) in the CSF. This neurotransmitter is released from a small number of neurons in the hypothalamus. Given the association of narcolepsy with the major histocompatibility antigen human leukocyte antigen DQB1*0602, it is thought that narcolepsy is an autoimmune process that leads to destruction of the hypocretin-secreting neurons in the hypothalamus. The classic symptom tetrad of narcolepsy is (1) cataplexy, (2) hypnagogic or hypnopompic hallucinations, (3) sleep paralysis, and (4) excessive daytime somnolence. Of these symptoms, cataplexy is the most specific for the diagnosis of narcolepsy. Cataplexy refers to the sudden loss of muscle tone in response to strong emotions. It most commonly occurs with laughter or surprise but may be associated with anger as well. Cataplexy can have a wide range of symptoms from mild sagging of the jaw lasting for a few seconds to a complete loss of muscle tone lasting several minutes. During this time, individuals are aware of their surroundings and are not unconscious. This symptom is present in 76% of individuals diagnosed with narcolepsy and is the most specific finding for the diagnosis. Hypnagogic and hypnopompic hallucinations and sleep paralysis can occur from any cause of chronic sleep deprivation, including sleep apnea and chronic insufficient sleep. Excessive daytime somnolence is present in 100% of individuals with narcolepsy but is not specific for the diagnosis because this symptom may be present with any sleep disorder as well as with chronic insufficient sleep. The presence of two or more REM periods occurring during a daytime multiple sleep latency test is suggestive but not diagnostic of narcolepsy. Other disorders that may lead to presence of REM during short daytime nap periods include sleep apnea, sleep phase delay syndrome, and insufficient sleep.

I-92.   **The answer is B.** (*Chap. 27; http://www.sleepfoundation.org/site/c.huIXKjM0IxF/ b.2417355/k.143E/2002_Sleep_in_America_Poll.htm, accessed May 12, 2011*) Insomnia is the most common sleep disorder in the population. In the 2002 Sleep in America Poll, 58% of respondents reported at least one symptom of insomnia on a weekly basis, and one-third of individuals experience these symptoms on a nightly basis. Insomnia is defined clinically as the inability to fall asleep or stay asleep, which leads to daytime sleepiness or poor daytime function. These symptoms occur despite adequate time and opportunity for sleep. Insomnia can be further characterized as primary or secondary. Primary insomnia occurs in individuals with an identifiable cause of insomnia and is often a long-standing diagnosis for many years. Within the category of primary insomnia is adjustment insomnia, which is typically of short duration with a well-defined stressor. Secondary causes of insomnia include comorbid medical or psychiatric conditions and can be related to caffeine or illegal and prescribed drugs. Obstructive sleep apnea is thought to affect as many as 10–15% of the population and is currently underdiagnosed in the United States. In addition, because of the rising incidence of obesity, obstructive sleep apnea is also expected to increase in incidence over the coming years. Obstructive sleep apnea occurs when there is ongoing effort to inspire against an occluded oropharynx during sleep. It is directly related to obesity and has an increased incidence in men and in older populations. Narcolepsy affects 1 in 4000 people and is caused by deficit of hypocretin (orexin) in the brain. Symptoms of narcolepsy include a sudden loss of tone in response to emotional stimuli (cataplexy), hypersomnia, sleep paralysis, and hallucinations with sleep onset and waking. Physiologically, there is intrusion or persistence of rapid eye movement sleep during wakefulness that accounts for the classic symptoms of narcolepsy. Restless legs syndrome is estimated to affect 1–5% of young to middle-aged adults and as many as 10–20% of elderly adults. Restless legs syndrome is marked by uncomfortable sensations in the legs that are difficult to describe. The symptoms have an onset with quiescence, especially at night, and are relieved with movement. Delayed sleep phase syndrome is a circadian rhythm disorder that commonly presents with a complaint of insomnia and accounts for as much as 10% of individuals referred to the sleep clinic for evaluation of insomnia. In delayed sleep phase syndrome, the intrinsic circadian rhythm is delayed such that sleep onset occurs much later than normal. When allowed to sleep according to the intrinsic circadian rhythm, individuals with delayed sleep phase syndrome sleep normally and do not experience excessive somnolence. This disorder is most common in adolescence and young adulthood.

I-93.   **The answer is C.** (*Chap. 27*) Parasomnias are abnormal behaviors or experiences that arise from slow-wave sleep. Also known as confusional arousals, the electroencephalogram during a parasomnia event frequently shows persistence of slow-wave (delta) sleep into arousal. Non–rapid eye movement (NREM) parasomnias may also include more complex behavior, including eating and sexual activity. Treatment of NREM parasomnias is usually not indicated, and a safe environment should be assured for the patient. When injury is likely to occur, treatment with a drug that decreases slow-wave sleep will treat the parasomnia. Typical treatment is a benzodiazepine. There are no typical parasomnias that arise from stage I or stage II sleep. REM parasomnias include nightmare disorder and REM-behavior disorder. REM-behavior disorder is increasingly recognized as associated with Parkinson's disease and other parkinsonian syndromes. This disorder is characterized by the absence of decreased muscle tone in REM sleep, which leads to the acting out of dreams, sometimes resulting in violence and injury.

I-94.   **The answer is E.** *(Chap. 28)* (See Figure I-94.) Bitemporal hemianopia is caused by a lesion at the optic chiasm because fibers there decussate into the contralateral optic tract. Crossed fibers are more damaged by compression than uncrossed fibers. This finding is usually caused by symmetric compression in the sellar region by a pituitary adenoma, meningioma, craniopharyngioma, glioma, or aneurysm. These lesions are often insidious and may be unnoticed by the patient. They will escape detection by the physician unless each eye is tested separately. Lesions anterior to the chiasm (retinal injury, optic nerve injury) will cause unilateral impairment and an abnormal pupillary response. Postchiasmic lesions (temporal, parietal, occipital cortex) cause homonymous lesions (similar field abnormalities in both eyes) that vary with location. Occlusion of the posterior cerebral artery supplying the occipital lobe is a common cause of total homonymous hemianopia.

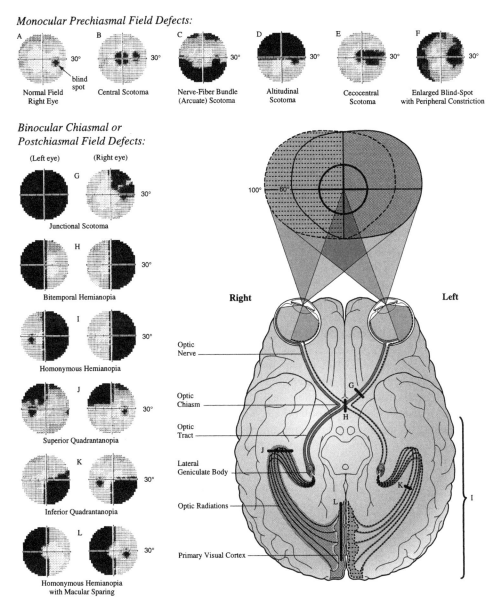

Monocular Prechiasmal Field Defects:

Binocular Chiasmal or Postchiasmal Field Defects:

FIGURE I-94

I-95.   **The answer is E.** *(Chap. 28)* The differential diagnosis of a red, painful eye is broad and includes corneal abrasion, subconjunctival hemorrhage, infective or allergic conjunctivitis (the most common cause of red, painful eye), keratoconjunctivitis sicca (medications, Sjogren's syndrome, sarcoidosis), keratitis (contact lens injury, trachoma, vitamin A deficiency), herpes infection, episcleritis (autoimmune, idiopathic), scleritis (autoimmune), uveitis, endophthalmitis, or acute angle-closure glaucoma. Uveitis requires slit-lamp examination for diagnosis. Anterior uveitis involving the iris is usually idiopathic but may be associated with sarcoidosis, ankylosing spondylitis, juvenile rheumatoid arthritis, inflammatory bowel disease, psoriasis, inflammatory arthritis, Behçet's disease, and a variety of infections. Posterior uveitis in the vitreous, retina, or choroid is more likely to be associated with a systemic disease or infection than anterior uveitis. Acute angle-closure glaucoma, although rare, is often misdiagnosed unless intraocular pressure is measured. Many physicians avoid dilating patients' pupils for fear of provoking acute angle-closure glaucoma. The risk is remote and rarely causes permanent vision loss. The value of a complete funduscopic examination outweighs the risk of this rare event. Transient ischemic attack (TIA) caused by temporary interruption of blood flow to the retina for more than a few seconds causes transient visual abnormality (amaurosis fugax). TIA is usually associated with atherosclerosis. If flow is restored quickly vision returns to normal.

I-96. **The answer is A.** *(Chap. 28)* Age-related macular degeneration is a major cause of painless, gradual bilateral central visual loss. It occurs as nonexudative (dry) or exudative (wet) forms. Recent genetic data have shown an association with the alternative complement pathway gene for complement factor H. The mechanism link for that association is unknown. The nonexudative form is associated with retinal drusen that leads to retinal atrophy. Treatment with vitamin C, vitamin E, beta-carotene, and zinc may retard the visual loss. Exudative macular degeneration, which is less common, is caused by neovascular proliferation and leakage of choroidal blood vessels. Acute visual loss may occur because of bleeding. Exudative macular degeneration may be treated with intraocular injection of a vascular endothelial growth factor antagonist (bevacizumab or ranibizumab). Blepharitis is inflammation of the eyelids usually related to acne rosacea, seborrheic dermatitis, or staphylococcal infection. Diabetic retinopathy, now a leading cause of blindness in the United States, causes gradual bilateral visual loss in patients with long-standing diabetes. Retinal detachment is usually unilateral and causes visual loss and an afferent pupillary defect.

I-97. **The answer is B.** *(Chap. 29)* A history of severe respiratory infection, including the common cold, influenza, pneumonia, or HIV, is the most common cause of long-lasting loss of smell. The mechanism, along with cases of chronic rhinosinusitis (another common cause) is likely related to permanent damage to the olfactory epithelium. Head trauma, causing shearing and scarring of olfactory fila at the cribiform plate, may cause anosmia. Fewer than 10% of patients with posttraumatic anosmia regain normal function. The severity of disease is associated with the likelihood of olfactory abnormality in trauma and chronic rhinosinusitis. Significant decrements in smell are present in more than 50% of people older than 65 years old. This finding may explain the common finding of loss of food flavor and nutritional deficiencies in elderly adults. Confirming popular wisdom studies have shown that at any age, women have a better ability to identify odorants than men (Figure I-97).

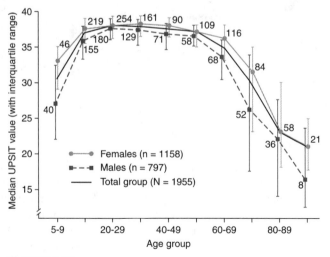

FIGURE I-97

I-98. **The answer is E.** *(Chap. 30)* Hearing loss is a common complaint, particularly in older individuals. In this age group, 33% have hearing loss to a degree that requires hearing aids. When evaluating hearing loss, the physician should attempt to determine whether the cause is conductive, sensorineural, or mixed. Sensorineural hearing loss results from injury of the cochlear apparatus or disruption of the neural pathways from the inner ear to the brain. The primary site of damage is the hair cells of the inner ear. Common causes of hair cell injury include prolonged exposure to loud noises, viral infections, ototoxic drugs, cochlear otosclerosis, Meniere's disease, and aging. In contrast, conductive hearing loss results from impairment of the external ear and auditory canal to transmit and amplify sound through the middle ear to the cochlea. Causes of conductive hearing loss include cerumen impaction, perforations of the tympanic membrane, otosclerosis, cholesteatomas, large middle ear effusions, and tumors of the external auditory canal or middle ear among others. The initial physical examination can often differentiate between conductive or sensorineural hearing loss. Examination of the external auditory canal can identify cerumen or foreign body impaction. On otoscopic examination, it is more important to assess the topography of the tympanic membrane than to look for the presence of a light reflex. Of particular attention is the area in the upper third of the tympanic membrane known as the pars flaccida. This area can develop chronic retraction pockets that are indicative of Eustachian tube dysfunction or a cholesteatoma, a benign tumor composed of keratinized squamous epithelium. Bedside tests with a tuning fork also are useful for differentiating conductive from sensorineural hearing loss. In the Rinne's test, air conduction is compared with bony conduction of sound. A tuning fork is placed over the mastoid process and then in front of the external ear. In conductive hearing loss, the intensity of sound is louder when placed on the bone, but in sensorineural hearing loss, the intensity is greatest at the external ear. In the Weber test, the tuning fork is placed in the midline of the head. In unilateral conductive hearing loss, the intensity of sound is loudest in the affected ear, but in unilateral sensorineural hearing loss, the intensity of sound is loudest in the unaffected ear. This patient reports left greater than right hearing loss that is suspected to be sensorineural in nature. Thus, the sound is expected to be greatest in the right ear on the Weber test. A more formal evaluation of hearing loss would include pure tone audiometry that plots hearing threshold versus frequency. Pure tone audiometry establishes the severity, type, and laterality of hearing loss. In this patient, high-frequency hearing loss would be expected based on his complaints of inability to hear the alarm tone of his digital watch.

I-99. **The answer is E.** *(Chap. 31)* Acute sinusitis is a common complication of upper respiratory tract infections and is defined as sinusitis lasting less than 4 weeks' duration. Acute sinusitis typically presents with nasal drainage and congestion, facial pain or pressure, and headache that is worse with lying down or bending forward. The presence of purulent drainage does not differentiate bacterial from viral causes of sinusitis. The vast majority of cases of acute sinusitis are caused by viral infection. However, when patients with acute sinusitis present to a medical professional, antibiotics are prescribed more than 85% of the time. Indeed, this should not be the preferred treatment because most cases improve without antibiotic therapy. Rather, the initial approach to a patient with acute sinusitis should be symptomatic treatment with nasal decongestants and nasal saline lavage. If a patient has a history of allergic rhinitis or chronic sinusitis, nasal glucocorticoids can be prescribed as well. Antibiotic therapy is recommended in adults for symptom duration longer than 7–10 days and in children longer than 10–14 days. In addition, any patient with concerning features such as unilateral or focal facial pain or swelling should be treated with antibiotics. The initial antibiotic of choice for acute sinusitis is amoxicillin 500 mg orally three times daily or 875 mg twice daily. If a patient has had exposure to antibiotics within the past 30 days or treatment failure, a respiratory fluoroquinolone can be give. Ten percent of individuals do not respond to initial antibiotic therapy. In these cases, one can consider referral to otolaryngology for sinus aspiration and culture. Radiologic imaging of the sinuses is not recommended for evaluation of acute disease unless the sinusitis is nosocomially acquired because the procedures (CT or radiography) do not differentiate between bacterial or viral causes.

I-100. **The answer is B.** *(Chap. 31)* Approximately 5–15% of all cases of acute pharyngitis in adults are caused by *Streptococcus pyogenes*. Appropriate identification and treatment of

S. pyogenes infection is needed because antibiotic therapy is recommended to decrease the small risk of acute rheumatic fever. In addition, treatment with antibiotics within 48 hours of onset of symptoms decreases symptom duration and, importantly, decreases transmission of streptococcal pharyngitis. In adults, the recommended diagnostic procedure by the Centers for Disease Control and Prevention and the Infectious Disease Society of America is a rapid antigen detection test for group A streptococci only. In children, however, the recommendation is to perform a throat culture for confirmation if the rapid screen result is negative to limit spread of disease and minimize potential complications. Throat culture generally is regarded as the most appropriate diagnostic method but cannot discriminate between colonization and infection. In addition, it takes 24–48 hours to get a result. Because most cases of pharyngitis at all ages are viral in origin, empiric antibiotic therapy is not recommended.

I-101.   **The answer is D.** *(Chap. 33)* Shortness of breath, or dyspnea, is a common presenting complaint in primary care. However, dyspnea is a complex symptom and is defined as the subjective experience of breathing discomfort that includes components of physical as well as psychosocial factors. A significant body of research has been developed regarding the language by which a patient describes dyspnea with certain factors being more common in specific diseases. Individuals with airways diseases (asthma, chronic obstructive pulmonary disease [COPD]) often describe air hunger, increased work of breathing, and the sensation of being unable to get a deep breath because of hyperinflation. In addition, individuals with asthma often complain of a tightness in the chest. Individuals with cardiac causes of dyspnea also describe chest tightness and air hunger but do not have the same sensation of being unable to draw a deep breath or have increased work of breathing. A careful history will also lead to further clues regarding the cause of dyspnea. Nocturnal dyspnea is seen in congestive heart failure or asthma, and orthopnea is reported in heart failure, diaphragmatic weakness, and asthma that is triggered by esophageal reflux. When discussing exertional dyspnea, it is important to assess if the dyspnea is chronic and progressive or episodic. Whereas episodic dyspnea is more common in myocardial ischemia and asthma, COPD and interstitial lung diseases present with a persistent dyspnea. Platypnea is a rare presentation of dyspnea in which a patient is dyspneic in the upright position and feels improved with lying flat. On physical examination of a patient with dyspnea, the physician should observe the patient's ability to speak and the use of accessory muscle or preference of the tripod position. As part of vital signs, a pulsus paradoxus may be measured with a value of greater than 10 mmHg common in asthma and COPD. Pulsus paradoxus greater than 10 mmHg may also occur in pericardial tamponade. Lung examination may demonstrate decreased diaphragmatic excursion, crackles, or wheezes that allow one to determine the cause of dyspnea. Further workup may include pulmonary function testing, chest radiography, chest CT, electrocardiography, echocardiography, or exercise testing, among others, to ascertain the cause of dyspnea.

I-102.   **The answer is B.** *(Chap. 34)* Chronic cough should not be diagnosed until consistently present for over 2 months. The duration of cough is a clue to its etiology. Acute cough (<3 weeks) is most commonly due to a respiratory tract infection, aspiration event, or inhalation of noxious chemicals or smoke. Subacute cough (3–8 weeks duration) is frequently the residuum from a tracheobronchitis, such as in pertussis or "post-viral tussive syndrome." Chronic cough (>8 weeks) may be caused by a wide variety of cardiopulmonary diseases, including those of inflammatory, infectious, neoplastic, and cardiovascular etiologies. In virtually all instances, evaluation of chronic cough merits a chest radiograph. The list of diseases that can cause persistent coughing without other symptoms and without detectable abnormality on physical examination is long. It includes serious illnesses such as Hodgkin's disease in young adults and lung cancer in an older population. An abnormal chest film leads to evaluation of the radiographic abnormality to explain the symptom of cough. A normal chest image provides valuable reassurance to the patient and the patient's family, who may have imagined the direst explanation for the cough. Chest PET-CT is often helpful in evaluation of solitary pulmonary nodules or suspected malignancy. Sinus CT should not be utilized in the initial evaluation of chronic cough without strong historical or physical examination of sinus disease or infection. While ACE-inhibitor medications are a common cause of chronic cough, measurement of ACE levels is not helpful clinically. Measurement of serum IgE may be a component of the comprehensive evaluation of patients with refractory asthma or suspected allergic bronchopulmonary aspergillosis. It is not helpful in the initial evaluation of cough in a patient without allergic history.

I-103.   **The answer is D.** *(Chap. 34)* It is commonly held that medications (most notably ACE-inhibitors); post-nasal drainage; gastroesophageal reflux; and asthma, alone or in combination, account for more than 90% of patients who have chronic cough and a normal or noncontributory chest radiograph. However, clinical experience does not support this contention, and strict adherence to this concept discourages the search for alternative explanations by both clinicians and researchers. Serious pulmonary diseases, including inflammatory lung diseases, chronic infections, and neoplasms, may remain occult on plain chest imaging and require additional testing for detection. Any patient with chronic unexplained cough who is taking an ACE inhibitor should be given a trial period off the medication, regardless of the timing of the onset of cough relative to the initiation of ACE inhibitor therapy. In most instances, a safe alternative is available; angiotensin-receptor blockers do not cause cough. Post-nasal drainage of any etiology can cause cough as a response to stimulation of sensory receptors of the cough-reflex pathway in the hypopharynx or aspiration of draining secretions into the trachea. Many patients with symptomatic post-nasal drip do not develop chronic cough. Linking gastroesophageal reflux to chronic cough poses similar challenges. It is thought that reflux of gastric contents into the lower esophagus may trigger cough via reflex pathways initiated in the esophageal mucosa. Reflux to the level of the pharynx with consequent aspiration of gastric contents causes a chemical bronchitis and possible pneumonitis that can elicit cough for days after the aspiration event. Reflux may also elicit no or minimal symptoms. Assigning the cause of cough to gastroesophageal reflux must be weighed against the observation that many people with chronic reflux (such as frequently occurs during pregnancy) do not experience chronic cough. Cough due to asthma in the absence of wheezing, shortness of breath, and chest tightness is referred to as "cough-variant asthma", and is more common in children than adults. Chronic eosinophilic bronchitis causes chronic cough with a normal chest radiograph. This condition is characterized by sputum eosinophilia in excess of 3% without airflow obstruction or bronchial hyperresponsiveness and is successfully treated with inhaled glucocorticoids. Treatment of chronic cough in a patient with a normal chest radiograph is often empiric and is targeted at the most likely cause or causes of cough as determined by history, physical examination, and possibly pulmonary-function testing. Therapy for post-nasal drainage depends on the presumed etiology (infection, allergy, or vasomotor rhinitis) and may include systemic antihistamines; antibiotics; nasal saline irrigation; and nasal pump sprays with corticosteroids, antihistamines, or anticholinergics. Antacids, histamine type-2 (H2) receptor antagonists, and proton-pump inhibitors are used to neutralize or decrease production of gastric acid in gastroesophageal reflux disease; dietary changes, elevation of the head and torso during sleep, and medications to improve gastric emptying are additional therapies. Cough-variant asthma typically responds well to inhaled glucocorticoids and intermittent use of inhaled beta-agonist bronchodilators. In this patient, the symptoms of heartburn and the timing of the cough with meals merits an empiric therapeutic trial directed toward reducing acid reflux. Empiric therapy for *H. pylori* eradication is not indicated at this time.

I-104.   **The answer is D.** *(Chap. 35)* When a patient presents for evaluation of hypoxia, it is important to consider the underlying mechanism of hypoxia in order to determine the etiology. The primary causes of hypoxia are related to respiratory disease and include ventilation/perfusion (V/Q) mismatch, hypoventilation, and intrapulmonary right-to-left shunting. Causes of hypoxia outside of the respiratory system include intracardiac right-to-left shunting, high-altitude hypoxia, anemic hypoxia, circulatory hypoxia, and carbon monoxide poisoning. In this patient, the mechanism of hypoxia can be narrowed to two possibilities—intracardiac versus intrapulmonary right-to-left shunting—quite easily because the patient failed to correct his hypoxia in response to 100% oxygen. The history of platypnea and orthodeoxia is suggestive that the likely cause is intrapulmonary rather than intracardiac shunting. The finding of a possible lung nodule on chest radiographs in the lower lung fields also is supportive of a pulmonary cause of shunting through an arteriovenous malformation, which can appear as a lung nodule on chest x-ray. An intracardiac right-to-left shunt is caused by congenital cardiac malformations and Eisenmenger syndrome. If there was an intracardiac cause of shunt, the cardiac examination would be expected to demonstrate a murmur and/or evidence of pulmonary hypertension.

V/Q mismatch is the most common cause of hypoxia and results from perfusion of areas of the lung that receive limited ventilation. Examples of V/Q mismatch include asthma, chronic obstructive pulmonary disease, and pulmonary embolus. Hypoxia caused by V/Q mismatch can be corrected with supplemental oxygen. Hypoventilation can be caused by multiple causes, including acute respiratory depression or chronic respiratory failure with elevations in $PaCO_2$. Hypoxia caused by hypoventilation is also correctable with oxygen but frequently has a normal alveolar–arterial oxygen gradient.

Causes of hypoxia outside the respiratory system are less common. High-altitude hypoxia becomes apparent when individuals travel to elevations greater than 3000 m. Anemic hypoxia is not associated with a decrease in PaO_2, but a decrease in hemoglobin does cause decreased oxygen-carrying capacity in the blood and relative tissue hypoxia if severe. Circulatory hypoxia refers to tissue hypoxia that occurs because of a decrease cardiac output that leads to greater tissue extraction of oxygen. As a result, the venous partial pressure of oxygen is reduced, and there is an increased arterial-mixed venous oxygen gradient.

I-105.   **The answer is C.** *(Chap. 35)* In the evaluation of cyanosis, the first step is to differentiate central from peripheral cyanosis. In central cyanosis, because the etiology is either reduced oxygen saturation or abnormal hemoglobin, the physical findings include bluish discoloration of both mucous membranes and skin. In contrast, peripheral cyanosis is associated with normal oxygen saturation but slowing of blood flow and an increased fraction of oxygen extraction from blood; subsequently, the physical findings are present only in the skin and extremities. Mucous membranes are spared. Peripheral cyanosis is commonly caused by cold exposure with vasoconstriction in the digits. Similar physiology is found in Raynaud's phenomenon. Peripheral vascular disease and deep venous thrombosis result in slowed blood flow and increased oxygen extraction with subsequent cyanosis. Methemoglobinemia causes abnormal hemoglobin that circulates systemically. Consequently, the cyanosis associated with this disorder is systemic. Other common causes of central cyanosis include severe lung disease with hypoxemia, right-to-left intracardiac shunting, and pulmonary arteriovenous malformations.

I-106.   **The answer is C.** *(Chap. e13)* Mitral valve prolapse is characterized by a midsystolic nonejection sound (click) followed by a late systolic murmur that crescendos and terminates with S2. A decrease in venous return induced by standing will move the click closer to S1 and increase the duration of the murmur. Squatting will increase venous return and shorten the duration of the murmur. The murmur of hypertrophic cardiomyopathy behaves in a similar fashion, but there would be no nonejection click, and left ventricular hypertrophy would be expected on electrocardiography (ECG). Aortic stenosis is best heard at the right second intercostal space radiating to the carotid and is crescendo–decrescendo in character. Congenital pulmonic stenosis is crescendo–decrescendo in character and is heard best in the second to third left intercostal space. If severe, there is a parasternal lift right ventricular overload on ECG. Tricuspid regurgitation causes a holosystolic, not midsystolic, murmur that increases with inspiration.

I-107.   **The answer is C.** *(Chap. e13)* Tricuspid regurgitation and mitral regurgitation (along with ventricular septal defect) cause holosystolic murmurs. These murmurs have their onset with S1 and terminate at or with S2. Whereas tricuspid regurgitation is heard best over the left sternal border, mitral regurgitation is heard best at the apex with radiation to the base or axilla. The onset of a murmur after S1 with a nonejection sound (click) is characteristic of mitral valve prolapse. Amyl nitrate decreases the intensity of mitral regurgitation and ventricular septal defect murmurs. Tricuspid regurgitation increases with inspiration. Wide splitting of S2 is characteristic of ventricular septal defects. Inaudible A2 at the ventricular apex is characteristic of mitral regurgitation. Because of the incompetent tricuspid valve, the murmur of tricuspid regurgitation is associated with prominent c-v waves and a sharp y-descent in the jugular venous pulse.

I-108.   **The answer is A.** *(Chap. e13)* Evaluating the splitting of the aortic (A2) and pulmonic (P2) components of the second heart sound (S2) during auscultation can be diagnostically useful. In normal conditions, P2 follows A2, and the splitting increases during inspiration. Reversed (or paradoxical) splitting of S2, when P2 precedes A2 during expiration (and they come closer together during inspiration), is attributable to a delay in A2 and is characteristic of severe aortic stenosis, hypertrophic obstructive cardiomyopathy, left bundle branch block, right ventricular pacing, or acute myocardial ischemia. Wide splitting of S2 is an accentuation of the physiologic pattern usually caused by delayed pulmonic valve closing (right bundle branch block, pulmonary stenosis, pulmonary hypertension) or early aortic valve closure (severe mitral regurgitation). Fixed splitting (no respiratory variation) with the murmur described is characteristic of an atrial septal defect. This is an important finding because it may be asymptomatic until the third or fourth decade of life and, if undiagnosed, may lead to severe pulmonary hypertension and Eisenmenger syndrome.

I-109.   **The answer is B.** *(Chap. 53)* This patient presents with complaints of diffuse hair loss that has been associated with increased stress as well as hormonal changes after pregnancy and delivery. On physical examination, there is diffuse shedding of normal hairs without scalp lesions or scarring consistent with a diagnosis of telogen effluvium. Telogen effluvium occurs when a stressor causes the typical asynchronous hair growth pattern to become synchronous. This can occur from physical or mental stress (high fever, severe infection) or hormonal changes. When the hair growth becomes more synchronous, more hairs enter the telogen (dying) phase at the same time. The patient may present with complaints of significant hair loss, but hair density to the examiner may appear normal. Broken hairs are not observed, and gentle pulling of the hair results in more than four hairs falling out. Telogen effluvium is reversible without treatment, and this patient has identifiable stressors that are related to the cause. Reassurance and observation are all that are recommended. Some medications can cause telogen effluvium. If identified, these should be discontinued. In addition, both hyper- and hypothyroidism can lead to the condition. One should consider evaluation for these and other metabolic disorders if the condition does not reverse or the patient has additional symptoms.

Other causes of nonscarring alopecia include androgenic alopecia, alopecia areata, tinea capitis, and traumatic alopecia. Androgenic alopecia is the cause of male and female pattern baldness. It does not typically result from androgen excess. Rather, it is associated with an increased sensitivity of the affected hairs to the effects of androgens. Androgenic alopecia can be treated with minoxidil, finasteride, or hair transplants. Alopecia areata is a condition of focal hair loss measuring about 2–5 cm in diameter. The surrounding tissue demonstrates increased T lymphocytes, and the treatment includes intralesional glucocorticoids or topical anthralin or tazarotene. Tinea capitis is also usually a focal area of hair loss related to an underlying superficial fungal infection. However, in severe cases, large plaques and pustules can develop. Treatment with oral griseofulvin or terbinafine with topical selenium sulfide or ketoconazole is usually effective in treating the disease. Traumatic alopecia presents with multiple broken hairs at sites of increased stress related to the use of hair care products, including rubber bands, curlers, or chemicals. It can also result from trichotillomania. Discontinuation of any offending practice or agent is all that is required to return the hair to normal. Counseling is typically required for those with trichotillomania.

I-110.   **The answer is D.** *(Chap. 55)* Immediate drug reactions rely on the release of mediators from mast cells or basophils, which can occur directly or through immunoglobulin E (IgE)–dependent activation of these cells. Anaphylactoid reactions that are the result of the direct mast cell degranulation do not require prior exposure to the drug or agent to cause the reaction as in this case. The major causes of anaphylactoid reactions are non-steroidal anti-inflammatory drugs and radiocontrast media. IgE-dependent drug reactions require prior exposure to the drugs to generate the appropriate antibodies, which are expressed on the surfaces of the sensitized cells. Upon reexposure to the drug, drug protein conjugates cross-link these IgE molecules to cause activation of the cells and release of inflammatory mediators. The major drugs classes that cause IgE-dependent reactions are penicillins and muscle relaxants. The symptoms of immediate drug reactions are similar regardless of whether they are caused by direct mast cell activation or IgE mechanisms and begin within minutes of drug exposure. The symptoms include pruritus, urticaria, nausea, vomiting, diarrhea, abdominal cramping, bronchospasm, laryngeal edema, and cardiovascular collapse.

Other causes of drug reactions include deposition of immune complexes and delayed hypersensitivity T-cell reactions. Both of these types of drug reactions cause delayed reactions. The clinical scenario associated with immune complex deposition is serum sickness, which typically occurs 6 days or more after exposure to the drug. However, if the patient has had a prior exposure to the drug, the symptoms could occur at an earlier time frame. Symptoms of serum sickness include fever arthritis, nephritis, neuritis, edema, and an urticarial rash. Delayed hypersensitivity reactions are the most common causes of allergic drug eruptions and include the mild morbilliform eruptions as well as toxic epidermal necrolysis and Stevens-Johnson syndrome. Drug-cell specific T cells have been demonstrated in these reactions directed against the native drug rather than its metabolites. Hepatic metabolism into toxic intermediate compounds may occur with some drug toxicity; the prototype for this phenomenon is acetaminophen toxicity and hepatic failure.

I-111.   **The answer is A.** (*Chap. 55*) Hypersensitivity syndromes can occur with many drugs, including phenytoin, carbamazepine, barbiturates, lamotrigine, minocycline, dapsone, allopurinol, and sulfonamides. This syndrome is also known as DRESS (drug reaction with eosinophilia and systemic symptoms) and presents with a diffuse purpuric and lichenoid rash associated with fever, facial and periorbital edema, generalized lymphadenopathy, leukocytosis, hepatitis, and occasionally nephritis or pneumonitis. Eosinophilia and atypical lymphocytosis can be seen. The reaction typically begins within 2–8 weeks after starting the drug but may persist for several weeks after cessation of the drug, especially if there is associated hepatitis. Mortality rates can be as high as 10% with DRESS, and it is important to recognize this as a drug reaction as immediate cessation of the offending agent is required. Mortality is highest in those with acute hepatitis. In addition to stopping the drug, treatment with systemic corticosteroids at prednisone doses of 1.5–2 mg/kg daily is recommended with a slow taper over 8–12 weeks. Topical steroids may also be helpful. Patients should be closely followed for resolution of symptoms, and the patient should be observed carefully for the late development of autoimmune thyroiditis, which can occur as long as 6 months after the initial presentation of the syndrome. Although it is important to treat the patients underlying seizure disorder, cross-reactions with other aromatic anticonvulsants can occur, and these compounds, including carbamazepine and barbiturates, can also lead to the syndrome.

I-112.   **The answer is E.** (*Chap. 56*) The photosensitivity reactions of phototoxicity or photoallergy can be related to both topical or systemic administration of drugs and require the absorption of energy by the drug to create a photosensitizer that can generate reactive oxygen species. Phototoxicity is a nonimmunologic reaction that leads to erythema resembling a sunburn. Photoallergy is a less common immunologic reaction that leads to a hypersensitivity syndrome characterized severe pruritus with eczematous dermatitis. This can progress to lichenification in sun-exposed areas. Drugs that can cause both photoallergy and phototoxicity are fluoroquinolones, sulfonamides, and sulfonylureas.

I-113.   **The answer is B.** (*Chap. 57*) The first step in diagnosing polycythemia vera is to document an elevated red blood cell (RBC) mass. A normal red blood cell (RBC) mass suggests spurious polycythemia. Next, serum erythropoietin (EPO) levels should be measured. If EPO levels are low, the diagnosis is polycythemia vera. Confirmatory tests include Janus kinase (JAK) 2 mutation analysis, leukocytosis, and thrombocytosis. Elevated EPO levels are seen in the normal physiologic response to hypoxia as well as in autonomous production of EPO. Further steps in the workup include evaluation for hypoxia with an arterial blood gas, consideration of smoker's polycythemia (elevated carboxyhemoglobin levels), and disorders of increased hemoglobin affinity for oxygen. Low serum EPO levels with low oxygen saturation suggest inadequate renal production (renal failure). High RBC mass and high EPO levels with normal oxygen saturation may be seen with autonomous EPO production, such as in renal cell carcinoma.

I-114. **The answer is E.** *(Chap. 58)* von Willebrand disease (VWD) is an inherited disorder of platelet adhesion that has several types. The most common type is inherited in an autosomal dominant fashion and is associated with low levels of qualitatively normal von Willebrand factor. As a disorder primary hemostasis associated with the development of a platelet plug, VWD is primarily associated with mucosal bleeding. General bleeding symptoms that are more common in VWD include prolonged bleeding after surgery or dental procedures, menorrhagia, postpartum hemorrhage, and large bruises. However, easy bruising and menorrhagia are common complaints and are not specific for VWD in isolation. Factors that raise concern for VWD in women with menstrual symptoms include iron-deficiency anemia, need for blood transfusion, passage of clots more than 1 inch in diameter, and need to change a pad or tampon more than hourly. Epistaxis is also a very common occurrence in the general population, but it is the most common complaint of males with VWD. Concerning features of epistaxis that may be more likely to indicate an underlying bleeding diathesis are lack of seasonal variation and bleeding that requires medical attention. Although most gastrointestinal bleeding in individuals with VWD is unrelated to the bleeding diathesis, VWD types 2 and 3 are associated with angiodysplasia of the bowel and gastrointestinal bleeding. Spontaneous hemarthroses or deep muscle hematomas are seen in clotting factor deficiencies and not seen VWD except severe VWD with associated decreased factor VIII levels less than 5%.

I-115. **The answer is B.** *(Chap. 58)* The activated partial thromboplastin time (aPTT) measures the integrity of the intrinsic and common coagulation pathways, and as such, is affected by all of the coagulation factors, except factor VII. The aPTT reagent contains phospholipids derived from animal or vegetable sources and includes an activator of the intrinsic coagulation system, such as nonparticulate ellagic acid or kaolin. The phospholipid reagent frequently varies from laboratory to laboratory. Thus, an aPTT measured in one hospital may differ from another. Isolated elevations in the aPTT can be related to factor deficiencies, heparin or direct thrombin inhibitors, lupus anticoagulant, or the presence of a specific factor inhibitor. To differentiate between the presence of factor deficiencies and inhibitors, mixing studies should be performed. Mixing studies are performed by mixing normal plasma and the patient's plasma in a 1:1 ratio. The aPTT and prothrombin time (PT) are incubated at 37°C, and levels are measured immediately and serially thereafter for about 2 hours. If the cause is an isolated factor deficiency, the aPTT should correct to normal values and remain normal throughout the incubation period. In the presence of an acquired inhibitor, the aPTT may or may not correct immediately, but upon incubation, the inhibitor becomes more active, and the aPTT will progressively prolong. In contrast, the aPTT does not correct immediately or with incubation in the presence of lupus anticoagulants. The presence of serious bleeding in the presence of mixing studies suggesting an inhibitor should further rule out lupus anticoagulant as a cause because the lupus anticoagulant typically presents with no symptoms or as a thrombotic disorder. The mixing studies do not, however, eliminate the presence of heparin as a cause of the prolonged aPTT. If heparin were present, the thrombin time, but not the reptilase time, would be prolonged. In this scenario, both values were normal, ruling out the presence of heparin or a direct thrombin inhibitor. Likewise, disseminated intravascular coagulation can be ruled out in the presence of normal fibrinogen levels. In serious vitamin K deficiency, both the PT and aPTT should be prolonged.

I-116. **The answer is E.** *(Chap. 59)* Lymphadenopathy has many causes, including infections, immunologic diseases, and malignancy among others. In the vast majority of cases, the cause of enlarged lymph nodes is a benign process. In the primary care practice, fewer than 1% of individuals will have malignancy, and in individuals referred for lymphadenopathy, this number rises only to 16%. Some features on history and physical examination lead to an increased likelihood that the cause of lymphadenopathy is malignant in origin. Malignancy is more common in individuals older than 50 years. Fevers and chills are more commonly present in benign respiratory illness but can be present in malignancy. Thus, fever is a nonspecific symptom. Likewise, generalized versus focal lymphadenopathy is also not specific. The site of lymph node enlargement can be important and raise the risk of malignancy. The presence of supraclavicular lymphadenopathy is never normal. These lymph nodes drain the thoracic cavity and retroperitoneal space and are most commonly enlarged in malignancy. However, infectious etiologies can also cause supraclavicular lymphadenopathy. The size and texture of the lymph nodes also provide important information. Nodes less than 1.0 cm × 1.0 cm are almost always benign, but lymph nodes greater than 2.0 cm in maximum diameter or with an area of 2.25 cm² (1.5 × 1.5 cm) are more likely to be malignant. Nodes containing metastatic cancer tend to be described as hard, fixed, and nontender. In lymphoma, however, the nodes can be tender because of rapid enlargement of the node with subsequent stretching of the capsule of the lymph nodes. Lymphomatous nodes are also frequently described as firm, rubbery, and mobile.

I-117. **The answer is F.** (*Chap. 59*) This patient's lymphadenopathy is benign. Inguinal nodes smaller than 2 cm are common in the population at large and need no further workup provided that there is no other evidence of disseminated infection or tumor and that the nodes have qualities that do not suggest tumor (not hard or matted). A practical approach would be to measure the nodes or even photograph them if visible and follow them serially over time. Occasionally, inguinal lymph nodes can be associated with sexually transmitted diseases. However, these are usually ipsilateral and tender, and evaluation includes bimanual examination and appropriate cultures, not necessarily pelvic ultrasonography. A total-body CT scan would be indicated if other pathologic nodes suggestive of lymphoma or granulomatous disease are present in other anatomic locations. Bone marrow biopsy would be indicated only if a diagnosis of lymphoma is made first.

I-118. **The answer is C.** (*Chap. 59*) Portal hypertension causes splenomegaly via passive congestion of the spleen. It generally causes only mild enlargement of the spleen because expanded varices provide some decompression for elevated portal pressures. Myelofibrosis necessitates extramedullary hematopoiesis in the spleen, liver, and even other sites such as the peritoneum, leading to massive splenomegaly caused by myeloid hyperproduction. Autoimmune hemolytic anemia requires the spleen to dispose of massive amounts of damaged red blood cells, leading to reticuloendothelial hyperplasia and frequently an extremely large spleen. Chronic myelogenous leukemia and other leukemias and lymphomas can lead to massive splenomegaly caused by infiltration with an abnormal clone of cells. Marginal zone lymphoma typically presents with splenomegaly. If a patient with cirrhosis or right heart failure has massive splenomegaly, a cause other than passive congestion should be considered.

I-119. **The answer is A.** (*Chap. 59*) The presence of Howell-Jolly bodies (nuclear remnants), Heinz bodies (denatured hemoglobin), basophilic stippling, and nucleated red blood cells (RBCs) in the peripheral blood implies that the spleen is not properly clearing senescent or damaged RBCs from the circulation. This usually occurs because of surgical splenectomy but is also possible when there is diffuse infiltration of the spleen with malignant cells. Hemolytic anemia can have various peripheral smear findings depending on the etiology of the hemolysis. Spherocytes and bite cells are an example of damaged RBCs that might appear because of autoimmune hemolytic anemia and oxidative damage, respectively. Disseminated intravascular coagulation is characterized by schistocytes and thrombocytopenia on smear with an elevated international normalized ratio and activated partial thromboplastin time as well. However, in these conditions, damaged RBCs are still cleared effectively by the spleen. Transformation to acute leukemia does not lead to splenic damage.

I-120. **The answer is A.** (*Chap. 59*) Splenectomy leads to an increased risk of overwhelming postsplenectomy sepsis, an infection that carries an extremely high mortality rate.

The most commonly implicated organisms are encapsulated. *Streptococcus pneumoniae*, *Haemophilus influenzae*, and sometime gram-negative enteric organisms are most frequently isolated. There is no known increased risk for any viral infections. Vaccination for *S. pneumoniae*, *H. influenzae*, and *Neisseria meningitidis* is indicated for any patient who may undergo splenectomy. The vaccines should be given at least 2 weeks before surgery. The highest risk of sepsis occurs in patients younger than 20 years of age because the spleen is responsible for first-pass immunity and younger patients are more likely to have primary exposure to implicated organisms. The risk is highest during the first 3 years after splenectomy and persists at a lower rate until death.

I-121.   **The answer is E.** *(Chap. 60)* Chronic granulomatous disease (CGD) is an inherited disorder of abnormal phagocyte function. Seventy percent of cases are inherited in an X-linked fashion with the other 30% being autosomal recessive. Affected individuals are susceptible to infectious with catalase-positive organisms, especially *Staphylococcus aureus*. Other organisms that can be seen include *Burkholderia cepacia*, *Aspergillus* spp., and *Chromobacterium violaceum*. Most individuals present in childhood, and infections commonly affect the skin, ears, lungs, liver, and bone. Excessive inflammatory reaction can lead to suppuration of lymph nodes, and granulomatous inflammation can be seen on lymph node biopsy and found in the gastrointestinal and genitourinary tracts. Aphthous ulcers and eczematous skin rash can also be seen. The underlying genetic defect in CGD is the inability of neutrophils and monocytes to generate the appropriate oxidative burst in response to infectious organisms. Several mutations can lead to the disease, and these affect one of the five subunits of the NADPH (nicotinamide adenine dinucleotide phosphate) oxidase enzyme. The test of choice to diagnose chronic granulomatous disease is the nitroblue tetrazolium dye test, which demonstrates lack of superoxide and hydrogen peroxide production in the face of an appropriate stimulus.

I-122.   **The answer is A.** *(Chap. 60)* Under normal or nonstress conditions, roughly 90% of the neutrophil pool is in the bone marrow, 2–3% in the circulation, and the remainder in the tissues. The circulating pool includes the freely flowing cells in the bloodstream and the others are marginated in close proximity to the endothelium. Most of the marginated pool is in the lung, which has a vascular endothelium surface area. Margination in the postcapillary venules is mediated by selectins that cause a low-affinity neutrophil–endothelial cell interaction that mediates "rolling" of the neutrophils along the endothelium. A variety of signals, including interleukin 1, tumor necrosis factor α, and other chemokines, can cause leukocytes to proliferate and leave the bone marrow and enter the circulation. Neutrophil integrins mediate the stickiness of neutrophils to endothelium and are important for chemokine-induced cell activation. Infection causes a marked increase in bone marrow production of neutrophils that marginate and enter tissue. Acute glucocorticoids increase neutrophil count by mobilizing cells from the bone marrow and marginated pool.

I-123.   **The answer is E.** *(Chap. 60)* Many drugs can lead to neutropenia, most commonly via retarding neutrophil production in the bone marrow. Of the list in the answer choices, trimethoprimsulfamethoxazole is the most likely culprit. Other common causes of drug-induced neutropenia include alkylating agents such as cyclophosphamide or busulfan, antimetabolites including methotrexate and 5-flucytosine, penicillin and sulfonamide antibiotics, antithyroid drugs, antipsychotics, and anti-inflammatory agents. Prednisone, when used systemically, often causes an increase in the circulating neutrophil count because it leads to demargination of neutrophils and bone marrow stimulation. Ranitidine, an H_2 blocker, is a well-described cause of thrombocytopenia but has not been implicated in neutropenia. Efavirenz is a nonnucleoside reverse transcriptase inhibitor whose main side effects include a morbilliform rash and central nervous system effects, including strange dreams and confusion. The presence of these symptoms does not require drug cessation. Darunavir is a new protease inhibitor that is well tolerated. Common side effects include a maculopapular rash and lipodystrophy, a class effect for all protease inhibitors.

I-124.   **The answer is E.** *(Chap. e49)* Mercury is one of the metals that is a significant cause of health concern because of low-level exposure in environmental and occupational exposures. The toxicity of low level organic mercury exposure (as manifested by neurobehavioral performance) is of increasing concern based on studies of the offspring of mothers who ingested mercury-contaminated fish. With respect to whether the consumption of fish by women during pregnancy is good or bad for offspring neurodevelopment, balancing the trade-offs of the beneficial effects of the omega-3-fatty acids (FAs) in fish versus the adverse effects of mercury contamination in fish has led to some confusion and inconsistency in public health recommendations. Overall, it appears that it is best for pregnant women to either limit fish consumption to species known to be low in mercury contamination but high in omega-3-FAs (e.g., sardines or mackerel) or to avoid fish and obtain omega-3-FAs through supplements or other dietary sources. Current evidence has not supported the recent contention that ethyl mercury, used as a preservative in multiuse vaccines administered in early childhood, has played a significant role in causing neurodevelopmental problems such as autism. Dimethylmercury, a compound only found in research labs, is "supertoxic"—a few drops of exposure via skin absorption or inhaled vapor can cause severe cerebellar degeneration and death. Acute mercury exposure can be assessed with serum levels, but chronic exposure is best assessed by assaying hair samples.

I-125.   **The answer is C.** *(Chap. 396)* This patient has the typical manifestations of ciguatera poisoning from ingested snapper, grouper, or barracuda. Ciguatera poisoning is the most common nonbacterial food poisoning associated with fish in the United States; most U.S. cases occur in Florida and Hawaii. The poisoning almost exclusively involves tropical and semitropical marine coral reef fish common in the Indian Ocean, the South Pacific, and the Caribbean Sea. Among reported cases, 75% (except in Hawaii) involve the barracuda, snapper, jack, or grouper. Most, if not all, ciguatoxins are unaffected by freeze drying, heat, cold, and gastric acid. None of the toxins affects the odor, color, or taste of fish. The onset of symptoms may come within 15–30 minutes of ingestion and typically takes place within 2–6 hours. Symptoms increase in severity over the ensuing 4–6 hours. Most victims develop symptoms within 12 hours of ingestion, and virtually all are afflicted within 24 hours. More than 150 symptoms have been reported, including abdominal pain, nausea, vomiting, diarrhea, chills, paresthesias, pruritus, tongue and throat numbness or burning, odontalgia or dental dysesthesias, and an extensive variety of neurologic findings. Bradycardia, hypotension, central respiratory failure, and coma may occur. Death is rare. Symptoms may persist for 48 hours and then generally resolve. A pathognomonic symptom is the reversal of hot and cold tactile perception, which develops in some persons after 3–5 days and may last for months. More severe reactions tend to occur in persons previously stricken with the disease. Therapy is supportive and symptom directed. Consumption of fish in ciguatera-endemic regions should be avoided. All oversized fish of any predacious reef species should be suspected of harboring ciguatoxin. Neither moray eels nor the viscera of tropical marine fish should ever be eaten.

I-126.   **The answer is B.** *(Chap. e50)* More than 5 million poison exposures occur in the United States each year. Most are acute, accidental (unintentional), involve a single agent, occur in the home, result in minor or no toxicity, and involve children younger than 6 years of age. Pharmaceuticals are involved in 47% of exposures and 84% of serious or fatal poisonings. Unintentional exposures can result from the improper use of chemicals at work or play; label misreading; product mislabeling; mistaken identification of unlabeled chemicals; uninformed self-medication; and dosing errors by nurses, pharmacists, physicians, parents, and elderly adults. Excluding the recreational use of ethanol, attempted suicide (deliberate self-harm) is the most common reported reason for intentional poisoning. Recreational use of prescribed and over-the-counter drugs for psychotropic or euphoric effects (abuse) or excessive self-dosing (misuse) are increasingly common and may also result in unintentional self-poisoning. About 20–25% of exposures require bedside health professional evaluation, and 5% of all exposures require hospitalization. Poisonings account for 5–10% of all ambulance transports, emergency department visits, and intensive care unit admissions. Up to 30% of psychiatric admissions are prompted by attempted suicide via overdosage. Overall, the mortality rate is low: fewer than 1% of all exposures. It is much higher (1–2%) in hospitalized patients with intentional (suicidal) overdose, who account for the majority of serious poisonings. Acetaminophen is the pharmaceutical agent most often implicated in fatal poisoning. Overall, carbon monoxide is the leading cause of death from poisoning, but this is not reflected in hospital or poison center statistics because patients with such poisoning are typically dead when discovered and are referred directly to medical examiners.

I-127.   **The answer is D.** *(Chap. e50)* Sympathetic toxidromes share many features, including increased pulse, blood pressure, neuromuscular activity, tremulousness, delirium, and agitation. In many cases, these syndromes can be subclassified according to other features or relative strengths of the above symptoms. Sympathomimetics such as cocaine and amphetamines cause extreme elevations in vital signs and organ damage caused by peripheral vasoconstriction, usually in the absence of hallucinations. Benzodiazepine and alcohol withdrawal syndromes present similarly, but hallucinations and often seizures are common in these conditions. Hot, dry, flushed skin; urinary retention; and absent bowel sounds characterize anticholinergic syndromes associated with antihistamines, antipsychotics, antiparkinsonian agents, muscle relaxants, and cyclic antidepressants. Nystagmus is a unique feature of ketamine and phencyclidine overdose.

I-128.   **The answer is A.** *(Chap. e50)* Lithium interferes with cell membrane ion transport, leading to nephrogenic diabetes insipidus and falsely elevated chloride. This can cause the appearance of low anion gap metabolic acidosis. Sequelae include nausea, vomiting, ataxia, encephalopathy, coma, seizures, arrhythmia, hyperthermia, permanent movement disorder, and encephalopathy. Severe cases are treated with bowel irrigation, endoscopic removal of long-acting formulations, hydration, and sometimes hemodialysis. Care should be taken because toxicity occurs at lower levels in chronic toxicity compared with acute toxicity. Salicylate toxicity leads to a normal osmolal gap as well as an elevated anion gap metabolic acidosis, respiratory alkalosis, and sometimes normal anion gap metabolic acidosis. Methanol toxicity is associated with blindness and is characterized by an increased anion gap metabolic acidosis, normal lactate and ketones, and a high osmolal gap. Propylene glycol toxicity causes an increased anion gap metabolic acidosis with elevated lactate and a high osmolal gap. The only electrolyte abnormalities associated with opiate overdose are compensatory to a primary respiratory acidosis.

I-129.   **The answer is B.** *(Chap. e50)* The clinical implications of understanding the difference between therapeutic drug dosing and overdosage are critical. Drug effects begin earlier, peak later, and last longer in the context of overdose compared with commonly referenced values. Therefore, if a patient has a known ingestion of a toxic dose of a dangerous substance and symptoms have not yet begun, then aggressive gut decontamination should ensue because symptoms are apt to ensue rapidly. The late peak and longer duration of action are important as well. A common error in practice is for patients to be released or watched less carefully after reversal of toxicity associated with an opiate agonist or benzodiazepine. However, the duration of activity of the offending toxic agent often exceeds the half-life of the antagonists, naloxone or flumazenil, requiring the administration of subsequent doses several hours later to prevent further central nervous system or physiologic depression.

I-130.   **The answer is E.** *(Chap. e50)* Gastric decontamination is controversial because few data are available to support or refute its use more than an hour after ingestion. It remains a very common practice in most hospitals. Syrup of ipecac is no longer endorsed for in-hospital use and is controversial even for home use, although its safety profile is well documented and therefore it likely poses little harm for ingestions when the history is clear and the indication strong. Activated charcoal is generally the decontamination method of choice because it is the least aversive and least invasive option available. It is effective in decreasing systemic absorption if given within 1 hour of poison ingestion. It may be effective even later after ingestion for drugs with significant anticholinergic effect (e.g., tricyclic antidepressants). Considerations are poor visibility of the gastrointestinal tract on endoscopy after charcoal ingestion and perhaps decreased absorption of oral drugs. Gastric lavage is the most invasive option and is effective, but it is occasionally associated with tracheal intubation and bowel wall perforation. It is also the least comfortable option for the patient. Moreover, aspiration risk is highest in those undergoing gastric lavage. All three of the most common options for decontamination carry at least a 1% risk of an aspiration event, which warrants special consideration in the patient with mental status change.

I-131.   **The answer is E.** *(Chap. e51)* Whereas acute mountain sickness (AMS) is the benign form of altitude illness, high-altitude cerebral edema (HACE) and high-altitude pulmonary edema (HAPE) are life threatening. Altitude illness is likely to occur above 2500 m but has been documented even at 1500–2500 m. The acclimation to altitude includes hyperventilation in response to the reduced inspired PO_2 initially followed by increased erythropoietin and 2,3-bisphosphoglycerate. AMS is characterized by nonspecific symptoms (headache, nausea, fatigue, and dizziness) with a paucity of physical findings developing 6–12 hours after ascent to a high altitude. AMS must be distinguished from exhaustion, dehydration, hypothermia, alcoholic hangover, and hyponatremia. The most important risk factors for the development of altitude illness are the rate of ascent and a history of high-altitude illness. Exertion is a risk factor, but lack of physical fitness is not. One protective factor in AMS is high-altitude exposure during the preceding 2 months. Children and adults seem to be equally affected, but people greater than 50 years of age may be less likely to develop AMS than younger people. Most studies reveal no gender difference in AMS incidence. Sleep desaturation—a common phenomenon at high altitude—is associated with AMS. Gradual ascent is the best approach to prevent AMS. Acetazolamide or dexamethasone beginning 1 day before ascent and continuing for 2–3 days is effective if rapid ascent is necessary. A double-blind placebo-controlled trial demonstrated no benefit on AMS from gingko biloba. Mild cases of AMS can be treated with rest; more serious cases are treated with acetazolamide and oxygen. Descent is therapeutic in all serious cases, including HACE and HAPE. Patients who have recovered from mild cases of AMS may reascend carefully after recovery; patients with HACE should not.

I-132.   **The answer is D.** *(Chap. e51)* High-altitude pulmonary edema (HAPE) is related to an enhanced or atypical pulmonary vascular response to hypoxia. It is not necessarily preceded by acute mountain sickness. HAPE develops within 2–4 days after arrival at high altitude; it rarely occurs after more than 4 or 5 days at the same altitude. A rapid rate of ascent, exercise, a history of HAPE, respiratory tract infections, and cold environmental temperatures are risk factors. Men are more susceptible than women. People with abnormalities of the cardiopulmonary circulation leading to pulmonary hypertension (e.g., patent foramen ovale, mitral stenosis, primary pulmonary hypertension, unilateral absence of the pulmonary artery) are at increased risk of HAPE even at moderate altitudes. Echocardiography is recommended when HAPE develops at relatively low altitudes (<3000 m) and whenever cardiopulmonary abnormalities predisposing to HAPE are suspected. The initial manifestation of HAPE may be a reduction in exercise tolerance greater than that expected at the given altitude. A dry, persistent cough may presage HAPE and may be followed by the production of blood-tinged sputum. Tachypnea and tachycardia, even at rest, are important markers as illness progresses. Crackles may be heard on auscultation but are not diagnostic. Fever and leukocytosis may occur. Descent and oxygen (to raise SaO_2 >90%) are the mainstays of therapy for HAPE. Nifedipine can be used as adjunctive therapy. Inhaled beta-agonists, which are safe and convenient to carry, are useful in the prevention of HAPE and may be effective in its treatment, although no trials have yet been carried out. Inhaled nitric oxide and expiratory positive airway pressure may also be useful therapeutic measures but may not be available in high-altitude settings. No studies have investigated phosphodiesterase-5 inhibitors in the treatment of HAPE, but reports have described their use in clinical practice. Patients with HAPE who have recovered may be able to reascend. In high-altitude cerebral edema, reascent after a few days is not advisable.

I-133.   **The answer is E.** *(Chap. e52)* Untreated pneumothorax has the risk of rapidly expanding and potentially causing tension upon decompression. Patients with extensive bullae should be considered carefully because they may have a similar risk. The effect of hyperbaric oxygen in patients with chronic CO_2 retention has not been studied. The other commonly quoted contraindication to hyperbaric oxygen therapy is a history of receiving bleomycin chemotherapy. Bleomycin is associated with a dose-dependent risk of pneumonitis, and this risk may be enhanced with hyperbaric oxygen exposure. There are reports of patients developing pneumonitis with high FIO_2 or hyperbaric therapy even years after receiving bleomycin. Radiation proctitis and carbon monoxide poisoning are clinical conditions in which hyperbaric oxygen therapy may be warranted. The indications for hyperbaric oxygen therapy are evolving with some advocating therapy for delayed radiation injury, wound therapy, myonecrosis, thermal injuries, and other conditions in which local hypoxia may occur or impaired oxygen delivery may be present.

I-134.   **The answer is D.** *(Chap. e52)* Because for every 10.1-m increase in depth of seawater, the ambient pressure (P_{amb}) increases by 1 standard atmosphere, at 20-m depth, a person is exposed to a P_{amb} of approximately 3 atmospheres absolute. Decompression sickness (DCS) is caused by the formation of bubbles from dissolved inert gas (usually nitrogen) during or after ascent (decompression) from a compressed gas dive. Deeper and longer dives increase the amount of dissolved inert gas, and more rapid ascent increases the potential for bubbles to form and affect end organs. Although variable, DCS usually does not occur unless the dive depth exceeds 7 m (1.7 atm absolute). DCS usually develops within 8–12 hours of ascent. The majority of patients present with mild symptoms, including musculoskeletal pain; fatigue; and minor neurologic manifestations, such as patchy paresthesias. A feared complication is cerebral arterial gas embolism (CAGE). To lessen the chance of gas bubbles entering the cerebral circulation, patients with DCS should remain in a horizontal posture. Initial first aid should include 100% oxygen to accelerate inert gas washout and resolution of bubbles. For patients with symptoms beyond mild DCS, recompression and hyperbaric oxygen therapy are generally recommended. If evacuated by air, the patient should be transported at low altitude by helicopter. After full recovery, diving can be restarted after at least 1 month.

I-135.   **The answer is B.** *(Chap. 268)* ALI and ARDS are both characterized by diffuse lung injury, bilateral radiographic infiltrates, and hypoxemia in the absence of left atrial hypertension. ALI is considered a less severe form of diffuse lung injury that may evolve to ARDS or warrant intensive therapy to forestall the progression. The distinction between ALI and ARDS is made by the magnitude of the PaO_2/FIO_2 ratio with ARDS defined as a ratio of 200 mmHg or below and ALI 300 mmHg or below. Many medical and surgical illnesses are associated with the development of ALI and ARDS, but most cases (>80%) are caused by a relatively small number of clinical disorders, namely, severe sepsis syndrome and bacterial pneumonia (40–50%), trauma, multiple transfusions, aspiration of gastric contents, and drug overdose. Among patients with trauma, pulmonary contusion, multiple bone fractures, and chest wall trauma or flail chest are the most frequently reported surgical conditions in ARDS, but head trauma, near drowning, toxic inhalation, and burns are rare causes. The risks of developing ARDS are increased in patients with more than one predisposing medical or surgical condition (e.g., the risk for ARDS increases from 25% in patients with severe trauma to 56% in patients with trauma and sepsis). Several other clinical variables have been associated with the development of ARDS. These include older age, chronic alcohol abuse, metabolic acidosis, and severity of critical illness.

I-136.   **The answer is D.** *(Chap. 268)* To date, despite intensive investigation of multiple pathophysiologically based therapies, the only intervention that decreased mortality in patients with ARDS was a low tidal volume (6 mL/kg ideal body weight) mechanical ventilation strategy. The rationale for this intervention is that overdistension of normal alveoli in patients with ARDS promotes further lung injury. Maintaining a normal or low left atrial filling pressure is also recommended therapy for patients with ARDS. It minimizes pulmonary edema and prevents further decrements in arterial oxygenation and lung compliance, improves pulmonary mechanics, and shortens intensive care unit stay and the duration of mechanical ventilation. Numerous studies have demonstrated that placing the patient in the prone position may improve oxygenation, but there has been no consistent mortality benefit. Other "lung protective" strategies of mechanical ventilation (high-frequency ventilation, high positive end-expiratory pressure, pressure-volume curve measurement) are under investigation. Inflammatory mediators and leukocytes are abundant in the lungs of patients with ARDS. Many attempts have been made to treat both early and late ARDS with glucocorticoids to reduce this potentially deleterious pulmonary inflammation. Few studies have shown any benefit. Current evidence does *not* support the use of high-dose glucocorticoids in the care of ARDS patients. Similarly, ARDS is characterized by a surfactant deficiency, but administration of exogenous surfactant has not yielded clinical results (in contrast to the dramatic benefit in neonatal lung injury). See Table I-137.

TABLE I-137   Evidence-Based Recommendations for Acute Respiratory Distress Syndrome Therapies

Treatment	Recommendation*
Mechanical ventilation	
Low tidal volume	A
Minimize left atrial filling pressures	B
High-PEEP or "open lung"	C
Prone position	C
Recruitment maneuvers	C
ECMO	C
High-frequency ventilation	D
Glucocorticoids	D
Surfactant replacement, inhaled nitric oxide, and other anti-inflammatory therapy (e.g., ketoconazole, PGE₁, NSAIDs)	D

*A, recommended therapy based on strong clinical evidence from randomized clinical trials; B, recommended therapy based on supportive but limited clinical data; C, indeterminate evidence: recommended only as alternative therapy; D, not recommended based on clinical evidence against efficacy of therapy.
Abbreviations: ECMO, extracorporeal membrane oxygenation; NSAID, nonsteroidal anti-inflammatory drug; PEEP, positive end-expiratory pressure; PGE_1, prostaglandin E_1.

I-137.   The answer is E. *(Chap. 268)* Recent mortality estimates for ARDS range from 26–44%. The mortality rate in ARDS is largely attributable to nonpulmonary causes, with sepsis and nonpulmonary organ failure accounting for more than 80% of deaths. Mortality caused by hypoxemic respiratory failure is not typical. The degree of hypoxemia during ARDS is also not a strong predictor of outcome. The major risk factors for ARDS mortality include age, preexisting chronic medical conditions or organ dysfunction, and severity of critical illness (number of organ failures). Patients with ARDS from direct lung injury (including pneumonia, pulmonary contusion, and aspiration) have nearly twice the mortality rate of those with indirect causes of lung injury, but surgical and trauma patients with ARDS, especially those without direct lung injury, have a better survival rate than other ARDS patients. The majority of patients recover nearly normal lung function with 1 year. One year after endotracheal extubation, more than one-third of ARDS survivors have normal spirometry values and diffusion capacity, and most of the remaining patients have only mild abnormalities in their pulmonary function. Unlike the risk for mortality, recovery of lung function is strongly associated with the extent of lung injury in early ARDS. When caring for ARDS survivors, it is important to be aware of the potential for a substantial burden of emotional and respiratory symptoms. There are significant rates of depression and posttraumatic stress disorder in ARDS survivors.

I-138.   The answer is D. *(Chap. 269)* Noninvasive ventilation (NIV) has been gaining more acceptance because it is effective in certain conditions, such as acute and chronic respiratory failure, and is associated with fewer complications, namely, pneumonia and tracheolaryngeal trauma. The major limitation to its widespread application has been patient intolerance because the tight-fitting mask required for NIV can cause both physical and emotional discomfort. In addition, NIV has had limited success in patients with acute hypoxemic respiratory failure, for whom endotracheal intubation and conventional mechanical ventilation remain the ventilatory method of choice. The most important group of patients who benefit from a trial of NIV are those with acute exacerbations of chronic obstructive pulmonary disease (COPD) leading to respiratory acidosis (pH <7.35). Experience from several well-conducted randomized trials has shown that in patients with ventilatory failure characterized by blood pH levels between 7.25 and 7.35, NIV is associated with low failure rates (15–20%) and good outcomes (intubation rate; length of stay in intensive care; and in some series, mortality rates). In more severely ill patients with pH below 7.25, the rate of NIV failure is inversely related to the severity of respiratory acidosis, with greater failure as the pH decreases. In patients with milder acidosis (pH >7.35), NIV is not better than conventional therapy that includes controlled oxygen delivery and pharmacotherapy for exacerbations of COPD (systemic corticosteroids; bronchodilators; and, if needed, antibiotics). The contraindications to NIV are listed in the Table I-139.

TABLE I-139   Contraindications for Noninvasive Ventilation

Cardiac or respiratory arrest

Severe encephalopathy

Severe gastrointestinal bleed

Hemodynamic instability

Unstable angina and myocardial infarction

Facial surgery or trauma

Upper airway obstruction

High-risk aspiration or inability to protect airways

Inability to clear secretions

I-139.   **The answer is A.** *(Chap. 269)* Modes of ventilation differ in how breaths are triggered, cycled, and limited. All modes allow determination of either the pressure or volume limit. Assist control and synchronized intermittent mandatory ventilation (SIMV) are volume cycled, in which a fixed volume is delivered to the patient by the machine using the necessary inspiratory pressure. Pressure control and pressure support are pressure cycled, in which a known pressure limit is imposed and volume delivered by the machine may vary. Continuous positive airway pressure does not alter pressure or deliver a fixed volume to the patient. Assist control and SIMV differ by the response to patient initiated breaths. Both will deliver a fixed volume when the patient does not initiate a breath. However, with SIMV, if the patient is breathing at a rate greater than set on the machine, each spontaneous breath is dependent completely on patient effort. On assist control, each patient initiated breath above the set rate is supported by the machine by delivering the set rate. In patients with a high respiratory rate, this can result in hyperventilation, and intrinsic PEEP because of inadequate time for exhalation of the full tidal volume. In the patient described, because each breath that is either initiated by the patient or the machine is at a set rate and a fixed volume, this is most consistent with the assist control mode of mechanical ventilation.

I-140.   **The answer is D.** *(Chap. 269)* Determining when an individual is an appropriate candidate for a spontaneous breathing trial is important for the care of mechanically ventilated patients. An important initial step in determining if a patient is likely to be successfully extubated is to evaluate the mental status of the patient. This can be difficult if the patient is receiving sedation, and it is recommended that sedation be interrupted on a daily basis for a short period to allow assessment of mental status. Daily interruption of sedation has been shown to decrease the duration of mechanical ventilation. If the patient is unable to respond to any commands or is completely obtunded, the individual is at high risk for aspiration and unlikely to be successfully extubated. In addition, the patient should be hemodynamically stable and the lung injury stable or improving. If these conditions are met, the patient should be on minimal ventilatory support. This includes the ability to maintain the pH between 7.35 and an SaO_2 greater than 90% while receiving an FIO_2 of 0.5 or less and a PEEP of 5 cmH_2) or less. The presence of rapid shallow breathing during a spontaneous breathing trial identifies patients who are less likely to be extubated successfully.

I-141. **The answer is B.** *(Chap. 269)* Patients initiated on mechanical ventilation require a variety of supportive measures. Sedation and analgesia with a combination of benzodiazepines and narcotics are commonly used to maintain patient comfort and safety while mechanically ventilated. Recent studies have shown the utility of minimizing sedation in critically ill patients. However, adequate pain control is an essential component of patient comfort. In addition, patients are immobilized and are thus at high risk for development of deep venous thrombosis and pulmonary embolus. Prophylaxis with unfractionated heparin or low-molecular-weight heparin should be administered subcutaneously. Prophylaxis against diffuse gastrointestinal mucosal injury is also indicated, particularly in individuals with neurologic insult and those with severe respiratory failure and adult respiratory distress syndrome. Gastric acid suppression can be managed with H_2-receptor antagonists, proton pump inhibitors, and sucralfate. It is also recommended that individuals who are expected to be intubated for more than 72 hours receive nutritional support. Prokinetic agents are often required. Frequent positional changes and close surveillance for skin breakdown should be instituted in all intensive care units to minimize development of decubitus ulcers. In the past, frequent ventilator circuit changes had been studied as a measure for prevention of ventilator-associated pneumonia, but they were ineffective and may even have increased the risk of ventilator-associated pneumonia.

I-142. **The answer is D.** *(Chap. 269)* Mechanical ventilation is frequently used to support ventilation in individuals with both hypoxemic and hypercarbic respiratory failure. Mechanical ventilators provide warm, humidified gas to the airways in accordance with preset ventilator settings. The ventilator serves as the energy source for inspiration, but expiration is a passive process, driven by the elastic recoil of the lungs and chest wall. PEEP may be used to prevent alveolar collapse on expiration. The physiologic consequences of PEEP include decreased preload and decreased afterload. Decreased preload occurs because PEEP decreases venous return to the right atrium and may manifest as hypotension, especially in an individual who is volume depleted. In addition, PEEP is transmitted to the heart and great vessels. This complicated interaction leads to a decrease in afterload and may be beneficial to individuals with depressed cardiac function. When using mechanical ventilation, the physician should also be cognizant of other potential physiologic consequences of the ventilator settings. Initial settings chosen by the physician include mode of ventilation, respiratory rate, fraction of inspired oxygen, and tidal volume if volume-cycled ventilation is used or maximum pressure if pressure-cycled ventilation is chosen. The respiratory therapist also has the ability to alter the inspiratory flow rate and waveform for delivery of the chosen mode of ventilation. These choices can have important physiologic consequences for the patient. In individuals with obstructive lung disease, it is important to maximize the time for exhalation. This can be done by decreasing the respiratory rate or decreasing the inspiratory time (decrease the inspiration-to-expiration ratio, prolong expiration), which is accomplished by increasing the inspiratory flow rate. Care must also be taken in choosing the inspired tidal volume in volume-cycled ventilatory modes because high inspired tidal volumes can contribute to development of acute lung injury caused by overdistention of alveoli.

I-143. **The answer is B.** *(Chap. 269)* Patients intubated for respiratory failure because of obstructive lung disease (asthma or chronic obstructive pulmonary disease) are at risk for the development of intrinsic positive end-expiratory pressure (auto-PEEP). Because these conditions are characterized by expiratory flow limitation, a long expiratory time is required to allow a full exhalation. If the patient is unable to exhale fully, auto-PEEP develops. With repeated breaths, the pressure generated from auto-PEEP continues to rise and impedes venous return to the right ventricle. This results in hypotension and increases the risk for pneumothorax. Both of these conditions should be considered when evaluating this patient. However, because breath sounds are heard bilaterally, pneumothorax is less likely, and tube thoracostomy is not indicated at this time. Development of auto-PEEP has most likely occurred in this patient because the patient is currently agitated and hyperventilating as the effects of the paralytic agent wear off. In AC mode ventilation, each respiratory effort delivers the full tidal volume of 550 mL, and there is a decreased time for exhalation, allowing auto-PEEP to occur. Immediate management of this patient should include disconnecting the patient from the ventilator to allow the patient to fully exhale and decreasing the auto-PEEP. A fluid bolus may temporarily increase the blood pressure but would not eliminate the underlying cause of the hypotension. After treatment of the auto-PEEP by disconnecting the patient from the ventilator, sedation is important to prevent further occurrence of auto-PEEP by decreasing the respiratory rate to the set rate of the ventilator. Sedation can be accomplished with a combination of benzodiazepines and narcotics or propofol. Initiation of vasopressor support is not indicated unless other measures fail to treat the hypotension and it is suspected that sepsis is the cause of hypotension.

I-144.   **The answer is A.** *(Chaps. 5 and 269)* To obtain a stable airway for invasive mechanical ventilation, patients must safely undergo endotracheal intubation. In most patients, paralytic agents are used in combination with sedatives to accomplish endotracheal intubation. Succinylcholine is a depolarizing neuromuscular blocking agent with a short half-life and is one of the most commonly used paralytic agents. However, because it depolarizes the neuromuscular junction, succinylcholine cannot be used in individuals with hyperkalemia because the drug may cause further increases in the potassium level and potentially fatal cardiac arrhythmias. Some conditions in which it is relatively contraindicated to use succinylcholine because of the risk of hyperkalemia include acute renal failure, crush injuries, muscular dystrophy, rhabdomyolysis, and tumor lysis syndrome. Acetaminophen overdose is not a contraindication to the use of succinylcholine unless concomitant renal failure is present.

I-145.   **The answers are 1-C; 2-B; 3-D; 4-A.** *(Chaps. 270, 271, and 272)* A variety of vasopressor agents are available for hemodynamic support. The effects of these medications depend on their effects on the sympathetic nervous system to produce changes in heart rate, cardiac contractility, and peripheral vascular tone. Stimulation of α_1 adrenergic receptors in the peripheral vasculature causes vasoconstriction and improves MAP by increasing systemic vascular resistance. The β_1 receptors are located primarily in the heart and cause increased cardiac contractility and heart rate. The β_2 receptors are found in the peripheral circulation and cause vasodilatation and bronchodilation. Phenylephrine acts solely as an α-adrenergic agonist. It is considered a second-line agent in septic shock and is often used in anesthesia to correct hypotension after induction of anesthesia. Phenylephrine is also useful for spinal shock. The action of dopamine depends on the dosage used. At high doses, dopamine has high affinity for the α receptor, but at lower doses (<5 µg/kg/min), it does not. In addition, dopamine acts at β_1 receptors and dopaminergic receptors. The effect on these receptors is greatest at lower doses. Norepinephrine and epinephrine affect both α and β_1 receptors to increase peripheral vascular resistance, heart rate, and contractility. Norepinephrine has less β_1 activity than epinephrine or dopamine and thus has less associated tachycardia. Norepinephrine and dopamine are the recommended first-line therapies for septic shock. Epinephrine is the drug of choice for anaphylactic shock. Dobutamine is primarily a β_1 agonist with lesser effects at the β_2 receptor. Dobutamine increases cardiac output through improving cardiac contractility and heart rate. Dobutamine may be associated with development of hypotension because of its effects at the β_2 receptor causing vasodilatation and decreased systemic vascular resistance.

I-146 and I-147.   **The answers are B and C, respectively.** *(Chap. 270)* Hypovolemic shock is the most common form of shock and occurs either because of hemorrhage or loss of plasma volume in the form of gastrointestinal, urinary, or insensible losses. Symptoms of hemorrhagic and nonhemorrhagic shock are indistinguishable. Mild hypovolemia is considered to be loss of less than 20% of the blood volume and usually presents with few clinical except save for mild tachycardia. Loss of 20–40% of the blood volume typically induces orthostasis. Loss of more than 40% of the blood volume leads to the classic manifestations of shock, which are marked tachycardia, hypotension, oliguria, and finally obtundation. Central nervous system perfusion is maintained until shock becomes severe. Oliguria is a very important clinical parameter that should help guide volume resuscitation. After assessing for an adequate airway and spontaneous breathing, initial resuscitation aims at reexpanding the intravascular volume and controlling ongoing losses. Volume resuscitation should be initiated with rapid IV infusion of isotonic saline or Ringer's lactate. In head-to-head trials, colloidal solutions have not added any benefit compared with crystalloid and in fact appeared to increase mortality for trauma patients. Hemorrhagic shock with ongoing blood losses and a hemoglobin of 10 g/dL or less should be treated with transfusion of packed red blood cells (PRBCs). After hemorrhage is controlled, transfusion of PRBCs should be performed only for hemoglobin of 7 g/dL or less. Patients who remain hypotensive after volume resuscitation have a very poor prognosis. Inotropic support and intensive monitoring should be initiated in these patients. An algorithm for the resuscitation of a patient in shock is shown in Figure I-148.

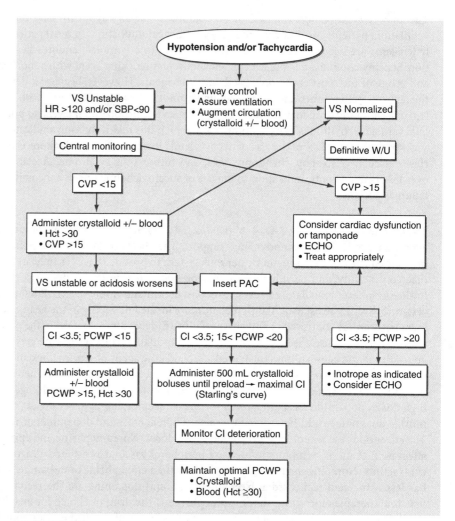

FIGURE I-148

I-148.   **The answer is D.** *(Chap. 270)* The patient is in cardiogenic shock from an ST-elevation myocardial infarction. Shock is a clinical syndrome in which vital organs do not receive adequate perfusion. Understanding the physiology underlying shock is a crucial factor in determining appropriate management. Cardiac output is the major determinant of tissue perfusion and is the product of stroke volume and heart rate. In turn, stroke volume is determined by preload, or ventricular filling, afterload, or resistance to ventricular ejection, and contractility of the myocardium. In this patient, the hypoxic and damaged myocardium has suddenly lost much of its contractile function, and stroke volume will therefore decrease rapidly, dropping cardiac output. Systemic vascular resistance will increase in order to improve return of blood to the heart and increase stroke volume. Central venous pressure is elevated as a consequence of increased vascular resistance, decreased cardiac output and poor forward flow, and neuroendocrine-mediated vasoconstriction. The pathophysiology of other forms of shock is shown in Table I-149 as a comparison.

TABLE I-149 Physiologic Characteristics of the Various Forms of Shock

Type of Shock	CVP and PCWP	Cardiac Output	Systemic Vascular Resistance	Venous O₂ Saturation
Hypovolemic	↓	↓	↑	↓
Cardiogenic	↑	↓	↑	↓
Septic				
Hyperdynamic	↓↑	↑	↓	↑
Hypodynamic	↓↑	↓	↑	↓↑
Traumatic	↓	↓↑	↑↓	↓
Neurogenic	↓	↓	↓	↓
Hypoadrenal	↓	↓	=↓	↓

Abbreviations: CVP, central venous pressure; PCWP, pulmonary capillary wedge pressure.

I-149.   **The answer is C.** *(Chap. 271)* The annual incidence of sepsis has increased to >700,000 individuals yearly in the United States, and sepsis accounts for more than 200,000 deaths yearly. Approximately two-thirds of the cases of sepsis occur in individuals with other significant comorbidities, and the incidence of sepsis increases with age and preexisting comorbidities. In addition, the incidence of sepsis is thought to be increasing as a result of several other factors. These include increased longevity of individuals with chronic disease, including AIDS, and increased risk for sepsis in individuals with AIDS. The practice of medicine has also influenced the risk of sepsis, with an increased risk of sepsis related to the increased use of antimicrobial drugs, immunosuppressive agents, mechanical ventilation, and indwelling catheters and other hardware.

I-150.   **The answer is B.** *(Chap. 271)* Sepsis is a systemic inflammatory response that develops in response to a microbial source. To diagnose the systemic inflammatory response syndrome (SIRS), a patient should have two or more of the following conditions: (1) fever or hypothermia; (2) tachypnea; (3) tachycardia; or (4) leukocytosis, leukopenia, or greater than 10% band forms. This patient fulfills the criteria for sepsis with septic shock because she meets these criteria for SIRS with the presence of organ dysfunction and ongoing hypotension despite fluid resuscitation. The patient has received 2 L of intravenous colloid and now has a central venous pressure of 18 cmH₂O. Ongoing large-volume fluid administration may result in pulmonary edema as the central venous pressure is quite high. At this point, fluid administration should continue but at a lower infusion rate. In this patient, who is receiving chronic glucocorticoids for an underlying inflammatory condition, stress-dose steroids should be administered because adrenal suppression will prevent the patient from developing the normal stress response in the face of SIRS. If the patient fails to respond to glucocorticoids, she should be started on vasopressor therapy. The diagnosis of adrenal insufficiency may be very difficult in critically ill patients. Whereas a plasma cortisol level of less than 15 µg/mL indicates adrenal insufficiency (inadequate production of cortisol), many experts now feel that the adrenocorticotropic hormone stimulation test is not useful for detecting less profound degrees of corticosteroid deficiency in patients who are critically ill. A single small study has suggested that norepinephrine may be preferred over dopamine for septic shock, but these data have not been confirmed in other trials. The "Surviving Sepsis" guidelines state that either norepinephrine or dopamine should be considered as a first-line agent for the treatment of septic shock. Transfusion of red blood cells in critically ill patients has been associated with a higher risk for development of acute lung injury, sepsis, and death. A threshold hemoglobin value of 7 g/dL has been shown to be as safe as a value of 10 g/dL and is associated with fewer complications. In this patient, a blood transfusion is not currently indicated, but it may be considered if the central venous oxygen saturation is below 70% to improve oxygen delivery to tissues. An alternative to blood transfusion in this setting is the use of dobutamine to improve cardiac output.

I-151.   **The answer is C.** *(Chap. 271)* Sepsis occurs as a result of the inflammatory reaction that develops in response to an infection. Microbial invasion of the bloodstream is not necessary for the development of severe sepsis. In fact, blood culture results are positive in only 20–40% of cases of severe sepsis and in only 40–70% of cases of septic shock. The systemic response to infection classically has been demonstrated by the response to lipopolysaccharide (LPS) or endotoxin. LPS binds to receptors on the surfaces of monocytes, macrophages, and neutrophils, causing activation of these cells to produce a variety of inflammatory mediators and cytokines, most notably tumor necrosis factor α (TNF-α). TNF-α stimulates leukocytes and vascular endothelial cells to release other cytokines (as well as additional TNF-α), to express cell-surface molecules that enhance neutrophil–endothelial adhesion at sites of infection, and to increase prostaglandin and leukotriene production. Whereas blood levels of TNF-α are not elevated in individuals with localized infections, they increase in most patients with severe sepsis or septic shock. Moreover, IV infusion of TNF-α can elicit the characteristic abnormalities of SIRS. Although TNF-α is a central mediator, it is only one of many proinflammatory molecules that contribute to innate host defense. Chemokines, most prominently interleukin-8 (IL-8) and IL-17, attract circulating neutrophils to the infection site. These and other proinflammatory cytokines probably interact synergistically with one another and with additional mediators to promote the process of complement activation and increase in procoagulant factors, cellular injury, and intravascular thrombosis. The nonlinearity and multiplicity of these interactions have made it difficult to interpret the roles played by individual mediators in both tissues and blood. This process is meant to wall off invading microorganisms to prevent infection from spreading to other tissues, but in cases of severe sepsis, this leads to tissue hypoxia and ongoing cellular injury. In addition, systemic hypotension develops as a reaction to inflammatory mediators and occurs despite increased levels of plasma catecholamines. Physiologically, this is manifested as a marked decrease in systemic vascular resistance despite evidence of increased sympathetic activation. Survival in sepsis has improved in the past decades largely because of advances in supportive care in the intensive care unit.

I-152.   **The answer is B.** *(Chap. 271)* As the mortality from sepsis has increased over the past 20 years, more research has been performed to attempt to limit mortality. Antimicrobial chemotherapy should be started as soon as samples of blood and other relevant sites have been obtained for culture. A large retrospective review of patients who developed septic shock found that the interval between the onset of hypotension and the administration of appropriate antimicrobial chemotherapy was the major determinant of outcome; a delay of as little as 1 hour was associated with lower survival rates. Empiric antibiotics should have broad coverage of gram-positive and -negative organisms. In general, combination therapy has no advantage over monotherapy with broad-spectrum antibiotics. Use of inappropriate antibiotics, defined on the basis of local microbial susceptibilities and published guidelines for empirical therapy, was associated with fivefold lower survival rates even among patients with negative culture results. Specific therapies have been developed to target the inflammatory response to sepsis, particularly the effect of the inflammatory response on the coagulation system. Unfortunately, none of the pathophysiologically oriented therapies has shown consistent benefit in sepsis. Recently, activated protein C (drotrecogin-α), which had been approved by the U.S. Food and Drug Administration for the treatment of septic shock, was removed from the market by its manufacturer after the European PROWESS-SHOCK trial failed to show a survival benefit. Bicarbonate therapy is commonly used when severe metabolic acidosis (pH <7.2) is present in septic shock. However, there is no evidence that bicarbonate improves hemodynamics, response to vasopressors, or outcomes in septic shock. In patients with septic shock, plasma vasopressin levels increase transiently but then decrease dramatically. Early studies found that vasopressin infusion can reverse septic shock in some patients, reducing or eliminating the need for catecholamine vasopressors. More recently, a randomized clinical trial that compared vasopressin plus norepinephrine with norepinephrine alone in 776 patients with pressor-dependent septic shock found no difference between treatment groups in the primary study outcome, 28-day mortality. Although some patients with sepsis may benefit from red blood cell transfusion, erythropoietin is not used to treat anemia in sepsis.

I-153.   **The answer is A.** *(Chap. 272)* Cardiogenic shock (CS) is characterized by systemic hypoperfusion caused by severe depression of the cardiac index (<2.2 L/min/m^2) and sustained systolic arterial hypotension (<90 mmHg) despite an elevated filling pressure (pulmonary capillary wedge pressure >18 mmHg). It is associated with in-hospital mortality rates above 50%. Acute myocardial infarction (MI) with left ventricular dysfunction is the most common cause of cardiogenic shock. Other complications of acute MI such as mitral regurgitation or free wall rupture are far less common. CS is the leading cause of death of patients hospitalized with MI. Early reperfusion therapy for acute MI decreases the incidence of CS. Shock typically is associated with ST-segment elevation MI and is less common with non–ST-segment elevation MI. In patients with acute MI, older age, female sex, prior MI, diabetes, and anterior MI location are all associated with an increased risk of CS. Shock associated with a first inferior MI should prompt a search for a mechanical cause. Reinfarction soon after MI increases the risk of CS. Two-thirds of patients with CS have flow-limiting stenoses in all three major coronary arteries, and 20% have stenosis of the left main coronary artery. CS may rarely occur in the absence of significant stenosis, as seen in LV apical ballooning/Takotsubo's cardiomyopathy.

I-154.   **The answer is E.** *(Chap. 272)* In patients with acute myocardial infarction and cardiogenic shock, percutaneous coronary intervention can improve mortality rate and outcomes. Stabilizing the patient in cardiogenic shock is an important first maneuver. Initial therapy is aimed at maintaining adequate systemic and coronary perfusion by raising systemic blood pressure with vasopressors and adjusting volume status to a level that ensures optimum left ventricular filling pressure. Decreased diastolic blood pressure is detrimental because it reduces coronary blood flow. However, vasopressor and inotropic agents have the potential to exacerbate the ischemic process by raising myocardial oxygen consumption, increasing heart rate, or increasing left ventricular afterload. Norepinephrine is associated with fewer adverse events, including arrhythmias, compared with dopamine. Dobutamine has greater inotropic than chronotropic action but may cause a reduction in blood pressure due to vasodilation. Aortic counterpulsation with an intraaortic balloon pump (IABP) is helpful in rapidly stabilizing patients because it is capable of augmenting both arterial diastolic pressure and cardiac output. The balloon is automatically inflated during early diastole, augmenting coronary blood flow, and it collapses in early systole, reducing the left ventricular afterload. IABP improves hemodynamic status temporarily in most patients with cardiogenic shock. In contrast to vasopressors and inotropic agents, myocardial O_2 consumption is reduced, ameliorating ischemia. IABP is contraindicated if aortic regurgitation is present or aortic dissection is suspected.

I-155.   **The answer is E.** *(Chap. 273)* The most common electrical mechanism for cardiac arrest is ventricular fibrillation, which is responsible for 50–80% of cardiac arrests. Severe persistent bradyarrhythmias, asystole, and pulseless electrical activity (PEA: organized electrical activity, unusually slow, without mechanical response, formerly called electromechanical dissociation) cause another 20–30%. Pulseless sustained ventricular tachycardia (a rapid arrhythmia distinct from PEA) is a less common mechanism. Acute low cardiac output states, having a precipitous onset also may present clinically as a cardiac arrest. These hemodynamic causes include massive acute pulmonary emboli, internal blood loss from a ruptured aortic aneurysm, intense anaphylaxis, and cardiac rupture with tamponade after myocardial infarction. Sudden deaths from these causes are not typically included in the category of sudden cardiac death.

I-156.   **The answer is A.** *(Chap. 273)* The probability of achieving successful resuscitation from cardiac arrest is related to the interval from onset of loss of circulation to institution of resuscitative efforts, the setting in which the event occurs, the mechanism (ventricular fibrillation, ventricular tachycardia, PEA, asystole), and the clinical status of the patient before the cardiac arrest. Return of circulation and survival rates as a result of defibrillation decrease almost linearly from the first minute to 10 minutes. After 5 minutes, survival rates are no better than 25–30% in out-of-hospital settings. Settings in which it is possible to institute prompt cardiopulmonary resuscitation (CPR) followed by prompt defibrillation provide a better chance of a successful outcome. However, the outcome in intensive care units (ICUs) and other in-hospital environments is heavily influenced by the patient's preceding clinical status. The immediate outcome is good for cardiac arrest occurring in

ICUs in the presence of an acute cardiac event or transient metabolic disturbance, but survival among patients with far-advanced chronic cardiac disease or advanced noncardiac diseases (e.g., renal failure, pneumonia, sepsis, diabetes, cancer) is low and not much better in the in-hospital than in the out-of-hospital setting. Survival from unexpected cardiac arrest in unmonitored areas in a hospital is not much better than that it is for witnessed out-of-hospital arrests. Because implementation of community response systems, survival from out-of-hospital cardiac arrest has improved, although it still remains low under most circumstances. Survival probabilities in public sites exceed those in the home environment. This may be because many patients with at home cardiac arrest have severe underlying cardiac disease. The success rate for initial resuscitation and survival to hospital discharge after an out-of-hospital cardiac arrest depends heavily on the mechanism of the event. Most cardiac arrests that are caused by ventricular fibrillation (VF) begin with a run of nonsustained or sustained ventricular tachycardia (VT), which then degenerates into VF. When the mechanism is pulseless VT, the outcome is best, VF is the next most successful, and asystole and PEA generate dismal outcome statistics. Advanced age also adversely influences the chances of successful resuscitation as well as outcomes after resuscitation.

I-157.   **The answer is D.** *(Chap. 274)* Alterations in consciousness are among the most common reasons for admission to the hospital and occur frequently in seriously ill patients. When evaluating a patient with an alteration in consciousness, one must have a framework for understanding the spectrum of arousability one may encounter. *Coma* is a frequently misunderstood term that refers to a deep sleeplike state from which a patient cannot be aroused. A stuporous patient can be aroused briefly with noxious stimuli, and drowsiness refers to a patient who can be aroused easily with maintenance of attention for brief periods. Other conditions that alter the ability of a patient to respond appropriately to stimuli and are often confused with coma. A vegetative state is an awake but unresponsive condition that can occur in a patient who has emerged from a coma and is associated with extensive bilateral cerebral damage. A patient in a vegetative state can open the eyes spontaneously and often track objects. In addition, the patient has retention of respiratory and autonomic functions as well as spontaneous movement of extremities. However, meaningful responses to stimuli do not occur, and a vegetative state is sometimes referred to as an "awake coma." This patient would be characterized as being in a persistent vegetative state because the duration of the vegetative state has been 1 year. At this point, the likelihood of meaningful recovery of mental faculties is almost zero. A minimally conscious state is a less severe manifestation of bilateral cerebral injury. A patient in a minimally conscious state may have rudimentary vocal or motor behaviors and minimal responses to external stimuli. Other conditions that may be misinterpreted as a coma include akinetic mutism, catatonia, abulia, and locked-in syndrome.

I-158.   **The answer is A.** *(Chap. 274)* Brain death occurs when all cerebral function has ceased but the patient continues to have cardiac activity while supported by artificial means. If an individual is determined to have brain death, life-sustaining therapies are withdrawn. Although this can occur without the consent of the family, certainly it is important to have open communication with the family to allow the withdrawal of care without conflict. Most hospitals have developed specific protocols to diagnose a patient with brain death. Three essential elements should be demonstrated for the diagnosis of brain death. First, the patient should widespread cortical damage with complete absence of response to all external stimuli. Second, the patient should have no evidence of brainstem function with loss of oculovestibular and corneal reflexes and absent pupillary reaction to light. Finally, there should be no evidence of medullary activity manifested by apnea. When a brain death examination is performed, the patient should not be receiving any medications that could alter consciousness. The bedside examination will confirm absence of responsiveness to stimuli and lack of brainstem function. Apnea testing is the final examination in the performance of the brain death examination. This test is important for documenting the absence of medullary function. For an apnea test result to be accurate, the carbon dioxide must be allowed to rise to a level that would stimulate respiration. When performing the test, the patient is preoxygenated with 100% oxygen, which is sustained throughout the test. At this point, ventilator support is stopped. In the absence of any respiration, carbon dioxide rises by 2–3 mmHg/min, and it is necessary for arterial partial pressure of carbon dioxide to rise to between 50–60 mmHg. If the patient has a normal $PaCO_2$ before beginning the apnea test, the test would typically need to continue for at least 5 minutes to be valid. The patient is observed for respiratory effort, and a $PaCO_2$ level is often measured at the end of the test to document that the rise in carbon dioxide is adequate to stimulate respiration. Some patients may have cardiovascular instability that makes the performance of apnea testing risky because one does not wish for the apnea test to lead to cardiovascular collapse. In this setting, an electroencephalogram demonstrating absence of electrical activity is used as an adjunctive diagnostic test. Newer methods of testing, including radionuclide brain scanning, cerebral angiography, and transcranial Doppler ultrasonography, may be used, but these tests are less well validated. In most cases, clinical evidence of brain death must be sustained for 6–24 hours before withdrawal of care.

I-159.   **The answer is E.** *(Chap. 274)* Foraminal herniation, which forces the cerebellar tonsils into the foramen magnum, leads to compression of the medulla and subsequent respiratory arrest. Central transtentorial herniation occurs when the medial thalamus compresses the midbrain as it moves through the tentorial opening; miotic pupils and drowsiness are the classic clinical signs. A locked-in state is usually caused by infarction or hemorrhage of the ventral pons; other causes include Guillain-Barré syndrome and use of certain neuromuscular blocking agents. Catatonia is a semi-awake state seen most frequently as a manifestation of psychotic disorders such as schizophrenia. Third-nerve palsies arise from an uncal transtentorial herniation in which the anterior medial temporal gyrus herniates into the anterior portion of the tentorial opening anterior to the adjacent midbrain. Coma may occur because of compression of the midbrain.

I-160.   **The answer is D.** *(Chap. 275)* Clinicians caring for critically ill individuals are often asked to determine prognosis after events that lead to anoxic-ischemic brain injury, including prolonged cardiac arrest, shock, and carbon monoxide poisoning. Lack of cerebral circulation for longer than 3–5 minutes most often results in at least minor permanent cerebral damage, which can be difficult to predict. In the early hours after an anoxic-ischemic event, family members often ask for guidance regarding prognosis, and the clinical examination over a period of 72 hours provides important clues to whether any meaningful recovery of cerebral function may occur. However, before performing the examination, the patient must be in a stable clinical state without medications or other clinical factors that would prevent an appropriate examination. In recent years, clinical trials have supported the use of induced hypothermia to improve neurologic outcomes after cardiac arrest, and current clinical practice is to lower body temperature to 33°C for 12–24 hours. To ensure patient comfort during induced hypothermia and prevent elevation in body temperature from shivering, the patient is heavily sedated and often paralyzed for the duration of the hypothermia and through the rewarming process. Given that this patient is hypothermic, sedated, and paralyzed, the clinical examination cannot be used to provide any prognostic information to the family at the present time.

    If the patient were not hypothermic, paralyzed, or sedated, the initial examination should assess for the presence of brainstem function to determine if brain death is present. If brainstem function was present, other clinical signs of poor prognosis in the first 1–3 days include the presence of status epilepticus, frequent myoclonus, lack of response on somatosensory evoked potentials, or a serum neuron specific enolase level greater than 33 µg/L. After 72 hours, the patient is often reassessed for the response to noxious stimuli and corneal or pupillary response. The absence of response or an extensor motor response only at this point in time predicts a 0–3% long-term likelihood of neurologic recovery.

I-161.   **The answer is C.** *(Chap. 275)* When a patient presents to the emergency department with a severe headache, the most immediately life-threatening diagnosis is SAH. The most common cause of SAH outside of trauma is rupture of a saccular aneurysm, and some patients may experience a sentinel bleed from a small rupture, providing a window of opportunity to definitively treat the aneurysm before a more substantial bleed.

The most common symptom of a SAH is a severe headache that is abrupt in onset (thunderclap headache). About 50% of individuals experience a sudden loss of consciousness caused by a rapid increase in intracranial pressure that is followed by the severe headache upon regaining consciousness. Other common characteristics associated with SAH are worsening of pain with exertion or bending forward, neck stiffness, and vomiting. In 95% of cases, blood in the subarachnoid space is visible on a noncontrasted CT scan of the head. However, if the event occurred more than 3 days previously as in this case, blood may not be seen. In this situation, the patient should undergo lumbar puncture to determine if red blood cells are present in the CSF without clearing. At this stage, the red blood cells will likely have undergone some degree of lysis with a resultant discoloration of the CSF to a characteristic yellow color called xanthochromia. The peak intensity of xanthochromia is at 48 hours, but it persists for 1–4 weeks. If the lumbar puncture demonstrates xanthochromia, then further evaluation would most likely consist of a conventional four-vessel cerebral angiography to localize the aneurysm and provide a potential method of treatment via endovascular techniques. CT angiography may be used as an alternative for localization but does not provide the opportunity for intervention. Lumbar puncture will also evaluate for meningitis and encephalitis, which are also possible in this case. Appropriate culture and polymerase chain reaction diagnostic tests should be included in the diagnostic evaluation.

I-162. **The answer is A.** *(Chap. 275)* This patient presents with an SAH caused by a ruptured anterior cerebral artery and has evidence of increased intracranial pressure with midline shift on a CT scan of the head. He has undergone aneurysm repair, and the care now should focus on the medical management of SAH. Some of the principles of the medical management of SAH include treatment of intracranial hypertension, management of blood pressure, prevention of vasospasm, and prevention of rebleeding. A patient who is unresponsive with evidence of intracranial hypertension should immediately undergo emergent ventriculostomy, which allows measurement of intracranial pressure (ICP) and can treat elevated ICP. Other strategies for treatment of elevated ICP include hyperventilation, mannitol, sedation, and hypernatremia. If a patient survives the initial aneurysmal bleed and the aneurysm is treated, the leading cause of morbidity and mortality after SAH is development of cerebral vasospasm. Vasospasms occur in about 30% of patients after SAH, typically between day 4 and 14, peaking at day 7. Efforts to prevent vasospasm include administration of nimodipine 60 mg orally every 4 hours. The mechanism of action is not clear. It may act to limit vasospasm but also likely prevents ischemia-induced cerebral injury as well. When administering the calcium channel blocker, it is important to prevent hypotension. Concurrent administration of vasopressors may be required. In addition, most patients also receive volume expansion. This therapy has commonly been known as "triple H" therapy for hypertension, hypervolemia, and hemodilution. Glucocorticoids are not used in the treatment of SAH. There is no evidence that they reduce cerebral edema or have a neuroprotective effect.

I-163. **The answer is D.** *(Chap. 275)* This patient has evidence of ICP and needs to be managed urgently. A variety of maneuvers may decrease ICP acutely. Hyperventilation causes vasoconstriction, reducing cerebral blood volume and decreasing ICP. However, this can be used only for a short period because the decrease in cerebral blood flow is of limited duration. Mannitol, an osmotic diuretic, is recommended in cases of increased ICP resulting from cytotoxic edema. Hypotonic fluids should be avoided. Instead, hypertonic saline is given to elevate sodium levels and prevent worsening of edema. A more definitive treatment to decrease ICP is to have a ventriculostomy placed by which excessive pressure can be relieved by draining CSF. Further decreases in MAP may worsen the patient's clinical status. The patient already has had more than a 20% reduction in MAP, which is the recommended reduction in cases of hypertensive emergency. In addition, the patient is exhibiting signs of increased ICP, which indicates that cerebral perfusion pressure (MAP – ICP) has been lowered. Paradoxically, the patient may need a vasopressor agent to increase MAP and thus improve cerebral perfusion. Finally, in cases of increased ICP, nitroprusside is not a recommended intravenous antihypertensive agent because it causes arterial vasodilation and may decrease cerebral perfusion pressure and worsen neurologic function.

I-164 and I-165. The answers are E and C, respectively. *(Chap. 276)* This clinical scenario describes an individual with superior vena cava (SVC) syndrome, which is an oncologic emergency. Eighty-five percent of cases of SVC syndrome are caused by either small cell or squamous cell cancer of the lung. Other causes of SVC syndrome include lymphoma, aortic aneurysm, thyromegaly, fibrosing mediastinitis, thrombosis, histoplasmosis, and Behçet's syndrome. The typical clinical presentation is dyspnea, cough, and facial and neck swelling. Symptoms are worsened by lying flat or bending forward. As the swelling progresses, it can lead to glossal and laryngeal edema with symptoms of hoarseness and dysphagia. Other symptoms can include headaches, nasal congestion, pain, dizziness, and syncope. In rare cases, seizures can occur from cerebral edema, although this is more commonly associated with brain metastases. On physical examination, dilated neck veins with collateralization on the anterior chest wall are frequently seen. There is also facial and upper extremity edema associated with cyanosis. The diagnosis of SVC syndrome is a clinical diagnosis. A pleural effusion is seen in about 25% of cases, more commonly on the right. A chest CT scan would demonstrate decreased or absent contrast in the central veins with prominent collateral circulation and would help elucidate the cause. Most commonly this would be mediastinal adenopathy or a large central tumor obstructing venous flow. The immediate treatment of SVC syndrome includes oxygen, elevation of the head of the bed, and administration of diuretics in combination with a low-sodium diet. Conservative treatment alone often provides adequate relief of symptoms and allows determination of the underlying cause of the obstruction. In this case, this would include histologic confirmation of cell type of the tumor to provide more definitive therapy. Radiation therapy is the most common treatment modality and can be used in an emergent situation if conservative treatment fails to provide relief to the patient.

I-166. **The answer is A** *(Chap. 276)* This patient presents with symptoms of spinal cord compression in the setting of known stage IV breast cancer. This represents an oncologic emergency because only 10% of patients presenting with paraplegia regain the ability to walk. Most commonly, patients develop symptoms of localized back pain and tenderness days to months before developing paraplegia. The pain is worsened by movement, cough, or sneezing. In contrast to radicular pain, the pain related to spinal cord metastases is worse with lying down. Patients presenting with back pain alone should have a careful examination to attempt to localize the lesion before development of more severe neurologic symptoms. In this patient with paraplegia, there is an definitive level at which sensation is diminished. This level is typically one to two vertebrae below the site of compression. Other findings include spasticity, weakness, and increased deep tendon reflexes. In those with autonomic dysfunction, bowel and bladder incontinence occur with decreased anal tone, absence of the anal wink and bulbocavernosus reflexes, and bladder distention. The most important initial step is the administration of high-dose intravenous corticosteroids to minimize associated swelling around the lesion and prevent paraplegia while allowing further evaluation and treatment. MRI should be performed of the entire spinal cord to evaluate for other metastatic disease that may require therapy. Although a brain MRI may be indicated in the future to evaluate for brain metastases, it is not required in the initial evaluation because the bilateral nature of the patient's symptoms and sensory level clearly indicate the spinal cord as the site of the injury. After an MRI has been performed, a definitive treatment plan can be made. Most commonly, radiation therapy is used with or without surgical decompression.

I-167 and I-168. The answers are B and E, respectively. *(Chap. 276)* Tumor lysis syndrome occurs most commonly in individuals undergoing chemotherapy for rapidly proliferating malignancies, including acute leukemias and Burkitt's lymphoma. In rare instances, it can be seen in chronic lymphoma or solid tumors. As the chemotherapeutic agents act on these cells, there is massive tumor lysis that results in release of intracellular ions and nucleic acids. This leads to a characteristic metabolic syndrome of hyperuricemia, hyperphosphatemia, hyperkalemia, and hypocalcemia. Acute kidney injury is frequent and can lead to renal failure, requiring hemodialysis if uric acid crystallizes within the renal tubules. Lactic acidosis and dehydration increase the risk of acute kidney injury. Hyperphosphatemia occurs because of the release of intracellular phosphate ions and causes a reciprocal reduction in serum calcium. This hypocalcemia can be profound, leading to neuromuscular irritability and tetany. Hyperkalemia can become rapidly life threatening and cause ventricular arrhythmia.

Knowing the characteristics of tumor lysis syndrome, one can attempt to prevent the known complications from occurring. It is important to monitor serum electrolytes very frequently during treatment. Laboratory studies should be obtained no less than three times daily, but more frequent monitoring is often needed. Allopurinol should be administered prophylactically at high doses. If allopurinol fails to control uric acid to less than 8 mg/dL, rasburicase, a recombinant urate oxidase, can be added at a dose of 0.2 mg/kg. Throughout this period, the patient should be well hydrated with alkalinization of the urine to a pH of greater than 7.0. This is accomplished by administration of intravenous normal or ½ normal saline at a dose of 3000 mL/m^2 daily with sodium bicarbonate. Prophylactic hemodialysis is not performed unless there is underlying renal failure before starting chemotherapy.

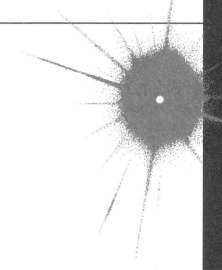

SECTION II
Nutrition

QUESTIONS

DIRECTIONS: Choose the **one best** response to each question.

II-1. What is the optimal percentage of daily caloric intake derived from carbohydrates?

A. <25%
B. 25–35%
C. 45–55%
D. 65–75%

II-2. When considering the nutritional requirements for an individual, what term is used to define the quantitative estimated nutrient intake?

A. Adequate intake
B. Dietary reference intakes
C. Estimated average requirement
D. Recommended daily allowance
E. Tolerable upper levels of nutrient intake

II-3. The resting energy expenditure is a rough estimate of total caloric needs in a state of energy balance. Of these two patients with stable weights, which person has the highest resting energy expenditure (REE): Patient A, a 40-year-old man who weighs 90 kg and is sedentary, or Patient B, a 40-year-old man who weighs 70 kg and is very active?

A. 40-year-old man who weighs 90 kg and is sedentary
B. 40-year-old man who weighs 70 kg and is very active
C. REE is the same for both patients
D. Not enough information given to calculate the REE

II-4. A new study has been published showing a benefit of 25 mg/d of vitamin X. The recommended estimated average requirement of vitamin X is 10 mg/d, two standard deviations below the amount published in the study. The tolerable upper limit of vitamin X is unknown. Your patient wants to know if it is safe to consume 25 mg/d of vitamin X. What is the most appropriate answer?

A. Two standard deviations above the estimated average requirement defines the tolerable upper limit.
B. 25 mg/d is probably too much vitamin X in 1 day.
C. 25 mg/d is statistically in a safe range of the estimated average requirement.
D. The study was not designed to assess safety and therefore should not influence practice.

II-5. A 36-year-old man is admitted from the emergency room with cellulitis of the right leg. He is homeless and is an alcoholic. He drinks a half-liter of vodka daily. He has no other significant medical history. You are concerned about his nutritional state, as he has limited caloric intake other than alcohol. Given his alcoholism and poor oral intake, he would be at risk of deficiency of all of the following vitamins EXCEPT:

A. Folate
B. Thiamine
C. Vitamin B_{12}
D. Vitamin C
E. Vitamin E

II-6. A 62-year-old man with a long-standing history of alcoholism is brought to the emergency department after being found wandering in a park without shirt or shoes in the winter. When asked about the circumstances that led to him being in the emergency room, he initially states that some men were chasing him. When you return to the room 20 minutes later, he does not recall meeting you and states that he was kicked out of his daughter's home without clothing. His daughter reports that he frequently seems confused and makes up stories all the time regarding his behavior. His only other complaint is a burning pain in his legs that is present at all times. He has no psychiatric history. He is college educated and worked as an accountant until his alcoholism led to the loss of his job. He typically drinks about 2 L of wine daily, but denies recent alcohol intake. On physical examination, he appears confused and oriented to name only. Vital signs are normal. Horizontal nystagmus is noted. He has a bilateral symmetric sensory neuropathy in a stocking-glove distribution. Deep tendon reflexes are depressed. His gait is widely based and ataxic. A fine resting tremor is present. His blood alcohol level is 0.02 g/dL. What is the most likely cause of the patient's current clinical condition?

A. Acute alcohol intoxication
B. Delirium tremens
C. Lead intoxication
D. Niacin deficiency
E. Thiamine deficiency

II-7. A 48-year-old man is diagnosed with carcinoid syndrome after presenting with diarrhea, flushing, and hypotension. With treatment, he experiences an appropriate response biochemically and with most of his symptoms; however, he continues to complain of diarrhea and mouth soreness. He also remains fatigued with a loss of appetite and irritability. On examination, you notice his tongue is bright red and somewhat enlarged, and is tender to the touch. Dermatologically, he has a red scaly rash on sun-exposed areas and around his neckline. What is the most likely vitamin or mineral deficiency in this patient?

A. Copper
B. Niacin
C. Riboflavin
D. Vitamin C
E. Zinc

II-8. Vitamin A deficiency is associated with an increased risk of which of the following?

A. Blindness
B. Mortality from dysentery
C. Mortality from malaria
D. Mortality from respiratory illness
E. All of the above

II-9. A 51-year-old alcoholic man is admitted to the hospital for upper gastrointestinal bleeding. From further history and physical examination, it becomes apparent that his bleeding is from gingival membranes. He is intoxicated and complains of fatigue. Reviewing his chart you find that he had a hemarthrosis evacuated 6 months ago and has been lost to follow-up since then. He takes no medications. Laboratory data show platelets of 250,000 and INR of 0.9. He also has a diffuse hemorrhagic eruption on his legs that is centered around hair follicles. What is the recommended treatment for this patient's underlying disorder?

A. Folate
B. Niacin
C. Thiamine
D. Vitamin C
E. Vitamin K

II-10. A 42-year-old male patient wants your opinion about vitamin E supplements. He has read that taking high doses of vitamin E can improve his sexual performance and slow the aging process. He is not vitamin E deficient. You explain to him that these claims are not based on good evidence. What other potential side effect should this patient be concerned about?

A. Deep venous thrombosis
B. Hemorrhage
C. Night blindness
D. Peripheral neuropathy
E. Retinopathy

II-11. You are seeing a pediatric patient from Djibouti in consultation who was admitted with a constellation of symptoms including diarrhea, alopecia, muscle wasting, depression, and a rash involving the face, extremities, and perineum. The child has hypogonadism and dwarfism. You astutely make the diagnosis of zinc deficiency, and laboratory tests confirm this (zinc level <70 µL/dL). What other clinical finding is this patient likely to manifest?

A. Dissecting aortic aneurysm
B. Hypochromic anemia
C. Hypoglycemia
D. Hypopigmented hair
E. Macrocytosis

II-12. When compared to kwashiorkor, which of the following statements is TRUE regarding marasmus or cachexia?

A. A diagnosis of marasmus or cachexia requires a more aggressive approach to nutritional replacement than kwashiorkor.
B. Individuals with marasmus or cachexia have a starved appearance, whereas those with kwashiorkor typically appear well nourished.
C. Marasmus and cachexia are associated with a higher risk of infection and poor wound healing compared to kwashiorkor.
D. Marasmus develops over a period of weeks, whereas kwashiorkor takes months or years to develop.
E. The albumin level is typically less than 2.8 g/dL in marasmus, but not in kwashiorkor.

II-13. Which of the following patients would be *least* likely to be at high risk of nutritional depletion?

A. A 21-year-old woman with a history of anorexia nervosa in remission for 1 year with a body mass index of 19.4 kg/m^2 admitted to the hospital with an asthma exacerbation

B. A previously healthy 28-year-old man admitted to the intensive care unit with third-degree burns covering 85% of his body surface area

C. A 32-year-old man with alcoholism admitted with acute pancreatitis who has been NPO for 6 days

D. A 41-year-old woman with short gut syndrome following resection of small bowel for a gastrointestinal stromal tumor admitted to the hospital with dehydration

E. A 55-year-old woman admitted to the hospital for right mastectomy for breast cancer who has recently lost weight from 91 kg to 79 kg unintentionally

II-14. You are caring for a 54-year-old woman in the intensive care unit who was admitted for treatment of severe sepsis and pneumonia. You would like to initiate enteral nutrition and plan to calculate basal energy expenditure for the patient. All of the following factors are used to determine the patient's caloric needs EXCEPT:

A. Age
B. Albumin
C. Gender
D. Height
E. Weight

II-15. A 19-year-old woman with anorexia nervosa undergoes surgery for acute appendicitis. The postoperative course is complicated by acute respiratory distress syndrome, and she remains intubated for 10 days. She develops wound dehiscence on postoperative day 10. Laboratory data show a white blood cell count of 4000/μL, hematocrit 35%, albumin 2.1 g/dL, total protein 5.8 g/dL, transferrin 54 mg/dL, and iron-binding capacity 88 mg/dL. You are considering initiating nutritional therapy on hospital day 11. Which of the following is true regarding the etiology and treatment of malnutrition in this patient?

A. She has marasmus and nutritional support should be started slowly.

B. She has kwashiorkor and nutritional support should be aggressive.

C. She has marasmic kwashiorkor, kwashiorkor predominant, and nutritional support should be aggressive.

D. She has marasmic kwashiorkor, marasmus predominant, and nutritional support should be slow.

II-16. After being stranded alone in the mountains for 8 days, a 26-year-old hiker is brought to the hospital for evaluation of self-amputation of his right wrist. He has not had anything to eat or drink for the past 6 days. Vital signs are within normal limits. Weight is 79.5 kg, which is 1.8 kg less than he weighed 6 months ago. His wound appears clean

and is not infected. Laboratory data show a creatinine of 2.5 mg/dL, blood urea nitrogen of 52 mg/dL, glucose 96 mg/dL, albumin 4.1 mg/dL, chloride 105 meq/L, and ferritin 173 ng/mL. Which of the following statements is true regarding his risk of malnourishment?

A. He has protein-calorie malnutrition due to the rate of weight loss.

B. He has protein-calorie malnutrition due to his elevated ferritin.

C. He is at risk, but a normal individual can tolerate 7 days of starvation.

D. He is not malnourished because he is not hypoglycemic after 6 days of no food or water.

II-17. A 65-year-old man is admitted for colectomy for stage III colon cancer. On the second postoperative day, he requires repeat exploratory laparotomy due to bleeding complications. It is now postoperative day 7 from the patient's original resection, and he has had no nutrition since prior to surgery. His body mass index prior to surgery was 28.7 kg/m^2, and he had normal nutritional status. He is clinically stable currently, but delirious and at high aspiration risk. He has bowel sounds present, and ileostomy output is good. What is recommended at the present time for this patient?

A. Continued NPO status as 5–7 days without nutritional support is acceptable for this patient

B. Initiation of a clear liquid diet supplemented with intravenous fluids with dextrose to maintain adequate intake

C. Placement of a central venous catheter and initiation of total parenteral nutrition

D. Placement of a nasogastric tube and initiation of enteral nutrition

E. Placement of a nasojejunal tube and initiation of enteral nutrition

II-18. All of the following statements regarding enteral feeding in critically ill patients are true EXCEPT:

A. Enteral feeding increases splanchnic blood flow.

B. Enteral feeding stimulates secretion of gastrointestinal hormones to promote trophic gut activity.

C. Enteral feeding stimulates IgA antibody release.

D. Enteral feeding decreases neuronal activity to the gut.

E. Seventy percent of nutrients utilized by the gut are directly derived from food within the lumen of the gut.

II-19. What body mass index is likely to be lethal in males?

A. <10 kg/m^2
B. 11 kg/m^2
C. 13 kg/m^2
D. 16 kg/m^2
E. 18.5 kg/m^2

II-20. A 43-year-old woman develops hemorrhagic pancreatitis with severe systemic inflammation response syndrome. She is intubated and sedated in the medical intensive care unit with acute respiratory distress syndrome, hypotension, and renal dysfunction. She has ongoing daily fevers to as high as 104.5°F (40.3°C). She is initiated on parenteral nutrition (PN) and develops hyperglycemia as high as 500 g/dL. She also has an increasingly positive fluid balance of more than 2 L daily. What is the most appropriate approach to management of PN in the context of this patient's hyperglycemia and fluid retention?

A. Addition of regular insulin to the PN formula
B. Limiting sodium to less than 40 meq/d
C. Limiting glucose to less than 200 g/d
D. Providing both glucose and fat to the PN mixture
E. All of the above

II-21. A 55-year-old woman with a history of diabetic gastroparesis is intubated and on mechanical ventilation after a stroke. When the patient was suctioned that morning, she coughed profusely, with thick green secretions. You are concerned about the possibility of aspiration as a cause of her worsening respiratory status. All of the following measures are useful in preventing aspiration pneumonia in an intubated patient EXCEPT:

A. Combined enteral and parenteral nutrition
B. Elevating the head of the bed to 30°
C. Feeding at a continuous rate
D. Holding feedings for gastric residuals of more than 500 mL
D. Post–ligament of Treitz feeding

II-22. All of the following statements regarding the influence of genetics on obesity are true EXCEPT:

A. Adopted children have body mass indices more similar to their biologic parents than their adoptive parents.
B. Decreased levels of leptin and resistance to leptin are associated with the development of obesity.
C. Heritability follows a Mendelian pattern.
D. Identical twins have more similar body mass indices when compared to dizygotic twins.
E. In humans with mutations of the *ob* gene, severe early-onset obesity is seen.

II-23. All of the following syndromes are associated with obesity EXCEPT:

A. Acromegaly
B. Cushing's syndrome
C. Hypothyroidism
D. Insulinoma
E. Prader-Willi syndrome

II-24. A 34-year-old woman sees her primary care physician for counseling regarding weight loss. She gained approximately 36 kg during her first pregnancy 6 years previously and has not lost this weight. Prior to that time, she maintained a weight of 70 kg at a height of 68 in (BMI 23.6 kg/m²). Her current weight is 110 kg (BMI 36.8 kg/m²). She has no medical history other than obesity. She is taking oral

contraceptive pills and does not smoke. What is the most effective strategy for weight loss in this individual?

A. A very low calorie diet (≤800 kcal/d) with a proprietary formula
B. Referral for bariatric surgery
C. A goal to attain her prepregnancy weight within 6 months
D. Initiation of an exercise plan of 150 minutes of moderate-intensity activity weekly without changing her dietary habits
E. Decrease calorie consumption by 500–1000 kcal/d to achieve a weight loss of 0.5–1 kg per week

II-25. A 44-year-old woman seeks evaluation for bariatric surgery. She has tried a variety of diets in the past, but failed to sustain weight loss. She is being treated for hypertension and hypercholesterolemia, and is concerned about developing diabetes mellitus if she does not lose weight. Her height is 65 in and weight is 122 kg (BMI 44.6 kg/m²). What advice would you provide her regarding the benefits and risks of bariatric surgical procedures?

A. A restrictive surgery is as effective as a restrictive-malabsorptive surgery.
B. A vertical-banded gastroplasty is the most effective restrictive surgical procedure.
C. All types of bariatric surgery are associated with micronutrient deficiencies that require lifelong supplementation.
D. The mean weight loss following bariatric surgery is 30–35%, and 60% of individuals are able to maintain weight loss at 6 years.
E. The mortality associated with bariatric surgery is about 2%.

II-26. A 21-year-old woman is evaluated for low body weight. The woman's concerned mother brought her to clinic, but the patient herself states that she is comfortable with her body weight and that she would be happier if she lost an additional 2–5 kg. She had a normal childhood and development. She has always been a high-achieving student and is currently enrolled in an honors program at her university. She has been on the dean's list each semester and will graduate with a dual degree in political science and international business in 6 months. When she enrolled in college, she had a height of 64 in and a weight of 57 kg (BMI 21.5 kg/m²). She had initially joined a sorority, but she no longer participates and states that she is more focused on her studies at this point. She is not in a romantic relationship and denies depression or anxiety. She has grown an additional inch since enrolling in college, and her current weight is 58 kg (BMI 17.5 kg/m²). She denies excessive dieting, but states that she controls her diet carefully. She reports daily exercise, stating that she runs or bikes for 60–120 minutes daily, and she feels this is an important stress release for her. She reports a normal diet and that she will occasionally eat an entire pizza or quart of ice cream when stressed. She denies purging. She cannot recall when her last menstrual period occurred, but states that these have been irregular throughout her life. On physical examination, the patient is wearing a sweater despite the outdoor temperature being more than 80°F. Her vital signs are BP 95/60, HR 58 bpm, RR 16/min, and oxygen saturation 99% on room air, and she is afebrile. She has salivary gland enlargement and soft, downy hair on her arms and chest. What is the most likely diagnosis?

A. Anorexia nervosa
B. Binge eating disorder
C. Bulimia nervosa
D. Hyperthyroidism
E. Patient is healthy and without a diagnosable medical condition

II-27. The patient in question II-26 undergoes an extensive laboratory evaluation prior to treatment. Her basic metabolic panel shows sodium of 132 meq/L, potassium 3.1 meq/L, chloride 94 meq/L, bicarbonate 28 meq/L, BUN 24 mg/dL, and creatinine 1.2 mg/dL. She also has an endocrine workup, which demonstrates a TSH of 0.4 μIU/mL, T_3 42 ng/mL, T_4 5.0 ng/mL, free T_4 0.8 ng/dL, and serum cortisol at 0800 of 28 μg/dL. Bone densitometry has a T-score of −2.7 at the hip and lumbar spine. What is the most appropriate treatment for this patient?

A. Alendronate 70 mg weekly plus combined estrogen/progesterone oral contraceptive pills
B. Doxepin 75 mg daily
C. Levothyroxine 50 μg daily
D. Psychological evaluation and treatment combined with supervised meals
E. All of the above

II-28. Which characteristic is more common in binge eating disorder than bulimia nervosa?

A. Frequent loss of control while eating, leading to consumption of large amounts of food in a short period of time
B. Higher prevalence in men compared to women
C. Obesity
D. Presence of menstrual cycle
E. Self-induced vomiting

II-29. You diagnose anorexia nervosa in one of your new clinic patients. When coordinating a treatment program with the psychiatrist, what characteristics would prompt consideration for inpatient treatment instead of scheduling an outpatient assessment?

A. Amenorrhea
B. Exaggeration of food intake
C. Irrational fear of gaining weight
D. Purging behavior
E. Weight <75% of expected body weight

II-30. You are counseling a patient who is recovering from long-standing anorexia nervosa (AN). She is a 22-year-old woman who suffered the effects of AN for 8 years with a nadir body mass index of 17 kg/m² and many laboratory abnormalities during that time. What characteristic of AN is least likely to improve despite successful lasting treatment of the disorder?

A. Amenorrhea
B. Delayed gastric emptying
C. Lanugo
D. Low bone mass
E. Salivary gland enlargement

II-31. An 80-year-old woman is evaluated for a complaint of involuntary weight loss. Her baseline weight at her clinic visit 6 months ago was 67 kg. She reports that her appetite began to decrease about 2 months ago when she noticed that food no longer had the same taste. Her daughter accompanies her to the visit and reports that her mother seems increasingly listless and withdrawn. Her daughter also notes that her mother seems more forgetful, and her home has become disorganized. The patient has a history of hypertension and peripheral vascular disease. She had a transient ischemic attack 6 years ago, but has never had a stroke. There have been no recent changes to any medications. Her weight in the clinic today is 60 kg. What is the appropriate approach for the evaluation of this patient's weight loss?

A. Ask the patient to return to the clinic in 1 month for repeat weight evaluation.
B. Order thyroid function tests.
C. Perform a Mini-Mental State Examination.
D. Reassure the patient and her daughter that this degree of weight loss is not abnormal.
E. Both B and C are correct.

ANSWERS

II-1.   **The answer is C.** *(Chap. 73)* Carbohydrates comprise the greatest percentage of calories in the diet as they are the major fuel source for the brain and most tissues. The brain requires 100 g/d of glucose, with the rest of the body requiring about 50 g/d of glucose. Although glucose can be derived from proteolysis or fats, carbohydrates remain the primary energy source of the body and should comprise 45–55% of the total caloric intake. Fats should comprise no more than 30% of caloric intake, and proteins typically should comprise about 15%.

II-2. **The answer is B.** *(Chap. 73)* Dietary reference intakes (DRIs) have supplanted the recommended daily allowances (RDAs) as the benchmark recommendations for determining nutrient intake in clinical practice. The RDAs outline the average intake that will meet the nutrient needs of nearly all healthy individuals of a specific age, life stage, sex, or physiologic condition. In contrast, the DRIs take a more comprehensive approach and also consider the estimated average requirement, adequate intake, and upper tolerable limit of intake. The estimated average intake is the amount of a nutrient estimated to meet the nutrient needs for half of the healthy individuals of a specific sex and age. Because this is a median value, it is generally not acceptable to set the estimated average intake as the benchmark for intake as, by definition, 50% of individuals would require more of the specific nutrient compared to this value. As stated above, the RDA is an estimated intake that would meet the nutrient needs of almost all healthy individuals and is defined as being two standard deviations above the estimated average requirement. Adequate intake is used in the place of RDAs when estimated average requirements are unable to be determined, thus preventing the calculation of an RDA. Adequate intake is determined based on observed or experimentally determined approximations of nutrient needs and is used for infants up to 1 year old, as well as for many minerals including calcium, manganese, chromium, and fluoride, among others. The tolerable upper limit of nutrient intake is the highest level of daily nutrient intake that is unlikely to cause adverse health effects. In many cases, there are insufficient data to determine a tolerable upper limit.

II-3. **The answer is B.** *(Chap. 73)* For patients with stable weights, REE can be calculated if the gender, weight, and activity level are provided. For males, REE = 900 + 10w, and for females, REE = 700 + 7w, where w is weight in kilograms. The REE is then adjusted for activity level by multiplying by 1.2 for sedentary, 1.4 for moderately active, and 1.8 for very active individuals. Patient A has an REE of 2160 kcal/d. Patient B has an REE of 2880 kcal/d. For a given weight, a higher level of activity increases the REE more than a 20-kg change in weight at a given level of activity.

II-4. **The answer is C.** *(Chap. 73)* The estimated average requirement (EAR) is the amount of a nutrient estimated to be adequate for half of the individuals of a specific age and sex. It is not useful clinically for estimating nutritional adequacy because it is a median requirement for a group: 50% of the individuals in a group fall below the requirement and 50% fall above it. A person taking the EAR of a vitamin has a 50% risk of inadequate intake. The recommended daily allowance (RDA) is defined statistically as two standard deviations above the EAR to ensure that the needs of most individuals are met. In this case the study used a dosage of two standard deviations above the EAR, which would be the RDA. Data on the tolerable upper limit of a vitamin are usually inadequate to establish a value for the upper limit of tolerability. The absence of a published tolerable upper limit does not imply that the risks are nonexistent.

II-5. **The answer is E.** *(Chap. 74)* Deficiencies of many vitamins and minerals are rare in developed countries except in individuals with alcoholism or chronic illness. Alcoholism in general is associated with decreased intake of nutrients and may be associated with malabsorption or impaired storage. Common vitamin deficiencies in those with alcoholism include thiamine and folate. Other vitamins that may be deficient in alcoholics are niacin, vitamin B$_6$, vitamin C, and vitamin A. Vitamin B12 deficiency is uncommon as the vitamin is widely available in the food supply. It can be found in meats, nuts, and cereal grains, and in low levels in fruits and vegetables. Dietary deficiency of vitamin E does not occur, and deficiency is found only in individuals with prolonged fat malabsorption or genetic abnormalities of vitamin E metabolism or transport.

II-6. **The answer is E.** *(Chap. 74)* Thiamine (vitamin B$_1$) is a water-soluble vitamin found in yeast, organ meat, pork, legumes, whole grains, beef, and nuts. It is generally more common in those with rice-based diets as rice contains little thiamine. In Western diets, the most common cause of thiamine deficiency is alcoholism and chronic illness. Alcohol interferes with the absorption of thiamine and with the synthesis of thiamine pyrophosphate. When thiamine deficiency is possible, one must take care to replenish thiamine whenever carbohydrates are administered, as failure to do so can precipitate lactic acidosis. Thiamine deficiency in its earliest stages produces anorexia and nonspecific symptoms. Prolonged deficiency results in beriberi, which is often characterized as wet or dry. In patients with wet beriberi, cardiovascular symptoms predominate with findings including cardiomegaly, tachycardia, and high-output heart failure. In dry beriberi, the symptoms are primarily neurologic with symmetric peripheral sensory and motor neuropathy, and diminished reflexes. Alcoholics also commonly have central nervous system findings that are frequently underdiagnosed and are attributed to the alcoholism. Wernicke encephalopathy manifests as horizontal nystagmus, ophthalmoplegia, cerebellar ataxia, and mental impairment. When memory loss and confabulation are present, the syndrome is known as Wernicke-Korsakoff syndrome.

II-7.   **The answer is B.** (*Chap. 74*) Niacin (vitamin B_3) has high bioavailability from beans, milk, meat, and eggs. Although the bioavailability from grains is lower, most flour is enriched with "free" niacin; thus deficiency of niacin is rare in Western diets. Niacin deficiency can be found in individuals with corn-based diets in some parts of China, Africa, and India; individuals with alcoholism; and individuals with genetic defects limiting the absorption of tryptophan. In addition, individuals with carcinoid syndrome are at increased risk of niacin deficiency because of an increased conversion of tryptophan to serotonin. Clinically, the syndrome of niacin deficiency is known as pellagra. Early symptoms of niacin deficiency are loss of appetite, generalized weakness, abdominal pain, and vomiting. Glossitis is characteristic of pellagra with a beefy red tongue. Pellagra also has many dermatologic manifestations including a characteristic skin rash appearing on sun-exposed areas. The rash is scaling and erythematous. The rash often forms a ring around the neck. The four *d's* of niacin deficiency—diarrhea, dermatitis, dementia, and death—are seen only in the most severe cases.

II-8.   **The answer is E.** (*Chap. 74*) Vitamin A, also known as retinol, is a fat-soluble vitamin that has biologically active metabolites, retinaldehyde, and retinoic acid, which are all important for good health. Collectively, these molecules are known as retinoids and are important for normal vision, cell growth and differentiation, and immunity. Vitamin A is found in its preformed state in liver, fish, and eggs, and it is often consumed as carotenoids from dark green and deeply colored fruits and vegetables. In developing countries, chronic vitamin A deficiency is endemic in many areas and is the most common cause of preventable blindness. In milder stages, vitamin A deficiency causes night blindness and conjunctival xerosis. This can progress to keratomalacia and blindness. Given the broad biologic functions of vitamin A, however, deficiency at any stage increases the risk of mortality from diarrhea, dysentery, measles, malaria, and respiratory disease. Vitamin A supplementation has been demonstrated to decrease childhood mortality by 23–34%.

II-9.   **The answer is D.** (*Chap. 74*) This patient has the classic perifollicular hemorrhagic rash of scurvy (vitamin C deficiency). In the United States, scurvy is primarily a disease of alcoholics and the elderly who consume less than 10 mg/d of vitamin C. In addition to nonspecific symptoms of fatigue, these patients also have impaired ability to form mature connective tissue and can bleed into various sites, including the skin and gingiva. A normal INR excludes symptomatic vitamin K deficiency. Thiamine, niacin, and folate deficiencies are also seen in patients with alcoholism. Thiamine deficiency may cause a peripheral neuropathy (beriberi). Folate deficiency causes macrocytic anemia and thrombocytopenia. Niacin deficiency causes pellagra, which is characterized by glossitis and a pigmented, scaling rash that may be particularly noticeable in sun-exposed areas.

II-10.   **The answer is B.** (*Chap. 74*) High doses of vitamin E (>800 mg/d) may reduce platelet aggregation and interfere with vitamin K metabolism. Doses greater than 400 mg/d may increase mortality from any cause. Vitamin E excess is not related to an increased risk of venous thrombosis. Peripheral neuropathy and a pigmented retinopathy may be seen in vitamin E deficiency. Vitamin A deficiency is a cause of night blindness.

II-11.   **The answer is D.** (*Chap. 74*) Hypozincemia is most commonly due to poor oral intake of zinc, although some medications can also inhibit zinc absorption (e.g., sodium valproate, penicillamine, ethambutol). Severe chronic zinc deficiency has been described among children from Middle Eastern countries as a cause of hypogonadism and dwarfism. Hypopigmented hair is also a part of this syndrome. Hypochromic anemia can be seen in a number of vitamin deficiency/excess disorders, including zinc toxicity and copper deficiency. Copper deficiency is also associated with dissecting aortic aneurysm. Hypoglycemia does not correlate with hypozincemia. Macrocytosis is associated with folate and vitamin B_{12} deficiency.

II-12.   **The answer is B.** *(Chap. 75)* Marasmus and cachexia both represent forms of prolonged starvation with decreased energy intake. The primary difference between marasmus and cachexia is that the starvation in marasmus is related to decreased caloric intake, whereas in cachexia the poor energy is relative and is associated with a chronic inflammatory state. Other than the cause of malnutrition, marasmus and cachexia have common features when compared to kwashiorkor, or protein-calorie malnutrition. Marasmus and cachexia develop over a course of months to years, resulting in an individual who appears starved with a weight less than 80% for height. In addition, there is evidence of muscle and fat wasting with decreased triceps skinfold and midarm muscle circumference. On laboratory examination, there are often few abnormalities. The albumin may be low, but does not fall below 2.8 g/dL in uncomplicated cases. The only finding may be a low creatinine-to-height index when the 24-hour urine creatinine is low (<60%) for normal values based on height. Despite the starved appearance, individuals with marasmus or cachexia are immunocompetent and are able to respond reasonably well to short-term stresses. As this is a chronic illness, the approach to treatment should be cautious support of nutritional needs. Overly aggressive nutritional repletion can lead to overfeeding syndromes and life-threatening hypophosphatemia. The oral and enteral routes are the preferred methods for improving nutrition.

In contrast, kwashiorkor, or protein-calorie malnutrition (PCM), occurs acutely over the course of weeks. In developed countries, the most common of PCM is acute, life-threatening illness such as trauma or sepsis. Pathophysiologically, the stresses of the acute illness lead to increased protein and calorie needs at a time when intake is often limited. Early in the course of PCM, the patient usually looks well nourished, so a high index of suspicion is required. Signs of PCM include edema, poor wound healing, easy hair pluckability, and skin breakdown. In addition, severe PCM is reflected in low levels of albumin, transferrin, or iron-binding capacity. Cellular immune function is decreased, and lymphopenia may be seen. Aggressive nutritional support is required to reverse the disorder, although mortality remains high.

II-13.   **The answer is A.** *(Chap. 75)* Several factors can help identify an individual who is at high risk of nutritional depletion upon hospital admission. The first factor to consider is the body mass index (BMI) and recent weight loss. If a patient is underweight (BMI <18.5 kg/m²) or has recently lost more than 10% of body weight, this would confer increased nutritional risk. Other general categories that increase nutritional risk include poor intake, excessive nutrient losses, hypermetabolic states, alcoholism, or medications that increase metabolic requirements. Poor oral intake can be related to current anorexia, food avoidance, or NPO status for more than 5 days, among others. Examples of excessive nutrient loss include malabsorption syndromes, enteric fistulae, draining wounds, or renal dialysis. Common hypermetabolic states are trauma, burns, sepsis, and prolonged febrile illness. The patient with anorexia in remission and a normal BMI would be least likely among these patients to have excessive nutritional risk.

II-14.   **The answer is B.** *(Chap. 75)* A patient's basal energy expenditure (BEE) can be calculated using the Harris-Benedict equation. The factors that are used for determining BEE are age, gender, height, and weight. The BEE for hospitalized patients is then adjusted by a factor of 1.1–1.4 depending on the severity of illness, with the highest values used for patients admitted with marked stress such as trauma or severe sepsis. The BEE serves as an estimate only. If it is important to have an exact calculation of energy expenditure, indirect calorimetry can be performed. Protein needs can also be calculated more definitively by the use of urine urea nitrogen (UUN) as an estimate of protein catabolism.

II-15.   **The answer is C.** *(Chap. 75)* The two major types of protein energy malnutrition are marasmus and kwashiorkor; differentiating the two is extremely important in the malnourished patient because it directly affects the choice of therapy. This patient has marasmic kwashiorkor due to the impact of her anorexia nervosa, the acute stressor of the surgery, and the 10 days of starvation. This patient has chronic starvation (marasmus) as well as the major sine qua non of kwashiorkor (i.e., reduced levels of serum proteins). She is kwashiorkor predominant because of the acute starvation and the severely low levels of serum proteins. Vigorous nutritional therapy is indicated for kwashiorkor.

II-16.   **The answer is C.** *(Chap. 75)* The energy stores in a healthy 70-kg man include approximately 15 kg as fat, 6 kg as protein, and 500 mg as glycogen. During the first day of a fast, most energy needs are met by consumption of liver glycogen. During longer fasting, resting energy expenditure will decrease by up to 25% (provided there is no ongoing inflammation). In the presence of water intake and no inflammation, a normal individual may fast for months. A well-nourished individual can tolerate approximately 7 days of starvation while experiencing a systemic response to inflammation. The hiker in this scenario has starved for 6 days and, except for mild acute renal failure, he has compensated well for his starvation. Greater than 10% weight loss in 6 months represents significant protein-calorie malnutrition. This person's ferritin is only mildly elevated, although a true systemic response to inflammation (SRI) does increase the rate of lean tissue loss. Moreover, there are no other indicators that he is experiencing the systemic inflammatory response syndrome (SIRS). SRI often causes hyperglycemia, not hypoglycemia.

II-17.   **The answer is E.** *(Chap. 76)* This patient would have at least a moderate systemic response to inflammation (SRI), as would be expected in the postoperative period. In such a situation, individuals benefit from adequate feeding by day 5–7. Picking the appropriate nutritional support should take into account the patient's overall clinical course. Generally, the enteral route is preferred to promote the ongoing health and immunologic barrier function of the gut, as long as there are no contraindications. Parenteral nutrition alone is generally only indicated for prolonged ileus, obstruction, or hemorrhagic pancreatitis. As this patient has bowel sounds and evidence of ileostomy output, he is not exhibiting ileus at the present time. Thus, enteral nutrition would be used. Given his delirium and aspiration risk, he should not be initiated on an oral diet, and nasogastric feeding is also contraindicated, as it is associated with a higher aspiration risk. The preferred feeding method would be the use of a nasojejunal feeding tube placed post–ligament of Treitz.

II-18.   **The answer is D.** *(Chap. 76)* When possible, at least a portion of the nutritional support given to a critically ill patient should be in the form of enteral nutrition. Use of the enteral route is particularly important for maintaining the overall health of the gastrointestinal tract. Seventy percent of the nutrients utilized by the bowel and its associated digestive organs are directly derived from food within the bowel lumen. Moreover, enteral feedings are important for maintaining the immunologic function of the gut as they stimulate the secretion of IgA and hormones to promote trophic activity of the gut. In addition, enteral feedings improve splanchnic blood flow and stimulate neuronal activity to prevent ischemia and ileus.

II-19.   **The answer is C.** *(Chap. 76)* It is important to understand the thresholds of body mass index (BMI) that indicate malnutrition. Normal BMI ranges between 20 and 25 kg/m², and a patient is considered underweight with likely moderate malnutrition at a BMI of 18.5 kg/m². Severe malnutrition is expected with a BMI of less than 16 kg/m². In men, a BMI of less than 13 kg/m² is lethal, and in women, the lethal BMI is less than 11 kg/m².

II-20.   **The answer is E.** *(Chap. 76)* The two most common problems with the use of parenteral nutrition (PN) are fluid retention and hyperglycemia. The fluid retention is greater than would be expected by the volume of PN and is linked to the hyperglycemia. The dextrose provided by PN is hypertonic and stimulates greater insulin secretion than is generated by meal feeding. Insulin itself has antinatriuretic and antidiuretic properties that exacerbate fluid and sodium retention. Strategies to minimize fluid and sodium retention include providing both glucose and fat as energy sources and limiting sodium intake to less than 40 meq daily. In addition, it is best to initiate feeding with less than 200 g glucose/day to assess glucose tolerance. Regular insulin can be added to the PN formula to maintain glycemic control. In addition to providing insulin with the PN formula, additional subcutaneous insulin may be given based on a sliding scale every 6 hours with about two-thirds of the total dose given during a 24-hour period added to the PN formula the next day. In more severe cases, intensive insulin support with a separate infusion of insulin should be used. If a patient has known insulin-dependent diabetes mellitus, the dose of insulin required is usually twice the usual outpatient dosage.

II-21.   **The answer is D.** *(Chap. 75)* Initiating enteral support is important in the critically ill, but does not come without complications. Tube malposition and aspiration are two of the most common complications of enteral feeding in the intensive care unit (ICU). Many patients in the ICU have delayed gastric emptying and also have alterations in mental status that increase the baseline risk of aspiration. This is further worsened in individuals who are intubated for mechanical ventilation. The act of suctioning alone induces coughing and gastric regurgitation. Endotracheal tubes are poor barriers to aspiration and may make aspiration worse by transiting across the vocal cords and epiglottis, two of the normal preventive mechanisms against aspiration. In the care of the ICU patient, measures should be taken to minimize the risk of aspiration. A primary measure is to keep the head of the bed elevated to more than 30°. In patients who are having difficulty tolerating full enteral nutrition, combining enteral and parenteral nutrition should be considered. Utilizing nurse-directed algorithms for formula advancement based on gastric residuals and patient tolerance is also important. Generally, feeding should not be held unless the residual is greater than 300 mL. Finally, the use of nasojejunal feeding tubes placed post–ligament of Treitz is a recent strategy to decrease the risk of aspiration. Neither nasogastric nor nasoduodenal tubes decrease the risk of aspiration.

II-22.   **The answer is C.** *(Chap. 77)* In 2007-2008, the National Health and Nutrition Examination Surveys (NHANES) found that 68% of the adult population of the United States was overweight or obese [body mass index (BMI) >25 kg/m^2]. Understanding the worsening of obesity in the United States requires understanding both the genetic and environmental factors that contribute to the development of obesity. It is clear that the rapid increase in obesity in the this county is far greater than can be attributed to changes in genetics. However, certain genetic factors certainly increase the risk of obesity. Obesity generally is inherited in a non-Mendelian pattern similar to that of height. Adopted children have BMIs more closely related to their biologic parents than their adopted parents. Likewise, monozygotic twins have BMIs more similar than dizygotic twins. Some of the genes that are known to play a role in the development of obesity include genes for leptin, proopiomelanocortin (POMC), and melanin-concentrating hormone, among others. Leptin is an important hormone in obesity. Produced by adipocytes, this hormone acts at the hypothalamus to decrease appetite and increase energy expenditure. In humans, mutations of the *ob* gene lead to decreased leptin production, and mutations of the *db* gene cause leptin resistance. The result of these mutations can be either decreased leptin production or resistance to leptin, which causes failure of the brain to recognize satiety. These mutations are generally associated with severe obesity beginning shortly after birth.

II-23.   **The answer is A.** *(Chap. 77)* Several syndromes have been recognized as being associated with the development of obesity. Prader-Willi syndrome falls into a category of syndromes of obesity associated with mental retardation. Individuals with Prader-Willi syndrome are of short stature with small hands and feet. They exhibit hyperphagia, obesity, and neurodevelopmental delay in association with hypogonadotropic hypogonadism. Endocrine abnormalities or abnormalities of the hypothalamus are also commonly associated with obesity. Patients with Cushing's syndrome have central obesity, hypertension, and glucose intolerance. Hypothyroidism is associated with obesity due to decreases in metabolic rate; however, it is a rare cause of obesity. Individuals with insulinoma often are obese, as they increase their caloric intake to try to prevent hypoglycemia episodes. Finally, individuals with hypothalamic dysfunction due to craniopharyngioma or other disorders lack the ability to respond to typical hormonal signals that indicate satiety, and therefore develop obesity. Acromegaly is not associated with obesity.

II-24.   **The answer is E.** *(Chap. 78)* With over 60% of the U.S. population being overweight or obese, the primary care physician should be monitoring weight and BMI at every visit and making recommendations for weight loss to prevent long-term complications of obesity, including hypertension, hypercholesterolemia, and diabetes mellitus. Despite the very simple concept that energy output needs to be greater than caloric intake, it is very difficult for individuals to achieve and sustain weight loss. One initial factor that predisposes an individual to fail at attempts to lose weight is failure to understand what is a reasonable goal and time frame for weight loss. The initial target for weight loss should be about 10% over 6 months. In this patient, that would be an approximately 24- to 25-lb weight loss over 6 months. She would not realistically be able to achieve her prepregnancy weight of 70 kg for at least 18–24 months. Many individuals find diet therapy difficult to sustain for an extended period, especially when a specific and limited diet is prescribed. It is more important for the individual to think of the dietary changes that occur concurrently with weight loss as a lifestyle change. To achieve a weight loss of 0.5–1 kg weekly, caloric intake needs to decrease by about 500–1000 kcal daily. The specific dietary intervention to undertake depends on personal factors. Studies show that low-carbohydrate, high-protein diets (Atkins, South Beach, etc.) lead to greater weight loss, improved satiety, and decreased coronary disease risk factors in the short term, but at 12 months there is no difference among diets. Very low calorie diets (≤800 kcal/d) are a very aggressive form of dietary therapy with proprietary formulas. These diets are designed to cause weight loss of 13–23 kg over a 3- to 6-month period and should be utilized only in individuals with obesity and medical comorbidities for whom conservative approaches have failed. In combination with dietary changes, it should also be recommended that individuals begin an exercise program. Although exercise alone can lead to some weight loss, it should not be the only strategy for losing weight. The recommended amount of physical activity is 150 minutes of moderate-intensity activity or 75 minutes of high-intensity activity weekly. Pharmacotherapy for obesity can be considered in individuals with a BMI greater than 30 kg/m^2. However, options for pharmacotherapy are limited at the present time. Many new medications are undergoing clinical trials and may play a role in weight loss in the future. Bariatric surgery should not be considered unless conservative strategies for weight loss have failed.

II-25.   **The answer is D.** (*Chap. 78*) Bariatric surgery should be considered for individuals who have a BMI of 40 kg/m^2 or greater, or a BMI of 35.0 kg/m^2 or greater if there are serious comorbid medical conditions including diabetes mellitus, hypertension, or hypercholesterolemia. Surgical weight loss therapy achieves weight loss through reducing the capability for calorie intake and may also cause malabsorption depending on the procedure chosen. There are two broad categories of weight loss procedures: restrictive and restrictive-malabsorptive. Restrictive surgeries decrease the size of the stomach to generate feelings of early satiety. The original procedure was the vertical-banded gastroplasty, but this procedure has been abandoned due to lack of effectiveness in long-term trials. It has been replaced by laparoscopic adjustable silicone gastric banding (LASGB). With this type of bariatric surgery, there is a subcutaneous reservoir into which saline can be injected or removed to change the size of the gastric opening. Restrictive-malabsorptive procedures include the Roux-en-Y gastric bypass, biliopancreatic diversion, and biliopancreatic diversion with duodenal switch. The Roux-en-Y procedure is the most common bypass procedure. The average weight loss following bariatric surgery is 30–35% of total body weight, and 60% of individuals are able to maintain this at 5 years. The restrictive-malabsorptive procedures achieve greater weight loss than restrictive procedures. Moreover, bariatric procedures lead to improvement in obesity-related comorbid conditions. The overall mortality rate from bariatric surgery is less than 1%, but increases with age and comorbid conditions. Approximately 5–15% of individuals develop stomal stenosis or marginal ulcers following the surgery that present as prolonged nausea and vomiting. Malabsorption does not occur following restrictive procedures. Individuals who have restrictive-malabsorptive procedures have an increased risk for micronutrient deficiency including vitamin B$_{12}$, iron, folate, calcium, and vitamin D. Lifelong supplementation of these vitamins will be required.

II-26 and II-27.   **The answers are A and D, respectively.** (*Chap. 79*) The patient in this scenario meets the criteria for the diagnosis of anorexia nervosa (AN). AN has a lifetime prevalence of about 1% in women. Although less common in males, the prevalence is rising in men as well. AN has a typical onset in late adolescence and young adulthood, although younger girls are being diagnosed as well. The etiology of AN is not known, although individuals with AN often have similar personality characteristics, with a tendency to more obsessional and perfectionist behavior. Patients with AN have an abnormal body image with an irrational fear of weight gain, despite being underweight. Weight loss is seen as a fulfilling accomplishment, and individuals with AN will have markedly decreased caloric intake and also excessive exercise. Despite this, those with AN will not complain of hunger. Although classically associated with bulimia nervosa, binge eating occurs in 25–50% of those with AN. As patients with AN become more obsessed with the eating disorder, they will become more socially isolated with an increased focus on exercise, dieting, and studying. Patients with AN often do not think they have a problem and only seek evaluation after pressure from family and friends. Amenorrhea is one of the diagnostic criteria. On physical examination, the patient will generally be underweight for height. Vital signs may show bradycardia and hypotension. Lanugo hair, acrocyanosis, and edema may be seen. Salivary gland enlargement may lead to a fullness of the face despite the overall starved appearance. On laboratory examination, anemia and leukopenia are common. The basic metabolic panel often demonstrates hyponatremia and hypokalemia with a metabolic alkalosis. BUN and creatinine may be slightly elevated despite the low muscle mass. Endocrine abnormalities are very common on laboratory examination and reflect hypothalamic dysfunction. Thyroid studies show a pattern characteristic of sick euthyroid syndrome [low thyroid-stimulating hormone (TSH), low T_4, low T_3, and elevated reverse T_3]. Gonadotropin-releasing hormone (GnRH) secretion is very low and associated with low levels of follicle-stimulating hormone (FSH) and luteinizing hormone (LH). Given the generally stressed state of the body, however, serum and urine cortisol may be elevated.

The primary treatment of AN requires intensive psychotherapy under the care of an experienced psychologist or psychiatrist along with careful medical follow-up. The goal of treatment is to restore body weight to 90% of predicted body weight or higher. For patients with significant electrolyte abnormalities or body weight less than 75% predicted, inpatient treatment is recommended. Nutrition is primarily accomplished through oral feeding. The initial caloric intake goal is about 1200–1800 kcal/d with close follow-up to observe for evidence of refeeding syndrome. The weight gain goal is 1–2 kg weekly with advancement of caloric goal to 3000–4000 kcal/d. As many patients resist weight gain and lie about oral intake, supervised mealtimes are required in both inpatient and outpatient settings. As part of therapy, individuals must confront issues with body image. No psychotropic medications have been demonstrated to improve outcomes in AN. Appetite stimulants also have no role in the treatment of AN. Doxepin is a tricyclic antidepressant that has mild appetite-stimulating properties; however, it has not been trialed in AN and has side effects that include prolongation of the QT interval and should be avoided. The endocrine abnormalities do not have to be treated either, as these cortisol and thyroid hormone levels will correct with adequate nutrition. Patients should receive calcium and vitamin D supplementation, but estrogens have no benefit on bone density in underweight patients. Bisphosphonates can yield improvements in bone density, but the risks of therapy in young individuals are felt to outweigh the benefits.

II-28.   **The answer is C.** *(Chap. 79)* Binge-eating disorder has a higher lifetime prevalence than bulimia nervosa or anorexia nervosa at about 4%. Although more men suffer from binge-eating disorder than other types of eating disorders, women with binge-eating disorder still outnumber men 2:1. Binge-eating disorder and bulimia nervosa share the common characteristic of episodes of eating a large amount of food in a short period of time with a feeling that the eating behavior is out of control. However, patients with binge-eating disorder do not exhibit inappropriate behaviors such as self-induced vomiting or the use of laxatives as a means to control the binge eating. Both binge-eating disorder and bulimia nervosa are associated with the presence of normal menstrual cycles in women. Individuals with binge-eating disorder are more likely to be obese and also have higher rates of anxiety and depression.

II-29.   **The answer is E.** *(Chap. 79)* Based on the American Psychiatric Association's practice guidelines, inpatient treatment or partial hospitalization is indicated for patients whose weight is less than 75% of expected for age and height, who have severe metabolic disturbances (e.g., electrolyte disturbances, bradycardia, hypotension), or who have serious concomitant psychiatric problems (e.g., suicidal ideation, substance abuse). There should be a low threshold for inpatient treatment if there has been rapid weight loss or if weight is less than 80% of expected. Amenorrhea, exaggeration of food intake, and fear of gaining weight are part of the diagnostic criteria for AN, and purging is not uncommon in this population. Weight restoration to 90% of predicted weight is the goal of nutritional therapy.

II-30.   **The answer is D.** *(Chap. 79)* Approximately 25–50% of patients with anorexia nervosa (AN) recover fully with few physiologic or psychological sequelae. However, many patients have persistent difficulties with weight maintenance, depression, and eating disturbances. Approximately 5% of patients with AN die per decade, usually due to the physical effects of chronic starvation or from suicide. Virtually all of the physiologic derangements associated with AN will improve with weight gain. One exception is the loss of bone mass, which may not recover fully when AN occurs during adolescence (i.e., during peak bone mass formation). Psychological health also improves with successful treatment, although these patients remain at risk for depression, recurrence, and development of bulimia nervosa.

II-31.   **The answer is E.** *(Chap. 80)* Involuntary weight loss (IWL) is a frequent finding in older individuals, affecting more than 25% of frail individuals older than 65 years. Clinically important weight loss is defined as a loss of more than 5% of body weight or more than 5 kg over the course of 6–12 months. In older individuals, weight loss is associated with hip fracture, pressure ulcers, decreased functional status, and death. There are many causes of IWL, with the most common categories being malignancy, chronic inflammatory or infectious disease, metabolic disorders, and psychiatric disorders. In older individuals, it is also important to consider neurologic disorders, including stroke leading to dysphagia, progressive vision loss, and dementia. IWL can be one of the earliest manifestations of Alzheimer's disease. An under-recognized cause of IWL is lack of access to food or inability to pay for food. When evaluating an individual for IWL, a complete physical examination, including a dental examination, should be performed to assess for obvious physical causes that would lead to weight loss. Medications may also lead to changes in appetite or weight loss. Patients should undergo age-appropriate cancer screening. In older individuals, a Mini-Mental State Examination, Mini-Nutritional Assessment, and assessment of performance of activities of daily living may be helpful. It may also be useful to observe the patient's eating. Depression in the elderly may also present with loss of appetite and should be assessed. Laboratory studies could include a complete blood count, comprehensive metabolic panel, thyroid function tests, and erythrocyte sedimentation rate and C-reactive protein. HIV testing is indicated if risk factors are identified.

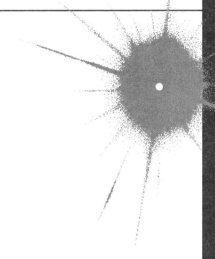

SECTION III
Oncology and Hematology

QUESTIONS

DIRECTIONS: Choose the **one best** response to each question.

III-1. For each patient choose the most likely peripheral blood smear:

(See Figure III-1)

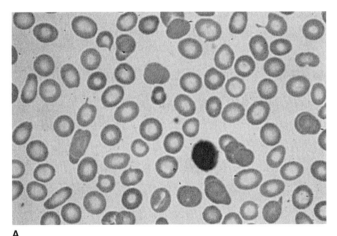

A

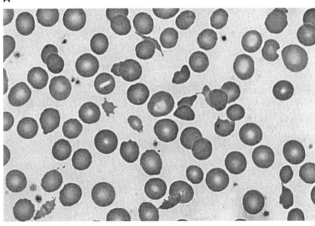

B

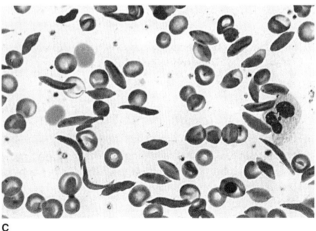

C

FIGURE III-1 (see Color Atlas)

1. A 22-year-old man with a hematocrit of 17%. He has sickle cell disease and is admitted with a vaso-occlusive crisis after an upper respiratory illness.

2. A 36-year-old woman with a hematocrit of 32%. She had a splenectomy 5 years ago after a motor vehicle crash.

3. A 55-year-old man with a hematocrit of 28%. He has advanced alcoholic liver disease with cirrhosis and is awaiting liver transplantation.

4. A 64-year-old woman with a hematocrit of 28%. She has heme-positive stool and a 2-cm adenomatous colonic polyp at colonoscopy.

5. A 72-year-old man a hematocrit of 33%. Four years ago, he received a mechanical prosthetic aortic valve because of aortic stenosis caused by a congenital bicuspid valve.

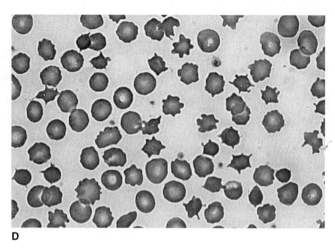

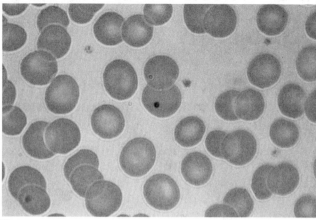

D

E

FIGURE III-1 (*Continued*)

III-2. A 39-year-old woman is evaluated for anemia. Her laboratory studies reveal a hemoglobin of 7.4 g/dL, hematocrit of 23.9%, mean corpuscular volume of 72 fL, mean cell hemoglobin of 25 pg, and mean cell hemoglobin concentration of 28%. The peripheral smear is shown in Figure III-2. Which of the following tests is most likely to be abnormal in this patient?

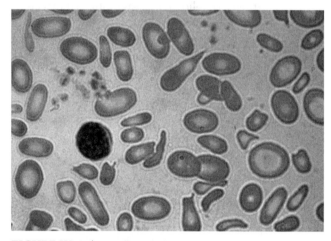

FIGURE III-2 (see Color Atlas)

A. Ferritin
B. Haptoglobin
C. Hemoglobin electrophoresis
D. Glucose-6-phosphate dehydrogenase
E. Vitamin B$_{12}$

III-3. A 62-year-old man is evaluated for anemia. He has a hemoglobin of 9.0 g/dL (normal hemoglobin value, 15 g/dL), hematocrit of 27.0% (normal hematocrit, 45%), mean cell volume of 88 fL, mean cell hemoglobin of 28 pg, and mean cell hemoglobin concentration of 30%. On peripheral blood smear, polychromatophilic macrocytes are seen. The reticulocyte count is 9%. What is the reticulocyte production index?

A. 0.54
B. 1.67
C. 2.7
D. 4.5
E. 5.4

III-4. You are asked to review the peripheral blood smear from a patient with anemia (Figure III-4). Serum lactate dehydrogenase is elevated, and there is hemoglobinuria. This patient is likely to have which physical examination finding?

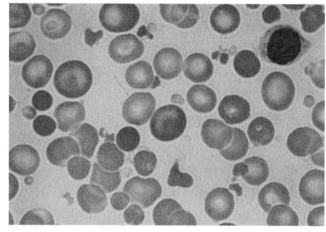

FIGURE III-4 (see Color Atlas)

A. Goiter
B. Heme-positive stools
C. Mechanical second heart sound
D. Splenomegaly
E. Thickened calvarium

III-5. In general, which of the following is the greatest risk factor for the development of cancer?

A. Age
B. Alcohol use
C. Cigarette smoking
D. Female sex
E. Obesity

III-6. Among women younger than 60 years of age who die from cancer, which of the following is the most common primary organ of origin?

A. Breast
B. Cervix
C. Colon
D. Bone marrow
E. Lung

III-7. A 68-year-old woman is diagnosed with stage II breast cancer. She has a history of severe chronic obstructive pulmonary disease with an FEV_1 of 32% predicted, coronary artery disease with prior stenting of the left anterior descending artery, peripheral vascular disease, and obesity. She continues to smoke 1 to 2 packs of cigarettes every day. She requires oxygen at 2 L/min continuously and is functionally quite limited. She currently is able to attend to all of her activities of daily living, including showering and dressing. She retired from her work as a waitress 10 years previously because of her lung disease. At home, she does attend to some of the household chores but is not able to use a vacuum. She goes out once or twice weekly to run typical errands and drives. She feels short of breath with most of these activities and often uses a motorized chart when out and about. How would you categorize her performance status and prognosis for treatment taking this into consideration?

A. She has an Eastern Cooperative Oncology Group (ECOG) grade of 1 and has a good prognosis with appropriate therapy.
B. She has an ECOG grade of 2 and has a good prognosis with appropriate therapy.
C. She has an ECOG grade of 3 and has a good prognosis with appropriate therapy.
D. She has an ECOG grade of 3 and has a poor prognosis despite therapy.
E. She has an ECOG grade of 4 and has a poor prognosis that precludes therapy.

III-8. Which of the following tumor markers is appropriately matched with the cell type cancer and can be followed during treatment as an adjunct to assess disease burden?

A. CA-125—Colon cancer
B. Calcitonin—Follicular carcinoma of the thyroid
C. CD30—Hairy cell leukemia
D. Human chorionic gonadotropin—Gestational trophoblastic disease
E. Neuron-specific enolase—Non–small cell carcinoma of the lung

III-9. Which of the following statements regarding current understanding of the genetic changes that must occur for a cell to become cancerous is TRUE?

A. Caretaker genes determine when a cell enters into a replicative phase and must acquire mutations to allow unregulated cell growth.
B. For a cell to become cancerous, it is estimated that a minimum of 20 mutations must occur.
C. For a tumor suppressor gene to become inactivated and allow unregulated cell growth, both copies of the gene must have mutations.
D. Oncogenes act in an autosomal recessive fashion.
E. Within a cancer, there are generally two to five cells of origin.

III-10. All the following conditions are associated with an increased incidence of cancer EXCEPT:

A. Down syndrome
B. Fanconi's anemia
C. von Hippel–Lindau syndrome
D. Neurofibromatosis
E. Fragile X syndrome

III-11. Cancer therapy is increasingly personalized with targeted small molecule therapies that are directed against specific signal transduction pathways that are commonly activated in a particular cell type of cancer. Which of the following therapies is correctly matched with its molecular target?

A. Bevacizumab—EGFR
B. Erlotinib—VEGF
C. Imatinib—Bcr-Abl
D. Rituximab—CD45
E. Sunitinib—RAF

III-12. Which of the following defines the term epigenetics?

A. Changes that alter the pattern of gene expression caused by mutations in the DNA code
B. Changes that alter the pattern of gene expression that persist across at least one cell division but are not caused by changes in the DNA code
C. Irreversible changes of the chromatin structure that regulates gene transcription and cell proliferation without permanent alteration of the DNA code

III-13. Which of the following patients with metastatic disease is potentially curable by surgical resection?

A. A 24-year-old man with a history of osteosarcoma of the left femur with a 1-cm metastasis to his right lower lobe referred for right lower lobectomy
B. A 56-year-old woman with a history of colon cancer with three metastases to the left lobe of the liver referred for left hepatic lobectomy
C. A 72-year-old man with metastatic prostate cancer to several vertebrae referred for orchiectomy
D. All of the above
E. None of the above

III-14. You are studying a new chemotherapeutic agent for use in advanced colorectal carcinoma and have completed a phase II clinical trial. Which of the following factors indicates that the drug is suitable for study in a phase III clinical trial?

A. Complete response rates of 10% to 15%
B. Increased disease-free survival rates by 1 month
C. Increased overall survival by 1 month
D. Partial response rate of 20% to 25%
E. Partial response rates of 50% or more

III-15. Match the following chemotherapeutic agents with their mechanisms of action:.

1. Cisplatin	A. Antimetabolite agent
2. Daunorubicin	B. Antimitotic agent
3. 5-Fluorouracil	C. Antitumor antibiotic
4. Gefitinib	D. DNA alkylator
5. Paclitaxel	E. Tyrosine kinase inhibitor

III-16. A 48-year-old woman with stage III breast cancer is undergoing chemotherapy with a regimen that includes doxorubicin. She presents 8 days after her last treatment to the emergency department with a fever of 104.1°F (40.1°C). She has chills, rigors, and a headache. Her chest radiograph, urinalysis, and tunneled intravenous catheter site show no obvious evidence of infection. Her white blood cell count upon presentation is 500/μL (0% neutrophils, 50% monocytes, 50% lymphocytes). Blood cultures are drawn peripherally and through the catheter. What is the next step in the treatment of this patient?

A. Broad-spectrum antibiotics with ceftazidime and vancomycin
B. Broad-spectrum antibiotics with ceftazidime, vancomycin, and voriconazole
C. Granulocyte-macrophage colony-stimulating factor after subsequent cycles of chemotherapy only
D. Granulocyte-macrophage colony-stimulating factor now and after subsequent cycles of chemotherapy
E. A and C
F. A and D

III-17. What is the most common side effect of chemotherapy?

A. Alopecia
B. Diarrhea
C. Febrile neutropenia
D. Mucositis
E. Nausea with or without vomiting

III-18. A 24-year-old woman is seen in follow-up 12 months after an allogeneic stem cell transplant for acute myeloid leukemia. She is doing well without evidence of recurrent disease but has had manifestations of chronic graft-versus-host disease. She should be administered all of the following vaccines EXCEPT:

A. Diphtheria–tetanus
B. Influenza
C. Measles, mumps, and rubella
D. Poliomyelitis via injection
E. 23-Valent pneumococcal polysaccharide

III-19. A 66-year-old woman has chronic lymphocytic leukemia with a stable white blood cell count of between 60,000 and 70,000/μL. She is currently hospitalized with pneumococcal pneumonia. This is the patient's third episode of pneumonia within the past 12 months. What finding on laboratory testing would be most likely in this patient?

A. Granulocytopenia
B. Hypogammaglobulinemia
C. Impaired T-cell function with normal T-lymphocyte counts
D. Low CD4 count
E. No specific abnormality is expected.

III-20. A 63-year-old man is treated with chemotherapy for stage IIIB adenocarcinoma of the lung with paclitaxel and carboplatin. He presents for evaluation of a fever of 38.3°C (100.9°F). He is found to have erythema at the exit site of his tunneled catheter, although the tunnel itself is not tender or red. Blood cultures are negative at 48 hours. His neutrophil count is 1,550/μL. What is the best approach to the management of this patient?

A. Removal of catheter alone
B. Treatment with ceftazidime and vancomycin
C. Treatment with topical antibiotics at the catheter site
D. Treatment with vancomycin alone
E. Treatment with vancomycin and removal of catheter

III-21. A 48-year-old woman presents to her physician with a complaint of an enlarging mole on her right lower extremity. She had noticed the area about 1 year previously and believes it has enlarged. She also notes that it recently has become itchy and occasionally bleeds. On physical examination, the lesion is located on the right mid-thigh. It measures 7.5 × 6 mm with irregular borders and a variegated hue with some areas appearing quite black. A biopsy confirms nodular melanoma. Which of the following is the best predictor of metastatic risk in this patient?

A. Breslow thickness
B. Clark level
C. Female gender
D. Presence of ulceration
E. Site of lesion

III-22. A 53-year-old man with a history of superficial spreading melanoma is diagnosed with disease metastatic to the lungs and bones. Genetic testing confirms the presence of the *BRAF V600E* mutation. What do you recommend for treatment of this patient?

A. Dacarbazine
B. Hospice care
C. Interleukin-2
D. Ipilimumab
E. Vemurafenib

III-23. A 65-year-old man presents to his primary care physician complaining of a hoarse voice for 6 months. He smokes 1 pack of cigarettes daily and drinks at least a six pack of beer daily. His physical examination reveals a thin man with a weak voice in no distress. No stridor is heard. The head and neck examination is normal. No cervical lymphadenopathy is present. He is referred to otolaryngology where a laryngeal lesion is discovered. Biopsy reveals squamous cell carcinoma. On imaging, the mass measures 2.8 cm. No suspicious lymphadenopathy is present on PET imaging. What is the best choice of therapy in this patient?

A. Concomitant chemotherapy and radiation therapy
B. Chemotherapy alone
C. Radiation therapy alone
D. Radical neck dissection alone
E. Radical neck dissection followed by concomitant chemotherapy and radiation

III-24. Which of the following statements is true with regard to the solitary pulmonary nodule?

A. A lobulated and irregular contour is more indicative of malignancy than a smooth one.
B. About 80% of incidentally found pulmonary nodules are benign.
C. Absence of growth over a period of 6 to 12 months is sufficient to determine if a solitary pulmonary nodule is benign.
D. Ground-glass nodules should be regarded as benign.
E. Multiple nodules indicate malignant disease.

III-25. A 64-year-old man seeks evaluation for a solitary pulmonary nodule that was found incidentally. He had presented to the emergency department for shortness of breath and chest tightness. A CT pulmonary angiogram did not show any evidence of pulmonary embolism. However, a 9-mm nodule is seen in the periphery of the left lower lobe. No enlarged mediastinal lymph nodes are present. He is a current smoker of 2 packs of cigarettes daily and has done so since the 16 years of age. He generally reports no functional limitation related to respiratory symptoms. His FEV_1 is 88% predicted, FVC is 92% predicted, and diffusion capacity is 80% predicted. He previously had a normal chest x-ray 3 years previously. What is the next best step in the evaluation and treatment of this patient?

A. Perform a bronchoscopy with biopsy for diagnosis.
B. Perform a combined PET and CT to assess for uptake in the nodule and assess for lymph node metastases.
C. Perform a follow-up CT scan in 3 months to assess for interval growth.
D. Refer the patient to radiation oncology for stereotactic radiation of the dominant nodule.
E. Refer the patient to thoracic surgery for video-assisted thoracoscopic biopsy and resection of lung nodule if malignancy is diagnosed.

III-26. A 62-year-old man presents to the emergency department complaining of a droopy right eye and blurred vision for the past day. The symptoms started abruptly, and he denies any antecedent illness. For the past 4 months, he has been complaining of increasing pain in his right arm and shoulder. His primary care physician has treated him for shoulder bursitis without relief. His medical history is significant for COPD and hypertension. He smokes 1 pack of cigarettes daily. He has chronic daily sputum production and has stable dyspnea on exertion. On physical examination, he has right eye ptosis with unequal pupils. On the right, his pupil is 2 mm and not reactive; on the left, the pupil is 4 mm and reactive. However, his ocular movements appear intact. His lung fields are clear to auscultation. On extremity examination, there is wasting of the intrinsic muscles of the hand. Which of the following would be most likely to explain the patient's constellation of symptoms?

A. Enlarged mediastinal lymph nodes causing occlusion of the superior vena cava
B. Metastases to the midbrain from small cell lung cancer
C. Paraneoplastic syndrome caused by antibodies to voltage-gated calcium channels
D. Presence of a cervical rib on chest radiography
E. Right apical pleural thickening with a mass-like density measuring 1 cm in thickness

III-27. A 55-year-old man presents with superior vena cava syndrome and is diagnosed with small cell lung cancer. Which of the following tests are indicated to properly stage this patient?

A. Bone marrow biopsy
B. CT scan of the abdomen
C. CT or MRI of the brain with intravenous contrast
D. Lumbar puncture
E. B and C
F. All of the above

III-28. As an oncologist you are considering treatment options for your patients with lung cancer, including small molecule therapy targeting the epidermal growth factor receptor (EGFR). Which of the following patients is most likely to have an EGFR mutation?

A. A 23-year-old man with a hamartoma
B. A 33-year-old woman with a carcinoid tumor
C. A 45-year-old woman who has never smoked with an adenocarcinoma
D. A 56-year-old man with a 100 pack-year history of tobacco with small cell lung carcinoma
E. A 76-year-old man with squamous cell carcinoma and a history of asbestos exposure

III-29. Given that most individuals with lung cancer present with advanced disease and have a high mortality, much research has investigated methods for early detection of lung cancer. Which of the following approaches is most likely to impact disease-related mortality from lung cancer?

A. Carefully design and implement low-dose chest CT screening in individuals with greater than 30 pack years of cigarette smoking

B. Continue annual screening with a chest x-ray for individuals with greater than 30 pack years of cigarette smoking

C. Do not recommend any screening because 30 years of research has not demonstrated any effect on mortality from lung cancer

D. Offer screening with low-dose CTs to all current or former smokers

E. Offer screening with combined PET and CT to individuals with greater than 30 pack years of tobacco use

III-30. A 34-year-old woman is seen by her internist for evaluation of right breast mass. This was noted approximately 1 week ago when she was showering. She has not had any nipple discharge or discomfort. She has no other medical problems. On examination, her right breast has a soft 1 cm × 2 cm mass in the right upper quadrant. There is no axillary lymphadenopathy present. The contralateral breast is normal. The breast is reexamined in 3 weeks, and the same findings are present. The cyst is aspirated, and clear fluid is removed. The mass is no longer palpable. Which of the following statements is true?

A. Breast MRI should be obtained to discern for residual fluid collection.

B. Mammography is required to further evaluate the lesion.

C. She should be evaluated in 1 month for recurrence.

D. She should be referred to a breast surgeon for resection.

E. She should not breastfeed any more children.

III-31. Which of the following women has the lowest risk of breast cancer?

A. A woman with menarche at 12 years, first child at 24 years, and menopause at 47 years

B. A woman with menarche at 14 years, first child at 17 years, and menopause at 52 years

C. A woman with menarche at 16 years, first child at 17 years, and menopause at 42 years

D. A woman with menarche at 16 years, first child at 32 years, and menopause at 52 years

E. They are all equal

III-32. Which of the following tumor characteristics confers a poor prognosis in patients with breast cancer?

A. Estrogen receptor positive

B. Good nuclear grade

C. Low proportion of cells in S-phase

D. Overexpression of erbB2 (HER-2/neu)

E. Progesterone receptor positive

III-33. A 56-year-old man presents to a physician with weight loss and dysphagia. He feels that food gets stuck in his mid-chest such that he no longer is able to eat meats. He reports his diet consists primarily of soft foods and liquids. The symptoms have progressively worsened over 6 months. During this time, he has lost about 50 lb. He occasionally gets pain in his mid-chest that radiates to his back and also occasionally feels that he regurgitates undigested foods. He does not have a history of gastroesophageal reflux disease. He does not regularly seek medical care. He is known to have hypertension but takes no medications. He drinks 500 cc or more of whiskey daily and smokes 1.5 packs of cigarettes per day. On physical examination, the patient appears cachectic with temporal wasting. He has a body mass index of 19.4 kg/m². His blood pressure is 198/110 mm Hg, heart rate is 110 beats/min, respiratory rate is 18 breaths/min, temperature is 37.4°C (99.2°F), and oxygen saturation is 93% on room air. His pulmonary examination shows decreased breath sounds at the apices with scattered expiratory wheezes. His cardiovascular examination demonstrates an S4 gallop with a hyperdynamic precordium. A regular tachycardia is present. Blood pressures are equal in both arms. Liver span is not enlarged. There are no palpable abdominal masses. What is the most likely cause of the patient's presentation?

A. Adenocarcinoma of the esophagus

B. Ascending aortic aneurysm

C. Esophageal stricture

D. Gastric cancer

E. Squamous cell carcinoma of the esophagus

III-34. A 64-year-old woman presents with complaints of a change in stool caliber for the past 2 months. The stools now have a diameter of only the size of her fifth digit. Over this same period, she feels she has to exert increasing strain to have a bowel movement and sometimes has associated abdominal cramping. She often has blood on the toilet paper when she wipes. During this time, she has lost about 20 lb. On physical examination, the patient appears cachectic with a body mass index of 22.5 kg/m². The abdomen is flat and nontender. The liver span is 12 cm to percussion. On digital rectal examination, a mass lesion is palpated approximately 8 cm into the rectum. A colonoscopy is attempted, which demonstrates a 2.5-cm sessile mass that narrows the colonic lumen. The biopsy confirms adenocarcinoma. The colonoscope is not able to traverse the mass. A CT scan of the abdomen does not show evidence of metastatic disease. Liver function test results are normal. A carcinoembryonic antigen level is 4.2 ng/mL. The patient is referred for surgery and undergoes rectosigmoidectomy with pelvic lymph node dissection. Final pathology demonstrates extension of the primary tumor into the muscularis propria but not the serosa. Of 15 lymph nodes removed, two are positive for tumor. What do you recommend for this patient after surgery?

A. Chemotherapy with a regimen containing 5-fluorouracil

B. Complete colonoscopy within 3 months

C. Measurement of CEA levels at 3-month intervals

D. Radiation therapy to the pelvis

E. All of the above

III-35. A healthy 62-year-old woman returns to your clinic after undergoing routine colonoscopy. Findings included two 1.3-cm sessile (flat-based), villous adenomas in her ascending colon that were removed during the procedure. What is the next step in management?

A.   Colonoscopy in 3 years
B.   Colonoscopy in 10 years
C.   CT scan of the abdomen
D.   Partial colectomy
E.   Reassurance

III-36. Which of the following should prompt investigation for hereditary nonpolyposis colon cancer screening in a 32-year-old man?

A.   Father, paternal aunt, and paternal cousin with colon cancer with ages of diagnosis of 54, 68, and 37 years, respectively
B.   Innumerable polyps visualized on routine colonoscopy
C.   Mucocutaneous pigmentation
D.   New diagnosis of ulcerative colitis
E.   None of the above

III-37. All of the following statements regarding pancreatic cancer are true EXCEPT:

A.   Alcohol consumption is not a risk factor for pancreatic cancer.
B.   Cigarette smoking is a risk factor for pancreatic cancer.
C.   Despite accounting for fewer than 5% of malignancies diagnosed in the United States, pancreatic cancer is the fourth leading cause of cancer death.
D.   If detected early, the 5-year survival is up to 20%.
E.   The 5-year survival rates for pancreatic cancer have improved substantially in the past decade.

III-38. A 65-year-old man is evaluated in clinic for 1 month of progressive painless jaundice and 10 lb of unintentional weight loss. His physical examination is unremarkable. A dual-phase contrast CT shows a suspicious mass in the head of the pancreas with biliary ductal dilation. Which of the following is the best diagnostic test to evaluate for suspected pancreatic cancer?

A.   CT-guided percutaneous needle biopsy
B.   Endoscopic ultrasound-guided needle biopsy
C.   ERCP with pancreatic juice sampling for cytopathology
D.   FDG-PET imaging
E.   Serum CA 19-9

III-39. A 63-year-old man complains of notable pink-tinged urine for the past month. At first he thought it was caused by eating beets, but has not cleared. His medical history is notable for hypertension and cigarette smoking. He does report some worsening urinary frequency and hesitancy over the past 2 years. Physical examination is unremarkable. Urinalysis is notable for gross hematuria with no white blood cells or casts. Renal function is normal. Which of the following statements regarding this patient is true?

A.   Cigarette smoking is not a risk for bladder cancer.
B.   Gross hematuria makes prostate cancer more likely than bladder cancer.
C.   If invasive bladder cancer with nodal involvement but no distant metastases is found, the 5-year survival is 20%.
D.   If superficial bladder cancer is found, intravesicular BCG may be used as adjuvant therapy.
E.   Radical cystectomy is generally recommended for invasive bladder cancer.

III-40. A 68-year-old man comes to his physician complaining of 2 months of increasing right flank pain with 1 month of worsening hematuria. He was treated for cystitis at a walk-in clinic 3 weeks ago with no improvement. He also reports poor appetite and 5 lb of weight loss. His physical examination is notable for a palpable mass in the right flank measuring greater than 5 cm. His renal function is normal. All of the following are true about this patient's likely diagnosis EXCEPT:

A.   Anemia is more common than erythrocytosis.
B.   Cigarette smoking increased his risk.
C.   If his disease has metastasized, with best therapy 5-year survival is greater than 50%.
D.   If his disease is confined to the kidney, 5-year survival is greater than 80%.
E.   The most likely pathology is clear cell carcinoma.

III-41. In the patient described above, imaging shows a 10-cm solid mass in the right kidney and multiple nodules in the lungs consistent with metastatic disease. Needle biopsy of a lung lesion confirms the diagnosis of renal cell carcinoma. Which of the following is recommended therapy?

A.   Gemcitabine
B.   Interferon-gamma
C.   Interleukin-2
D.   Radical nephrectomy
E.   Sunitinib

III-42. Which of the following has been shown in randomized trials to reduce the future risk of pancreatic cancer diagnosis?

A.   Finasteride
B.   Selenium
C.   Testosterone
D.   Vitamin C
E.   Vitamin E

III-43. A 54-year-old man is evaluated in an executive health program. On physical examination, he is noted to have an enlarged prostate with a right lobe nodule. He does not recall his last digital rectal examination and has never had prostate-specific antigen (PSA) tested. Based on this evaluation, which of the following is next recommended?

A.   Bone scan to evaluate for metastasis
B.   PSA
C.   PSA now and in 3 months to measure PSA velocity
D.   Repeat digital rectal examination in 3 months
E.   Transrectal ultrasound-guided biopsy

III-44. Which of the following statements describes the relationship between testicular tumors and serum markers?

- A. Pure seminomas produce α-fetoprotein (AFP) or beta human chorionic gonadotropin (β-hCG) in more than 90% of cases.
- B. More than 40% of nonseminomatous germ cell tumors produce no cell markers.
- C. Both β-hCG and AFP should be measured in following the progress of a tumor.
- D. Measurement of tumor markers the day after surgery for localized disease is useful in determining the completeness of the resection.
- E. β-hCG is limited in its usefulness as a marker because it is identical to human luteinizing hormone.

III-45. A 32-year-old man presents complaining of a testicular mass. On examination, you palpate a 1 cm × 2 cm painless mass on the surface of the left testicle. A chest x-ray shows no lesions, and a CT scan of the abdomen and pelvis shows no evidence of retroperitoneal adenopathy. The α-fetoprotein (AFP) level is elevated at 400 ng/mL. Beta human chorionic gonadotropin (β-hCG) is normal, as is lactate dehydrogenase (LDH). You send the patient for an orchiectomy. The pathology comes back as seminoma limited to the testis alone. The AFP level declines to normal at an appropriate interval. What is the appropriate management at this point?

- A. Radiation to the retroperitoneal lymph nodes
- B. Adjuvant chemotherapy
- C. Hormonal therapy
- D. Retroperitoneal lymph node dissection (RPLND)
- E. Positron emission tomography (PET) scan

III-46. Which of the following statements regarding the relationship between ovarian cancer and *BRCA* gene mutations is true?

- A. Most women with *BRCA* mutations have a family history that is strongly positive for breast or ovarian cancer (or both).
- B. More than 30% of women with ovarian cancer have a somatic mutation in either *BRCA1* or *BRCA2*.
- C. Prophylactic oophorectomy in patients with *BRCA* mutations does not protect against the development of breast cancer.
- D. Screening studies with serial ultrasound and serum CA-125 tumor marker studies are effective in detecting early stage disease.
- E. Women with known mutations in a single *BRCA1* or *BRCA2* allele have a 75% lifetime risk of developing ovarian cancer.

III-47. All of the following statements regarding the diagnosis of uterine cancer are true EXCEPT:

- A. Five-year survival after surgery in disease confined to the corpus is approximately 90%.
- B. Endometrial carcinoma is the most common gynecologic malignancy in the United States.
- C. Most women present with amenorrhea.
- D. Tamoxifen is associated with an increased risk of endometrial carcinoma.
- E. Unopposed estrogen exposure is a risk factor for developing endometrial carcinoma.

III-48. A 73-year-old man presents to the clinic with 3 months of increasing back pain. He localizes the pain to the lumbar spine and states that the pain is worst at night while he is lying in bed. It is improved during the day with mobilization. Past history is notable only for hypertension and remote cigarette smoking. Physical examination is normal. Laboratory studies are notable for an elevated alkaline phosphatase. A lumbar radiogram shows a lytic lesion in the L3 vertebra. Which of the following malignancies is most likely?

- A. Gastric carcinoma
- B. Non–small cell lung cancer
- C. Osteosarcoma
- D. Pancreatic carcinoma
- E. Thyroid carcinoma

III-49. A primary tumor of which of these organs is the *least likely* to metastasize to bone?

- A. Breast
- B. Colon
- C. Kidney
- D. Lung
- E. Prostate

III-50. A 22-year-old man comes into clinic because of a swollen leg. He does not remember any trauma to the leg, but the pain and swelling began 3 weeks ago in the anterior shin area of his left foot. He is a college student and is active in sports daily. A radiograph of the right leg shows a destructive lesion with a "moth-eaten" appearance extending into the soft tissue and a spiculated periosteal reaction. Codman's triangle (a cuff of periosteal bone formation at the margin of the bone and soft tissue mass) is present. Which of the following are the most likely diagnosis and optimal therapy for this lesion?

- A. Chondrosarcoma; chemotherapy alone is curative
- B. Chondrosarcoma; radiation with limited surgical resection
- C. Osteosarcoma; preoperative chemotherapy followed by limb-sparing surgery
- D. Osteosarcoma; radiation therapy
- E. Plasma cell tumor; chemotherapy

III-51. A 42-year-old man presented to the hospital with right upper quadrant pain. He was found to have multiple masses in the liver that were found to be malignant on H&E staining of a biopsy sample. Your initial history, physical examination, and laboratory tests, including prostate-specific antigen, are unrevealing. Lung, abdominal, and pelvic

CT scans are unremarkable. He is an otherwise healthy individual with no chronic medical problems. Which immunohistochemical markers should be obtained from the biopsy tissue?

A. α-Fetoprotein
B. Cytokeratin
C. Leukocyte common antigen
D. Thyroglobulin
E. Thyroid transcription factor 1

III-52. A 52-year-old woman is evaluated for abdominal swelling with a computed tomogram that shows ascites and likely peritoneal studding of tumor but no other abnormality. Paracentesis shows adenocarcinoma but cannot be further differentiated by the pathologist. A thorough physical examination, including breast and pelvic examination, shows no abnormality. CA-125 levels are elevated. Pelvic ultrasonography and mammography findings are normal. Which of the following statements is true?

A. Compared with other women with known ovarian cancer at a similar stage, this patient can be expected to have a less than average survival.
B. Debulking surgery is indicated.
C. Surgical debulking plus cisplatin and paclitaxel is indicated.
D. Bilateral mastectomy and bilateral oophorectomy will improve survival.
E. Fewer than 1% of patients with this disorder will remain disease free 2 years after treatment.

III-53. A 29-year-old man is found on routine chest radiography for life insurance to have left hilar adenopathy. CT scanning confirms enlarged left hilar and paraaortic nodes. He is otherwise healthy. Besides biopsy of the lymph nodes, which of the following is indicated?

A. Angiotensin-converting enzyme (ACE) level
B. β-hCG
C. Thyroid-stimulating hormone (TSH)
D. PSA
E. C-reactive protein

III-54. An 81-year-old man is admitted to the hospital for altered mental status. He was found at home, confused and lethargic, by his son. His medical history is significant for metastatic prostate cancer. The patient's medications include periodic intramuscular goserelin injections. On examination, he is afebrile. Blood pressure is 110/50 mm Hg, and the pulse rate is 110 beats/min. He is lethargic and minimally responsive to sternal rub. He has bitemporal wasting, and his mucous membranes are dry. On neurologic examination, he is obtunded. The patient has an intact gag reflex and withdraws to pain in all four extremities. Rectal tone is normal. Laboratory values are significant for a creatinine of 4.2 mg/dL, a calcium level of 14.4 meq/L, and an albumin of 2.6 g/dL. All the following are appropriate initial management steps EXCEPT:

A. Normal saline
B. Pamidronate
C. Furosemide when the patient is euvolemic
D. Calcitonin
E. Dexamethasone

III-55. A 55-year-old man is found to have a serum calcium of 13.0 mg/dL after coming to clinic complaining of fatigue and thirst for the past month. A chest radiograph demonstrates a 4-cm mass in the right lower lobe. Which of the following serum tests is most likely to reveal the cause of his hypercalcemia?

A. Adrenocorticotropic hormone (ACTH)
B. Antidiuretic hormone (ADH)
C. Insulin-like growth factor
D. Parathyroid hormone (PTH)
E. Parathyroid hormone related protein (PTH-rp)

III-56. A 55-year-old woman presents with progressive incoordination. Physical examination is remarkable for nystagmus, mild dysarthria, and past pointing on finger-to-nose testing. She also has an unsteady gait. MRI reveals atrophy of both lobes of the cerebellum. Serologic evaluation reveals the presence of anti-Yo antibody. Which of the following is the most likely cause of this clinical syndrome?

A. Non–small cell cancer of the lung
B. Small cell cancer of the lung
C. Breast cancer
D. Non-Hodgkin's lymphoma
E. Colon cancer

III-57. All of the following conditions may be associated with a thymoma EXCEPT:

A. Erythrocytosis
B. Hypogammaglobulinemia
C. Myasthenia gravis
D. Polymyositis
E. Pure red blood cell aplasia

III-58. A 52-year-old woman has been having worsening cough for the past month. She is a nonsmoker and has no known health problems. The cough is nonproductive and present throughout the day and night. It worsens when lying on her back. She has also noticed some upper chest pain and dyspnea on exertion for the past week. A chest radiograph shows a large mass (>5 cm) confined to the anterior mediastinum. Which of the following diagnoses is most likely?

A. Hodgkin's lymphoma
B. Non-Hodgkin's lymphoma
C. Teratoma
D. Thymoma
E. Thyroid carcinoma

III-59. All the following are suggestive of iron-deficiency anemia EXCEPT:

A. Koilonychia
B. Pica
C. Decreased serum ferritin
D. Decreased total iron-binding capacity (TIBC)
E. Low reticulocyte response

III-60. A 24-year-old man with a history of poorly treated chronic ulcerative colitis is found to have anemia with a hemoglobin of 9 g/dL and a reduced mean corpuscular volume. His ferritin is 250 µg/L. Which of the following is the most likely cause of his anemia?

A. Folate deficiency
B. Hemoglobinopathy
C. Inflammation
D. Iron deficiency
E. Sideroblastic anemia

III-61. All of the following statements regarding the anemia of chronic kidney disease are true EXCEPT:

A. The degree of anemia correlates with the stage of chronic kidney disease.
B. Erythropoietin levels are reduced.
C. Ferritin is reduced.
D. It is typically normocytic and normochromic.
E. Reticulocytes are decreased.

III-62. All of the following statements regarding the utility of hydroxyurea in patients with sickle cell disease are true EXCEPT:

A. It is effective in reducing painful crises.
B. It produces a chimeric state with partial production of hemoglobin A by the bone marrow.
C. It should be considered in patients with repeated acute chest syndrome episodes.
D. Its mechanism involves increasing production of fetal hemoglobin.
E. The major adverse effect is a reduction in white blood cell count.

III-63. Which of the following is the most cost-effective test to evaluate a patient for suspected cobalamin (vitamin B$_{12}$) deficiency?

A. Red blood cell folate
B. Serum cobalamin
C. Serum homocysteine
D. Serum methylmalonate
E. Serum pepsinogen

III-64. A patient being evaluated for anemia has the peripheral blood smear shown in Figure III-64. Which of the following is the most likely cause of the anemia?

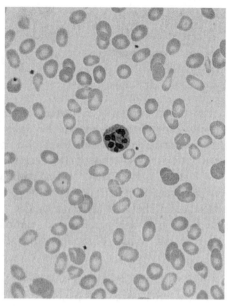

FIGURE III-64 (see Color Atlas)

A. Acute lymphocytic leukemia
B. Autoantibodies to ADAMTS-13
C. Cobalamin deficiency
D. Epstein-Barr virus infection
E. Iron deficiency

III-65. Patients from which of the following regions need not be screened for glucose-6-phosphate dehydrogenase (G6PD) deficiency when starting a drug that carries a risk for G6PD-mediated hemolysis?

A. Brazil
B. Russia
C. Southeast Asia
D. Southern Europe
E. Sub-Saharan Africa
F. None of the above

III-66. A 36-year-old African American woman with systemic lupus erythematosus presents with the acute onset of lethargy and jaundice. On initial evaluation, she is tachycardic and hypotensive, appears pale, is dyspneic, and is somewhat difficult to arouse. Physical examination reveals splenomegaly. Her initial hemoglobin is 6 g/dL, white blood cell count is 6300/µL, and platelets are 294,000/µL. Her total bilirubin is 4 g/dL, reticulocyte count is 18%, and haptoglobin is not detectable. Renal function is normal, as is urinalysis. What would you expect on her peripheral blood smear?

A. Macrocytosis and polymorphonuclear leukocytes with hypersegmented nuclei
B. Microspherocytes
C. Schistocytes
D. Sickle cells
E. Target cells

III-67. A 22-year-old pregnant woman of northern European descent presents 3 months into her first pregnancy with extreme fatigue, pallor, and icterus. She reports being previously healthy. On evaluation her hemoglobin is 8 g/dL with a normal mean corpuscular volume and an elevated mean corpuscular hemoglobin concentration, reticulocyte count is 9%, indirect bilirubin is 4.9 mg/dL, and serum haptoglobin is not detectable. Her peripheral smear is shown in Figure III-67. Her physical examination is notable for splenomegaly and a normal 3-month uterus. What is the most likely diagnosis?

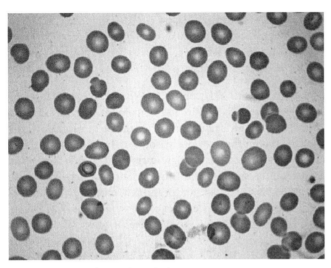

FIGURE III-67 (see Color Atlas)

A. Colonic polyp
B. G6PD deficiency
C. Hereditary spherocytosis
D. Parvovirus B19 infection
E. Thrombotic thrombocytopenic purpura

III-68. The triad of portal vein thrombosis, hemolysis, and pancytopenia suggests which of the following diagnoses?

A. Acute promyelocytic leukemia
B. Hemolytic uremic syndrome (HUS)
C. Leptospirosis
D. Paroxysmal nocturnal hemoglobinuria (PNH)
E. Thrombotic thrombocytopenic purpura (TTP)

III-69. All of the following laboratory values are consistent with an intravascular hemolytic anemia EXCEPT:

A. Increased haptoglobin
B. Increased lactate dehydrogenase (LDH)
C. Increased reticulocyte count
D. Increased unconjugated bilirubin
E. Increased urine hemosiderin

III-70. Which of the following hemolytic anemias can be classified as extracorpuscular?

A. Elliptocytosis
B. Paroxysmal nocturnal hemoglobinuria
C. Pyruvate kinase deficiency
D. Sickle cell anemia
E. Thrombotic thrombocytopenic purpura

III-71. A 34-year-old woman with a medical history of sickle cell anemia presents with a 5-day history of fatigue, lethargy, and shortness of breath. She denies chest pain and bone pain. She has had no recent travel. Of note, the patient's 4-year-old daughter had a "cold" 2 weeks before the presentation. On examination, the woman has pale conjunctiva, is anicteric, and is mildly tachycardic. Abdominal examination is unremarkable. Laboratory studies show a hemoglobin of 3 g/dL; her baseline is 8 g/dL. The white blood cell count and platelets are normal. Reticulocyte count is undetectable. Total bilirubin is 1.4 mg/dL. Lactic dehydrogenase is at the upper limits of the normal range. Peripheral blood smear shows a few sickled cells but a total absence of reticulocytes. The patient is given a transfusion of 2 units of packed red blood cells and admitted to the hospital. A bone marrow biopsy shows a normal myeloid series but an absence of erythroid precursors. Cytogenetics are normal. What is the most appropriate next management step?

A. Make arrangements for exchange transfusion.
B. Tissue type her siblings for a possible bone marrow transplant.
C. Check parvovirus titers.
D. Start prednisone and cyclosporine.
E. Start broad-spectrum antibiotics.

III-72. Aplastic anemia has been associated with all of the following EXCEPT:

A. Carbamazepine therapy
B. Methimazole therapy
C. Nonsteroidal anti-inflammatory drugs
D. Parvovirus B19 infection
E. Seronegative hepatitis

III-73. A 23-year-old man presents with diffuse bruising. He otherwise feels well. He takes no medications, does not use dietary supplements, and does not use illicit drugs. His medical history is negative for any prior illnesses. He is a college student and works as a barista in a coffee shop. A blood count reveals an absolute neutrophil count of 780/μL, hematocrit of 18%, and platelet count of 21,000/μL. Bone marrow biopsy reveals hypocellularity with a fatty marrow. Chromosome studies of peripheral blood and bone marrow cells are performed that exclude Fanconi's anemia and myelodysplastic syndrome. The patient has a fully histocompatible brother. Which of the following is the best therapy?

A. Antithymocyte globulin plus cyclosporine
B. Glucocorticoids
C. Growth factors
D. Hematopoietic stem cell transplant
E. Red blood cell and platelet transfusion

III-74. A 73-year-old man has complained of fatigue and worsening dyspnea on exertion for the past 2 to 3 months. His medical history is only notable for hypertension and hypercholesterolemia. He is an active golfer who notes that lately he has difficulty walking 18 holes. His handicap has increased by 5 strokes over this time period. Physical examination reveals normal vital signs and is unremarkable except for pallor. His laboratory examination is remarkable for a hematocrit of 25% with a platelet count of 185,000/μL and low normal white cell count. There are no circulating blasts. These abnormalities were not present 1 year ago. Bone marrow reveals a hypercellular marrow with fewer than 5% blasts and the 5q-cytogenetic abnormality. All of the following statements regarding this patient's condition are true EXCEPT:

A. He has myelofibrosis.
B. He is most likely to die as a result of leukemic transformation.
C. His median survival is more than 12 months.
D. Lenalidomide is effective in reversing the anemia.
E. Only stem cell transplantation offers a cure.

III-75. All of the following are considered myeloproliferative disorders in the WHO classification system EXCEPT:

A. Chronic myelogenous leukemia (bcr-abl positive)
B. Essential thrombocytosis
C. Mastocytosis
D. Polycythemia vera
E. Primary effusion lymphoma

III-76. Which of the following statements regarding polycythemia vera is correct?

A. An elevated plasma erythropoietin level excludes the diagnosis.
B. Transformation to acute leukemia is common.
C. Thrombocytosis correlates strongly with thrombotic risk.
D. Aspirin should be prescribed to all of these patients to reduce thrombotic risk.
E. Phlebotomy is used only after hydroxyurea and interferon have been tried.

III-77. A 68-year-old man seeks evaluation for fatigue, weight loss, and early satiety that have been present for about 4 months. On physical examination, his spleen is noted to be markedly enlarged. It is firm to touch and crosses the midline. The lower edge of the spleen reaches to the pelvis. His hemoglobin is 11.1 g/dL and hematocrit is 33.7%. The leukocyte count is 6200/μL and platelet count is 220,000/μL. The white cell count differential is 75% polymorphonuclear leukocytes, 8% myelocytes, 4% metamyelocytes, 8% lymphocytes, 3% monocytes, and 2% eosinophils. The peripheral blood smear shows teardrop cells, nucleated red blood cells, and immature granulocytes. Rheumatoid factor is positive. A bone marrow biopsy is attempted, but no cells are able to be aspirated. No evidence of leukemia or lymphoma is found. What is the most likely cause of the splenomegaly?

A. Chronic primary myelofibrosis
B. Chronic myelogenous leukemia
C. Rheumatoid arthritis
D. Systemic lupus erythematosus
E. Tuberculosis

III-78. A 50-year-old woman presents to your clinic for evaluation of an elevated platelet count. The latest complete blood count is white blood cells (WBC), 7000/μL; hematocrit, 34%; and platelets, 600,000/μL. All the following are common causes of thrombocytosis EXCEPT:

A. Iron-deficiency anemia
B. Essential thrombocytosis
C. Chronic myeloid leukemia
D. Myelodysplasia
E. Pernicious anemia

III-79. A 38-year-old woman is referred for evaluation of an elevated hemoglobin and hematocrit that was discovered during an evaluation of recurrent headaches. Until about 8 months previously, she was in good health, but she developed increasingly persistent headaches with intermittent vertigo and tinnitus. She was originally prescribed sumatriptan for presumed migraine headaches but did not experience relief of her symptoms. A CT scan of the brain showed no evidence of mass lesion. During evaluation of her headaches, she was found to have a hemoglobin of 17.3 g/dL and a hematocrit of 52%. Her only other symptom is diffuse itching after hot showers. She is a nonsmoker. She has no history pulmonary or cardiac disease. On physical examination, she appears well. Her body mass index is 22.3 kg/m^2. Vitals signs are blood pressure of 148/84 mm Hg, heart rate of 86 beats/min, respiratory rate of 12 breaths/min, and SaO$_2$ of 99% on room air. She is afebrile. The physical examination, including full neurologic examination, is normal. There are no heart murmurs. There is no splenomegaly. Peripheral pulses are normal. Laboratory studies confirm elevated hemoglobin and hematocrit. She also has a platelet count of 650,000/μL. Leukocyte count is 12,600/μL with a normal differential. Which of the following tests should be performed next in the evaluation of this patient?

A. Bone marrow biopsy
B. Erythropoietin level
C. Genetic testing for JAK2 V617F mutation
D. Leukocyte alkaline phosphatase
E. Red blood cell mass and plasma volume determination

III-80. A 45-year-old man is evaluated by his primary care physician for complaints of early satiety and weight loss. On physical examination, his spleen is palpable 10 cm below the left costal margin and is mildly tender to palpation. His laboratory studies show a leukocyte count of 125,000/μL with a differential of 80% neutrophils, 9% bands, 3% myelocytes, 3% metamyelocytes, 1% blasts, 1% lymphocytes, 1% eosinophils, and 1% basophils. Hemoglobin is 8.4 g/dL, hematocrit is 26.8%, and platelet count is 668,000/μL. A bone marrow biopsy demonstrates increased cellularity with an increased myeloid to erythroid ratio. Which of the following cytogenetic abnormalities is most likely to be found in this patient?

A. Deletion of a portion of the long arm of chromosome 5, del(5q)
B. Inversion of chromosome 16, inv(16)
C. Reciprocal translocation between chromosomes 9 and 22 (Philadelphia chromosome)
D. Translocations of the long arms of chromosomes 15 and 17
E. Trisomy 12

III-81. All of the following statements regarding the epidemiology of and risk factors for acute myeloid leukemias are true EXCEPT:

A. Anticancer drugs such as alkylating agents and topoisomerase II inhibitors are the leading cause of drug-associated myeloid leukemias.
B. Individuals exposed to high-dose radiation are at risk for acute myeloid leukemia, but individuals treated with therapeutic radiation are not unless they are also treated with alkylating agents.
C. Men have a higher incidence of acute myeloid leukemia than women.
D. The incidence of acute myeloid leukemia is greatest in individuals younger than 20 years of age.
E. Trisomy 21 (Down syndrome) is associated with an increased risk of acute myeloid leukemia.

III-82. A 56-year-old woman is diagnosed with chronic myelogenous leukemia, Philadelphia chromosome positive. Her presenting leukocyte count was 127,000/μL, and her differential shows less than 2% circulating blasts. Her hematocrit is 21.1% at diagnosis. She is asymptomatic except for fatigue. She has no siblings. What is the best initial therapy for this patient?

A. Allogeneic bone marrow transplant
B. Autologous stem cell transplant
C. Imatinib mesylate
D. Interferon-α
E. Leukapheresis

III-83. A 48-year-old woman is admitted to the hospital with anemia and thrombocytopenia after complaining of profound fatigue. Her initial hemoglobin is 8.5 g/dL, hematocrit is 25.7%, and platelet count is 42,000/μL. Her leukocyte count is 9540/μL, but 8% blast forms are noted on peripheral smear. A chromosomal analysis shows a reciprocal translocation of the long arms of chromosomes 15 and 17, t(15;17), and a diagnosis of acute promyelocytic leukemia is made. The induction regimen of this patient should include which of the following drugs?

A. Arsenic
B. Cyclophosphamide, daunorubicin, vinblastine, and prednisone
C. Rituximab
D. Tretinoin
E. Whole-body irradiation

III-84. The patient in question III-83 is started on the appropriate induction regimen. Two weeks after initiation of treatment, the patient develops acute onset of shortness of breath, fever, and chest pain. Her chest radiograph shows bilateral alveolar infiltrates and moderate bilateral pleural effusions. Her leukocyte count is now 22,300/μL, and she has a neutrophil count of 78%, bands of 15%, and lymphocytes 7%. She undergoes bronchoscopy with lavage that shows no bacterial, fungal, or viral organisms. What is the most likely diagnosis in this patient?

A. Arsenic poisoning
B. Bacterial pneumonia
C. Cytomegalovirus pneumonia
D. Radiation pneumonitis
E. Retinoic acid syndrome

III-85. A 76-year-old man is admitted to the hospital with complaints of fatigue for 4 months and fever for the past 1 week. His temperature has been as high as 38.3°C at home. During this time, he intermittently has had a 5.5-kg weight loss, severe bruising with minimal trauma, and an aching sensation in his bones. He last saw his primary care physician 2 months ago and was diagnosed with anemia of unclear etiology at that time. He has a history of a previous left middle cerebral artery cerebrovascular accident, which has left him with decreased functional status. At baseline, he is able to ambulate in his home with the use of a walker and is dependent on a caregiver for assistance with his activities of daily living. His vital signs are blood pressure of 158/86 mm Hg, heart rate of 98 beats/min, respiratory rate of 18 breaths/min, SaO₂ 95%, and temperature of 38°C. He appears cachectic with temporal muscle wasting. He has petechiae on his hard palate. He has no lymph node enlargement. On cardiovascular examination, there is a II/VI systolic ejection murmur present. His lungs are clear. The liver is enlarged and palpable 6 cm below the right costal margin. In addition, the spleen is also enlarged, with a palpable spleen tip felt about 4 cm below the left costal margin. There are multiple hematomas and petechiae present in the extremities. Laboratory examination reveals the following: hemoglobin, 5.1 g/dL; hematocrit, 15%; platelets, 12,000/μL; and white blood cell (WBC) count, 168,000/μL with 45% blast forms, 30% neutrophils, 20% lymphocytes, and 5% monocytes. Review of the peripheral blood smear confirms acute myeloid leukemia (M1 subtype, myeloblastic leukemia without maturation) with complex chromosomal abnormalities on cytogenetics. All of the following confer a poor prognosis for this patient EXCEPT:

A. Advanced age
B. Complex chromosomal abnormalities on cytogenetics
C. Hemoglobin below 7 g/dL
D. Prolonged interval between symptom onset and diagnosis
E. WBC count above 100,000/μL

III-86. The evaluation in a newly diagnosed case of acute lymphoid leukemia should routinely include all of the following EXCEPT:

A. Bone marrow biopsy
B. Cell-surface phenotyping
C. Cytogenetic testing
D. Lumbar puncture
E. Plasma viscosity

III-87. All of the following infectious agents have been associated with development of a lymphoid malignancy EXCEPT:

A. *Helicobacter pylori*
B. Hepatitis B
C. Hepatitis C
D. HIV
E. Human herpes virus 8 (HHV8)

III-88. A 64-year-old man with chronic lymphoid leukemia and chronic hepatitis C presents for his yearly follow-up. His white blood cell count is stable at 83,000/μL, but his hematocrit has dropped from 35% to 26%, and his platelet count also dropped from 178,000/μL to 69,000/μL. His initial evaluation should include all of the following EXCEPT:

A. AST, ALT, and prothrombin time
B. Bone marrow biopsy
C. Coombs test
D. Peripheral blood smear
E. Physical examination

III-89. During a routine visit, a 68-year-old woman complains of 3 months of fatigue, abdominal fullness, and bilateral axillary adenopathy. On physical examination, vital signs are normal, and she has bilateral palpable axillary and cervical adenopathy and an enlarged spleen. A complete blood count is notable for a white cell count of 88,000 with 99% lymphocytes. A peripheral smear is shown in Figure III-89. Which of the following is the most likely diagnosis?

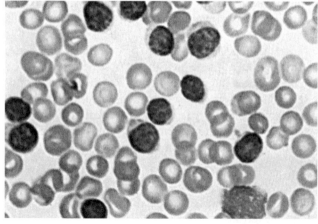

FIGURE III-89 (see Color Atlas)

A. Acute lymphoblastic leukemia
B. Acute myelogenous leukemia
C. Chronic lymphocytic lymphoma
D. Hairy cell leukemia
E. Mononucleosis

III-90. Which of the following carries the best disease prognosis with appropriate treatment?

A. Burkitt's lymphoma
B. Diffuse large B-cell lymphoma
C. Follicular lymphoma
D. Mantle cell lymphoma
E. Nodular sclerosing Hodgkin's disease

III-91. A 27-year-old man seeks medical attention for enlarging nodules in his neck. He reports they are nontender and have been growing for more than 1 month. At first he thought they were caused by a sore throat, but over the past 3 weeks he has felt well with no fever, chills, throat pain, or other associated symptoms. He notes a slightly diminished appetite but no weight loss. He works as a video game developer, does not smoke or use illicit drugs, and is sexually active with numerous female partners. He has never been tested for HIV. A lymph node biopsy is performed and is shown in Figure III-91. Which of the following is the most likely diagnosis?

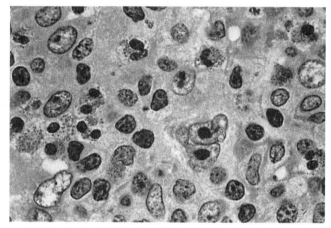

FIGURE III-91 (see Color Atlas)

A. Burkitt's lymphoma
B. Cat scratch disease
C. CMV infection
D. Hodgkin's disease
E. Non-Hodgkin's lymphoma

III-92. Which of the following is the most likely finding in a patient with a "dry" bone marrow aspiration?

A. Chronic myeloid leukemia
B. Hairy cell leukemia
C. Metastatic carcinoma infiltration
D. Myelofibrosis
E. Normal bone marrow

III-93. All of the following statements are true regarding the criteria to diagnose hypereosinophilic syndrome EXCEPT:

A. Increased bone marrow eosinophils must be demonstrated.

B. It is not necessary to have increased circulating eosinophils.

C. Primary myeloid leukemia must be excluded.

D. Reactive eosinophilia (e.g., parasitic infection, allergy, collagen vascular disease) must be excluded.

E. There must be less than 20% myeloblasts in blood or bone marrow.

III-94. All of the following statements regarding mastocytosis are true EXCEPT:

A. Elevated serum tryptase suggests aggressive disease.

B. Eosinophilia is common.

C. It is often associated with myeloid neoplasm.

D. More than 90% of cases are confined to the skin.

E. Urticaria pigmentosa is the most common clinical manifestation.

III-95. A 58-year-old man is evaluated in the emergency department for sudden onset cough with yellow sputum production and dyspnea. Aside from systemic hypertension, he is otherwise healthy. His only medication is amlodipine. Chest radiograph shows a right upper lobe alveolar infiltrate, and laboratory test results are notable for a blood urea nitrogen of 53 mg/dL, creatinine of 2.8 mg/dL, calcium of 12.3 mg/dL, total protein of 9 g/dL, and albumin of 3.1 g/dL. Sputum culture grows *Streptococcus pneumonia*. Which of the following tests will confirm the underlying condition predisposing him to pneumococcal pneumonia?

A. Bone marrow biopsy

B. Computed tomography of the chest, abdomen, and pelvis with contrast

C. HIV antibody

D. Sweat chloride testing

E. Videoscopic swallow study

III-96. A 64-year-old African American man is evaluated in the hospital for congestive heart failure, renal failure, and polyneuropathy. Physical examination on admission was notable for these findings and raised waxy papules in the axilla and inguinal region. Admission laboratories showed a blood urea nitrogen of 90 mg/dL and a creatinine of 6.3 mg/dL. Total protein was 9.0 g/dL with an albumin of 3.2 g/dL. Hematocrit was 24%, and white blood cell and platelet counts were normal. Urinalysis was remarkable for 3+ proteinuria but no cellular casts. Further evaluation included an echocardiogram with a thickened left ventricle and preserved systolic function. Which of the following tests is most likely to diagnose the underlying condition?

A. Bone marrow biopsy

B. Electromyogram (EMG) with nerve conduction studies

C. Fat pad biopsy

D. Right heart catheterization

E. Renal ultrasonography

III-97. A 75-year-old man is hospitalized for treatment of a deep venous thrombosis. He had recently been discharged from the hospital about 2 months ago. At that time, he had been treated for community-acquired pneumonia complicated by acute respiratory failure requiring mechanical ventilation. He was hospitalized for 21 days at that time and had discharged from a rehabilitation 2 weeks ago. On the day before admission, he developed painful swelling of his left lower extremity. Lower extremity Doppler ultrasonography confirmed an occlusive thrombus of his deep femoral vein. After an initial bolus, he is started on a continuous infusion of unfractionated heparin at 1600 U/hr because he has end-stage renal disease on hemodialysis. His activated partial thromboplastin time is maintained in the therapeutic range. On day 5, it is noted that his platelets have fallen from 150,000/μL to 88,000/μL. What is the most appropriate action at this time?

A. Continue heparin infusion at the current dose and assess for anti-heparin/platelet factor 4 antibodies.

B. Stop all anticoagulation while awaiting results of anti-heparin/platelet factor 4 antibodies.

C. Stop heparin infusion and initiate argatroban.

D. Stop heparin infusion and initiate enoxaparin.

E. Stop heparin infusion and initiate lepirudin.

III-98. A 48-year-old woman is evaluated by her primary care physician for a complaint of gingival bleeding and easy bruising. She has noted the problem for about 2 months. Initially, she attributed it to aspirin that she was taking intermittently for headaches, but she stopped all aspirin and nonsteroidal anti-inflammatory drug use 6 weeks ago. Her only medical history is an automobile accident 12 years previously that caused a liver laceration. It required surgical repair, and she did receive several transfusions of red blood cells and platelets at that time. She currently takes no prescribed medications and otherwise feels well. On physical examination, she appears well and healthy. She has no jaundice or scleral icterus. Her cardiac and pulmonary examination results are normal. The abdominal examination shows a liver span of 12 cm to percussion, and the edge is palpable 1.5 cm below the right costal margin. The spleen tip is not palpable. There are petechiae present on her extremities and hard palate with a few small ecchymoses on her extremities. A complete blood count shows a hemoglobin of 12.5 g/dL, hematocrit of 37.6%, white blood cell count of 8400/μL with a normal differential, and a platelet count of 7500/μL. What tests are indicated for the workup of this patient's thrombocytopenia?

A. Antiplatelet antibodies

B. Bone marrow biopsy

C. Hepatitis C antibody

D. Human immunodeficiency antibody

E. C and D

F. All of the above

III-99. A 54-year-old woman presents acutely with alterations in mental status and fever. She was well until 4 days previously when she began to develop complaints of myalgia and fever. Her symptoms progressed rapidly, and today her husband noted her to be lethargic and unresponsive when he awakened. She has recently felt well otherwise. Her only current medication is atenolol 25 mg daily for hypertension. On physical examination, she is responsive only to sternal rub and does not vocalize. Her vital signs are blood pressure of 165/92 mm Hg, heart rate of 114 beats/min, temperature of 38.7°C (101.7°F), respiratory rate of 26 breaths/min, and oxygen saturation of 92% on room air. Her cardiac examination shows a regular tachycardia. Her lungs have bibasilar crackles. The abdominal examination is unremarkable. No hepatosplenomegaly is present. There are petechiae on the lower extremities. Her complete blood count has a hemoglobin of 8.8 g/dL, hematocrit of 26.4%, white blood cell count of 10.2/μL (89% polymorphonuclear cells, 10% lymphocytes, 1% monocytes), and a platelet count of 54,000/μL. A peripheral blood smear is shown in Figure III-99. Her basic metabolic panel has a sodium of 137 meq/L, potassium of 5.4 meq/L, chloride of 98 meq/L, bicarbonate of 18 meq/L, BUN of 89 mg/dL, and creatinine of 2.9 mg/dL. Which statement most correctly describes the pathogenesis of the patient's condition?

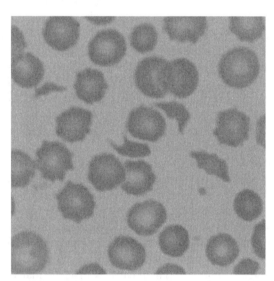

FIGURE III-99 (see Color Atlas)

A. Development of autoantibodies to a metalloproteinase that cleaves von Willebrand factor
B. Development of autoantibodies to the heparin-platelet factor 4 complex
C. Direct endothelial toxicity initiated by an infectious agent
D. Inherited disorder of platelet granule formation
E. Inherited disorder of von Willebrand factor that precludes binding with factor VIII

III-100. What is the best initial treatment for this patient?

A. Acyclovir 10 mg/kg intravenously every 8 hours
B. Ceftriaxone 2 g intravenously daily plus vancomycin 1 g intravenously twice daily
C. Hemodialysis
D. Methylprednisolone 1 g intravenously
E. Plasma exchange

III-101. Which of the following statements regarding hemophilia A and B is TRUE?

A. Individuals with factor VIII deficiency have a more severe clinical course than those with factor IX deficiency.
B. Levels of factor VIII or IX need to be measured before administration of replacement therapy in patients presenting with acute bleeding to calculate the appropriate dose of factor.
C. Primary prophylaxis against bleeding is never indicated.
D. The goal level of factor VIII or IX is greater than 50% in the setting of large-volume bleeding episodes.
E. The life expectancy of individuals with hemophilia is about 50 years.

III-102. A 24-year-old man is admitted to the hospital with circulatory collapse in the setting of disseminated meningococcemia. He is currently intubated, sedated, and on mechanical ventilation. He has received over 6 L of intravenous saline in the past 6 hours but remains hypotensive, requiring treatment with norepinephrine and vasopressin at maximum doses. He is making less than 20 mL of urine each hour. Blood is noted to be oozing from all of IV sites. His endotracheal secretions are blood tinged. His laboratory studies show a white blood cell count of 24,300/μL (82% neutrophils, 15% bands, 3% lymphocytes), hemoglobin of 8.7 g/dL, hematocrit of 26.1%, and platelets of 19,000/μL. The international normalized ratio is 3.6, the activated partial thromboplastin time is 75 seconds, and fibrinogen is 42 mg/dL. The lactate dehydrogenase level is 580 U/L, and the haptoglobin is less than 10 mg/dL. The peripheral smear shows thrombocytopenia and schistocytes. All of the following treatments are indicated in this patient EXCEPT:

A. Ceftriaxone 2 g intravenously twice daily
B. Cryoprecipitate
C. Fresh-frozen plasma
D. Heparin
E. Platelets

III-103. All the following are vitamin K–dependent coagulation factors EXCEPT:

A. Factor X
B. Factor VII
C. Protein C
D. Protein S
E. Factor VIII

III-104. A 31-year-old man with hemophilia A is admitted with persistent gross hematuria. He denies recent trauma and any history of genitourinary pathology. The examination is unremarkable. Hematocrit is 28%. All the following are treatments for hemophilia A EXCEPT:

A. Desmopressin (DDAVP)
B. Fresh-frozen plasma
C. Cryoprecipitate
D. Recombinant factor VIII
E. Plasmapheresis

III-105. All of the following statements regarding the lupus anticoagulant (LA) are true EXCEPT:

A. LAs typically prolong the activated partial thromboplastin time.
B. A 1:1 mixing study will not correct in the presence of LAs.
C. Bleeding episodes in patients with LAs may be severe and life threatening.
D. Female patients may experience recurrent midtrimester abortions.
E. LAs may occur in the absence of other signs of systemic lupus erythematosus.

III-106. All the following cause prolongation of the activated partial thromboplastin time that does not correct with a 1:1 mixture with pooled plasma EXCEPT:

A. Lupus anticoagulant
B. Factor VIII inhibitor
C. Heparin
D. Factor VII inhibitor
E. Factor IX inhibitor

III-107. You are evaluating a 45-year-old man with an acute upper gastrointestinal (GI) bleed in the emergency department. He reports increasing abdominal girth over the past 3 months associated with fatigue and anorexia. He has not noticed any lower extremity edema. His medical history is significant for hemophilia A diagnosed as a child with recurrent elbow hemarthroses in the past. He has been receiving infusions of factor VIII for most of his life and received his last injection earlier that day. His blood pressure is 85/45 mm Hg with a heart rate of 115 beats/min. His abdominal examination is tense with a positive fluid wave. Hematocrit is 21%. Renal function and urinalysis are normal. His activated partial thromboplastin time is minimally prolonged, his international normalized ratio is 2.7, and platelets are normal. Which of the following is most likely to yield a diagnosis for the cause of his GI bleeding?

A. Factor VIII activity level
B. *Helicobacter pylori* antibody test
C. Hepatitis B surface antigen
D. Hepatitis C RNA
E. Mesenteric angiogram

III-108. You are managing a patient with suspected disseminated intravascular coagulopathy (DIC). The patient has end-stage liver disease awaiting liver transplantation and was recently in the intensive care unit with *Escherichia coli* bacterial peritonitis. You suspect DIC based on a new upper gastrointestinal bleed in the setting of oozing from venipuncture sites. Platelet count is 43,000/μL, international normalized ratio is 2.5, hemoglobin is 6 mg/dL, and D-dimer is elevated to 4.5. What is the best way to distinguish between new-onset DIC and chronic liver disease?

A. Blood culture
B. Elevated fibrinogen degradation products
C. Prolonged aPTT
D. Reduced platelet count
E. Serial laboratory analysis

III-109. All of the following genetic mutations are associated with an increased risk of deep venous thrombosis EXCEPT:

A. Factor V Leiden mutation
B. Glycoprotein 1b platelet receptor
C. Heterozygous protein C deficiency
D. Prothrombin 20210G
E. Tissue plasminogen activator

III-110. A 76-year-old man presents to an urgent care clinic with pain in his left leg for 4 days. He also describes swelling in his left ankle, which has made it difficult for him to ambulate. He is an active smoker and has a medical history remarkable for gastroesophageal reflux disease, deep venous thrombosis (DVT) 9 months ago that resolved, and well-controlled hypertension. Physical examination is revealing for 2+ edema in his left ankle. A D-dimer is ordered and is elevated. Which of the following makes D-dimer less predictive of DVT in this patient?

A. Age older than 70 years
B. History of active tobacco use
C. Lack of suggestive clinical symptoms
D. Negative Homan's sign on examination
E. Previous DVT in the past year

III-111. A 22-year-old woman comes to the emergency department complaining of 12 hours of shortness of breath. The symptoms began toward the end of a long car ride home from college. She has no medical history, and her only medication is an oral contraceptive. She smokes occasionally, but the frequency has increased recently because of examinations. On physical examination, she is afebrile with respiratory rate of 22 breaths/min, blood pressure of 120/80 mm Hg, heart rate of 110 beats/min, and oxygen saturation on room air of 92%. The rest of her physical examination findings are normal. A chest radiograph and complete blood count are normal. Her serum pregnancy test result is negative. Which of the following is the indicated management strategy?

A. Check D-dimer and, if normal, discharge with non-steroidal anti-inflammatory therapy.
B. Check D-dimer and, if normal, obtain lower extremity ultrasound.
C. Check D-dimer and, if abnormal, treat for deep venous thrombosis/pulmonary embolism.
D. Check D-dimer and, if abnormal, obtain a contrast multislice computed tomography scan of the chest.
E. Obtain a contrast multislice computed tomography scan of the chest.

III-112. All of the anticoagulant or antiplatelet drugs listed are correctly matched with their mechanisms of action EXCEPT:

A. Abciximab—Glycoprotein IIb/IIIa receptor inhibitor
B. Clopidogrel—Adenosine diphosphate receptor blockade
C. Enoxaparin—Direct thrombin inhibition
D. Rivaroxaban—Factor Xa inhibition
E. Warfarin—Inhibition of production of the vitamin K–dependent clotting factors

III-113. A 66-year-old woman is prescribed clopidogrel and aspirin after implantation of a bare metal stent in her right coronary artery. Two weeks after the procedure, the woman presents to the emergency department with acute-onset chest pain and electrocardiographic changes consistent with an acute inferior myocardial infarction. Emergent cardiac catheterization confirms in-stent restenosis. The patient insists she has been adherent to her prescribed therapy. Which of the following statements most correctly described the most likely cause of the patient's restenosis despite her current therapy?

A. She likely has aspirin resistance and should be treated with higher doses of aspirin to prevent a recurrence.
B. She likely has clopidogrel resistance caused by a genetic polymorphism of the CYP pathway.
C. She should have been treated with low-molecular-weight heparin to prevent this complication.
D. She should have been treated with warfarin to prevent this complication.
E. Because she has demonstrated resistance to clopidogrel, switching to prasugrel would not be useful to prevent further complications.

III-114. A 48-year-old woman is diagnosed with a deep venous thrombosis of her left lower extremity. When considering initial anticoagulant therapy, all of the following are advantages of low-molecular-weight heparins over heparin EXCEPT:

A. Better bioavailability
B. Dose-dependent clearance
C. Longer half-life after subcutaneous injection
D. Lower risk of heparin-induced thrombocytopenia
E. Predictable anticoagulant effect

ANSWERS

III-1. **The answers are 1—C, 2—E, 3—D, 4—A, and 5—B.** *(Chap. e17)* Patients with homozygous sickle cell disease have red blood cells (RBCs) that are less pliable and more "sticky" than normal RBCs. Vaso-occlusive crisis is often precipitated by infection, fever, excessive exercise, anxiety, abrupt changes in temperature, hypoxia, or hypertonic dyes. Peripheral blood smear will show the typical elongated, crescent-shaped RBCs. There is also a nucleated RBC at the bottom of the figure, which may occur attributable to increased bone marrow production. Howell-Jolly bodies, small nuclear remnants normally removed by the intact spleen, are seen in RBCs in patients after splenectomy and with maturation or dysplastic disorders characterized by excess production. Acanthocytes are contracted dense RBCs with irregular membrane projections that vary in width and length. They are seen in patients with severe liver disease and abetalipoproteinemia and in rare patients with McLeod blood group. Iron deficiency, often caused by chronic stool blood loss in patients with colonic polyps or adenocarcinoma, causes a hypochromic microcytic anemia characterized by small, pale RBCs (a small lymphocyte is present on the smear to assess RBC size). RBCs are never hyperchromic; if more than the normal amount of hemoglobin is made, the cells get larger, not darker. Fragmented red cells, or schistocytes, are helmet-shaped cells that reflect microangiopathic hemolytic anemia (e.g., thrombotic thrombocytopenic purpura, disseminated intravascular coagulation, hemolytic uremic syndrome, scleroderma crisis) or shear damage from a prosthetic heart valve.

III-2.   **The answer is A.** *(Chap. 57)* This patient with anemia demonstrates a low mean cell volume, low mean cell hemoglobin, and low mean cell hemoglobin concentration. The peripheral smear demonstrates microcytic and hypochromic cells, which would be expected given these laboratory findings. In addition, there is marked variation in size (anisocytosis) and shape (poikilocytosis). These findings are consistent with severe iron-deficiency anemia, and serum ferritin would be expected to be less than 10 to 15 μg/L. A low haptoglobin level would be seen in cases of hemolysis, which can be intravascular or extravascular in origin. In intravascular hemolysis, the peripheral smear would be expected to show poikilocytosis with the presence of schistocytes (fragmented red blood cells [RBCs]). In extravascular hemolysis, the peripheral smear would typically shows spherocytes. Hemoglobin electrophoresis is used to determine the presence of abnormal hemoglobin variants. Sickle cell anemia is the most common form and demonstrates sickled RBCs. Thalassemias are also common inherited hemoglobinopathies. The peripheral smear in thalassemia often shows target cells. Glucose-6-phosphate dehydrogenase deficiency leads to oxidant-induced hemolysis with presence of bite cells or blister cells. Vitamin B_{12} deficiency leads to macrocytosis, which is not consistent with this case.

III-3.   **The answer is C.** *(Chap. 57)* The reticulocyte index and reticulocyte production index are useful in the evaluation of anemia to determine the adequacy of bone marrow response to the anemia. A normal reticulocyte count is 1% to 2%, and in the presence of anemia, this would be expected to rise to more than two to three times the normal value (the reticulocyte index). The reticulocyte index is calculated as Reticulocyte count × (Patient's hemoglobin/Normal hemoglobin). In this case, the reticulocyte index would be 5.4%. A second correction is further necessary in this patient given the presence of polychromatophilic macrocytes on peripheral smear. This finding indicates premature release of reticulocytes from the bone marrow ("shift cells"), and thus these cells have a longer life span. It is recommended to further divide the reticulocyte index by a factor of 2, which is known as the reticulocyte production index. In this case, the value would be 2.7%.

III-4.   **The answer is C.** *(Chap. 57)* This blood smear shows fragmented red blood cells (RBCs) of varying size and shape. In the presence of a foreign body within the circulation (prosthetic heart valve, vascular graft), RBCs can become destroyed. Such intravascular hemolysis will also cause serum lactate dehydrogenase to be elevated and hemoglobinuria. In isolated extravascular hemolysis, there is no hemoglobin or hemosiderin released into the urine. The characteristic peripheral blood smear in splenomegaly is the presence of Howell-Jolly bodies (nuclear remnants within red blood cells). Certain diseases are associated with extramedullary hematopoiesis (e.g., chronic hemolytic anemias), which can be detected by an enlarged spleen, thickened calvarium, myelofibrosis, or hepatomegaly. The peripheral blood smear may show teardrop cells or nucleated RBCs. Hypothyroidism is associated with macrocytosis, which is not demonstrated here. Chronic gastrointestinal blood loss will cause microcytosis, not schistocytes.

III-5.   **The answer is A.** *(Chap. 81)* Although cigarette smoking is the greatest modifiable risk factor for the development of cancer, the most significant risk factor for cancer in general is age. Two-thirds of all cancers are diagnosed in individuals older than 65 years, and the risk of developing cancer between the ages of 60 and 79 years is one in three in men and one in five in women. In contrast, the risk of cancer between birth and age 49 years is one in 70 for boys and men and one in 48 for girls and women. Overall, men have a slightly greater risk of developing cancer than women (44% vs. 38% lifetime risk).

III-6.   **The answer is A.** *(Chap. 81)* The cause of cancer death differs across the life span. In women who are younger than 20 years of age, the largest cause of cancer death is leukemia. Between the ages of 20 and 59 years, breast cancer becomes the leading cause of cancer death. However, lung cancer is the leading cause of cancer death after the age of 60 years and is overall the number one cause of cancer death in women.

III-7. **The answer is B.** *(Chap. 81)* Although tumor burden is certainly a major factor in determining cancer outcomes, it is also important to consider the functional status of the patient when considering the therapeutic plan. The physiologic stresses of undergoing surgical interventions, radiation therapy, and chemotherapy can exhaust the limited reserves of a patient with multiple medical problems. It is clearly difficult to adequately measure the physiologic reserves of a patient, and most oncologists use performance status measures as a surrogate. Two of the most commonly used measures of performance status are the Eastern Cooperative Oncology Group (ECOG) and Karnofsky performance status. The ECOG scale provides a grade between 0 (fully active) and 5 (dead). Most patients are considered to have adequate reserve for undergoing treatment if the performance status is 0 to 2, with a grade 2 indicating someone who is ambulatory and capable of all self-care but unable carry out work activities. These individuals are up and about more than 50% of waking hours. A grade 3 performance score indicates someone who is capable of only limited self-care and is confined to a bed or chair more than 50% of waking hours. The Karnofsky score ranges from 0 (dead) to 100 (normal) and is graded at 10-point intervals. A Karnofsky score of less than 70 also indicates someone with poor performance status.

III-8. **The answer is D.** *(Chap. 81)* Tumor markers are proteins produced by tumor cells that can be measured in the serum or urine. These markers are neither sensitive nor specific enough to be useful for diagnosis or screening of cancer. However, in an individual with a known malignancy, rising or falling levels may be helpful for determining disease activity and response to therapy. Common tumor markers with associated diseases are shown in Table III-8 below. Of the tumor pairs listed, only human chorionic gonadotropin is correctly paired with its association with gestational trophoblastic disease.

TABLE III-8   Tumor Markers

Tumor Markers	Cancer	Nonneoplastic Conditions
Hormones		
Human chorionic gonadotropin	Gestational trophoblastic disease, gonadal germ cell tumor	Pregnancy
Calcitonin	Medullary cancer of the thyroid	
Catecholamines	Pheochromocytoma	
Oncofetal Antigens		
α-Fetoprotein	Hepatocellular carcinoma, gonadal germ cell tumor	Cirrhosis, hepatitis
Carcinoembryonic antigen	Adenocarcinomas of the colon, pancreas, lung, breast, ovary	Pancreatitis, hepatitis, inflammatory bowel disease, smoking
Enzymes		
Prostatic acid phosphatase	Prostate cancer	Prostatitis, prostatic hypertrophy
Neuron-specific enolase	Small cell cancer of the lung, neuroblastoma	
Lactate dehydrogenase	Lymphoma, Ewing's sarcoma	Hepatitis, hemolytic anemia, many others
Tumor-Associated Proteins		
Prostate-specific antigen	Prostate cancer	Prostatitis, prostatic hypertrophy
Monoclonal immunoglobulin	Myeloma	Infection, MGUS
CA-125	Ovarian cancer, some lymphomas	Menstruation, peritonitis, pregnancy
CA 19-9	Colon, pancreatic, breast cancer	Pancreatitis, ulcerative colitis
CD30	Hodgkin's disease, anaplastic large cell lymphoma	—
CD25	Hairy cell leukemia, adult T-cell leukemia or lymphoma	—

Abbreviation: MGUS, monoclonal gammopathy of uncertain significance.

III-9. **The answer is C.** *(Chap. 83)* Cancer occurs when a single cell acquires a series of genetic mutations that allow the cell to proliferate without regulation. The clonal nature of cancer is a key feature that allows a malignancy to be differentiated from hyperplasia, in which polyclonality is seen. Significant research has occurred over the past decades that allows us to understand the genetic causes of cancer in greater detail, and new research is providing a growing knowledge of cancer of any number of cell types with the hopes that future therapies can be personalized to the mutations that are present in the individual cancer. Based on laboratory research, it is thought that five to 10 mutations are needed for a cell to transform into a malignant cancer, although often many more mutations can be seen. The major genes involved in cancer are oncogenes and tumor suppressor genes. Both of these types of genes contribute to the malignant phenotype by leading to unregulated cell division or the ability to avoid programmed cell death. Oncogenes require only a single mutation to become activated and act in an autosomal dominant fashion. In contrast, tumor suppressor genes require both copies of the allele to become inactivated to lose their protective effects against unregulated cell growth. Caretaker genes are a subset of tumor suppressor genes and have no direct effect on cell growth. These genes function to help the cell protect the integrity of its genome by repairing DNA defects that occur.

III-10. **The answer is E.** *(Chap. 83)* A small proportion of cancers occur in patients with a genetic predisposition. Roughly 100 syndromes of familial cancer have been reported. Recognition allows for genetic counseling and increased cancer surveillance. Down syndrome, or trisomy 21, is characterized clinically by a variety of features, including moderate to severe learning disability, facial and musculoskeletal deformities, duodenal atresia, congenital heart defects, and an increased risk of acute leukemia. Fanconi's anemia is a condition that is associated with defects in DNA repair. There is a higher incidence of cancer, with leukemia and myelodysplasia being the most common cancers. von Hippel–Lindau syndrome is associated with hemangioblastomas, renal cysts, pancreatic cysts and carcinomas, and renal cell cancer. Neurofibromatosis (NF) types I and II are both associated with increased tumor formation. NF II is more associated with schwannoma. Both carry a risk of malignant peripheral nerve sheath tumors. Fragile X is a condition associated with chromosomal instability of the X chromosome. These patients have mental retardation; typical morphologic features, including macro-orchidism and prognathia; behavioral problems; and occasionally seizures. Increased cancer incidence has not been described.

III-11. **The answer is C.** *(Chap. 84)* Cancer treatment is undergoing a revolution with an increasing number of therapies that are directed specifically against signal transduction pathways. These pathways are often activated in cancer cells and contribute to the malignant phenotype of the cell. One commonly affected signal transduction pathway is that of tyrosine kinase. Typically, tyrosine kinase is only active for a very short period. However, in malignant cells, the tyrosine kinase pathway can be constitutively activated through mutation, gene amplification, or gene translocation. Small molecule therapy that can inhibit a tyrosine kinase pathway can lead to decreased proliferation of malignant cells, decreased survival, and impeded angiogenesis. Examples of targeted small molecule therapies and their molecular targets can be found in Table III-11 on the next page. These include drugs as well as monoclonal antibodies. Among the first small molecule therapies to be used in malignancy was imatinib, which has dramatically changed therapy in chronic myeloid leukemia. This drug targets the activated tyrosine kinase pathway activated by the Bcr-Abl mutation that is present in this disease.

Bevacizumab is a monoclonal antibody targeted against pathways in vascular endothelial growth factor (VEGF) and is used in lung and colon cancer. It had previously been used for breast cancer, but the U.S. Food and Drug Administration has recommended against its use in breast cancer as of November 2011 (www.fda.gov, accessed December 1, 2011). Erlotinib and gefitinib are active against tumors carrying mutations of the epidermal growth factor receptor (EGFR), especially in lung cancer. Rituximab has been used for many years and is an anti-CD20. Its most common use is in B-cell lymphomas and leukemias, but it is undergoing trials for use in autoimmune disease as well. Sunitinib and sorafenib both have activity against a large number of kinases. Whereas sunitinib targets c-Kit, VEGFR-2, PDGFR-β, and Fit-3, sorafenib targets RAF, VEGFR-2, PDGFR-α/β, Fit-3, and c-Kit.

TABLE III-11   Some Molecularly Targeted Agents Approved by the U.S. Food and Drug Administration for the Treatment of Cancer

Drug	Molecular Target	Disease	Mechanism of Action
All-*trans* retinoic acid (ATRA)	PML-RAR-α oncogene	Acute promyelocytic leukemia M3 AML; t(15;17)	Inhibits transcriptional repression by PML-RAR-α
Imatinib (Gleevec)	Bcr-Abl, c-Abl, c-Kit, PDGFR-α/β	Chronic myeloid leukemia; GIST	Blocks ATP binding to tyrosine kinase active site
Dasatinib (Sprycel)			
Nilotinib (Tasigna)			
Sunitinib (Sutent)	c-Kit, VEGFR-2, PDGFR-β, Flt-3	GIST; renal cell cancer	Inhibits activated c-Kit and PDGFR in GIST; inhibits VEGFR in RCC
Sorafenib (Nexavar)	RAF, VEGFR-2, PDGFR-α/β, Flt-3, c-Kit	RCC; hepatocellular carcinoma	Targets VEGFR pathways in RCC; possible activity against BRAF in melanoma, colon cancer, and others
Erlotinib (Tarceva)	EGFR	Non–small cell lung cancer; pancreatic cancer	Competitive inhibitor of the ATP-binding site of the EGFR
Gefitinib (Iressa)	EGFR	Non–small cell lung cancer	Inhibitor of EGFR tyrosine kinase
Bortezomib (Velcade)	Proteasome	Multiple myeloma	Inhibits proteolytic degradation of multiple cellular proteins
Monoclonal Antibodies			
Trastuzumab (Herceptin)	HER2/neu (ERBB2)	Breast cancer	Binds HER2 on tumor cell surface and induces receptor internalization
Cetuximab (Erbitux)	EGFR	Colon cancer, squamous cell carcinoma of the head and neck	Binds extracellular domain of EGFR and blocks binding of EGF and TGF-α; induces receptor internalization; potentiates the efficacy of chemotherapy and radiotherapy
Panitumumab (Vectibix)	EGFR	Colon cancer	Similar to cetuximab; likely to be very similar in clinical activity
Rituximab (Rituxan)	CD20	B-cell lymphomas and leukemias that express CD20	Multiple potential mechanisms, including direct induction of tumor cell apoptosis and immune mechanisms
Alemtuzumab (Campath)	CD52	Chronic lymphocytic leukemia and CD52-expressing lymphoid tumors	Immune mechanisms
Bevacizumab (Avastin)	VEGF	Colon, lung, breast cancers; data pending in other tumors	Inhibits angiogenesis by high-affinity binding to VEGF

Abbreviations: AML, acute myeloid leukemia; EGFR, epidermal growth factor receptor; Flt-3, fms-like tyrosine kinase-3; GIST, gastrointestinal stromal tumor; PDGFR, platelet-derived growth factor receptor; PML-RAR-α, promyelocytic leukemia-retinoic acid receptor-alpha; RCC, renal cell cancer; t(15;17), translocation between chromosomes 15 and 17; TGF-α, transforming growth factor-alpha; VEGFR, vascular endothelial growth factor receptor.

III-12.   **The answer is B.** *(Chap. 84)* *Epigenetics* is a term that refers to changes in the chromatin structure of the cell that lead to alterations in gene expression without underlying changes in the DNA code. As such, these changes are potentially reversible and may be targets for cancer therapy. An example of an important epigenetic change is hypermethylation of promoter regions (so-called CpG islands) in tumor suppressor genes that lead to the inactivation of one allele of the gene.

III-13. **The answer is A.** *(Chap. 85)* Generally, when metastatic disease is observed, surgical interventions do not change the outcome of a particular cancer. However, in a few instances, one should consider surgery as potentially curative. One example is metastatic osteosarcoma to the lung, which can be cured by resection of the lung lesion. There are other instances in which surgery may be effective in patients with metastatic disease. In non–small cell lung cancer, individual with a solitary brain metastasis at the time of diagnosis may also be treated with resection of the brain and lung lesions in a staged fashion. In colon cancer with liver metastases, hepatic lobectomy may produce long-term disease-free survival in as many as 25% of individuals if fewer than five lesions are observed in a single hepatic lobe. Another role for surgical resection in metastatic disease is to remove the source of hormone production that can stimulate cancer growth. This is occasionally recommended in prostate cancer, although antiandrogen therapy is most commonly used.

III-14. **The answer is D.** *(Chap. 85)* Clinical trials in cancer drug discovery follows a stepwise process before the drug is determined to be safe and effective for treatment of a specific cancer. Before proceeding to trials in human, cancer drugs must demonstrate antitumor activity with a specific dose and interval in animal trials. After this, drugs enter phase I trials to establish safe dosage range and side effects in humans. Clinical antitumor effect is observed, but phase II trials enroll a larger group of people to more rigorously quantify antitumor effects in humans. Further side effect data is collected as well. The dose given in phase II trials is the maximal tolerated dose determined in phase I trials. Although phase I trials often given escalating doses of an agent, phase II trials use a fixed dose, and the drug is given to only a very select and homogeneous group of patients. An agent is determined to be "active" and may proceed to a phase III trial if there is a partial regression rate of at least 20% to 25% with reversible non–life-threatening side effects. Phase III trials enroll the largest numbers of patients and often compare the drug with standard therapies for the particular cancer. Phase IV trials occur after release of the drug and are called postmarketing studies. These trials provide important information about risks, benefits, and optimal use in the general population of patients with a particular cancer, which can often be quite different than those patients enrolled in a clinical trial.

III-15. **The answers are 1—D, 2—C, 3—A, 4—E, and 5—B.** *(Chap. 85)* Cancer chemotherapy typically requires actively dividing cells to exert their actions to kill the cancer cells. The mechanism of action of the majority of chemotherapeutic agents can be broadly categorized as those affecting DNA, those affecting microtubules, and molecularly targeted agents. Within each of these broad categories, several common families of drugs operating have distinct mechanisms of action. DNA alkylating agents are cell cycle phase nonspecific agents that covalently modify DNA bases and lead to cross-linkage of DNA strands. These cells become unable to complete normal cell division. Examples of common DNA alkylating agents are cyclophosphamide, chlorambucil, dacarbazine, and the platinum agents (carboplatin, cisplatin, and oxaliplatin). Antitumor antibiotics are naturally occurring substances typically produced by bacteria that bind to DNA directly and cause free radical damage that leads to DNA breakage. Included in this group are topoisomerase poisons that are derived from plants that prevent DNA unwinding and replication. Examples of agents in this category are bleomycin, etoposide, topotecan, irinotecan, doxorubicin, daunorubicin, and mitoxantrone. Other drugs that are common anticancer agents affect DNA indirectly, especially through interference in the synthesis of purines or pyrimidines. This category of agents is known as antimetabolites and includes methotrexate, azathioprine, 5-fluorouracil, cytosine arabinoside, gemcitabine, fludarabine, asparaginase, and pemetrexed, among others.

 Chemotherapeutics agents that target the microtubules interfere with cell division by inhibiting the mitotic spindle. These antimitotic agents include vincristine, vinblastine, vinorelbine, paclitaxel, and docetaxel, among others.

 Molecularly targeted agents are relatively new agents for the treatment of malignancy. When compared with traditional cancer chemotherapy, these agents are directed against specific proteins within cells that are important in cell signal processing. There are many different types of molecularly targeted agents with the largest class being tyrosine kinase inhibitors. Commonly used tyrosine kinase inhibitors include imatinib, gefitinib, erlotinib, sorafenib, and sunitinib. All-*trans* retinoic acid is another example of a molecularly targeted agent that attaches to the promyelocytic leukemia–retinoic acid receptor fusion protein to stimulate differentiation of the promyelocytes to mature granulocytes. Other categories of targeted agents include histone deacetylase inhibitors and mTOR (mammalian target of rapamycin) inhibitors.

III-16. **The answer is E.** *(Chap. 85)* Myelosuppression predictably occurs after administration of a variety of chemotherapeutic agents. Antimetabolites and anthracyclines (including doxorubicin) typically cause neutropenia between 6 and 14 days after administration of the agent. Febrile neutropenia is diagnosed based on a single temperature greater than 38.5°C or three temperatures greater than 38.0°C. Treatment of febrile neutropenia conventionally includes initiation of treatment with broad-spectrum antibiotics. If there is no obvious site of infection, then coverage for *Pseudomonas aeruginosa* is recommended. Active antibiotics include third- or fourth-generation cephalosporins (including ceftazidime), antipseudomonal penicillins, carbapenems, and aminoglycosides. Vancomycin should be considered in this patient because of her tunneled intravenous catheter despite the apparent lack of cutaneous infection and would be continued until culture demonstrated the absence of a resistant organism. There is no need for an antifungal agent because this patient has not had prolonged neutropenia, and this is the first fever recorded. Moreover, given the chemotherapy given, the expected duration of neutropenia is expected to be relatively brief. In many instances such as this, oral antibiotics such as ciprofloxacin can be given.

There is no role for granulocyte transfusions in the treatment. However, the use of colony-stimulating factors often is considered. These agents have historically been overused, and the American Society of Clinical Oncology has developed practice guidelines to assist in determining which patients should receive colony-stimulating factors. Briefly, there is no evidence for benefit in either febrile or afebrile neutropenic patients, and they should not routinely be used in acute myeloid leukemia or myelodysplastic syndromes. The only therapeutic use is in individuals who have undergone bone marrow or stem cell transplantation to speed myeloid recovery. The primary use of colony-stimulating factors is in the setting of prevention. Because this patient has now experienced an episode of febrile neutropenia, she should be given colony-stimulating factors beginning 24 to 72 hours after chemotherapy administration, and the medication should continue until the neutrophil count is 10,000/μL or greater. Colony-stimulating factors may be given after the first cycle of chemotherapy if the likelihood of febrile neutropenia is greater than 20%, if the patient has preexisting neutropenia or active infection, if the patient is older than 65 years of age and is being treated for lymphoma, or if the patient has a poor performance status or has had extensive prior chemotherapy.

III-17. **The answer is E.** *(Chap. 85)* Nausea with or without vomiting is the most common side effect of chemotherapy. It can be anticipatory in nature, acute, or occur more than 24 hours after administration. Patients at increased risk of nausea include younger patients, women, and those with a history of motion or morning sickness. The chemotherapeutic agents used also alter the risk of nausea and vomiting. Highly emetogenic drugs include high-dose cyclophosphamide and cisplatin. Low-risk drugs include fluorouracil, taxanes, and etoposide. In patients receiving high-risk regimens, prophylactic treatment with a combination of medications acting at different sites is recommended. Typically, the regimen would include a serotonin antagonist such as dolasetron, a neurokine receptor antagonist such are aprepitant, and potent corticosteroids such as dexamethasone.

III-18. **The answer is C.** *(Chap. 86)* Patients who have undergone allogeneic stem cell transplant remain at risk for infectious complications for an extended period despite engraftment and apparent return of normal hematopoietic capacity. Individuals with graft-versus-host disease (GVHD) often require immunosuppressive treatment that further increases their infectious risk. Prevention of infection is the goal in these individuals, and the clinician should ensure appropriate vaccinations for all patients who have undergone intensive chemotherapy, have been treated for Hodgkin's disease, or have undergone hematopoietic stem cell transplant. No vaccines except influenza should be given before 12 months after transplant. Then the only vaccines that should be given are inactivated vaccines. Therefore, oral vaccine for poliomyelitis and the varicella zoster vaccine are contraindicated. The measles, mump, and rubella vaccine is also a live virus vaccine, but can be safely given after 24 months if the patient does not have

GVHD. Other recommended vaccines include diphtheria–tetanus, inactivated poliomyelitis (by injection), *Haemophilus influenzae* type B, hepatitis B, and 23-valent pneumococcal polysaccharide vaccine. Meningococcal vaccination is recommended in splenectomized patients and in those living in endemic areas, including college dormitories.

III-19. **The answer is B.** *(Chap. 86)* Specific malignancies are associated with underlying immune dysfunction and infection with specific organisms. Chronic lymphocytic leukemia and multiple myeloma may have an associated hypogammaglobulinemia. Individuals with these disorders are at risk of infections with *Streptococcus pneumoniae, Haemophilus influenzae,* and *Neisseria meningitidis.* Although immunoglobulin therapy is effective, it is more cost effective to give prophylactic antibiotics in these patients. Acute myeloid or lymphocytic leukemias often have an associated neutropenia and may present with overwhelming infection from extracellular bacteria and fungi, especially if the duration of neutropenia is prolonged. Patients with lymphomatous disorders often have abnormal T-cell function despite normal numbers of T cells. Moreover, most patients also receive treatment with high doses of glucocorticoids that further impair T-cell function. These individuals have an increased risk of infection with intracellular pathogens and may contract pneumonia with *Pneumocystis jiroveci.*

III-20. **The answer is D.** *(Chap. 86)* Clinicians are often faced with treatment decisions regarding catheter-related infections in patients who are immunocompromised from cancer and chemotherapy. Because many patients require several weeks of chemotherapy, tunneled catheters are often placed, and determining the need for catheter removal is an important consideration. When blood culture results are positive or there is evidence of infection along the track of the tunnel, catheter removal is recommended. When the erythema is limited to the exit site only, then it is not necessary to remove the catheter unless the erythema fails to respond to treatment. The recommended treatment for an exit site infection should be directed against coagulase-negative staphylococci. In the options presented, vancomycin alone is the best option for treatment. There is no need to add therapy for gram-negative organisms because the patient does not have neutropenia and has negative culture results.

III-21. **The answer is A.** *(Chap. 87)* The staging criteria for melanoma include the thickness of the lesion, the presence of ulceration, and the presence and number of involved lymph nodes. Of these, the single best predictor of metastatic risk is the Breslow thickness, particularly greater than 4 mm, although the other factors also provide additional predictive value. Other factors that predict survival in melanoma are younger age, gender with female sex predicting a better survival, and anatomic site with favorable sites being the forearm and leg. The Clark level defined melanoma based on the layer of skin to which a melanoma had invaded, but this has been found to be not predictive of metastatic risk.

III-22. **The answer is E.** *(Chap. 87, Chapman PB et al: N Engl J Med 2011; 364: 2507-2516)* Treatment of metastatic melanoma has largely shown very little improvements on mortality in this disease. The median survival after diagnosis of metastatic disease is typically 6 to 15 months. Until August 2011, the only Food and Drug Administration (FDA)–approved chemotherapy for the treatment of metastatic disease was dacarbazine, although response rates are about 20% or less. Interleukin-2 therapy has also been attempted alone or in combination with interferon-α. This therapy has lead to long-term disease-free survival in about 5% of treated patients but is associated with significant toxicity that limits its usefulness. Interleukin-2 should only be administered to patients with good performance status and at centers experienced in the treatment of IL-2 toxicity. Most recently in August 2011, the FDA approved the drug vemurafenib (PLX4032) for the treatment of metastatic melanoma. This drug targets *BRAF*, which is a common mutation in melanoma that results in constitutive activation of the mitogen-activated protein (MAP) kinase pathway. Vemurafenib has specifically demonstrated to have the best activity against the BRAF V600E mutation, the most common kinase mutation in metastatic melanoma. Data published in 2011 demonstrated that individuals with this specific mutation have response rates of 48% to the drug compared with only 5% for dacarbazine. Furthermore, the 6-month survival was 84% in the vemurafenib group compared with only 64% in the dacarbazine group. Ipilimumab is another promising new therapy for the treatment of metastatic melanoma. This treatment is a monoclonal antibody that blocks cytotoxic T-cell antigen 4 (CTLA-4), and a recent clinical trial demonstrated improved overall survival rates in patients treated with ipilimumab plus dacarbazine compared with dacarbazine alone (Robert C et al: *N Engl J Med* 2011; 364: 2517-25).

III-23. **The answer is C.** *(Chap. 88)* Head and neck cancers account for about 3% of all malignancies in the United States and comprise a varied site of tumors, including those of the nasopharynx, oropharynx, hypopharynx, and larynx. Squamous cell history is the predominant cell type at all sites, but there are different risk factors by site. Nasopharyngeal cancers are rare in the United States but are endemic in the Mediterranean and Far East, where they are associated with Epstein-Barr virus infection. Oropharyngeal cancers are associated with tobacco use, especially smokeless tobacco, and increasing numbers of oropharyngeal cancers are found to be associated with human papilloma virus (HPV). The association with HPV virus infection, particularly serotypes 16 and 18, characterizes these oropharyngeal cancers as a form of sexually transmitted disease and is associated with oral sexual practices and an increased number of sexual partners. However, the predominant risk factors for head and neck cancers, particularly those of the hypopharynx and larynx, are alcohol and tobacco use. Cancers of the larynx often present with the subacute onset of hoarseness that does not resolve over time, but symptoms of head and neck cancer can be rather nonspecific. In more advanced cases, pain, stridor, dysphagia, odynophagia, and cranial neuropathies can occur. Diagnosis of head and neck cancer should include computed tomography of the head and neck and endoscopic examination under anesthesia to perform biopsies. Positron emission tomography scans may be used as adjunctive therapy. The staging of head and neck cancers follows a TNM staging guideline. This patient would be staged as T2N0M0 based on a tumor size without evidence of lymph node involvement or distant metastatic disease. With this designation, the patient's overall stage would be stage II and classified as localized disease. The intent of therapy at this stage of disease is cure of cancer, and the overall 5-year survival is 60% to 90%. The choice of therapy for laryngeal cancer is radiation therapy to preserve the voice. Surgical therapy could be chosen by the patient as well but is less desirable. In locally or regionally advanced disease, patients can still be approached with curative intent, but this requires multimodality therapy with surgery followed by concomitant chemotherapy and radiation treatment.

III-24. **The answer is A.** *(Chap. 89)* Solitary pulmonary nodules are frequent causes of referral to a pulmonologist, but most solitary pulmonary nodules are benign. In fact, more than 90% of incidentally identified nodules are of benign origin. Features that are more likely to be present in a malignant lesion are size larger than 3 cm, eccentric calcification, rapid doubling time, and lobulated and irregular contour. Ground-glass appearance on computed tomography can be either malignant or benign. Among malignant lesions, it is seen more commonly in bronchoalveolar cell carcinoma. When multiple pulmonary nodules are identified, it most commonly represents prior granulomatous disease from healed infections. If multiple nodules are malignant in origin, it usually indicates disease metastatic to the lung but can be simultaneous lung primary lesions or lesions metastatic from a primary lung cancer. Many incidentally identified nodules are too small to be diagnosed by biopsy and are nonspecific in nature. In this situation, it is prudent to follow the lesions for 2 years, especially in a patient who is high risk for lung cancer to allow for a proper doubling time to occur. If the lesion remains stable for 2 years, it is most likely benign, although some slow-growing tumors such bronchoalveolar cell carcinoma can have a slower growth rate.

III-25. **The answer is E.** *(Chap. 89)* The evaluation and treatment of solitary pulmonary nodules is important to understand. This patient has a long smoking history with a new nodule that was not apparent by chest radiography 3 years previously. This should be assumed to be a malignant nodule, and definitive diagnosis and treatment should be attempted. The option for diagnostic and staging procedures include positron emission tomography (PET) and computed tomography (CT), bronchoscopic biopsy, percutaneous needle biopsy, and surgical biopsy with concomitant resection if positive. PET and CT would be low yield in this patient given the small size of the primary lesion (<1 cm) and the lack of enlarged mediastinal lymph nodes. Likewise, bronchoscopy would not provide a good yield because the lesion is very peripheral in origin, and a negative biopsy for malignancy would not be definitive. Appropriate approaches would be to either perform a percutaneous needle biopsy with CT guidance or perform a surgical biopsy with definitive resection if positive. Because this patient has preserved lung function, surgical biopsy and resection is a good treatment option. A repeat CT scan assessing for interval growth would only be appropriate if the patient declined further workup at this time. Referral for treatment with radiation therapy is not appropriate in the absence of tissue diagnosis of malignancy, and surgical resection is the preferred primary treatment because the patient has no contraindications to surgical intervention.

III-26. **The answer is E.** *(Chap. 89)* Pancoast syndrome results from apical extension of a lung mass into the brachial plexus with frequent involvement of the eighth cervical and first and second thoracic nerves. As the tumor continues to grow, it will also involve the sympathetic ganglia of the thoracic chain. The clinical manifestations of a Pancoast tumor include shoulder and arm pain and Horner's syndrome (ipsilateral ptosis, miosis, and anhidrosis). Often, the shoulder and arm pain presents several months before diagnosis. The most common cause of Pancoast syndrome is an apical lung tumor, usually non–small cell lung cancer. Other causes include mesothelioma and infection, among others. Although midbrain lesions can cause Horner's syndrome, other cranial nerve abnormalities would be expected.

Enlarged mediastinal lymph nodes and masses in the middle mediastinum can occlude the superior vena cava (SVC), leading to SVC syndrome. Individuals with SVC syndrome typically present with dyspnea and have evidence of facial and upper extremity swelling. Eaton Lambert myasthenic syndrome is caused by antibodies to voltage-gated calcium channels and is characterized by generalized weakness of muscles that increases with repetitive nerve stimulation. Cervical ribs can cause thoracic outlet syndrome by compression of nerves or vasculature as they exit the chest. This typically presents with ischemic symptoms to the affected limb, but intrinsic wasting of the muscles of the hand can be seen because of neurologic compromise.

III-27. **The answer is E.** *(Chap. 89)* At the time of diagnosis, 70% of small cell lung cancers have metastasized. In contrast to non–small cell lung cancer, small cell lung cancer is staged as limited or extensive disease based on the spread of disease in the body rather than size of the tumor burden or extent of lymph node involvement. Common sites of metastases in small cell lung cancer are thoracic lymph nodes, brain, adrenal glands, and liver. All patients diagnosed with small cell lung cancer should undergo chest and abdominal computed tomography (CT) scans as well as CT or magnetic resonance imaging (MRI) imaging of the brain. If bone pain is present, radionuclide bone scans should be performed. Bone marrow biopsies are not typically indicated as isolated bone marrow metastases are rare. If there are signs of spinal cord compression or leptomeningeal involvement, imaging of the spine by MRI or CT and lumbar puncture are indicated, respectively.

III-28. **The answer is C.** *(Chap. 89)* Mutations of the epidermal growth factor receptor (EGFR) have recently been recognized as important mutations that affect the response of non–small cell lung cancers to treatment with EGFR tyrosine kinase inhibitors. Initial studies of erlotinib in all patients with advanced non–small cell lung cancer failed to show a treatment benefit; however, when only patients with EGFR mutations were considered, treatment with anti-EGFR therapy improved progression-free and overall survival. Patients who are more likely to have EGFR mutations are women, nonsmokers, Asians, and those with adenocarcinoma histopathology.

III-29. **The answer is B.** *(Chap. 89, N Engl J Med 2011; 365: 395-409)* Screening for lung cancer in high-risk individuals has been investigated for many years. Screening trials require large numbers of participants that can be followed for long periods of time and are expensive to conduct. Until 2011, no screening trial had been able to demonstrate any decrease in lung cancer mortality. Previous screening modalities have been primarily chest radiographs with or without sputum cytology. In June 2011, the main results of the National Lung Cancer Screening Trial (NLST) were published in the *New England Journal of Medicine*. The trial enrolled more than 50,000 individuals with a greater than 30 pack-year history of cigarette smoking and randomized the individuals to yearly chest radiographs or low-dose computed

tomography (CT) scans for a period of 3 years. Outcomes in the individuals continued to be followed for a total of almost 8 years, when the trial was stopped early. Individuals receiving low-dose CT scans demonstrated a 20% mortality reduction from lung cancer compared with those receiving chest radiographs alone, and more individuals receiving CT scans were diagnosed at early stages of disease. A caveat in broadly applying these results in clinical practice is that more than 90% of positive scans proved to be false positives. At this point, more research on the cost effectiveness of CT scans and the appropriate population to which to offer scans needs to be done before widespread screening is recommended.

III-30. **The answer is C.** *(Chap. 90)* The patient has a breast cyst. This has a benign feel on examination, and aspiration of the mass showed nonbloody fluid with resolution of the mass. If there were residual mass or bloody fluid, mammography and biopsy would be the next step. In patients such as this with nonbloody fluid in whom aspiration clears the mass, reexamination in 1 month is indicated. If the mass recurs, then aspiration should be repeated. If fluid recurs, mammography and biopsy would be indicated at that point. There is no indication at this point to refer for advanced imaging or surgical evaluation. Breastfeeding is not affected by the presence of a breast cyst.

III-31. **The answer is C.** *(Chap. 90)* Breast cancer risk is related to many factors, but age of menarche, age of first full-term pregnancy, and age at menopause together account for 70% to 80% of all breast cancer risk. The lowest risk patients have the shortest duration of total menses (i.e., later menarche and earlier menopause), as well as an early first full-term pregnancy. Specifically, the lowest risks are menarche at age 16 years old or older, first pregnancy by the age of 18 years, and menopause that begins 10 years before the median age of menopause of 52 years. Thus, patient C meets these criteria.

III-32. **The answer is D.** *(Chap. 90)* Pathologic staging remains the most important determinant of overall prognosis. Other prognostic factors have an impact on survival and the choice of therapy. Tumors that lack estrogen or progesterone receptors are more likely to recur. The presence of estrogen receptors, particularly in postmenopausal women, is also an important factor in determining adjuvant chemotherapy. Tumors with a high growth rate are associated with early relapse. Measurement of the proportion of cells in S-phase is a measure of the growth rate. Tumors with more than the median number of cells in S-phase have a higher risk of relapse and an improved response rate to chemotherapy. Histologically, tumors with a poor nuclear grade have a higher risk of recurrence than do tumors with a good nuclear grade. At the molecular level, tumors that overexpress erbB2 (HER-2/neu) or that have a mutated p53 gene portend a poorer prognosis for patients. The overexpression of erbB2 is also useful in designing optimal treatment regimens, and a human monoclonal antibody to erbB2 (Herceptin) has been developed.

III-33. **The answer is E.** *(Chap. 91)* Esophageal cancer is an uncommon gastrointestinal malignancy with a high mortality rate because most patients do not present until advanced disease is present. The typical presenting symptoms of esophageal cancer are dysphagia with significant weight loss. Dysphagia is typically fairly rapidly progressive over a period of weeks to months. Dysphagia initially in only to solid foods but progresses to include semisolids and liquids. For dysphagia to occur, an estimated 60% of the esophageal lumen must be occluded. Weight loss occurs because of decreased oral intake in addition to the cachexia that is common with cancer. Associated symptoms may include pain with swallowing that can radiate to the back, regurgitation or vomiting of undigested food, and aspiration pneumonia. The two major cell types of esophageal cancer in the United States are adenocarcinoma and squamous cell carcinoma, which have different risk factors. Individuals with squamous cell carcinomas typically have a history of both tobacco and alcohol abuse, but those with adenocarcinoma more often have a history of long-standing gastroesophageal reflux disease and Barrett's esophagitis. Among those with a history of alcohol and tobacco abuse, there is an increased risk with increased intake and interestingly is more associated with whiskey drinking compared with wine or beer. Other risk factors for squamous cell carcinoma of the esophagus include ingestion of nitrites, smoked opiates, fungal toxins in pickled vegetables, and physical insults that include long-standing ingestion of very hot tea or lye.

III-34.   **The answer is E.** *(Chap. 91)* Colorectal cancer is the second most common cause of cancer death in the United States, and the mortality rate related to the disease has been decreasing in recent years. When colorectal cancer is identified, patients should be referred for surgical intervention because proper staging and prognosis cannot be determined without pathologic specimens if there is no gross evidence of metastatic disease. The preoperative workup to assess for metastatic or synchronous disease includes a complete colonoscopy if possible, chest radiography, liver function testing, carcinoembryonic antigen (CEA) testing, and computed tomography of the abdomen. Staging of colorectal cancer follows a TNM staging system. However, the T staging is not based on absolute size of the tumor rather it is based upon the extension of the tumor through the colonic wall. T1 tumors can extend into the submucosa but not beyond, T2 tumors extend into the muscularis propria, and T3 tumors involve the serosa and beyond. Nodal metastases are graded as N1 (one to three lymph nodes positive) and N2 (≥four lymph nodes positive). This patient's stage of cancer would be T2N1M0 and would be staged as a stage III cancer. Despite the relatively advanced stage, the overall 5-year survival rate would be 50% to 70% because of improvements in overall care of the patient with colorectal cancer. Because the patient had an occluding lesion that prevents preoperative colonoscopy, the patient needs to have a complete colonoscopy performed within the first several months after surgery and every 3 years thereafter. Serial measurements of CEA every 3 months have also been advocated by some specialists. Annual CT scanning may be performed for the first 3 years after resection, although the utility of the practice is debated. Radiation therapy to the pelvis is recommended for all patients with rectal cancer because it reduces the local recurrence rate, especially in stage II and III tumors. When postoperative radiation therapy is combined with chemotherapeutic regimens containing 5-fluorouracil, the local recurrence rate is further reduced and overall survival is increased as well.

III-35.   **The answer is A.** *(Chap. 91)* Most colorectal cancers arise from adenomatous polyps. Only adenomas are premalignant, and only a minority of these lesions becomes malignant. Most polyps are asymptomatic, causing occult bleeding in fewer than 5% of patients. Sessile (flat-based) polyps are more likely to become malignant than pedunculated (stalked) polyps. Histologically, villous adenomas are more likely to become malignant than tubular adenomas. The risk of containing invasive carcinoma in the polyp increases with size with less than 2% in polyps smaller than 1.5 cm, 2% to 10% in polyps 1.5 to 2.5 cm, and 10% in polyps larger than 2.5 cm. This patient had two polyps that were high risk based on histology (villous) and appearance (sessile) but only moderate risk by size (<1.5 cm). Polyps, particularly those larger than 2.5 cm in size, sometimes contain cancer cells but usually progress to cancer quite slowly over an approximate 5-year period. Patients with adenomatous polyps should have a follow-up colonoscopy or radiographic study in 3 years. If no polyps are found on initial study, the test (endoscopic or radiographic) should be repeated in 10 years. Computed tomography is only warranted for staging if there is a diagnosis of colon cancer, not for the presence of polyps alone.

III-36.   **The answer is A.** *(Chap. 91)* A strong family history of colon cancer should prompt consideration for hereditary nonpolyposis colon cancer (HNPCC), or Lynch syndrome, particularly if diffuse polyposis is not noted on colonoscopy. HNPCC is characterized by (1) three or more relatives with histologically proven colorectal cancer, one of whom is a first-degree relative and of the other two, at least one with the diagnosis before age 50 years, and (2) colorectal cancer in at least two generations. The disease is an autosomal dominant trait and is associated with other tumors, including in the endometrium and ovary. The proximal colon is most frequently involved, and cancer occurs with a median age of 50 years, 15 years earlier than in sporadic colon cancer. Patients with HNPCC are recommended to receive biennial colonoscopy and pelvic ultrasonography beginning at age 25 years. Innumerable polyps suggest the presence of one of the autosomal dominant polyposis syndromes, many of which carry a high malignant potential. These include familial adenomatous polyposis, Gardner's syndrome (associated with osteomas, fibromas, epidermoid cysts), or Turcot's syndrome (associated with brain cancer). Peutz-Jeghers syndrome is associated with mucocutaneous pigmentation and hamartomas. Tumors may develop in the ovary, breast, pancreas, and endometrium; however, malignant colon cancers are not common. Ulcerative colitis is strongly associated with development of colon cancer, but it is unusual for colon cancer to be the presenting finding in ulcerative colitis. Patients are generally symptomatic from their inflammatory bowel disease long before cancer risk develops.

III-37. **The answer is E.** *(Chap. 93)* Pancreatic cancer is the fourth leading cause of cancer death in the United States despite representing only 3% of all newly diagnosed malignancies. Infiltrating ductal adenocarcinomas account for the vast majority of cases and arise most frequently in the head of pancreas. At the time of diagnosis, 85% to 90% of patients have inoperable or metastatic disease, which is reflected in the 5-year survival rate of only 5% for all stages combined. An improved 5-year survival of up to 20% may be achieved when the tumor is detected at an early stage and when complete surgical resection is accomplished. Over the past 30 years, 5-year survival rates have not improved substantially. Cigarette smoking may be the cause of up to 20% to 25% of all pancreatic cancers and is the most common environmental risk factor for this disease. Other risk factors are not well established because of inconsistent results from epidemiologic studies, but they include chronic pancreatitis and diabetes. Alcohol does not appear to be a risk factor unless excess consumption gives rise to chronic pancreatitis.

III-38. **The answer is B.** *(Chap. 93)* Dual-phase, contrast-enhanced spiral computed tomography (CT) is the imaging modality of choice to visualize suspected pancreatic masses. In addition to imaging the pancreas, it also provides accurate visualization of surrounding viscera, vessels, and lymph nodes. In most cases, this study can determine surgical resectability. There is no advantage of magnetic resonance imaging (MRI) over CT in predicting tumor resectability, but selected cases may benefit from MRI to characterize the nature of small indeterminate liver lesions and to evaluate the cause of biliary dilatation when no obvious mass is seen on CT. Preoperative confirmation of malignancy is not always necessary in patients with radiologic appearances consistent with operable pancreatic cancer. Endoscopic ultrasound-guided needle biopsy is the most effective technique to evaluate the mass for malignancy. It has an accuracy of approximately 90% and has a smaller risk of intraperitoneal dissemination compared with CT-guided percutaneous biopsy. Endoscopic retrograde cholangiopancreatography (ERCP) is a useful method for obtaining ductal brushings, but the diagnostic value of pancreatic juice sampling is only 25% to 30%. CA 19-9 is elevated in approximately 70% to 80% of patients with pancreatic carcinoma, but ERCP is not recommended as a routine diagnostic or screening test because its sensitivity and specificity are inadequate for accurate diagnosis. Preoperative CA 19-9 levels correlate with tumor stage and prognosis. It is also an indicator of asymptomatic recurrence in patients with completely resected tumors. Fluorodeoxyglucose positron emission tomography (FDG-PET) should be considered before surgery for detecting distant metastases.

III-39. **The answer is D.** *(Chap. 94)* Bladder cancer is the fourth most common cancer in men and the thirteenth most common cancer in women. Cigarette smoking has a strong association with bladder cancer, particularly in men. The increased risk persists for at least 10 years after quitting. Bladder cancer is a small cause of cancer deaths because most detected cases are superficial with an excellent prognosis. Most cases of bladder cancer come to medical attention by the presence of gross hematuria emanating from exophytic lesions. Microscopic hematuria is more likely caused by prostate cancer than bladder cancer. Cystoscopy under anesthesia is indicated to evaluate for bladder cancer. In cases of superficial disease, bacille Calmette-Guérin (BCG) is an effective adjuvant to decrease recurrence or treat unresectable superficial disease. In the United States, cystectomy is generally recommended for invasive disease. Even invasive cancer with nodal involvement has a greater than 40% 10-year survival after surgery and adjuvant therapy.

III-40 and III-41. **The answers are C and E, respectively.** *(Chap. 94)* The incidence of renal cell carcinoma continues to rise and is now nearly 58,000 cases annually in the United States, resulting in 13,000 deaths. The male-to-female ratio is 2 to 1. Incidence peaks between the ages of 50 and 70 years, although this malignancy may be diagnosed at any age. Many environmental factors have been investigated as possible contributing causes; the strongest association is with cigarette smoking. Risk is also increased for patients who have acquired cystic disease of the kidney associated with end-stage renal disease and for those with tuberous sclerosis. Most renal cell carcinomas are clear cell tumors (60%) with papillary and chromophobic tumors less common. Clear cell tumors account for more than 80% of patients who develop metastases. The classic triad of hematuria, flank pain, and a palpable mass is only present in 10% to 20% of patients initially. Most cases currently are found as incidental findings on computed tomography or ultrasonography done for different reasons. The increasing number of incidentally discovered low-stage tumors has contributed to an improved 5-year survival. The paraneoplastic phenomenon of erythrocytosis caused by increased production of erythropoietin is only found in 3% of cases; anemia caused by advanced disease is far more common. Stage 1 and 2 tumors are confined to the kidney and have a greater than 80% survival after radical nephrectomy. Stage 4 tumors with distant metastases have a 50year survival of 10%. Renal cell carcinoma is notably resistant to traditional chemotherapeutic agents. Cytokine therapy with interleukin-2 or interferon-gamma produces regression in 10% to 20% of patients with metastatic disease. Recently, the advent of antiangiogenic medications has changed the treatment of advance renal cell carcinoma. Sunitinib was demonstrated to be superior to interferon-gamma, and it (or sorafenib) is now first-line therapy for patients with advanced metastatic disease.

III-42.   **The answer is A.** *(Chap. 95)* The results from several large double-blind, randomized chemoprevention trials have established 5 alpha-reductase inhibitors as the predominant therapy to reduce the future risk of a prostate cancer diagnosis. Randomized placebo-controlled trials have shown that finasteride and dutasteride reduce the period prevalence of prostate cancer. Trials of selenium, vitamin C, and vitamin E have shown no benefit versus placebo.

III-43.   **The answer is E.** *(Chap. 95)* As shown in Figure III-43, transrectal ultrasound-guided biopsy is recommended for men with either an abnormal digital rectal examination (DRE)

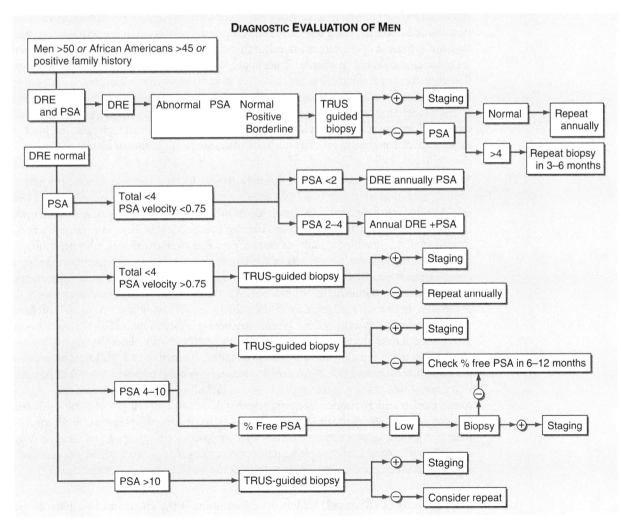

FIGURE III-43

or abnormal serum prostate-specific antigen (PSA) results. Twenty-five percent of men with a PSA above 4 ng/mL and abnormal DRE results have cancer, as do 17% of men with a PSA of 2.5 to 4 ng/mL and normal DRE results.

III-44. **The answer is C.** *(Chap. 96)* Ninety percent of persons with nonseminomatous germ cell tumors produce either α-fetoprotein (AFP) or beta human chorionic gonadotropin (β-hCG); in contrast, persons with pure seminomas usually produce neither. These tumor markers are present for some time after surgery; if the presurgical levels are high, 30 days or more may be required before meaningful postsurgical levels can be obtained. The half-lives of AFP and β-hCG are 6 days and 1 day, respectively. After treatment, unequal reduction of β-hCG and AFP may occur, suggesting that the two markers are synthesized by heterogeneous clones of cells within the tumor; thus, both markers should be followed. β-hCG is similar to luteinizing hormone except for its distinctive beta subunit.

III-45. **The answer is D.** *(Chap. 96)* Testicular cancer occurs most commonly in the second and third decades of life. The treatment depends on the underlying pathology and the stage of the disease. Germ cell tumors are divided into seminomatous and nonseminomatous subtypes. Although the pathology of this patient's tumor was seminoma, the presence of α-fetoprotein (AFP) is suggestive of occult nonseminomatous components. If there are any nonseminomatous components, the treatment follows that of a nonseminomatous germ cell tumor. This patient therefore has a clinical stage I nonseminomatous germ cell tumor. Because his AFP returned to normal after orchiectomy, there is no obvious occult disease. However, between 20% and 50% of these patients will have disease in the retroperitoneal lymph nodes. Numerous trials have indicated no overall survival difference in this cohort between observation and retroperitoneal lymph node dissection (RPLND). Because of the potential side effects of RPLND, the choice of surveillance or RPLND is based on the pathology of the primary tumor. If the primary tumor shows no evidence for lymphatic or vascular invasion and is limited to the testis, then either option is reasonable. If lymphatic or vascular invasion is present or the tumor extends into the tunica, spermatic cord, or scrotum, then surveillance should not be offered. Either approach should cure more than 95% of patients. Radiation therapy is the appropriate choice for stage I and stage II seminoma. It has no role in nonseminomatous lesions. Adjuvant chemotherapy is not indicated in early-stage testicular cancer. Hormonal therapy is effective for prostate cancer and receptor-positive breast cancer but has no role in testicular cancer. Positron emission tomography may be used to locate viable seminoma in residua which mandates surgical excision or biopsy.

III-46. **The answer is A.** *(Chap. 97)* Approximately 10% of women with ovarian cancer have a somatic mutation in one of two DNA repair genes, *BRCA1* (chromosome 17q12-21) or *BRCA2* (chromosome 13q12-13). Individuals inheriting a single copy of a mutant allele have a very high incidence of breast and ovarian cancer. Most of these women have a family history that is notable for multiple cases of breast or ovarian cancer (or both), although inheritance through male members of the family can camouflage this genotype through several generations. The most common malignancy in these women is breast carcinoma, although women harboring germ-line *BRCA1* mutations have a marked increased risk of developing ovarian malignancies in their forties and fifties with a 30% to 50% lifetime risk of developing ovarian cancer. Women harboring a mutation in *BRCA2* have a lower penetrance of ovarian cancer with perhaps a 20% to 40% chance of developing this malignancy, with onset typically in their fifties or sixties. Women with a *RCA2* mutation also are at slightly increased risk of pancreatic cancer. Screening studies in this select population suggest that current screening techniques, including serial evaluation of the CA-125 tumor marker and ultrasound, are insufficient at detecting early-stage and curable disease, so women with these germ-line mutations are advised to undergo prophylactic removal of their ovaries and fallopian tubes typically after completing childbearing and ideally before ages 35 to 40 years. Early prophylactic oophorectomy also protects these women from subsequent breast cancer with a reduction of breast cancer risk of approximately 50%.

III-47. **The answer is C.** *(Chap. 97)* Endometrial carcinoma is the most common gynecologic malignancy in the United States. Most are adenocarcinomas. Development of these tumors is a multistep process with estrogen playing an important early role in driving endometrial gland proliferation. Relative overexposure to this class of hormones is a risk factor for the subsequent development of endometrial tumors. In contrast, progestins drive glandular maturation and are protective. Hence, women with high endogenous or pharmacologic exposure to estrogens, especially if unopposed by progesterone, are at high risk for endometrial cancer. Obese women, women treated with unopposed estrogens, and women with estrogen-producing tumors (e.g., granulosa cell tumors of the ovary) are at higher risk for endometrial cancer. In addition, treatment with tamoxifen, which has anti-estrogenic effects in breast tissue but estrogenic effects in uterine epithelium, is associated with an increased risk of endometrial cancer. The majority of women with tumors of the uterine corpus present with postmenopausal vaginal bleeding caused by shedding of the malignant endometrial lining. Premenopausal women often present with atypical bleeding between typical menstrual cycles. These signs typically bring a woman to the attention of a health care professional, and hence the majority of women present with early-stage disease in which the tumor is confined to the uterine corpus. For patients with disease confined to the uterus, hysterectomy with removal of the fallopian tubes and ovaries results in approximately 90% 5-year survival.

III-48. **The answer is B.** (*Chap. 98*) Bone pain resulting from metastatic lesions may be difficult to distinguish from degenerative disease, osteoporosis, or disk disease in elderly individuals. Generally, these patients present with insidious worsening localized pain without fevers or signs of infection. In contrast to pain related to disk disease, the pain of metastatic disease is worse when the patient is lying down or at night. Neurologic symptoms related to metastatic disease constitute an emergency. Lung, breast, and prostate cancers account for approximately 80% of bone metastases. Thyroid carcinoma, renal cell carcinoma, lymphoma, and bladder carcinoma may also metastasize to bone. Metastatic lesions may be lytic or blastic. Most cancers cause a combination of both, although prostate cancer is predominantly blastic. Either lesion may cause hypercalcemia, although lytic lesions more commonly do this. Lytic lesions are best detected with plain radiography. Blastic lesions are prominent on radionuclide bone scans. Treatment and prognosis depend on the underlying malignancy. Bisphosphonates may reduce hypercalcemia, relieve pain, and limit bone resorption.

III-49. **The answer is B.** (*Chap. 98*) Metastatic tumors of bone are more common than primary bone tumors. Prostate, breast, and lung primaries account for 80% of all bone metastases. Tumors from the kidney, bladder, and thyroid and lymphomas and sarcomas also commonly metastasize to bone. Metastases usually spread hematogenously. In decreasing order, the most common sites of bone metastases include the vertebrae, proximal femur, pelvis, ribs, sternum, proximal humerus, and skull. Pain is the most common symptom. Hypercalcemia may occur with bone destruction. Lesions may be osteolytic, osteoblastic, or both. Osteoblastic lesions are associated with a higher level of alkaline phosphatase. Colon cancer typically metastasizes initially via lymphatic spread, making the liver and lungs common sites of secondary disease.

III-50. **The answer is C.** (*Chap. 98*) The most common malignant tumors of bone are plasma cell tumors related to multiple myeloma. The bone lesions are lytic lesions caused by increased osteoclast activity without osteoblastic new bone formation. Of the nonhematopoietic tumors, the most common are osteosarcoma, chondrosarcoma, Ewing's sarcoma, and malignant fibrous histiocytoma. Osteosarcomas account for 45% of bone sarcomas and produce osteoid (unmineralized bone) or bone. They typically occur in children, adolescents, and adults up to the third decade of life. The "sunburst" appearance of the lesion and Codman's triangle in this young man are indicative of an osteosarcoma. Whereas osteosarcomas have a predilection for long bones, chondrosarcomas are more often found in flat bones, especially the shoulder and pelvic girdles. Osteosarcomas are radioresistant. Long-term survival with combined chemotherapy and surgery is 60% to 80%. Chondrosarcomas account for 20% to 25% of bone sarcomas and are most common in adults in the fourth to sixth decades of life. They typically present indolently with pain and swelling. They are often difficult to distinguish from benign bone lesions. Most chondrosarcomas are chemoresistant, and the mainstay of therapy is resection of the primary as well as metastatic sites.

III-51. **The answer is B.** *(Chap. 99)* Patients with cancer from an unknown primary site present a common diagnostic dilemma. Initial evaluation should include history, physical examination, appropriate imaging, and blood studies based on gender (e.g., prostate-specific antigen in men, mammography in women). Immunohistochemical staining of biopsy samples using antibodies to specific cell components may help elucidate the site of the primary tumor. Although many immunohistochemical stains are available, a logical approach is represented in Figure III-51. Additional tests may be helpful based on the appearance under light microscopy or the results of the cytokeratin stains. In cases of cancer of unknown primary, cytokeratin staining is usually the first branch point from which the tumor lineage is determined. Cytokeratin is positive in carcinoma because all epithelial tumors contain this protein. Subsets of cytokeratin, such as CK7 and CK20, may be useful to determine the likely etiology of the primary tumor. Leukocyte common antigen, thyroglobulin, and thyroid transcription factor 1 are characteristic of lymphoma, thyroid cancer, and lung or thyroid cancer, respectively. α-Fetoprotein staining is typically positive in germ cell, stomach, and liver carcinoma.

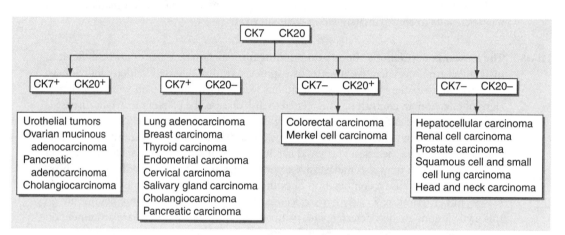

FIGURE III-51

III-52. **The answer is C.** *(Chap. 99)* The patient presents with symptoms suggestive of ovarian cancer. Although her peritoneal fluid is positive for adenocarcinoma, further speciation cannot be done. Surprisingly, the physical examination and imaging do not show a primary source. Although the differential diagnosis of this patient's disorder includes gastric cancer or another gastrointestinal malignancy and breast cancer, peritoneal carcinomatosis is most commonly caused by ovarian cancer in women even when the ovaries are normal at surgery. Elevated CA-125 levels or the presence of psammoma bodies is further suggestive of an ovarian origin, and such patients should receive surgical debulking and carboplatin or cisplatin plus paclitaxel. Patients with this presentation have a similar stage-specific survival compared with other patients with known ovarian cancer. Ten percent of patients with this disorder, also known as primary peritoneal papillary serous carcinoma, will remain disease free 2 years after treatment.

III-53. **The answer is B.** *(Chap. 99)* The patient is a young man with asymmetric hilar adenopathy. The differential diagnosis would include lymphoma; testicular cancer; and, less likely, tuberculosis or histoplasmosis. Because of his young age, testicular examination and ultrasonography would be indicated, as would measurement of α-fetoprotein (AFP) or beta human chorionic gonadotropin (β-hCG), which are generally markedly elevated. In men with carcinoma of unknown primary source, AFP and β-hCG should be checked because the presence of testicular cancer portends an improved prognosis compared with possible primary sources. Biopsy would show lymphoma. The ACE level may be elevated but is not diagnostic of sarcoidosis. Sarcoidosis should not be considered likely in the presence of asymmetric hilar adenopathy. Thyroid disorders are not likely to present with unilateral hilar adenopathy. Finally, prostate-specific antigen is not indicated in this age category, and C-reactive protein would not differentiate any of the disorders mentioned above. Biopsy is clearly the most important diagnostic procedure.

III-54. **The answer is E.** *(Chap. 100)* Hypercalcemia is a common oncologic complication of metastatic cancer. Symptoms include confusion, lethargy, change in mental status, fatigue, polyuria, and constipation. Regardless of the underlying disease, the treatment is similar. These patients are often dehydrated because hypercalcemia may cause nephrogenic diabetes insipidus and are often unable to take fluids orally. Therefore, the primary management entails reestablishment of euvolemia. Often hypercalcemia resolves with hydration alone. Patients should be monitored for hypophosphatemia. Bisphosphonates are now the mainstay of therapy because they stabilize osteoclast resorption of calcium from the bone. However, their effects may take 1 to 2 days to manifest. Care must be taken in cases of renal insufficiency because rapid administration of pamidronate may exacerbate renal failure. When euvolemia is achieved, furosemide may be given to increase calciuresis. Nasal or subcutaneous calcitonin further aids the shift of calcium out of the intravascular space. Since the advent of bisphosphonates, calcitonin is only used in severe cases of hypercalcemia because of its rapid effect. Glucocorticoids may be useful in patients with lymphoid malignancies because the mechanism of hypercalcemia in these conditions is often related to excess hydroxylation of vitamin D. However, in this patient with prostate cancer, dexamethasone will have little effect on the calcium level and may exacerbate the altered mental status.

III-55. **The answer is E.** *(Chap. 100)* A variety of hormones are produced ectopically by tumors that may cause symptomatic disease. Eutopic production of parathyroid hormone (PTH) by the parathyroid gland is the most common cause of hypercalcemia. Hypercalcemia may rarely be produced by ectopic hyperparathyroid production but is most often caused by parathyroid hormone related protein (PTH-rp) production by squamous cell (head and neck, lung, skin), breast, genitourinary, and gastrointestinal tumors. This protein can be measured as a serum assay. Antidiuretic hormone (ADH), causing hyponatremia, is commonly produced by lung (squamous, small cell), gastrointestinal, genitourinary, and ovary tumors. Adrenocorticotropic hormone (ACTH), causing Cushing's syndrome, is commonly produced by tumors in the lung (small cell, bronchial carcinoid, adenocarcinoma, squamous), thymus, pancreatic islet, and medullary thyroid carcinoma. Insulin-like growth factor secreted by mesenchymal tumors, sarcomas, and adrenal, hepatic, gastrointestinal, kidney, or prostate tumors may cause symptomatic hypoglycemia.

III-56. **The answer is C.** *(Chap. 101)* One of the better characterized paraneoplastic neurologic syndromes is cerebellar ataxia caused by Purkinje cell drop-out in the cerebellum; it is manifested by dysarthria, limb and gait ataxia, and nystagmus. Radiologic imaging reveals cerebellar atrophy. Many antibodies have been associated with this syndrome, including anti-Yo, anti-Tr, and antibodies to the glutamate receptor. Although lung cancer, particularly small cell cancer, accounts for a large number of patients with neoplasm-associated cerebellar ataxia, those with the syndrome who display anti-Yo antibodies in the serum typically have breast or ovarian cancer. Cerebellar ataxia may also be seen in Hodgkin's lymphoma in association with anti-Tr antibodies.

III-57. **The answer is A.** *(Chap. e20)* About 40% of patients with thymoma have another systemic autoimmune illness related to the thymoma. About 30% of patients with thymoma have myasthenia gravis, 5% to 8% have pure red blood cell (RBC) aplasia, and about 5% have hypogammaglobulinemia. Thymectomy results in the resolution of pure RBC aplasia in about 30% of patients but rarely benefits patients with hypogammaglobulinemia. Among patients with myasthenia gravis, about 10% to 15% have a thymoma. Thymectomy produces at least some symptomatic improvement in about 65% of patients with myasthenia gravis. In one large series, thymoma patients with myasthenia gravis had a better long-term survival from thymoma resection than did those without myasthenia gravis. Thymoma more rarely may be associated with polymyositis, systemic lupus erythematosus, thyroiditis, Sjögren's syndrome, ulcerative colitis, pernicious anemia, Addison's disease, scleroderma, and panhypopituitarism. In one series, 70% of patients with thymoma were found to have another systemic illness. Erythrocytosis caused by ectopic production of erythropoietin is often seen in conjunction with renal cell and hepatocellular carcinomas.

III-58. **The answer is D.** *(Chap. e20)* Thymoma is the most common cause of an anterior mediastinal mass in adults, accounting for about 40% of all mediastinal masses. The other major causes of anterior mediastinal masses are lymphomas, germ cell tumors, and substernal thyroid tumors. Carcinoid tumors, lipomas, and thymic cysts also may produce radiographic masses. After combination chemotherapy for another malignancy, teenagers and young adults may develop a rebound thymic hyperplasia in the first few months after treatment. Granulomatous inflammatory diseases (tuberculosis, sarcoidosis) can produce thymic enlargement. Thymomas are most common in the fifth and sixth decades of life, are uncommon in children, and are distributed evenly between men and women. About 40% to 50% of patients are asymptomatic; masses are detected incidentally on routine chest radiographs. When symptomatic, patients may have cough, chest pain, dyspnea, fever, wheezing, fatigue, weight loss, night sweats, or anorexia. Occasionally, thymomas may obstruct the superior vena cava. After a mediastinal mass has been detected, a surgical procedure is required for definitive diagnosis. An initial mediastinoscopy or limited thoracotomy can be undertaken to get sufficient tissue to make an accurate diagnosis. Fine-needle aspiration is poor at distinguishing between lymphomas and thymomas but is more reliable in diagnosing germ cell tumors and metastatic carcinoma. Thymomas and lymphomas require sufficient tissue to examine the tumor architecture to ensure an accurate diagnosis and obtain prognostic information. Thymomas are epithelial tumors, and all of them have malignant potential. It is not worthwhile to try to divide them into benign and malignant forms. Staging systems are based on degree of invasiveness and correlate with prognosis. About 65% of thymomas are encapsulated and noninvasive, and about 35% are invasive. Tumors that are encapsulated and non-invasive (stage 1) have a 96% 5-year survival after complete resection surgery.

III-59. **The answer is D.** *(Chap. 103)* Iron-deficiency anemia is a condition consisting of anemia and clear evidence of iron deficiency. It is one of the most prevalent forms of malnutrition. Globally, 50% of anemia is attributable to iron deficiency and accounts for approximately 841,000 deaths annually worldwide. Africa and parts of Asia bear 71% of the global mortality burden; North America represents only 1.4% of the total morbidity and mortality associated with iron deficiency. Initially, a state of negative iron balance occurs during which iron stores become slowly depleted. Serum ferritin may decrease, and the presence of stainable iron on bone marrow preparation decreases. When iron stores are depleted, serum iron begins to fall. Total iron-binding capacity (TIBC) starts to increase, reflecting the presence of circulating unbound transferrin. When the transferrin saturation falls to 15% to 20%, hemoglobin synthesis is impaired. The peripheral blood smear reveals the presence of microcytic and hypochromic red blood cells. Reticulocytes may also become hypochromic. Reticulocyte numbers are reduced relative to the level of anemia, reflecting a hypoproduction anemia secondary to iron deficiency. Clinically, these patients exhibit the usual signs of anemia, which are fatigue, pallor, and reduced exercise capacity. Cheilosis and koilonychia are signs of advanced tissue iron deficiency. Some patients may experience pica, a desire to ingest certain materials, such as ice (pagophagia) and clay (geophagia).

III-60. **The answer is C.** *(Chap. 103)* (See Table III-60 on the following page.) The differential diagnosis of microcytic anemia includes iron deficiency, hemoglobinopathy (e.g., thalassemia), myelodysplastic syndromes (including sideroblastic anemia), and chronic inflammation. Inflammation can be distinguished from iron deficiency because iron deficiency typically includes a very low ferritin level (<50 μg/L) and iron binding saturation, but in inflammation, they are normal or increased. Any chronic inflammatory state may cause a hypoproliferative anemia caused by inadequate marrow utilization of iron related to hyperproduction of a number of cytokines, including tumor necrosis factor, interferon-gamma, and inter-leukin-1. The anemia of chronic disease may be normocytic/normochromic or microcytic. Serum iron and iron binding are normal to high in thalassemia and sideroblastic anemia. Folate deficiency causes macrocytic anemia.

TABLE III-60   Diagnosis of Microcytic Anemia

Test	Iron Deficiency	Inflammation	Thalassemia	Sideroblastic Anemia
Smear	Micro/hypo	Normal micro/hypo	Micro/hypo with targeting	Variable
SI	<30	<50	Normal to high	Normal to high
TIBC	>360	<300	Normal	Normal
Percent saturation	<10	10–20	30–80	30–80
Ferritin (μg/L)	<15	30–200	50–300	50–300
Hemoglobin pattern on electrophoresis	Normal	Normal	Abnormal with β-thalassemia; can be normal with α-thalassemia	Normal

Abbreviations: SI, serum iron; TIBC, total iron-binding capacity.

III-61.   **The answer is C.** *(Chap. 103)* Progressive chronic kidney disease (CKD) is usually associated with a moderate to severe hypoproliferative anemia. The level of the anemia correlates with the stage of CKD. Red blood cells (RBCs) are typically normocytic and normochromic, and reticulocytes are decreased. The anemia is primarily caused by a fail-ure of erythropoietin (EPO) production by the diseased kidney and a reduction in RBC survival. Polycystic kidney disease shows a smaller degree of EPO deficiency for a given level of renal failure. By contrast, patients with diabetes or myeloma have more severe EPO deficiency for a given level of renal failure. Assessment of iron status provides infor-mation to distinguish the anemia of CKD from other forms of hypoproliferative anemia and to guide management. Patients with the anemia of CKD usually present with normal serum iron, total iron-binding capacity, and ferritin levels. However, those maintained on chronic hemodialysis may develop iron deficiency from blood loss through the dialysis procedure. EPO therapy is effective in correcting the anemia of CKD. Iron must be replen-ished in patients with concomitant iron deficiency to ensure an adequate response to EPO therapy.

III-62.   **The answer is B.** *(Chap. 104,* N Engl J Med *2009; 361:2309-2317)* The most significant recent advance in the therapy of sickle cell anemia has been the introduction of hydroxy-urea as a mainstay of therapy for patients with severe symptoms. Hydroxyurea increases fetal hemoglobin and may exert beneficial effects on red blood cell (RBC) hydration, vascular wall adherence, and suppression of the granulocyte and reticulocyte counts. Hemoglobin F levels increase in most patients within a few months. Hydroxyurea should be considered in patients experiencing repeated episodes of acute chest syndrome or with more than three crises per year requiring hospitalization. The utility of this agent for reducing the incidence of other complications (priapism, retinopathy) is under evalua-tion, as are the long-term side effects. Hydroxyurea offers broad benefits to most patients whose disease is severe enough to impair their functional status, and it may improve survival. The main adverse effect is a reduction in white blood cell (WBC) count; dosage should be titrated to maintain a WBC count at 5000 to 8000/μL. WBCs and reticulocytes may play a major role in the pathogenesis of sickle cell crisis, and their suppression may be an important benefit of hydroxyurea therapy. A recent study demonstrated that non-myeloablative bone marrow transplantation in patients with sickle cell disease could pro-duce a stable chimera that corrected RBC counts and reversed the sickle cell phenotype.

III-63.   **The answer is B.** *(Chap. 105)* Serum cobalamin is measured by an enzyme-linked immu-nosorbent assay test and is the most cost-effective test to rule out deficiency. Normal serum levels are typically above 200 ng/L. In patients with megaloblastic anemia caused by cobalamin deficiency, the level is usually less than 100 ng/L. In general, the more severe the deficiency, the lower the serum cobalamin level. In patients with spinal cord damage caused by the deficiency, levels are very low even in the absence of anemia. Borderline low levels may occur in pregnancy in patients with megaloblastic anemia caused by folate deficiency. In patients with cobalamin deficiency sufficient to cause anemia or neuropathy, the serum methylmalonate (MMA) level is increased. Serum MMA and homocysteine levels have been proposed for the early diagnosis of cobalamin deficiency even in the absence of hematologic abnormalities or subnormal levels of serum cobalamin. Serum MMA levels fluctuate, however, in patients with renal failure. Mildly elevated serum MMA or homocysteine levels occur in up to 30% of apparently healthy volunteers and 15% of elderly subjects. These findings bring into question the exact cutoff points for normal MMA and homocysteine levels. It is also unclear at present whether these mildly increased metabolite levels have clinical consequences. Serum homocysteine is increased in both early cobalamin and folate deficiency but may also be increased in other conditions (e.g., chronic renal disease; alcoholism; smoking; pyridoxine deficiency; hypothyroidism; and therapy with steroids, cyclosporine, and other drugs). The red blood cell folate assay is a test of body folate stores. It is less affected than the serum assay by recent diet and traces of hemolysis. Subnormal levels occur in patients with megaloblastic anemia caused by folate deficiency but also in nearly two-thirds of patients with severe cobalamin deficiency. False-normal results may occur if a folate-deficient patient has received a recent blood transfusion or if a patient has an increased reticulocyte count. Serum pepsinogen may be low in patients with pernicious anemia.

III-64.   **The answer is C.** *(Chap. 105)* The peripheral blood smear shows hypochromasia, macrocytosis, and a hypersegmented (>five lobes) neutrophil. These findings are typical for a megaloblastic anemia as seen in cobalamin or folate deficiency. The mean corpuscular volume is typically greater than 100 fL, and there is significant anisocytosis and poikilocytosis. There may also be leukopenia and thrombocytopenia that correlate with the degree of deficiency. Other less common causes of megaloblastic anemia include therapy with drugs that interfere with folate metabolism (methotrexate) or DNA synthesis (hydroxyurea, AZT, cytosine arabinoside, 6-mercaptopurine) and some cases of acute myeloblastic leukemia or myelodysplasia. Autoantibodies to ADAMTS-13 are associated with thrombotic thrombocytopenic purpura, which causes a microangiopathic hemolytic anemia. Epstein-Barr virus infection is associated with large atypical lymphocytes, not hypersegmented neutrophils. Iron-deficiency anemia causes a microcytic hypochromic anemia.

III-65.   **The answer is B.** *(Chap. 106)* Red blood cells (RBCs) use glutathione produced by the hexose monophosphate shunt to compensate for increased production of reactive oxygen species (oxidant stress), usually induced by drugs or toxins. Defects in glucose-6-phosphate dehydrogenase (G6PD) are the most common congenital hexose monophosphate shunt defect. If the RBC is unable to maintain an adequate level of glutathione during oxidant stress, hemoglobin precipitates in the RBC, producing Heinz bodies. Because the G6PD gene is on the X chromosome, almost all affected patients are males. G6PD deficiency is widely distributed throughout regions that are currently or were once highly malarial endemic. It is common in males of African, African American, Sardinian, and Sephardic descent. In most persons with G6PD deficiency, there is no evidence of symptomatic disease. However, infection, ingestion of fava beans, or exposure to an oxidative agent (drug or toxin) can trigger an acute hemolytic event. Bite cells, Heinz bodies, and bizarre poikilocytes may be evident on smear. The drugs that most commonly precipitate a G6PD crisis include dapsone, sulfamethoxazole, primaquine, and nitrofurantoin. The anemia is often severe with rapid onset after drug ingestion, and renal failure can occur.

III-66.   **The answer is B.** *(Chaps. 106 and 319)* This patient's lupus and her rapid development of truly life-threatening hemolytic anemia are both very suggestive of autoimmune hemolytic anemia. Diagnosis is made by a positive Coombs test documenting antibodies to the red cell membrane, but smear will often show microspherocytes, indicative of the damage incurred to the red cells in the spleen. Schistocytes are typical for microangio-pathic hemolytic anemias such as hemolytic uremic syndrome (HUS) or thrombotic thrombocytopenic purpura. The lack of thrombocytopenia makes these diagnoses considerably less plausible. Macrocytosis and polymorphonuclear leukocytes with hypersegmented nuclei are very suggestive of vitamin B_{12} deficiency, which causes more chronic, non–life-threatening anemia. Target cells are seen in liver disease and thalassemias. Sickle cell anemia is associated with aplastic crises, but this patient has no known diagnosis of sickle cell disease and is showing evidence of erythropoietin response based on the presence of elevated reticulocyte count.

III-67.   **The answer is C.** *(Chap. 106)* The peripheral blood smear shows microspherocytes, small densely staining red blood cells (RBCs) that have lost their central pallor characteristic of hereditary spherocytosis. Spherocytosis is almost the only condition with an increased mean corpuscular hemoglobin concentration. Hereditary spherocytosis is a heterogeneous RBC membranopathy that can be either congenital (usually autosomal dominant) or acquired; it is characterized by predominantly extravascular hemolysis in the spleen caused by defects in membrane structural proteins. This spleen-mediated hemolysis leads to the conversion of classic biconcave RBCs on smear to spherocytes. Splenomegaly is common. This disorder can be severe, depending on the site of mutation, but is often overlooked until some stressor such as pregnancy leads to a multifactorial anemia, or an infection such as parvovirus B19 transiently eliminates RBC production altogether. Acute treatment is with transfusion. Glucose-6-phosphate dehydrogenase (G6PD) deficiency is a cause of hemolysis that is usually triggered by the presence of an offending oxidative agent. The peripheral blood smear may show Heinz bodies. Parvovirus infection may cause a pure RBC aplasia. The presence of active reticulocytosis and laboratory findings consistent with hemolysis are not compatible with that diagnosis. Chronic gastrointestinal blood loss, such as caused by a colonic polyp, would cause a microcytic, hypochromic anemia without evidence of hemolysis (indirect bilirubin, haptoglobin abnormalities).

III-68.   **The answer is D.** *(Chap. 106)* Each of the listed diagnoses has a rather characteristic set of laboratory findings that are virtually diagnostic for the disease once the disease has progressed to a severe stage. The combination of portal vein thrombosis, hemolysis, and pancytopenia is typical for paroxysmal nocturnal hemoglobinuria (PNH). PNH is a rare disorder characterized by hemolytic anemia (particularly at night), venous thrombosis, and deficient hematopoiesis. It is a stem cell–derived intracorpuscular defect. Anemia is usually moderate in severity, and there is often concomitant granulocytopenia and thrombocytopenia. Venous thrombosis occurs much more commonly than in the population at large. The intraabdominal veins are often involved, and patients may present with Budd-Chiari syndrome. Cerebral sinus thrombosis is a common cause of death in patients with PNH. The presence of pancytopenia and hemolysis should raise suspicion for this diagnosis even before the development of a venous thrombosis. In the past, PNH was diagnosed by abnormalities on the Ham or sucrose lysis test; however, currently flow cytometry analysis of glycosylphosphatidylinositol (GPI) linked proteins (e.g., CD55 and CD59) on red blood cells and granulocytes is recommended. Hemolytic uremic syndrome (HUS) and thrombotic thrombocytopenic purpura (TTP) both cause hemolysis and thrombocytopenia, as well as fevers. Cerebrovascular events and mental status change occur more commonly in TTP, and renal failure is more common in HUS. Severe leptospirosis, or Weil's disease, is notable for fevers, hyperbilirubinemia, and renal failure. Conjunctival suffusion is another helpful clue. Acute promyelocytic leukemia is notable for anemia, thrombocytopenia, and either elevated or a decreased white blood cell count, all in the presence of disseminated intravascular coagulation.

III-69.   **The answer is A.** *(Chap. 106)* Haptoglobin is an α-globulin normally present in serum. It binds specifically to the globin portion of hemoglobin, and the complex is cleared by the mononuclear cell phagocytosis. Haptoglobin is reduced in all hemolytic anemias because it binds free hemoglobin. It can also be reduced in cirrhosis and so is not diagnostic of hemolysis outside of the correct clinical context. Assuming normal bone marrow and iron stores, the reticulocyte count will be elevated as well to try to compensate for the increased red blood cell (RBC) destruction of hemolysis. Release of intracellular contents from the RBC (including hemoglobin and lactate dehydrogenase) induces heme metabolism, producing unconjugated bilirubinemia. If the haptoglobin system is overwhelmed, the kidney will filter free hemoglobin and reabsorb it in the proximal tubule for storage of iron by ferritin and hemosiderin. Hemosiderin in the urine is a marker of filtered hemoglobin by the kidneys. In massive hemolysis, free hemoglobin may be excreted in urine.

III-70.   **The answer is E.** *(Chap. 106)* Hemolytic anemias may be classified as intracorpuscular or extracorpuscular. In intracorpuscular disorders, the patient's red blood cells (RBCs) have an abnormally short life span because of an intrinsic RBC factor. In extracorpuscular disorders, the RBC has a short life span because of a nonintrinsic RBC factor. Thrombotic thrombocytopenic purpura (TTP) is an acquired disorder in which red blood cell and platelet destruction occur not because of defects of these cell lines but rather as a result of microangiopathy leading to destructive shear forces on the cells. Other clinical signs and symptoms include fever; mental status change; and, less commonly, renal impairment. Most acquired adult cases of TTP are associated with autoantibodies to ADAMTS-13 (or von Willebrand factor–cleaving protease). All cases of hemolysis in conjunction with thrombocytopenia should be rapidly ruled out for TTP by evaluation of a peripheral smear for schistocytes because plasmapheresis is lifesaving. Other causes of extravascular hemolytic anemia include hypersplenism, autoimmune hemolytic anemia, disseminated intravascular coagulation, and other microangiopathic hemolytic anemias. The other four disorders listed in the question all refer to some defect of the RBC itself that leads to hemolysis. Elliptocytosis is a membranopathy that leads to varying degrees of destruction of the RBC in the reticuloendothelial system. Sickle cell anemia is a congenital hemoglobinopathy classified by recurrent pain crises and numerous long-term sequelae that is caused by a well-defined β-globin mutation. Pyruvate kinase deficiency is a rare disorder of the glycolytic pathway that causes hemolytic anemia. Paroxysmal nocturnal hemoglobinuria (PNH) is a form of acquired hemolysis caused by an intrinsic abnormality of the RBCs. It also often causes thrombosis and cytopenias. Bone marrow failure is a feared association with PNH.

III-71.   **The answer is C.** *(Chap. 107)* Pure red blood cell aplasia (PRCA) is a condition characterized by the absence of reticulocytes and erythroid precursors. A variety of conditions may cause PRCA. It may be idiopathic. It may be associated with certain medications, such as trimethoprim–sulfamethoxazole (TMP-SMX) and phenytoin. It can be associated with a variety of neoplasms, either as a precursor to a hematologic malignancy such as leukemia or myelodysplasia or as part of an autoimmune phenomenon, as in the case of thymoma. Infections also may cause PRCA. Parvovirus B19 is a single-strand DNA virus that is associated with erythema infectiosum, or fifth disease in children. It is also associated with arthropathy and a flulike illness in adults. It is thought to attack the P antigen on proerythroblasts directly. Patients with a chronic hemolytic anemia, such as sickle cell disease, or with an immunodeficiency are less able to tolerate a transient drop in reticulocytes because their red blood cells do not survive in the peripheral blood for an adequate period. In this patient, her daughter had an illness before the appearance of her symptoms. It is reasonable to check her parvovirus immunoglobulin M (IgM) titers. If the results are positive, a dose of intravenous Ig is indicated. Because her laboratory test results and smear are not suggestive of dramatic sickling, an exchange transfusion is not indicated. Immunosuppression with prednisone, cyclosporine, or both may be indicated if another etiology of the PRCA is identified. However, that would not be the next step. Similarly, a bone marrow transplant might be a consideration in a young patient with myelodysplasia or leukemia, but there is no evidence of that at this time. Antibiotics have no role in light of her normal white blood cell count and the lack of evidence for a bacterial infection.

III-72.   **The answer is D.** *(Chap. 107)* Aplastic anemia is defined as pancytopenia with bone marrow hypocellularity. Aplastic anemia may be acquired, iatrogenic (chemotherapy), or genetic (e.g., Fanconi's anemia). Acquired aplastic anemia may be caused by drugs or chemicals (expected toxicity or idiosyncratic effects), viral infections, immune diseases, paroxysmal nocturnal hemoglobinuria, pregnancy, or idiopathic causes. Aplastic anemia from idiosyncratic drug reactions (including those listed as well others, including as quinacrine, phenytoin, sulfonamides, or cimetidine) are uncommon but may be encountered given the wide usage of some of these agents. In these cases, there is usually not a dose-dependent response; the reaction is idiosyncratic. Seronegative hepatitis is a cause of aplastic anemia, particularly in young men who recovered from an episode of liver inflammation 1 to 2 months earlier. Parvovirus B19 infection most commonly causes pure red blood cell (RBC) aplasia, particularly in patients with chronic hemolytic states and high RBC turnover (e.g., sickle cell anemia).

III-73. **The answer is D.** *(Chap. 107)* This patient has aplastic anemia. In the absence of drugs or toxins that cause bone marrow suppression, it is most likely that he has an immune-mediated injury. Growth factors are not effective in the setting of hypoplastic bone marrow. Transfusion should be avoided unless emergently needed to prevent the development of alloantibodies. Glucocorticoids have no efficacy in aplastic anemia. Immunosuppression with antithymocyte globulin and cyclosporine is a therapy with proven efficacy for this autoimmune disease with a response rate of up to 70%. Relapses are common, and myelodysplastic syndrome or leukemia may occur in approximately 15% of treated patients. Immunosuppression is the treatment of choice for patients without suitable bone marrow transplant donors. Bone marrow transplantation is the best current therapy for young patients with matched sibling donors. Allogeneic bone marrow transplants from matched siblings result in long-term survival in more than 80% of patients, with better results in children than adults. The effectiveness of androgens has not been verified in controlled trials, but occasional patients will respond or even demonstrate blood count dependence on continued therapy. Sex hormones upregulate telomerase gene activity in vitro, possibly also their mechanism of action in improving marrow function. For patients with moderate disease or those with severe pancytopenia in whom immunosuppression has failed, a 3 to 4-month trial is appropriate.

III-74. **The answer is B.** *(Chap. 107)* Myelodysplasia, or the MDSs, are a heterogeneous group of hematologic disorders broadly characterized by cytopenias associated with a dysmorphic (or abnormal appearing) and usually cellular bone marrow and by consequent ineffective blood cell production. The mean onset of age is after 70 years. MDS is associated with environmental exposures such as radiation and benzene; other risk factors have been reported inconsistently. Secondary MDS occurs as a late toxicity of cancer treatment, usually with a combination of radiation and the radiomimetic alkylating agents such as busulfan, nitrosourea, or procarbazine (with a latent period of 5–7 years) or the DNA topoisomerase inhibitors (2 years). Both acquired aplastic anemia after immunosuppressive treatment and Fanconi's anemia can evolve into MDS. MDS is a clonal hematopoietic stem cell disorder leading to impaired cell proliferation and differentiation. Cytogenetic abnormalities are found in approximately half of patients, and some of the same specific lesions are also seen in frank leukemia. Anemia dominates the early course. Most symptomatic patients complain of the gradual onset of fatigue and weakness, dyspnea, and pallor, but at least half the patients are asymptomatic, and their MDS is discovered only incidentally on routine blood counts. Previous chemotherapy or radiation exposure is an important historic fact. Fever and weight loss should point to a myeloproliferative rather than myelodysplastic process. About 20% of patients have splenomegaly. Bone marrow is typically hypercellular. Median survival varies from months to years, depending on the number of blasts in marrow and the specific cytogenetic abnormality. Isolated 5q- is associated with a median survival in years. Most patients die as a result of complications of pancytopenia and not because of leukemic transformation; perhaps one-third will succumb to other diseases unrelated to their MDS. Precipitous worsening of pancytopenia, acquisition of new chromosomal abnormalities on serial cytogenetic determination, increase in the number of blasts, and marrow fibrosis are all poor prognostic indicators. The outlook in therapy-related MDS, regardless of type, is extremely poor, and most patients progress within a few months to refractory acute myeloid leukemia. Historically, the therapy of MDS has been unsatisfactory. Only stem cell transplantation offers cure.

Survival rates of 50% at 3 years have been reported, but older patients are particularly prone to develop treatment-related mortality and morbidity. Results of transplant using matched unrelated donors are comparable, although most series contain younger and more highly selected cases. However, multiple new drugs have been approved for use in MDS. Several regimens appear to not only improve blood counts but also to delay onset of leukemia and to improve survival.

Lenalidomide, a thalidomide derivative with a more favorable toxicity profile, is particularly effective in reversing anemia in MDS patients with 5q- syndrome; a high proportion of these patients become transfusion independent.

III-75. **The answer is E.** *(Chap. 108)* The World Health Organization's classification of the chronic myeloproliferative diseases (MPDs) includes eight disorders, some of which are rare or poorly characterized but all of which share an origin in a multipotent hematopoietic progenitor cell, overproduction of one or more of the formed elements of the blood without significant dysplasia, a predilection to extramedullary hematopoiesis or myelofibrosis, and transformation at varying rates to acute leukemia. Within this broad classification, however, significant phenotypic heterogeneity exists. Some diseases such as chronic myelogenous leukemia (CML), chronic neutrophilic leukemia (CNL), and chronic eosinophilic leukemia (CEL) express primarily a myeloid phenotype, but in others, such as polycythemia vera (PV), primary myelofibrosis (PMF), and essential thrombocytosis (ET), erythroid or megakaryocytic hyperplasia predominates. The latter three disorders, in contrast to the former three, also appear capable of transforming into each other. Such phenotypic heterogeneity has a genetic basis. CML is the consequence of the balanced translocation between chromosomes 9 and 22 [t(9;22)(q34;11)], CNL has been associated with a t(15;19) translocation, and CEL occurs with a deletion or balanced translocations involving the *PDGFR-alpha* gene. By contrast, to a greater or lesser extent, PV, PMF, and ET are characterized by expression of a *JAK2* mutation, V617F, that causes constitutive activation of this tyrosine kinase that is essential for the function of the erythropoietin and thrombopoietin receptors but not the granulocyte colony-stimulating factor receptor. This essential distinction is also reflected in the natural history of CML, CNL, and CEL, which is usually measured in years, and their high rate of transformation into acute leukemia. By contrast, the natural history of PV, PMF, and ET is usually measured in decades, and transformation to acute leukemia is uncommon in the absence of exposure to mutagenic agents. Primary effusion lymphoma is not a myeloproliferative disease. It is one of the diseases (Kaposi's sarcoma, multicentric Castleman's disease) associated with infection with human herpes virus-8, particularly in immunocompromised hosts.

III-76. **The answer is A.** *(Chap. 108)* Polycythemia vera (PV) is a clonal disorder that involves a multipotent hematopoietic progenitor cell. Clinically, it is characterized by a proliferation of red blood cells (RBCs), granulocytes, and platelets. The precise etiology is unknown. Unlike chronic myelogenous leukemia, no consistent cytogenetic abnormality has been associated with the disorder. However, a mutation in the autoinhibitory, pseudokinase domain of the tyrosine kinase JAK2—that replaces valine with phenylalanine (V617F), causing constitutive activation of the kinase—appears to have a central role in the pathogenesis of PV. Erythropoiesis is regulated by the hormone erythropoietin. Hypoxia is the physiologic stimulus that increases the number of cells that produce erythropoietin. Erythropoietin may be elevated in patients with hormone-secreting tumors. Levels are usually "normal" in patients with hypoxic erythrocytosis. In PV, however, because erythrocytosis occurs independently of erythropoietin, levels of the hormone are usually low. Therefore, an elevated level is *not* consistent with the diagnosis. PV is a chronic, indolent disease with a low rate of transformation to acute leukemia, especially in the absence of treatment with radiation or hydroxyurea. Thrombotic complications are the main risk for PV and correlate with the erythrocytosis. Thrombocytosis, although sometimes prominent, does not correlate with the risk of thrombotic complications. Salicylates are useful in treating erythromelalgia but are not indicated in asymptomatic patients. There is no evidence that thrombotic risk is significantly lowered with their use in patients whose hematocrits are appropriately controlled with phlebotomy. Phlebotomy is the mainstay of treatment. Induction of a state of iron deficiency is critical to prevent a reexpansion of the RBC mass. Chemotherapeutics and other agents are useful in cases of symptomatic splenomegaly. Their use is limited by side effects, and there is a risk of leukemogenesis with hydroxyurea.

III-77. **The answer is A.** *(Chap. 108)* Chronic primary myelofibrosis (PMF) is the least common myeloproliferative disorder and is considered a diagnosis of exclusion after other causes of myelofibrosis have been ruled out. The typical patient with PMF presents in the sixth decade of life, and the disorder is asymptomatic in many patients. Fevers, fatigue, night sweats, and weight loss may occur in PMF, but these symptoms are rare in other myeloproliferative disorders. However, no signs or symptoms are specific for the diagnosis of PMF. Often marked splenomegaly is present and may extend across the midline and to the pelvic brim. A peripheral blood smear demonstrates the typical findings of myelofibrosis, including teardrop-shaped red blood cells (RBCs), nucleated RBCs, myelocytes, and metamyelocytes that are indicative of extramedullary hematopoiesis. Anemia is usually mild, and platelet and leukocyte counts are often normal. About 50% of patients with PMF have the *JAK2 V617F* mutation. Bone marrow aspirate is frequently unsuccessful because the extent of marrow fibrosis makes aspiration impossible. When a bone marrow biopsy is performed, it demonstrates hypercellular marrow with trilineage hyperplasia and increased number of megakaryocytes with large dysplastic nuclei. Interestingly, individuals with PMF often have associated autoantibodies, including rheumatoid factor, antinuclear antibodies, or a positive Coombs test results. To diagnose someone as having PMF, it must be shown that he or she does not have another myeloproliferative disorder or hematologic malignancy that is the cause of myelofibrosis. The most common disorders that present in a similar fashion to PMF are polycythemia vera and chronic myelogenous leukemia. Other nonmalignant disorders that can cause myelofibrosis include HIV infection, hyperparathyroidism, renal osteodystrophy, systemic lupus erythematosus, tuberculosis, and bone marrow replacement in other cancers such as prostate and breast cancer. In the patient described here, there is no other identifiable cause of myelofibrosis; thus, chronic PMF can be diagnosed.

III-78. **The answer is E.** *(Chap. 108)* Thrombocytosis may be "primary" or "secondary." Essential thrombocytosis is a myeloproliferative disorder that involves a multipotent hematopoietic progenitor cell. Unfortunately, no clonal marker can reliably distinguish it from more common nonclonal, reactive forms of thrombocytosis. Only 50% of patients with essential (primary) thrombocytosis have the *JAK2 V617F* mutation. Therefore, the diagnosis is one of exclusion. Common causes of secondary thrombocytosis include infection, inflammatory conditions, malignancy, iron deficiency, hemorrhage, and postsurgical states. Other myeloproliferative disorders, such as CML and myelofibrosis, may result in thrombocytosis. Similarly, myelodysplastic syndromes, particularly the 5q-syndrome, may cause thrombocytosis. Pernicious anemia caused by vitamin B_{12} deficiency does not typically cause thrombocytosis. However, correction of B_{12} deficiency or folate deficiency may cause a "rebound" thrombocytosis. Similarly, cessation of chronic ethanol use may also cause rebound thrombocytosis.

III-79. **The answer is E.** *(Chap. 108)* In a patient presenting with an elevated hemoglobin and hematocrit, the initial step in the evaluation is to determine whether erythrocytosis represents a true elevation in red blood cell (RBC) mass or whether spurious erythrocytosis is present because of plasma volume contraction. (See Figure III-79.) This step may be not necessary, however, in individuals with hemoglobin greater than 20 g/dL. After absolute erythrocytosis has been determined by measurement of RBC mass and plasma volume, the cause of erythrocytosis must be determined. If there is not an obvious cause of the erythrocytosis, an erythropoietin level should be checked. An elevated erythropoietin level suggests hypoxia or autonomous production of erythropoietin as the cause of erythrocytosis. However, a normal erythropoietin level does not exclude hypoxia as a cause. A low erythropoietin level should be seen in the myeloproliferative disorder polycythemia vera (PV), the most likely cause of erythrocytosis in this patient. PV is often discovered incidentally when elevated hemoglobin is found during testing for other reasons. When symptoms are present, the most common complaints are related to hyperviscosity of the blood and include vertigo, headache, tinnitus, and transient ischemic attacks. Patients may also complain of pruritus after showering. *Erythromelalgia* is the term give to the symptoms complex of burning, pain, and erythema in the extremities and is associated with thrombocytosis in PV. Isolated systolic hypertension and splenomegaly may be found. In addition to elevated red RBC mass and low erythropoietin levels, other laboratory findings in PV include thrombocytosis and leukocytosis with abnormal leukocytes present. Uric acid levels and leukocyte alkaline phosphatase may be elevated but are not diagnostic for PV. Approximately 30% of individuals with PV are homozygous for the *JAK2 V617F* mutation, and more than 90% are heterozygous for this mutation. This mutation located on the short arm of chromosome 9 causes constitutive activation of the Janus kinase (JAK) protein, a tyrosine kinase that renders erythrocytes resistant to apoptosis and allows them to continue production independently from erythropoietin. However, not every patient with PV expresses this mutation, and approximately 50% of patients with chronic myelofibrosis and essential thrombocytosis express this mutation. Thus, it is not recommended as an initial diagnostic test for PV but may be used for confirmatory purposes. Bone marrow biopsy provides no specific information in PV and is not recommended.

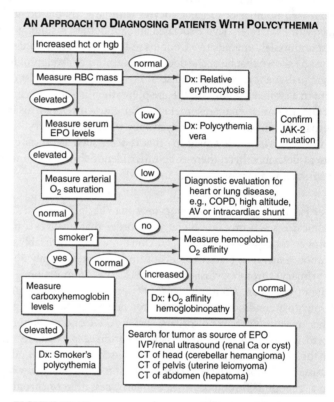

FIGURE III-79

III-80. **The answer is C.** *(Chap. 109)* This patient presents with typical findings of chronic myelogenous leukemia (CML), which has an incidence of 1.5 per 100,000 people yearly. The typical age of onset is in the mid-forties, and there is a slight male predominance. Half of individuals are asymptomatic at the time of diagnosis. If symptoms are present, they are typically nonspecific and include fatigue and weight loss. Occasionally, patients have symptoms related to splenic enlargement such as early satiety and left upper quadrant pain. Laboratory findings are suggestive of CML. A high leukocyte count of 100,000/μL is typical, with a predominant granulocytic differential, including neutrophils, myelocytes, metamyelocytes, and band forms. The circulating blast count should be less than 5%. Anemia and thrombocytosis are also common. The bone marrow demonstrates nonspecific increase in cellularity with an increase in the myeloid-to-erythroid ratio. The diagnosis of CML is established by identifying a clonal expansion of a hematopoietic stem cell possessing a reciprocal translocation between chromosomes 9 and 22. This translocation results in the head-to-tail fusion of the breakpoint cluster region (*BCR*) gene on chromosome 22q11 with the *ABL1* (named after the Abelson murine leukemia virus) gene located on chromosome 9q34. The bcr-abl fusion protein results in constitutive activation of abl tyrosine kinase enzyme that prevents apoptosis and leads to increased survival of the cells containing the mutation. Ultimately, untreated CML develops into an accelerated phase with increasing numbers of mutations and leads to acute blast crisis. The deletion of the long arm of chromosome 5 is present in some individuals with acute myeloid leukemias and is associated with older age at diagnosis. The inversion of chromosome 16 is typically present in acute myelomonocytic leukemia (M4 subtype). The translocation of the long arms of chromosomes 15 and 17 is the mutation associated with acute promyelocytic anemia that results in arrest of cellular differentiation that can be treated with pharmacologic doses of ATRA (all-*trans* retinoic acid). Finally, trisomy 12 is one of several mutations that may result in the development of chronic lymphocytic leukemia.

III-81. **The answer is D.** *(Chap. 109)* The acute myeloid leukemias (AMLs) are a group of hematologic malignancies derived from hematologic stem cells that have acquired chromosomal mutations that prevent differentiation into mature myeloid cells. The specific chromosomal abnormalities predict in which stage of differentiation the cell is arrested and are associated with the several subtypes of AML that have been identified. In the United States, more than 16,000 new cases of AML are diagnosed yearly, and the numbers of new cases of AML has increased in the past 10 years. Men are diagnosed with AML more frequently than women (4.6 cases per 100,000 population vs. 3.0 cases per 100,000, respectively). In addition, older age is associated with increased incidence of AML, with an incidence of 18.6 cases per 100,000 population in those older than 65 years of age. AML is uncommon in adolescents. Other known risk factors for the development of AML include hereditary genetic abnormalities, radiation and chemical exposures, and drugs. The most common hereditary abnormality linked to AML is trisomy 21 (Down syndrome). Other hereditary syndromes associated with an increase of AML include diseases associated with defective DNA repair such as Fanconi's anemia and ataxia telangiectasia. Survivors of the atomic bomb explosions in Japan were found to have a high incidence of AML as have survivors of other high-dose radiation exposures. However, therapeutic radiation is not associated with an increased risk of AML unless the patient was also treated concomitantly with alkylating agents. Anticancer drugs are the most common causes of drug-associated AML. Of the chemotherapeutic agents, alkylating agents and topoisomerase II inhibitors are the drugs most likely to be associated with AML.

III-82. **The answer is C.** *(Chap. 109)* The goal of therapy in chronic myelogenous leukemia (CML) is to achieve prolonged, durable, nonneoplastic, nonclonal hematopoiesis, which entails the eradication of any residual cells containing the *BCR-ABL1* transcript. Hence, the goal is complete molecular remission and cure. Therapy of CML has changed in recent years because of the presence of a proven curative treatment (allogeneic transplantation) that has significant toxicity and a targeted treatment (imatinib) with outstanding outcome based on 8-year follow-up data. New tyrosine kinase inhibitors are becoming available, making this a dynamic topic. Many experts currently recommend initiating therapy with a tyrosine kinase inhibitor and reserving allogeneic transplantation for those who develop drug resistance. Imatinib mesylate is a tyrosine kinase inhibitor that acts to decrease the activity of the bcr-abl fusion protein that results from the reciprocal translocation of chromosomes 9 and 22 (Philadelphia chromosome). It acts as a competitive inhibitor of the abl kinase at its ATP binding site and thus leads to inhibition of tyrosine phosphorylation of proteins in *bcr-abl* signal transduction. In newly diagnosed CML, imatinib results in a complete hematologic remission in 95% of patients initially and 76% at 18 months. Low-risk patients have a higher durable remission rate. All imatinib-treated patients who achieved major molecular remission (26%), defined as 3 log or greater reduction in *BCR-ABL1* transcript level at 18 months compared with pretreatment level, were progression free at 5 years. There is a consensus that molecular responses can be used as a treatment goal in CML. Imatinib, taken orally, has limited side effects that include nausea, fluid retention, diarrhea, and skin rash and is usually well tolerated. Interferon-α was previously the first-line chemotherapy if bone marrow transplant was not an option, but it has been replaced by imatinib mesylate. Autologous stem cell transplant is not currently used for treatment of CML because there is no reliable way to select residual normal hematopoietic progenitor cells. Leukopheresis is used for control of leukocyte counts when the patient is experiencing complications such as respiratory failure or cerebral ischemia related to the high white blood cell count.

III-83 and III-84. The answers are D and E, respectively. *(Chap. 109)* Treatment of acute promyelocytic leukemia (PML) is an interesting example of how understanding the function of the protein produced by the genetic abnormality can be used to develop a treatment for the disease. The translocation of the long arms of chromosomes 15 and 17, t(15;17), results in the production of a chimeric protein called promyelocytic leukemia (Pml)/retinoic acid receptor α (Rar-α). The Pml-Rar-α fusion protein suppresses gene transcription and arrests differentiation of the cells in an immature state, leading to promyelocytic leukemia. Pharmacologic doses of the ligand of the Rar-α receptor, tretinoin, stimulate the cells to resume differentiation. With use of tretinoin, the leukemic cells differentiate to mature neutrophils and undergo subsequent apoptosis. Tretinoin plus concurrent anthracycline-based chemotherapy appears to be among the most effective treatments for APL, leading to complete remission (CR) rates of 90% to 95%. The primary side effect of tretinoin is the development of retinoic acid syndrome. The onset of retinoic acid syndrome from ATRA (all-*trans* retinoic acid) is usually within the first 3 weeks of treatment. Typical symptoms are chest pain, fever, and dyspnea. Hypoxia is common, and chest radiography usually shows diffuse alveolar infiltrates with pleural effusions. Pericardial effusions may also occur. The cause of retinoic acid syndrome is possibly related to the adhesion of the differentiated leukemia cells to the pulmonary endothelium or the release of cytokines by these cells to cause vascular leak. The mortality rate for patients with retinoic acid syndrome is 10%. High-dose glucocorticoid therapy is usually effective in the treatment of retinoic acid syndrome. Arsenic trioxide has antileukemic activity and may be used in tretinoin refractory cases. It is also under investigation for combination chemotherapy. Cyclophosphamide, daunorubicin, vinblastine, and prednisone are the constituents of the combination chemotherapy commonly known as CHOP, which is indicated for the treatment of B-cell lymphomas. Rituximab is most commonly used as a treatment of B-cell non-Hodgkin's lymphoma and a variety of autoimmune disorders. Rituximab is a monoclonal antibody directed against the CD20 cell-surface molecule of B lymphocytes. It has no current role in the treatment of acute myeloid leukemias. Whole-body irradiation is used primarily before bone marrow transplant to ensure complete eradication of cancerous leukemic cells in the bone marrow.

III-85. The answer is C. *(Chap. 109)* Patients with acute leukemia frequently present with nonspecific symptoms of fatigue and weight loss. In addition, weight loss and anorexia are also common. About half have had symptoms for more than 3 months at the time of presentation. Fever is present in only about 10% of patients at presentation, and 5% have evidence of abnormal hemostasis. On physical examination, hepatomegaly, splenomegaly, sternal tenderness, and evidence of infection or hemorrhage are common presenting signs. Laboratory studies are confirmatory with evidence of anemia, thrombocytopenia, and leukocytosis often present. The median presenting leukocyte count at presentation is 15,000/μL. About 20% to 40% have presenting leukocyte counts less than 5000/μL, and another 20% have counts greater than 100,000/μL. Review of the peripheral smear confirms leukemia in most cases. If Auer rods are seen, the diagnosis of acute myeloid leukemia (AML) is virtually certain. Thrombocytopenia (platelet count <100,000/μL) is seen in more than 75% of individuals with AML. After the diagnosis of AML has been confirmed, rapid evaluation and treatment should be undertaken. The general health of the cardiovascular, pulmonary, hepatic, and renal systems should be evaluated because chemotherapy has adverse effects that may cause organ dysfunction in any of these systems. Overall, chromosome findings at diagnosis are currently the most important independent prognostic factor. Patients with t(15;17) have a very good prognosis (~85% cured), and those with t(8;21) and inv(16) have a good prognosis (~55% cured), but those with no cytogenetic abnormality have a moderately favorable outcome (~40% cured). Patients with a complex karyotype, t(6;9), inv(3), or –7, have a very poor prognosis. Among the prognostic factors that predict poor outcomes in AML, age at diagnosis is one of the most important because individuals of advanced age tolerate induction chemotherapy poorly. In addition, advanced age is more likely to be associated with multiple chromosomal abnormalities that predict poorer response to chemotherapy, although some chromosomal markers predict a better response to chemotherapy. Poor performance status independent of age also decreases survival in AML. Responsiveness to chemotherapy and survival are also worse if the leukocyte count is greater than 100,000/μL or the antecedent course of symptoms is prolonged. Anemia, leukopenia, or thrombocytopenia present for more than 3 months is a poor prognostic indicator. However, there is no absolute degree of anemia or thrombocytopenia that predicts worse outcomes.

III-86. **The answer is E.** *(Chap. 110)* Viscosity testing is typically reserved for cases of multiple myeloma in which paraproteins (particularly immunoglobulin M) can lead to vascular sludging and subsequent tissue ischemia. Acute lymphoid leukemia (ALL) can lead to end-organ abnormalities in kidney and liver; therefore, routine chemistry tests are indicated. A lumbar puncture must be performed in cases of newly diagnosed ALL to rule out spread of disease to the central nervous system. Bone marrow biopsy reveals the degree of marrow infiltration and is often necessary for classification of the tumor. Immunologic cell-surface marker testing often identifies the cell lineage involved and the type of tumor, information that is often impossible to discern from morphologic interpretation alone. Cytogenetic testing provides prognostic information on the disease natural history. In ALL, prognosis depends on the genetic characteristics of the tumor, the patient's age, the white cell count, and the patient's overall clinical status and major organ function.

III-87. **The answer is B.** *(Chap. 110)* Hepatitis B and C are both common causes of cirrhosis and are strongly associated with the development of hepatocellular carcinoma. Hepatitis C, but not hepatitis B, can also lead to a lymphoplasmacytic lymphoma, often in the spleen, that resolves with cure of hepatitis C. Epstein-Barr virus has been associated with a large number of lymphoid malignancies, including posttransplant lymphoproliferative disease (PTLD), Hodgkin's disease, central nervous system lymphoma, and Burkitt's lymphoma. *Helicobacter pylori* infection is necessary and sufficient for gastric mucosa-associated lymphoid tissue (MALT) lymphoma development, and cure can be achieved with eradication of the organism in some cases. HHV8 is a known cause of body cavity lymphoma, including primary pleural lymphoma. In addition to those listed, HTLV-1 is associated with adult T-cell lymphoma or leukemia. Other disorders associated with lymphoma include celiac sprue, autoimmune disease, and biologic therapies for autoimmune disease. Celiac sprue has been associated with gastrointestinal tract lymphoma. Many collagen vascular diseases (e.g., Sjogren's) and anti–tumor necrosis factor therapies have been associated with the development of lymphoma.

III-88. **The answer is B.** *(Chap. 110)* Autoimmune hemolytic anemia and thrombocytopenia are common, and a peripheral blood smear and a Coombs test help evaluate their presence. Hypersplenism is also seen in chronic lymphoid leukemia (CLL) as the spleen sequesters large numbers of circulating blood cells and enlarges. Hence, a careful left upper quadrant examination looking for a palpable splenic tip is the standard of care in this situation. This patient is at risk of hepatic decompensation as well, given his hepatitis C that can also cause anemia and thrombocytopenia. Bone marrow infiltration of tumor cells can lead to cytopenias in CLL. However, this is in effect a diagnosis of exclusion. After these three possibilities have been ruled out, a bone marrow biopsy is a reasonable next step. This initial evaluation before presuming spread of CLL is critical for therapy because each possibility requires different therapy (glucocorticoids or rituximab for hemolysis, hepatology referral for liver failure, and splenectomy for symptomatic hypersplenism).

III-89. **The answer is C.** *(Chap. 110)* The peripheral smear shows increased numbers of small, well-differentiated, normal-appearing lymphocytes characteristic of chronic lymphocytic leukemia, the most common leukemia or lymphoma in adults. Common presenting complaints typically include fatigue, frequent infections, new lymphadenopathy, and abdominal complaints relating to splenomegaly. Hairy cell leukemia is a rare disease that presents predominantly in older men. Typical presentation involves pancytopenia, although occasional patients will have a leukemic presentation. Splenomegaly is usual. The malignant cells appear to have "hairy" projections on light and electron microscopy. Patients with this disorder are prone to unusual infections, including infection by *Mycobacterium avium intracellulare*, and to vasculitic syndromes. Hairy cell leukemia is responsive to chemotherapy with cladribine with clinical complete remissions in the majority of patients and frequent long-term disease-free survival.

III-90. **The answer is E.** *(Chap. 110)* Classical Hodgkin's disease carries a better prognosis than all types of non-Hodgkin's lymphoma. Patients with good prognostic factors can achieve cure with extended field radiation alone, but those with a higher risk disease often achieve cure with high-dose chemotherapy and sometimes radiation. The chance of cure is so high (>90%) that many protocols are now considering long-term sequelae of current therapy such as carcinomas, hypothyroidism, premature coronary disease, and constrictive pericarditis in those receiving radiation therapy. A variety of chemotherapy regimens are effective with long-term disease-free survival in patients with advanced disease achieved in more than 75% of patients who lack systemic symptoms and in 60% to 70% of patients with systemic symptoms.

III-91. **The answer is D.** *(Chap. 110)* The large cell with a bilobed nucleus and prominent nucleoli giving an "owl's eyes" appearance near the center of the field is a Reed-Sternberg cell, confirming the diagnosis of Hodgkin's disease. Hodgkin's disease occurs in 8000 patients in the United States each year, and the disease does not appear to be increasing in frequency. Most patients present with palpable lymphadenopathy that is nontender; in most patients, these lymph nodes are in the neck, supraclavicular area, and axilla. More than half the patients have mediastinal adenopathy at diagnosis, and this is sometimes the initial manifestation. Subdiaphragmatic presentation of Hodgkin's disease is unusual and more common in older men. One-third of patients present with fevers, night sweats, or weight loss, which are B symptoms in the Ann Arbor staging classification. Occasionally, Hodgkin's disease can present as a fever of unknown origin. This is more common in older patients who are found to have mixed cellularity Hodgkin's disease in an abdominal site. Rarely, the fevers persist for days to weeks followed by afebrile intervals and then recurrence of the fever (Pel-Ebstein fever). The differential diagnosis of a lymph node biopsy suspicious for Hodgkin's disease includes inflammatory processes, mononucleosis, non-Hodgkin's lymphoma, phenytoin-induced adenopathy, and nonlymphomatous malignancies.

III-92. **The answer is E.** *(Chap. e20)* A "dry tap" is defined as the inability to aspirate bone marrow and is reported in approximately 5% of attempts. It is rare in the case of normal bone marrow. The differential diagnosis includes metastatic carcinoma infiltration (17%); chronic myeloid leukemia (15%); myelofibrosis (14%); hairy cell leukemia (10%); acute leukemia (10%); and lymphomas, including Hodgkin's disease (9%).

III-93. **The answer is B.** *(Chap. e20)* The diagnostic criteria for chronic eosinophilic leukemia and the hypereosinophilic syndrome first requires the presence of persistent eosinophilia *greater than* 1500/µL in blood, increased marrow eosinophils, and less than 20% myeloblasts in blood or marrow. Additional disorders that must be excluded include all causes of reactive eosinophilia, primary neoplasms associated with eosinophilia (e.g., T-cell lymphoma, Hodgkin's disease, acute lymphoid leukemia, mastocytosis, chronic myelogenous leukemia, acute myeloid leukemia [AML], myelodysplasia, and myeloproliferative syndromes), and T-cell reaction with increased interleukin-5 or cytokine production. If these entities have been excluded and the myeloid cells show a clonal chromosome abnormality and blast cells (>2%) are present in peripheral blood or are increased in marrow (but <20%), then the diagnosis is chronic eosinophilic leukemia. Patients with hypereosinophilic syndrome and chronic eosinophilic leukemia may be asymptomatic (discovered on routine testing) or present with systemic findings such as fever, shortness of breath, new neurologic findings, or rheumatologic findings. The heart, lungs, and central nervous system are most often affected by eosinophil-mediated tissue damage.

III-94. **The answer is D.** *(Chap. e21)* Mastocytosis is a proliferation and accumulation of mast cells in one or more organ systems. Only the skin is involved in approximately 80% of cases with the other 20% being defined as systemic mastocytosis caused by the involvement of another organ system. The most common manifestation of mastocytosis is cutaneous urticaria pigmentosa, a maculopapular pigmented rash involving the papillary dermis. Other cutaneous forms include diffuse cutaneous mastocytosis (almost entirely in children) and mastocytoma. Clinical manifestations of systemic mastocytosis are related to either cellular infiltration of organs or release of histamine, proteases, eicosanoids, or heparin from mast cells. Therefore, signs and symptoms may include constitutional symptoms, skin manifestations (pruritus, dermatographia, rash), mediator-related symptoms (abdominal pain, flushing, syncope, hypertension, diarrhea), and bone related symptoms (fracture, pain, arthralgia). In a recent series, 40% of patients with systemic mastocytosis had an associated myeloid neoplasm, most commonly myeloproliferative syndrome, chronic myelogenous leukemia, and myelodysplastic syndrome. Eosinophilia was present in approximately one-third of patients. Elevated serum tryptase, bone marrow involvement, splenomegaly, skeletal involvement, cytopenia, and malabsorption predict more aggressive disease and a worse prognosis. Many patients with systemic mastocytosis have an activating mutation of c-Kit, a kinase inhibited by imatinib; however, the mutation appears relatively resistant to this agent.

III-95. **The answer is A.** *(Chap. 111)* The patient presents with pneumococcal pneumonia and evidence of hypercalcemia, renal failure, and a wide protein gap suggestive of an M protein. These findings are classic for multiple myeloma. Although the patient appears to be making large quantities of immunoglobulins, they are in fact generally monoclonal, and patients actually have functional hypogammaglobulinemia related to both decreased production and increased destruction of normal antibodies. This hypogammaglobulinemia predisposes patients to infections, most commonly pneumonia with pneumococcus or *Staphylococcus aureus* or gram-negative pyelonephritis. Bone marrow biopsy would confirm the presence of clonal plasma cells and define the quantity, which will help define treatment options. A serum protein electrophoresis would also be indicated to prove the presence of the M protein suspected by the wide protein gap. Although HIV may be associated with kidney injury, both acute and chronic, hypercalcemia would be an unusual feature. There is no clinical history of aspiration, and the location of infiltrate, upper lobe, is unusual for aspiration. Sweat chloride testing is not indicated because there is no suspicion for cystic fibrosis. Because solid organ malignancy is not suspected, computed tomography of the body is unlikely to be helpful.

III-96. **The answer is A.** *(Chap. 112)* This patient presents with a multisystem illness involving the heart, kidneys, and peripheral nervous system. The physical examination is suggestive of amyloidosis with classic waxy papules in the folds of his body. The laboratory test results are remarkable for renal failure of unclear etiology with significant proteinuria but no cellular casts. A possible etiology of the renal failure is suggested by the elevated gamma globulin fraction and low hematocrit, bringing to mind a monoclonal gammopathy perhaps leading to renal failure through amyloid AL deposition. This could also account for the enlarged heart seen on the echocardiography and the peripheral neuropathy. The fat pad biopsy is generally reported to be 60% to 80% sensitive for amyloid; however, it would not allow a diagnosis of this patient's likely myeloma. A right heart catheterization probably would prove that the patient has restrictive cardiomyopathy secondary to amyloid deposition; however, it too would not diagnose the underlying plasma cell dyscrasia. Renal ultrasonography, although warranted to rule out obstructive uropathy, would not be diagnostic. Similarly, the electromyographic and nerve conduction studies would not be diagnostic. The bone marrow biopsy is about 50% to 60% sensitive for amyloid, but it would allow evaluation of the percent of plasma cells in the bone marrow and allow the diagnosis of multiple myeloma to be made. Multiple myeloma is associated with amyloid AL in approximately 20% of cases. Light chains most commonly deposit systemically in the heart, kidneys, liver, and nervous system, causing organ dysfunction. In these organs, biopsy would show the classic eosinophilic material that, when exposed to Congo red stain, has a characteristic apple-green birefringence.

III-97. **The answer is C.** *(Chap. 115)* Heparin-induced thrombocytopenia (HIT) is a clinical diagnosis that must not be missed because life-threatening thrombosis can occur if not treated appropriately. The cause of HIT is the formation of antibodies to the complex of heparin and platelet factor 4 (PF4). This complex is able to activate platelets, monocytes, and endothelial cells. Many patients exposed to heparin will develop antibodies to the heparin–PF4 complex, but only a few of these will progress to develop thrombocytopenia or thrombocytopenia with thrombosis (HITT). The typical patient will develop evidence of HIT 5 to 14 days after exposure to heparin, although it can occur within 5 days in individuals exposed to heparin within about the previous 100 days as would be expected in this patient given his recent hospitalization. The nadir platelet count is typically greater than 20,000/μL. When HIT is suspected, one should not delay treatment for laboratory testing because no currently available test has adequate sensitivity or specificity for the diagnosis. The antiheparin/PF4 antibody test result is positive in many individuals who have been exposed to heparin regardless of whether HIT is present. The platelet activation assay is more specific but less sensitive for HIT. As soon as HIT is suspected, heparin should be discontinued and replaced with an alternative form of anticoagulation to protect against development of new thromboses. Low-molecular-weight heparins (LMWHs) such as enoxaparin are not appropriate treatment options in individuals with HIT. Although heparin is 10 times more likely to cause HIT, LMWHs also cause the illness and should not be used. The primary agents used for HIT in the United States are the direct thrombin inhibitors argatroban and lepirudin. Argatroban is the preferred agent for this patient because of his renal failure. The drug is not excreted by the kidneys, and no dosage adjustment is required. In contrast, lepirudin is markedly increased in renal failure, and a significant dosage adjustment is required. Danaparoid has previously been used frequently for HIT and HITT, but this medication is no longer available in the United States. Other anticoagulants that are used for treatment of HITT include bivalirudin and fondaparinux, but these also are not currently approved for use in the United States.

III-98. **The answer is E.** *(Chap. 115)* This patient presents with symptoms of thrombocytopenia, including bleeding gums and easy bruising. The only finding on physical examination may be petechiae at points of increased venous pressure, especially in the feet and ankles. The laboratory findings confirm thrombocytopenia but show no abnormalities in other cell lines. When evaluating isolated thrombocytopenia, one must initially consider whether an underlying infection or medication is causing the platelet count to fall. There is a long list of medications that are implicated in thrombocytopenia, including aspirin, acetaminophen, penicillins, H$_2$ blockers, heparin, and many others. This patient discontinued all medications over 6 weeks previously, and the platelet count would be expected to recover if a medication reaction were the cause. She gives no signs of any acute infection. Thus, the most likely diagnosis is immune thrombocytopenia purpura (ITP). This disorder is also known as idiopathic thrombocytopenia purpura and refers to an immune-mediated destruction of platelets and possible inhibition of platelet release from megakaryocytes. ITP can truly be idiopathic, or it can be secondary to an underlying disorder, including systemic lupus erythematosus (SLE), HIV, or chronic hepatitis C virus (HCV) infection. The platelet count can be quite low (<5000/μL) in patients with ITP and usually presents with mucocutaneous bleeding. Laboratory testing for ITP should include a peripheral smear that typically demonstrates large platelets with otherwise normal morphology. Initial testing should evaluate for secondary causes of ITP, including HIV antibodies, HCV antibodies, serologic testing for SLE, serum protein electrophoresis, and immunoglobulins. If anemia is also present, a direct Coombs test is indicated to assess whether there is a combined autoimmune hemolytic anemia with ITP (Evans syndrome). Antiplatelet antibody testing is not recommended because these tests have low sensitivity and specificity for ITP. In addition, bone marrow biopsy is typically not performed unless there are other abnormalities that are not explained by ITP or the patient has failed to respond to usual therapy.

III-99 and III-100. **The answers are A and E, respectively.** *(Chap. 115)* This patient presents with the classic pentad of thrombotic thrombocytopenic purpura (TTP), which is fever, neurologic symptoms, acute renal failure, thrombocytopenia, and microscopic angiopathic hemolytic anemia (MAHA). Although this is the classic presentation, it is not necessary to have all five characteristics for an individual to be diagnosed with TTP. In recent years, the pathogenesis of inherited and idiopathic TTP has been discovered to be attributable to a deficiency of or antibodies directed against the ADAMTS-13 protein. The ADAMTS-13 protein is a metalloproteinase that cleaves von Willebrand factor (VWF). In the absence of ADAMTS-13, ultra-large VWF multimers circulate in the blood and can cause pathogenic platelet adhesion and activation, resulting in microvascular ischemia and microangiopathic hemolytic anemia. However, it appears as if there is a necessary inciting event because not all individuals with an inherited deficiency of ADAMTS-13 develop TTP. Some drugs have been implicated as causative agents in TTP. Ticlopidine and possibly clopidogrel cause TTP by inducing antibody formation. Other drugs, including mitomycin C, cyclosporine, and quinine, can cause TTP by causing direct endothelial toxicity.

A diagnosis of TTP can be made based on clinical factors. It should be differentiated from disseminated intravascular coagulation, which causes MAHA but has a predominant coagulopathy. Hemolytic uremic syndrome also causes MAHA and appears very similar to TTP in clinical presentation, although neurologic symptoms are less prominent. Often a preceding diarrheal illness alerts one to hemolytic syndrome as the cause of MAHA. It is important to make a prompt and correct diagnosis because the mortality rate for patients with TTP without treatment is 85% to 100%, decreasing to 10% to 30% with treatment. The primary treatment for TTP remains plasma exchange. Plasma exchange should be continued until the platelet count returns to the normal range and there is no further evidence of hemolysis for at least 2 days. Glucocorticoids can be used as adjunctive treatment in TTP but are not effective as the sole therapy. Recent research suggests that rituximab may be useful in primary treatment of TTP. However, relapse is common with rituximab.

III-101. The answer is D. *(Chap. 116)* The hemophilias are X-linked inherited disorders that cause deficiency of factor VIII (hemophilia A) or factor 9 (hemophilia B). The hemophilias affect about one in 10,000 males worldwide with hemophilia A responsible for 80% of cases. Clinically, there is no difference between hemophilia A and B. The disease presentation largely depends on the residual activity of factor VIII or factor IX. Severe disease is typically seen when factor activity is less than 1%, and moderate disease appears when the levels range between 1% and 5%. The clinical manifestation of moderate and severe disease is commonly bleeding into the joints, soft tissues, and muscles that occurs after minimal trauma or even spontaneously. When factor activity is greater than 25%, bleeding would occur only after major trauma or surgery, and the diagnosis may not be made unless a prolonged activated partial thromboplastin time is seen on routine laboratory examination. To make a definitive diagnosis, one would need to measure specific levels of factor VIII and IX. Without treatment, life expectancy is limited, but given the changes in therapy since the 1980s, life span is about 65 years. Early treatment of hemophilia required the use of pooled plasma that was used to make factor concentrates. Given the large number of donors required to generate the factor concentrates and the frequent need for transfusion in some individuals, bloodborne pathogens such as HIV and hepatitis C are among the leading cause of death in patients with hemophilia. In the 1990s, recombinant factor VIII and IX were developed. Primary prophylaxis is given to individuals with baseline factor activity levels of less than 1% to prevent spontaneous bleeding, especially hemarthroses. Although this strategy is highly recommended, only about 50% of eligible patients receive prophylactic therapy because of the high costs and need for regular intravenous infusions. When an individual is suspected of having a bleed, the treatment should begin as soon as possible and not delayed until factor activity levels return. Factor concentrates should be given to raise the activity level to 50% for large hematomas or deep muscle bleeds, and an individual may require treatment for a period of 7 days or more. For milder bleeds, including uncomplicated hemarthrosis, the goal factor activity level is 30% to 50% with maintenance of levels between 15% and 25% for 2 to 3 days after the initial transfusions. In addition to treatment with factor concentrates, care should be taken to avoid medications that inhibit platelet function. DDAVP, a desmopressin analogue, can be given as adjunctive therapy for acute bleeding episodes in hemophilia A because this may cause a transient rise in factor VIII levels and von Willebrand factor because of release from endothelial cells. This medication is typically only useful in mild to moderate disease. Antifibrinolytic drugs such as tranexamic acid or ε-amino caproic acid are helpful in promoting hemostasis for mucosal bleeding.

III-102. The answer is D. *(Chap. 116)* Disseminated intravascular coagulation (DIC) is a consumptive coagulopathy that is characterized by diffuse intravascular fibrin formation that overcomes the body's natural anticoagulant mechanisms. DIC is most commonly associated with sepsis, trauma, or malignancy or in obstetric complications. The pathogenesis of

DIC is not completely elucidated, but it involves intravascular exposure to phospholipids from damaged tissue, hemolysis, and endothelial damage. This leads to stimulation of pro-coagulant pathways with uncontrolled thrombin generation and microvascular ischemia. A secondary hyperfibrinolysis subsequently occurs. The primary clinical manifestations of DIC are bleeding at venipuncture sites, petechiae, and ecchymoses. Severe gastrointestinal and pulmonary hemorrhage can occur. The clinical diagnosis of DIC is based on laboratory findings in the appropriate clinical setting, such as severe sepsis. Although there is no single test for DIC, the common constellation of findings is thrombocytopenia (<100,000/μL), elevated prothrombin time and activated partial thromboplastin time, evidence of micro-angiopathic hemolytic anemia, and elevated fibrin degradation productions and D-dimer. The fibrinogen level may be less than 100 mg/dL but often does not decrease acutely unless the DIC is very severe. The primary treatment of DIC is to treat the underlying cause, which in this case would be antibiotic therapy directed against *Neisseria meningitidis*. For patients such as this one who are experiencing bleeding related to the DIC, attempts to correct the coagulopathy should be undertaken. Platelet transfusions and fresh-frozen plasma (FFP) should be given. In addition, cryoprecipitate is indicated as the fibrinogen level is less than 100 mg/dL. In general, 10 U of cryoprecipitate are required for every 2 to 3 units of FFP. In acute DIC, heparin is not been demonstrated to be helpful and may increase bleeding. Low-dose heparin therapy (5–10 U/kg) is used for chronic low-grade DIC such as that seen in acute promyelocytic leukemia or removal of a dead fetus.

III-103. **The answer is E.** *(Chap. 116)* Vitamin K is a fat-soluble vitamin that plays an essential role in hemostasis. It is absorbed in the small intestine and stored in the liver. It serves as a cofactor in the enzymatic carboxylation of glutamic acid residues on prothrombin-complex proteins. The three major causes of vitamin K deficiency are poor dietary intake, intestinal malabsorption, and liver disease. The prothrombin complex proteins (factors II, VII, IX, and X and protein C and protein S) all decrease with vitamin K deficiency. Factor VII and protein C have the shortest half-lives of these factors and therefore decrease first. Therefore, vitamin K deficiency manifests with prolongation of the prothrombin time first. With severe deficiency, the activated partial thromboplastin time will be prolonged as well. Factor VIII is not influenced by vitamin K.

III-104. **The answer is E.** *(Chap. 116)* Hemophilia A results from a deficiency of factor VIII. Replacement of factor VIII is the centerpiece of treatment. Cessation of aspirin or nonsteroidal anti-inflammatory drugs is highly recommended. Fresh-frozen plasma (FFP) contains pooled plasma from human sources. Cryoprecipitate refers to FFP that is cooled, resulting in the precipitation of material at the bottom of the plasma. This product contains about half the factor VIII activity of FFP in a tenth of the volume. Both agents are therefore reasonable treatment options. DDAVP (desmopressin) causes the release of a number of factors and von Willebrand factor from the liver and endothelial cells. This may be useful for patients with mild hemophilia. Recombinant or purified factor VIII (i.e., Humate P) is indicated in patients with more severe bleeding. Therapy may be required for weeks, with levels of factor VIII kept at 50%, for postsurgical or severe bleeding. Plasmapheresis has no role in the treatment of patients with hemophilia A.

III-105. **The answer is C.** *(Chap. 116)* Lupus anticoagulants (Las) cause prolongation of coagulation tests by binding to phospholipids. Although most often encountered in patients with systemic lupus erythematosus, they may also develop in normal individuals. The diagnosis is first suggested by prolongation of coagulation tests. Failure to correct with incubation with normal plasma confirms the presence of a circulating inhibitor. Contrary to the name, patients with LA activity have normal hemostasis and are not predisposed to bleeding. Instead, they are at risk for venous and arterial thromboembolisms. Patients with a history of recurrent unplanned abortions or thrombosis should undergo lifelong anticoagulation. The presence of LAs or anticardiolipin antibodies without a history of thrombosis may be observed because many of these patients will not go on to develop a thrombotic event.

III-106. **The answer is D.** *(Chap. 116)* The activated partial thromboplastin time (aPTT) involves the factors of the intrinsic pathway of coagulation. Prolongation of the aPTT reflects either a deficiency of one of these factors (factor VIII, IX, XI, XII, and so on) or inhibition of the activity of one of the factors or components of the aPTT assay (i.e., phospholipids). This may be further characterized by the "mixing study" in which the patient's plasma is mixed with pooled plasma. Correction of the aPTT reflects a deficiency of factors that are replaced by the pooled sample. Failure to correct the aPTT reflects the presence of a factor inhibitor or phospholipid inhibitor. Common causes of a failure to correct include the presence of heparin in the sample, factor inhibitors (factor VIII inhibitor being the most common), and the presence of antiphospholipid antibodies. Factor VII is involved in the extrinsic pathway of coagulation. Inhibitors to factor VII would result in prolongation of the prothrombin time.

III-107. **The answer is D.** *(Chap. 116)* This patient presents with a significant upper gastrointestinal (GI) bleed with a prolonged prothrombin time (PT). Hemophilia should not cause a prolonged PT. This and the presence of ascites raise the possibility of liver disease and cirrhosis. The contamination of blood products in the 1970s and 1980s resulted in widespread transmission of HIV and hepatitis C virus (HCV) within the hemophilia population receiving factor infusions. It is estimated in 2006, that more than 80% of hemophilia patients older than 20 years old are infected with HCV. Viral inactivation steps were introduced in the 1980s, and recombinant factor VIII and IX were first produced in the 1990s. HCV is the major cause of morbidity and the second leading cause of death in patients exposed to older factor concentrates. Patients develop cirrhosis and complications that include ascites and variceal bleeding. End-stage liver disease requiring a liver transplant is curative for the cirrhosis and the hemophilia (the liver produces factor VIII). Hepatitis B was not transmitted in significant numbers to patients with hemophilia. Diverticular disease or peptic ulcer disease would not explain the prolonged PT. Patients with inadequately repleted factor VIII levels are more likely to develop hemarthroses than GI bleeds, and the slightly prolonged activated partial thromboplastin time makes this unlikely.

III-108. **The answer is E.** *(Chap. 116)* The differentiation between disseminated intravascular coagulation (DIC) and severe liver disease is challenging. Both entities may manifest with similar laboratory findings, which are elevated fibrinogen degradation products, prolonged activated partial thromboplastin time and prothrombin time, anemia, and thrombocytopenia. When suspecting DIC, these tests should be repeated over a period of 6 to 8 hours because abnormalities may change dramatically in patients with severe DIC. In contrast, these test results should not fluctuate as much in patients with severe liver disease. Bacterial sepsis with positive blood cultures is a common cause of DIC but is not diagnostic.

III-109. **The answer is B.** *(Chap. 117)* Venous thrombosis occurs through activation of the coagulation cascade primarily through the exposure to tissue factor, and the genetic factors that contribute to a predisposition to venous thrombosis typically are polymorphisms affecting procoagulant or fibrinolytic pathways. In contrast, arterial thrombosis occurs in the setting a platelet activation, and the genetic predisposition for arterial thrombosis includes mutations that affect platelet receptors or redox enzymes. The most common inherited risk factors for venous thrombosis are the factor V Leiden mutation and prothrombin 20210 mutation. Other mutations predisposing an individual to venous thrombosis include inherited deficiency of protein C or S and mutations of fibrinogen, tissue plasminogen activator, thrombomodulin, or plasminogen activator inhibitor. The glycoprotein 1b platelet receptor mutation would increase the risk of arterial, but not venous, thrombosis.

III-110. **The answer is A.** *(Chap. 117)* D-Dimer is a degradation product of cross-linked fibrin and is elevated in conditions of ongoing thrombosis. Low concentrations of D-dimer are considered to indicate the absence of thrombosis. Patients older than the age of 70 years frequently have elevated D-dimers in the absence of thrombosis, making this test less predictive of acute disease. Clinical symptoms are often not present in patients with deep venous thrombosis (DVT) and do not affect interpretation of a D-dimer. Tobacco use, although frequently considered a risk factor for DVT, and previous DVT should not affect the predictive value of D-dimer. Homan's sign, calf pain elicited by dorsiflexion of the foot, is not predictive of DVT and is unrelated to D-dimer.

III-111. The answer is E. *(Chaps. 117 and 262)* The clinical probability of pulmonary embolism (PE) can be delineated into low to high likelihood using the clinical decision rule shown in Table III-111 below. In those with a score of 3 or less, PE is low or moderately likely, and a D-dimer test should be performed. A normal D-dimer result combined with a low to moderate clinical probability of PE identifies patients who do not need further testing or anticoagulation therapy. Those with either a likely clinical probability (score >3) or an abnormal D-dimer (with unlikely clinical probability) require an imaging test to rule out PE. Currently, the most attractive imaging method to detect PE is the multislice computed tomography (CT). It is accurate and, if the result is normal, safely rules out PE. This patient has a clinical probability score of 4.5 because of her resting tachycardia and the lack of an alternative diagnosis at least as likely as PE. Therefore, there is no indication for measuring D-dimer, and she should proceed directly to multislice CT of the chest. If this cannot be performed expeditiously, she should receive one dose of low-molecular-weight heparin while awaiting the test.

TABLE III-111   Clinical Decision Rules

Low Clinical Likelihood of Deep Venous Thrombosis if Point Score Is Zero or Less; Moderate-Likelihood Score Is 1 to 2; High-Likelihood Score Is 3 or Greater	
Clinical Variable	Score
Active cancer	1
Paralysis, paresis, or recent cast	1
Bedridden for >3 days; major surgery <12 weeks	1
Tenderness along distribution of deep veins	1
Entire leg swelling	1
Unilateral calf swelling >3 cm	1
Pitting edema	1
Collateral superficial nonvaricose veins	1
Alternative diagnosis at least as likely as DVT	−2
High Clinical Likelihood of Pulmonary Embolism if Point Score Exceeds 4	
Clinical Variable	Score
Signs and symptoms of DVT	3.0
Alternative diagnosis less likely than PE	3.0
Heart rate >100 beats/min	1.5
Immobilization >3 days; surgery within 4 weeks	1.5
Prior PE or DVT	1.5
Hemoptysis	1.0
Cancer	1.0

Abbreviations: DVT, deep venous thrombosis; PE, pulmonary embolism.

III-112. The answer is C. *(Chap. 118)* In recent years, a variety of new anticoagulant and antiplatelet drugs have been developed for clinical use. Platelets play an important role in arterial thrombosis, particularly in coronary artery and cerebrovascular disease. Aspirin is the most widely used antiplatelet drug worldwide. Aspirin exerts its effects through inhibition of cyclooxygenase-1. Other commonly used oral antiplatelet agents are clopidogrel and dipyridamole. Clopidogrel is in a class of agents called thienopyridines along with ticlopidine. Thienopyridines act to block a specific adenosine diphosphate receptor ($P2Y_{12}$) and inhibit platelet aggregation. Dipyridamole inhibits phosphodiesterase to decrease the breakdown of cyclic adenosine monophosphate (cAMP) to decrease platelet aggregation. Intravenous antiplatelet agents have also become increasingly important in the treatment of acute coronary syndromes. All of the intravenous agents act to inhibit platelet aggregation by blocking the glycoprotein (GP) IIb/IIIa receptor. The three agents in clinical use as GP IIb/IIIa inhibitors are abciximab, eptifibatide, and tirofiban.

Anticoagulant agents are primarily used for the prevention and treatment of venous thrombosis. Many anticoagulants are available and act by a variety of mechanisms. Heparin has been used for many years but requires frequent monitoring to be used safely. More recently, low-molecular-weight heparins (LMWHs) have been introduced. These agents are given subcutaneously and generally preferred in many instances over heparin given a more predictable anticoagulant effect. Both heparin and the LMWHs are indirect thrombin inhibitors that act primarily through activation of antithrombin. When activated, antithrombin inhibits clotting enzymes, especially thrombin and factor Xa. Fondaparinux is a newer anticoagulant that inhibits only factor Xa, although it is a synthetic analogue of the pentasaccharide sequence in heparin that binds antithrombin. However, it is too short to bridge antithrombin to thrombin. The direct thrombin inhibitors bind directly to thrombin (rather than antithrombin) to exert their activity. The direct thrombin inhibitors include lepirudin, argatroban, and bivalirudin. The most commonly used oral anticoagulant is warfarin, which inhibits the production of vitamin K–dependent clotting factors. Given the need for frequent monitoring and extensive drug interactions, developing other oral anticoagulants that are safe and effective has been desired for many years. No oral drug has yet been introduced into the market. However, several are in the final stages of development. These include two factor Xa inhibitors (rivaroxaban and apixaban) and one factor IIa inhibitor (dabigatran etexilate).

III-113. **The answer is B.** *(Chap. 118)* After implantation of a bare metal coronary artery stent, aspirin and clopidogrel are recommended for at least 4 weeks to decrease the risk of in-stent restenosis. This patient, however, developed the complication despite adherence to her therapy. This generally suggests resistance to clopidogrel with a decreased ability of clopidogrel to inhibit platelet aggregation. There is a known genetic component to clopidogrel resistance related to specific genetic polymorphisms of the CYP isoenzymes. Up to 25% of whites, 30% of African Americans, and 50% of Asians may carry an allele that renders them resistant to clopidogrel. These polymorphisms are less important in the activation of prasugrel. Thus, in individuals who have evidence of clopidogrel resistance, switching to prasugrel should be considered.

Aspirin resistance is a more controversial subject. It is defined simply in clinical terms as failure of aspirin to prevent ischemic vascular events. Biochemically, aspirin resistance can be defined by failure of usual doses of the drug to produce inhibitory effects on platelet function. However, resistance to aspirin is not reversed by higher doses of aspirin or adding another antiplatelet agent. Because the primary mechanism of arterial thrombosis is platelet aggregation, the anticoagulant agents warfarin and low-molecular-weight heparin are not indicated.

III-114. **The answer is B.** *(Chap. 118)* Low-molecular-weight heparins (LMWHs) have largely replaced heparin for most indications if a patient does not have any contraindications to therapy. LMWHs have better bioavailability and longer half-lives after subcutaneous injection. Thus, they can be given at routine intervals for both prophylaxis and treatment. In addition, dosing of LMWHs is simplified because these drugs have a dose-independent clearance, and predictable anticoagulant effects means that monitoring of anticoagulant effect is not required in most patients. Finally, LMWHs have a lower risk of heparin-induced thrombocytopenia, which is important in both short- and long-term administration.

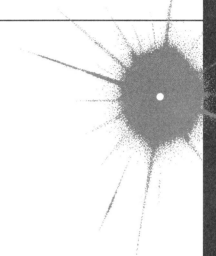

SECTION IV
Infectious Diseases

QUESTIONS

DIRECTIONS: Choose the **one best** response to each question.

IV-1. Deficits in the complement membrane attack complex (C5-8) are associated with infections of what variety?

A. Catalase-positive bacteria
B. *Neisseria meningitis*
C. *Pseudomonas aeruginosa*
D. *Salmonella* spp.
E. *Streptococcus pneumoniae*

IV-2. A 48-year-old man is admitted to the intensive care unit for treatment of septic shock for an uncertain cause. He was well until 1 day before admission. His family reports that he developed myalgias and fevers at that time. He had no other specific complaints but reportedly had decreased oral intake and generalized malaise. He was brought to the hospital by ambulance this morning when he was lethargic and unresponsive at home. Upon arrival of emergency medical services, his initial blood pressure was 60/40 mmHg with a heart rate of 142 beats/min. He was tachypneic with a respiratory rate of 32 breaths/min with an oxygen saturation of 75% on room air, and his initial temperature was 104.9°F (40.5°C). He was intubated and placed on mechanical ventilation. The patient received 1 L of normal saline before arrival in the emergency department but continues to have hypotension (blood pressure, 75/40 mmHg). Ongoing volume resuscitation is ordered, and the patient is initiated on norepinephrine to maintain adequate blood pressure. The patient has a history of hypertension and hyperlipidemia. He takes amlodipine 10 mg daily and atorvastatin 20 mg daily. His only other history is an automobile accident at age 20 years, requiring exploratory laparotomy and splenectomy. Blood, sputum, and urine cultures are obtained. What are the most appropriate empiric antibiotics for the treatment of this patient?

A. Ceftriaxone and vancomycin
B. Ceftriaxone, ampicillin, and vancomycin
C. Ceftriaxone, vancomycin, and amphotericin B
D. Clindamycin, gentamicin, and vancomycin
E. Clindamycin and quinine

IV-3. A 32-year-old woman is admitted to the hospital complaining of right thigh pain. She is treated empirically with oxacillin intravenously for a cellulitis. The admitting physician notes that the degree of pain appears to be disproportionate to the amount of overlying cellulitis. Over the course of the next 24 hours, the patient develops profound septic shock complicated by hypotension, acute renal failure, and evidence of disseminated intravascular coagulation. A CT scan of her right leg demonstrates a collection of fluid with gas in the deep fascia of her right leg. Emergent surgical evacuation is planned. What changes to the patient's antibiotic therapy would be recommended?

A. Continue oxacillin and add clindamycin.
B. Continue oxacillin and add clindamycin and gentamicin.
C. Discontinue oxacillin and add clindamycin, vancomycin, and gentamicin.
D. Discontinue oxacillin and add piperacillin/tazobactam and vancomycin.
E. Discontinue oxacillin and add vancomycin and gentamicin.

IV-4. Which type of bite represents a potential medical emergency in a febrile asplenic patient?

A. Cat bite
B. Dog bite
C. Fish bite
D. Human bite

IV-5. One goal of immunization programs is to eliminate a specific disease. In 2010, indigenous transmission of which of the following diseases had been eliminated in the United States?

A. Diphtheria
B. Mumps
C. Pertussis
D. Varicella
E. None of the above

IV-6. A 63-year-old man has chronic obstructive pulmonary disease and presents to your office for routine follow-up. He has no complaints currently and feels well. He is being managed with tiotropium 18 μg once daily with albuterol metered-dose inhaler as needed. His most recent forced expiratory volume in 1 second (FEV_1) was 55% predicted, and he is not on oxygen. He has received one dose of pneumococcal vaccine 5 years previously. He is asking if he should receive another dose of pneumococcal vaccine. According to the guidelines of the Centers for Disease Control and Prevention, what is your recommendation?

A. He does not require further vaccination unless his FEV_1 drops below 50% predicted.
B. He does not require further vaccination until he reaches age 65 years.
C. He should be revaccinated today.
D. He should be revaccinated 10 years after his initial vaccine.
E. No further vaccination is recommended because a single dose is all that is required.

IV-7. In which of the following patients is it appropriate to administer the vaccination against herpes zoster?

A. A 35-year-old woman who has never had varicella-zoster infection who is 12 weeks pregnant with her first child
B. A 54-year-old man who has never had varicella-zoster infection and is otherwise healthy
C. A 62-year-old man with HIV on antiretroviral therapy with a CD4+ lymphocyte count of 450/μL
D. A 64-year-old woman with dermatomyositis-associated interstitial lung disease treated with prednisone 20 mg daily and azathioprine 150 mg daily
E. A 66-year-old woman who was recently diagnosed with non-Hodgkin lymphoma

IV-8. A 39-year-old woman received a liver transplant 2 years ago and is maintained on prednisone, 5 mg, and cyclosporine, 8 mg/kg per day. She has had two episodes of rejection since transplant, as well an episode of cytomegalovirus syndrome and *Nocardia* pneumonia. She intends on taking a 2-week gorilla-watching trip to Rwanda and seeks your advice regarding her health while abroad. Which of the following potential interventions is strictly contraindicated?

A. Malaria prophylaxis
B. Meningococcal vaccine
C. Rabies vaccine
D. Typhoid purified polysaccharide vaccine
E. Yellow fever vaccine

IV-9. A 19-year-old woman comes to your office after being bitten by a bat on the ear while camping in a primitive shelter. She is unable to produce a vaccination record. On physical examination, she is afebrile and appears well. There are two small puncture marks on the pinna of her left ear. What is an appropriate vaccination strategy in this context?

A. Intravenous ribavirin
B. No vaccination
C. Rabies immunoglobulins
D. Rabies inactivated virus vaccine
E. Rabies inactivated virus vaccine plus immuno-globulins

IV-10. Which of the following immunizations is required for entry into many countries in sub-Saharan Africa?

A. Hepatitis A
B. Cholera
C. Meningococcus
D. Typhoid fever
E. Yellow fever

IV-11. A 48-year-old woman is traveling to Haiti with a humanitarian aid group. What is the recommended prophylaxis against malaria for this patient?

A. Atovaquone–proguanil
B. Chloroquine
C. Doxycycline
D. Mefloquine
E. Any of the above can be used

IV-12. A 46-year-old man wishes to travel to Kenya for a 2-week vacation. He is HIV positive and is taking antiretroviral therapy. His last CD4+ count was 625/μL and viral load was undetectable. His nadir CD4+ count was 250/μL. He has never had an AIDS-defining illness. In addition to HIV, he has a history of hypertension and is known to have proteinuria caused by to HIV-associated nephropathy. What is your recommendation to this patient regarding his travel plans?

A. He should not receive the live measles vaccine before travel.
B. He should receive the yellow fever vaccine before travel.
C. He will be required to show proof of HIV testing upon entry into the country.
D. His likelihood of response to the influenza vaccine would be less than 50%.
E. With a CD4+ count greater than 500/μL, he is at no greater risk during travel than persons without HIV.

IV-13. Which of the following is the most common cause of native valve infective endocarditis in the community?

A. Coagulase-negative staphylococci
B. Coagulase-positive staphylococci
C. Enterococci
D. Fastidious gram-negative coccobacilli
E. Non-enterococcal streptococci

IV-14. All of the following are minor criteria in the Duke criteria for the clinical diagnosis of infective endocarditis EXCEPT:

A. Immunologic phenomena (glomerulonephritis, Osler nodes, Roth spots)

B. New valvular regurgitation on transthoracic echocardiogram

C. Predisposing condition (heart condition, intravenous drug use)

D. Temperature >380°C

E. Vascular phenomena (arterial emboli, septic pulmonary emboli, Janeway lesions, and so on)

IV-15. Which of the following patients should receive antibiotic prophylaxis to prevent infective endocarditis?

A. A 23-year-old woman with known mitral valve prolapse undergoing a gingival surgery

B. A 24-year-old woman who had an atrial septal defect completely corrected 22 years ago who is undergoing elective cystoscopy for painless hematuria

C. A 30-year-old man with a history of intravenous drug use and prior endocarditis undergoing operative drainage of a prostatic abscess

D. A 45-year-old man who received a prosthetic mitral valve 5 years ago undergoing routine dental cleaning

E. A 63-year-old woman who received a prosthetic aortic valve 2 years ago undergoing screening colonoscopy

IV-16. A 38-year-old homeless man presents to the emergency department with a transient ischemic attack characterized by a facial droop and left arm weakness lasting 20 minutes and left upper quadrant pain. He reports intermittent subjective fevers, diaphoresis, and chills for the past 2 weeks. He has had no recent travel or contact with animals. He has taken no recent antibiotics. Physical examination reveals a slightly distressed man with disheveled appearance. His temperature is 38.2°C, heart rate is 90 beats/min, and blood pressure is 127/74 mmHg. He has poor dentition. Cardiac examination reveals an early diastolic murmur over the left third intercostal space. His spleen is tender and 2 cm descended below the costal margin. He has tender painful red nodules on the tips of the third finger of his right hand and on the fourth finger of his left hand that are new. He has nits evident on his clothes consistent with body louse infection. His white blood cell count is 14,500/μL with 5% band forms and 93% polymorphonuclear cells. Blood cultures are drawn followed by empirical vancomycin therapy. These cultures remain negative for growth 5 days later. He remains febrile but hemodynamically stable but does develop a new lesion on his toe similar to those on his fingers on hospital day 3. A transthoracic echocardiogram reveals a 1-cm mobile vegetation on the cusp of his aortic valve and moderate aortic regurgitation. A CT scan of the abdomen shows an enlarged spleen with wedge-shaped splenic and renal infarctions. What test should be sent to confirm the most likely diagnosis?

A. *Bartonella* serology

B. Epstein-Barr virus (EBV) heterophile antibody

C. HIV polymerase chain reaction (PCR)

D. Peripheral blood smear

E. Q fever serology

IV-17. In a patient with bacterial endocarditis, which of the following echocardiographic lesions is most likely to lead to embolization?

A. 5-mm mitral valve vegetation

B. 5-mm tricuspid valve vegetation

C. 11-mm aortic valve vegetation

D. 11-mm mitral valve vegetation

E. 11-mm tricuspid valve vegetation

IV-18. A patient is admitted with fevers, malaise, and diffuse joint pains. His initial blood cultures reveal methicillin-resistant *Staphylococcus aureus* (MRSA) in all culture bottles. He has no arthritis on examination, and his renal function is normal. Echocardiogram shows a 5-mm vegetation on the aortic valve. He is initiated on IV vancomycin at 15 mg/kg every 12 hours. Four days later, the patient remains febrile, and cultures remain positive for MRSA. In addition to a search for embolic foci of infection, which of the following changes would you make to his treatment regimen?

A. No change.

B. Add gentamicin.

C. Add rifampin.

D. Check the vancomycin serum peak and trough levels and consider tid dosing.

E. Discontinue vancomycin, start daptomycin.

IV-19. All of the following organisms may cause bullae as a manifestation of their infection except:

A. *Clostridium perfringens*

B. *Sporothrix schenckii*

C. *Staphylococcus aureus*

D. *Streptococcus pyogenes*

E. *Vibrio vulnificus*

IV-20. A 24-year-old man with no past medical history is brought to the emergency department complaining of left-sided chest pain for 2 days. He reports the skin over his left chest is tender and swollen. He has no history of HIV risk behavior and works as a landscaper. His physical examination is notable for a heart rate of 110 beats/min, blood pressure of 108/62 mmHg, and temperature of 101.8°F. He has pain and swelling of the left chest. His electrocardiogram is normal. A noncontrast CT scan of the chest (Figure IV-20) is obtained. Which of the following organisms is most likely causing his illness?

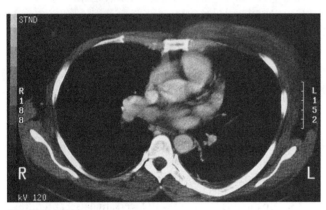

FIGURE IV-20

A. Coxsackie virus A16
B. *Mycobacterium tuberculosis*
C. *Rickettsia akari*
D. *Streptococcus pyogenes*
E. Varicella-zoster virus

IV-21. All of the following statements regarding the etiology and epidemiology of osteomyelitis are true EXCEPT:

A. After a foot puncture, 30% to 40% of patients with diabetes develop osteomyelitis.
B. In patients with prosthetic joints, *Staphylococcus aureus* bacteremia will cause osteomyelitis in 25% to 30% of cases.
C. Mycobacterium tuberculosis is an uncommon cause of osteomyelitis.
D. The foremost bacterial cause of osteomyelitis is *Staphylococcus aureus*.
E. The morbidity and economic consequences of MRSA osteomyelitis are greater than for MSSA osteomyelitis.

IV-22. A 79-year-old man has had a diabetic foot ulcer overlying his third metatarsal head for 3 months but has not been compliant with his physician's request to offload the affected foot. He presents with dull, throbbing foot pain and subjective fevers. Examination reveals a putrid-smelling wound notable also for a pus-filled 2.5-cm-wide ulcer. A metal probe is used to probe the wound, and it detects bone as well as a 3-cm deep cavity. Gram stain of the pus shows gram-positive cocci in chains, gram-positive rods, gram-negative diplococci, enteric-appearing gram-negative rods, tiny pleomorphic gram-negative rods, and a predominance of neutrophils. Which of the following empirical antibiotic regimens is recommended while blood and drainage cultures are processed?

A. Ampicillin–sulbactam, 1.5 g IV q4h
B. Clindamycin, 600 mg PO tid
C. Linezolid, 600 mg IV bid
D. Metronidazole, 500 mg PO qid
E. Vancomycin, 1 g IV bid

IV-23. A 45-year-old man with a history of alcoholism and presumed cirrhosis is brought to the emergency department by his friend complaining of 2 to 3 days of increasing lethargy and confusion. He has not consumed alcohol in the past 2 years. He currently takes no medications and works at home as a video game designer. He has no risk factors for HIV. He was referred by his primary care physician for a liver transplant evaluation and is scheduled to begin his evaluation next month. His vital signs included blood pressure of 90/60 mmHg, heart rate of 105 beats/min, temperature of 38.5°C, and respiratory rate of 10 breaths/min with O$_2$ saturation of 97% on room air. He is somnolent but is able to answer questions accurately. His skin is notable for many spider telangiectasias and palmar erythema. He has a distended diffusely tender abdomen with a positive fluid wave. Paracentesis reveals slightly cloudy fluid with WBC 1000/μL and 40% neutrophils. His blood pressure increases to 100/65 mmHg, and his heart rate decreases to 95 beats/min after 1 L of intravenous fluids. Which of the following statements regarding his condition and treatment is true?

A. Fever is present in more than 50% of cases.
B. Initial empiric therapy should include metronidazole or clindamycin for anaerobes.
C. The diagnosis of primary (spontaneous) bacterial peritonitis is not confirmed because the percentage of neutrophils in the peritoneal fluid is less than 50%.
D. The mostly causative organism for his condition is enterococcus.
E. The yield of peritoneal fluid cultures for diagnosis is greater than 90%.

IV-24. A 48-year-old woman with a history of end-stage renal disease caused by diabetic renal disease is admitted to the hospital with 1 day of abdominal pain and fever. She has been on continuous ambulatory peritoneal dialysis (CAPD) for the past 6 months. She reports that for the past day she has had poor return of dialysate and is feeling bloated. She has had complications from her diabetes, including retinopathy and peripheral neuropathy. She is uncomfortable but not toxic. Her vital signs include a temperature of 38.8°C, blood pressure of 130/65 mmHg, heart rate of 105 beats/min, and respiratory rate of 15 breaths/min with room air O$_2$ saturation of 98%. Her abdomen is slightly distended and diffusely tender with rebound tenderness. A sample of dialysate reveals WBC 400/μL with 80% neutrophils. Empiric intraperitoneal antibiotic therapy should include:

A. Cefoxitin
B. Fluconazole
C. Metronidazole
D. Vancomycin
E. Voriconazole

IV-25. A 77-year-old man presents to the hospital with 1 week of fever, chills, nausea, and right upper quadrant pain. His temperature is 39°C, and he appears toxic. His blood pressure is 110/70 mmHg, heart rate is 110 beats/min, and respiratory rate is 22 breaths/min with room air O₂ saturation 92%. He has diminished breath sounds at the right base and diffuse tenderness in the right upper quadrant. He has a history of cholelithiasis but has declined elective cholecystectomy. His CT scan of the abdomen is shown in Figure IV-25A. Which of the following statements regarding his condition or therapy is true?

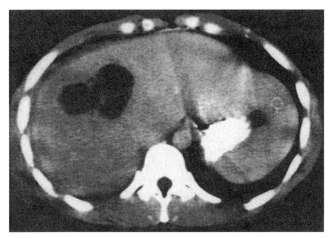

FIGURE IV-25A

A. Concomitant bacteremia is rare (<10%).
B. He should receive empiric antibiotics targeting *Candida* species.
C. He should receive empiric antibiotics targeting anaerobic organisms.
D. He should undergo percutaneous drainage.
E. His serum alkaline phosphatase is most likely normal.

IV-26. A 41-year-old man with hepatitis C–associated ascites presents with acute abdominal pain. Physical examination is notable for temperature of 38.3°C, heart rate of 115 beats/min, blood pressure of 88/48 mmHg, respiratory rate of 16 breaths/min, and oxygen saturation of 99% on room air. The patient is in moderate discomfort and is lying still. He is alert and oriented. His lungs are clear. Cardiac examination is unremarkable. His abdomen is diffusely tender with distant bowel sounds, mild guarding, and no rebound tenderness. Laboratory studies reveal a leukocyte count of 11,630/μL with 94% neutrophils, hematocrit of 29%, and platelet count of 24,000/μL. Paracentesis reveals 658 PMNs/μL, total protein of 1.2 g/dL, and glucose of 24 mg/dL and Gram stain showing gram-negative rods, gram-positive cocci in chains, gram-positive rods, and yeast forms. All of the following are indicated EXCEPT:

A. Abdominal radiograph
B. Broad-spectrum antibiotics
C. Drotrecogin alfa
D. Intravenous fluid
E. Surgical consultation

IV-27. Enteric pathogens can produce diarrheal illness through a variety of mechanisms that lead to specific clinical characteristics. All of the following are characteristics of diarrhea caused by *Vibrio cholerae* EXCEPT:

A. Disease localized to the proximal small intestine
B. Fecal leukocytes
C. Fecal lactoferrin
D. Toxin production
E. Watery diarrhea

IV-28. A 46-year-old woman travels to a rural area of Guatemala. Three days after arrival, she develops watery diarrhea with severe abdominal cramping. She reports two unformed stools daily for the past 2 days. She has noticed no blood in the stool and has not experienced a fever. What is the most likely cause of the patient's illness?

A. *Campylobacter jejuni*
B. Enterotoxigenic *Escherichia coli*
C. *Giardia lamblia*
D. Norovirus
E. *Shigella* spp.

IV-29. For the case above, which of the following treatments would you recommend?

A. Azithromycin 10 mg/kg on day 1 with 5 mg/kg on days 2 and 3 if the diarrhea persists
B. Ciprofloxacin 500 mg three times daily for 5 days
C. Ciprofloxacin 750 mg once
D. Loperamide 4 mg once followed by 2 mg after passage of each unformed stool
E. Oral rehydration therapy only

IV-30. Two hours after attending a company picnic, many individuals who attended the picnic develop an acute gastrointestinal illness. Food poisoning caused by *Staphylococcus aureus* is suspected. All of the following characteristics would be a common feature of food poisoning due to this organism EXCEPT:

A. Abdominal cramping
B. Diarrhea
C. Fever
D. Vomiting

IV-31. You are the on-call physician practicing in a suburban community. You receive a call from a 28-year-old woman with a past medical history significant for sarcoidosis who is currently taking no medications. She is complaining of an acute onset of crampy diffuse abdominal pain and multiple episodes of emesis that are nonbloody. She has not had any lightheadedness with standing or loss of consciousness. When questioned further, the patient states that her last meal was 5 hours previously, when she joined her friends for lunch at a local Chinese restaurant. She ate from the buffet, which included multiple poultry dishes and fried rice. What should you do for this patient?

A. Ask the patient to go to the nearest emergency department for resuscitation with IV fluids.

B. Initiate antibiotic therapy with azithromycin.

C. Reassure the patient that her illness is self-limited and no further treatment is necessary if she can maintain adequate hydration.

D. Refer the patient for CT to assess for appendicitis.

E. Refer the patient for admission for IV vancomycin and ceftriaxone because of her immunocompromised state resulting from sarcoidosis.

IV-32. Which of the following is a common manifestation of *Clostridium difficile* infection?

A. Fever
B. Nonbloody diarrhea
C. Adynamic ileus
D. Recurrence after therapy
E. All of the above

IV-33. All of the following patients should be treated for *Clostridium difficile* infection EXCEPT:

A. A 57-year-old nursing home resident with diarrhea for 2 weeks and pseudomembranes found on colonoscopy with no evidence of toxin A or B in the stool

B. A 63-year-old woman with fever, leukocytosis, adynamic ileus, and a positive PCR for *C. difficile* in the stool

C. A 68-year-old woman with recent course of antibiotics admitted to the medical intensive care unit after presentation to the emergency department with abdominal pain and diarrhea. She was found to have severe abdominal tenderness with absent bowel sounds, systemic hypotension, and colonic wall thickening on CT of the abdomen.

D. A 75-year-old woman who received recent therapy with amoxicillin for an upper respiratory tract infection and now has two loose bowel movements per day for the past 3 days

IV-34. A 78-year-old woman with dementia has been living in a nursing home for 5 years. She was been seen by her primary care provider for evaluation of diarrhea 4 weeks ago. At that time, a stool sample was positive by PCR for *Clostridium difficile*, and she was treated with oral metronidazole with some improvement in her symptoms.

However, she has had five loose bowel movements per day starting 4 days ago and now has abdominal tenderness. Stool PCR remains positive. Which of the following is the most appropriate therapy?

A. Fecal transplantation
B. IV immunoglobulin
C. Oral metronidazole
D. Oral nitazoxanide
E. Oral vancomycin

IV-35. Which of the following antibiotics has the weakest association with the development of *Clostridium difficile*–associated disease?

A. Ceftriaxone
B. Ciprofloxacin
C. Clindamycin
D. Moxifloxacin
E. Piperacillin/tazobactam

IV-36. All of the following are common causes of urethritis in men EXCEPT:

E. *Gardnerella vaginalis*
B. *Mycoplasma genitalium*
C. *Neisseria gonorrhoeae*
D. *Trichomonas vaginalis*
E. *Ureaplasma urealyticum*

IV-37. A 25-year-old woman presents with 2 days of urinary frequency, urgency, and pelvic discomfort. She has no pain in her vulva on urination. She has no other medical problems and does not have fevers. She is sexually active. A microscopic examination of her urine shows pyuria but no pathogens. After 24 hours, her urine culture does not grow any pathogens. Which of the following tests will likely confirm her diagnosis?

A. Cervical culture
B. Clue cells on microscopy of vaginal secretions
C. Nucleic acid amplification test of urine for *C. trachomatis*
D. Physical examination of the vulva and vagina
E. Vaginal pH ≥5.0

IV-38. Which of the following diagnostic features characterizes bacterial vaginosis?

A. Scant vaginal secretions, erythema of vaginal epithelium, and clue cells

B. Vaginal fluid pH >4.5, clue cells, and profuse mixed microbiota on microscopic examination

C. Vaginal fluid pH ≥5.0, motile trichomonads on microscopic exam, and fishy odor with 10% KOH

D. Vaginal fluid pH <4.5, lactobacilli predominate on microscopic examination, and scant clear secretions

E. Vaginal fluid pH <4.5, clue cells, and profuse mixed microbiota on microscopic examination

IV-39. Which of the following is most likely to be identified in a woman seen at a sexually transmitted disease clinic with mucopurulent cervicitis?

A. *Chlamydia trachomatis*
B. Herpes simplex virus
C. *Neisseria gonorrhoeae*
D. *Trichomonas vaginalis*
E. No organism identified

IV-40. A 19-year-old woman is seen in the emergency department for pelvic pain. She reports 1 week of pain but has developed more severe pain on the right side of her lower abdomen over the past day with accompanying fever. Additionally, she reports pain in her right upper abdomen for the past day that is worsened by deep breathing. She is sexually active with multiple partners and only reports a past medical history of asthma. Examination is notable for fever, normal breath sounds, mild tachycardia, and a tender right upper quadrant without rebound, guarding, or masses. Pelvic examination shows a normal cervical appearance, but cervical motion tenderness and adnexal tenderness are present. No masses are palpated. A urine pregnancy test result is negative and leukocytosis is present, but otherwise renal and liver function laboratory study results are normal. Which of the following is true regarding her right upper quadrant tenderness?

A. Acute cholecystitis is likely present; a tech HIDA scan should be ordered to confirm the diagnosis.
B. If a liver biopsy were performed, herpes simplex virus could be cultured from the liver tissue.
C. Laproscopic examination would show inflammation of her liver capsule.
D. Plasma PCR is indicated for diagnosis of acute hepatitis C virus (HCV) infection as the etiology of her hepatitis.
E. CT scan of the chest would confirm the presence of septic pulmonary emboli.

IV-41. A 23-year-old college student is seen in the student health clinic for evaluation of multiple genital ulcers that he noted developing over the past week. They started as pustules and after suppuration are now ulcers. The ulcers are extremely tender and occasionally bleed. Examination shows multiple bilateral deep ulcers with purulent bases that bleed easily. They are exquisitely tender but are soft to palpation. Which of the following organisms are likely to be found on culture of the lesions?

A. *Haemophilus ducreyi*
B. Herpes simplex virus
C. Human immunodeficiency virus
D. *Neisseria gonorrhoeae*
E. *Treponema pallidum*

IV-42. All of the following infections associated with sexual activity correlate with increased acquisition of HIV infection in women EXCEPT:

A. Bacterial vaginosis
B. Chlamydia
C. Gonorrhea
D. Herpes simplex virus-2
E. *Trichomonas vaginalis*
F. All of the above are associated with increased acquisition

IV-43. After leaving which of the following patient's room would the use of alcohol-based hand rub be inadequate?

A. A 54-year-old man with quadriplegia admitted with a urinary tract infection caused by extended-spectrum β-lactamase–producing bacteria
B. A 78-year-old nursing home resident with recent antibiotic use and *Clostridium difficile* infection
C. A 35-year-old woman with advanced HIV and cavitary pulmonary tuberculosis
D. A 20-year-old renal transplant recipient with varicella pneumonia
E. A 40-year-old man with MRSA furunculosis

IV-44. During the first 2 weeks after solid organ transplantation, which family of infection is most common?

A. Cytomegalovirus and Epstein-Barr virus reactivation
B. Humoral immunodeficiency–associated infections (e.g., meningococcemia, invasive *Streptococcus pneumoniae* infection)
C. Neutropenia-associated infection (e.g., aspergillosis, candidemia)
D. T-cell deficiency–associated infections (e.g., *Pneumocystis jiroveci*, nocardiosis, cryptococcosis)
E. Typical hospital-acquired infections (e.g., central line infection, hospital-acquired pneumonia, urinary tract infection)

IV-45. A 22-year-old woman underwent cadaveric renal transplantation 3 months ago for congenital obstructive uropathy. After a demanding college examination schedule during which she forgot to take some of her medications, she is admitted to the hospital with a temperature of 102°F, arthralgias, lymphopenia, and a rise in creatinine from her baseline of 1.2 mg/dL to 2.4 mg/dL. Which of the following medications did she most likely forget?

A. Acyclovir
B. Isoniazid
C. Itraconazole
D. Trimethoprim–sulfamethoxazole
E. Valganciclovir

IV-46. Which of the following pathogens are cardiac transplant patients at unique risk for acquiring from the donor heart early after transplant when compared to other solid organ transplant patients?

A. *Cryptococcus neoformans*
B. Cytomegalovirus
C. *Pneumocystis jiroveci*
D. *Staphylococcus aureus*
E. *Toxoplasma gondii*

IV-47. A 43-year-old woman undergoes allogeneic stem cell transplantation for acute myelogenous leukemia. Two weeks after the date of her transplantation, she is admitted to the hospital with a temperature of 101.1°F, pulse of 115 beats/min, blood pressure of 110/83 mmHg, and oxygen saturation of 89% on room air. Her white blood cell count is 500/μL, and 20% are polymorphonuclear cells. Because of hypoxia and infiltrates on plain chest radiograph, a CT scan is ordered. She is found to have diffuse nodules and masses, some with a halo sign. Which of the following tests is most likely to be diagnostic of her disease?

A. Microscopic examination of buffy coat
B. Plasma CMV viral load
C. Serum galactomannan antigen test
D. Sputum culture
E. Urine Legionella assay

IV-48. Which of the following antibiotics inhibit cell wall synthesis?

A. Ciprofloxacin, metronidazole, and quinupristin/dalfopristin
B. Rifampin, sulfamycin, and clindamycin
C. Tetracycline, daptomycin, and azithromycin
D. Tobramycin, chloramphenicol, and linezolid
E. Vancomycin, bacitracin, and penicillin

IV-49. A 23-year-old college student is admitted to the hospital with a fever and painful, erythematous purulent nodules on his forearm. He is an avid weightlifter and other than depression treated with citalopram has been otherwise healthy. These lesions have been present for approximately 1 week, and his primary care physician attempted to treat him with clindamycin as an outpatient. After admission, he develops hypotension and evidence of systemic inflammatory response syndrome, prompting transfer to the medical intensive care unit. There, dopamine is started, linezolid is administered, and hydrocortisone and fludrocortisone are given for possible adrenal insufficiency in the context of septic shock. After 6 hours, he develops an agitated delirium with diaphoresis, tachycardia, a temperature of 103.4°F, and diarrhea. His examination is notable for tremor; muscular rigidity; hyperreflexia; and clonus, especially in the lower extremities. Which of the following drug–drug interactions is most likely the culprit of this clinical syndrome?

A. Citalopram–dopamine
B. Citalopram–linezolid
C. Dopamine–fludrocortisone
D. Dopamine–linezolid
E. Fludrocortisone–linezolid

IV-50. All of the following statements regarding pneumococcus are true EXCEPT:

A. Asymptomatic colonization does not occur.
B. Infants (younger than 2 years old) and elderly adults are at greatest risk of invasive disease.
C. Pneumococcal vaccination has impacted the epidemiology of disease.
D. The likelihood of death within 24 hours of hospitalization for patients with invasive pneumococcal pneumonia has not changed since the introduction of antibiotics.
E. There is a clear association between prior viral upper respiratory infection and secondary pneumococcal pneumonia.

IV-51. A 75-year-old man who resides at a nursing home is brought to the hospital for altered mental status over 1 day. He has a history of Parkinson's disease and COPD. Staff noticed that he was somnolent and confused on the day of admission. In the emergency department, his temperature is 38.5°C, blood pressure is 95/65 mmHg, heart rate is 105 beats/min, respiratory rate is 24 breaths/min, and room air oxygen saturation is 85%. He has egophony over the right posterior lung field. His chest radiograph is shown in Figure IV-51. All of the statements regarding this patient are true EXCEPT:

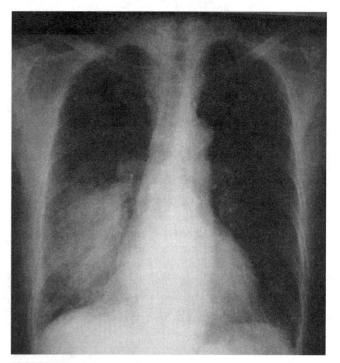

FIGURE IV-51

A. Blood cultures are unlikely (<30%) to be positive.
B. His radiograph demonstrates lobar consolidation.
C. Meningitis is the most common focal complication.
D. Penicillin may be appropriate therapy.
E. Urinary antigen testing could be diagnostic.

IV-52. A 19-year-old college student is brought to the emergency department by friends from his dormitory for confusion and altered mental status. They state that many students have upper respiratory tract infections. He does not use alcohol or illicit drugs. His physical examination is notable for confusion, fever, and a rigid neck. Cerebrospinal fluid (CSF) examination reveals a white blood cell count of 1800 cells/µL with 98% neutrophils, glucose of 1.9 mmol/L (35 mg/dL), and protein of 1.0 g/L (100 mg/dL). Which of the following antibiotic regimens is most appropriate as initial therapy?

A. Ampicillin plus vancomycin
B. Ampicillin plus gentamicin
C. Cefazolin plus doxycycline
D. Cefotaxime plus doxycycline
E. Cefotaxime plus vancomycin

IV-53. In addition to antibiotics, which of the following adjunctive therapies should be administered to improve the chance of a favorable neurologic outcome in the patient in question IV-52?

A. Dexamethasone
B. Dilantin
C. Gabapentin
D. L-Dopa
E. Parenteral nutrition

IV-54. Which of the following biochemical tests distinguishes *S. aureus* from *S. epidermidis*?

A. Catalase
B. Coagulase
C. Lactose fermentation
D. Oxidase
E. Urease

IV-55. A 30-year-old woman with end-stage renal disease who receives her dialysis through a tunneled catheter in her shoulder presents with fever and severe low back pain. On examination, she is uncomfortable and diaphoretic but hemodynamically stable. She has a soft 2/6 early systolic flow murmur. Her line site is red and warm with no pustular exudates. She is very tender over her lower back. Neurologically, she is completely intact. There is no evidence of Janeway lesions, Osler nodes, or Roth spots. Her white count is 16,700/µL with 12% bands. Immediate evaluation should include all of the following EXCEPT:

A. Admission to the hospital
B. MRI of the lumbar spine
C. Removal of her dialysis catheter
D. Transthoracic echocardiogram
E. Two sets of blood cultures followed by empiric therapy with vancomycin plus cefepime

IV-56. A 30-year-old healthy woman presents to the hospital with severe dyspnea, confusion, productive cough, and fevers. She had been ill 1 week earlier with a flulike illness characterized by fever, myalgias, headache, and malaise.

Her illness almost entirely improved without medical intervention until 36 hours ago, when she developed new rigors followed by progression of the respiratory symptoms. On initial examination, her temperature is 39.6°C, pulse is 130 beats/min, blood pressure is 95/60 mmHg, respiratory rate is 40 breaths/min, and oxygen saturation is 88% on 100% face mask. On examination, she is clammy, confused, and very dyspneic. Lung examination reveals amphoric breath sounds over her left lower lung fields. She is intubated and resuscitated with fluid and antibiotics. Chest CT scan reveals necrosis of her left lower lobe. Blood and sputum cultures grow *Staphylococcus aureus*. This isolate is likely to be resistant to which of the following antibiotics?

A. Doxycycline
B. Linezolid
C. Methicillin
D. Trimethoprim–sulfamethoxazole (TMP/SMX)
E. Vancomycin

IV-57. In the patient described above, all of the following may be efficacious therapy EXCEPT:

A. Daptomycin
B. Linezolid
C. Quinupristin/dalfopristin
D. Telavancin
E. Vancomycin

IV-58. Which of the following organisms is most likely to cause infection of a shunt implanted for the treatment of hydrocephalus?

A. *Bacteroides fragilis*
B. *Corynebacterium diphtheriae*
C. *Escherichia coli*
D. *Staphylococcus aureus*
E. *Staphylococcus epidermidis*

IV-59. A 42-year-old man with poorly controlled diabetes (HbA1c, 13.3%) presents with thigh pain and fever over several weeks. Physical examination reveals erythema and warmth over the thigh with notable woody, nonpitting edema. There are no cutaneous ulcers. CT of the thigh reveals several abscesses located between the muscle fibers of the thigh. Orthopedics is consulted to drain and culture the abscesses. Which of the following is the most likely pathogen?

A. *Clostridium perfringens*
B. Group A streptococcus
C. Polymicrobial flora
D. *Staphylococcus aureus*
E. *Streptococcus milleri*

IV-60. A 19-year-old woman from Guatemala presents to your office for a routine screening physical examination. At age 4 years, she was diagnosed with acute rheumatic fever. She does not recall the specifics of her illness and remembers only that she was required to be on bed rest for 6 months. She has remained on penicillin V orally at a dose of 250 mg bid since that time. She asks if she can safely discontinue this medication. She has had only one other flare of her disease, at age 8 years, when she stopped taking penicillin at the time of her emigration to the United States. She is currently working as a day care provider. Her physical examination is notable for normal point of maximal impulse (PMI) with a grade III/VI holosystolic murmur that is heard best at the apex of the heart and radiates to the axilla. What do you advise the patient to do?

A. An echocardiogram should be performed to determine the extent of valvular damage before deciding if penicillin can be discontinued.
B. Penicillin prophylaxis can be discontinued because she has had no flares in 5 years.
C. She should change her dosing regimen to IM benzathine penicillin every 8 weeks.
D. She should continue on penicillin indefinitely because she had a previous recurrence, has presumed rheumatic heart disease, and is working in a field with high occupational exposure to group A streptococcus.
E. She should replace penicillin prophylaxis with polyvalent pneumococcal vaccine every 5 years.

IV-61. A 36-year-old man is brought to the hospital by his wife because of a rapidly worsening skin infection. The patient has a history of type 1 diabetes, and his last documented HbA1c was 5.5%. His wife reports that he had a small insect bite on his calf a few days ago with some redness. Over the course of today, he has developed severe thigh pain initially with no redness, but over the past hour, he has had worsening pain and swelling with some mottling of the skin. He also reports that he feels like his thigh and calf are numb. He is febrile and tachycardic. Physical examination reveals marked tenderness and tenseness of the right leg from the thigh down. There is some redness and mottling. A femoral and posterior tibial pulse are present. CT scan of the leg shows extensive inflammation of the fascial planes but no evidence of muscle inflammation. Which of the following organisms is most likely responsible for his infection?

A. *Clostridium difficile*
B. *Staphylococcus aureus*
C. *Staphylococcus epidermidis*
D. *Streptococcus pneumonia*
E. *Streptococcus pyogenes*

IV-62. A 24-year-old woman is brought to the hospital by her husband with fever and severe abdominal pain. She lives in rural Pennsylvania and home delivered a child 2 days ago. She did not receive routine prenatal care. Her labor was difficult with delivery over 18 hours after membrane rupture. Her baby has been feeding well over the past 48 hours and has had no fever. The patient noticed she had low-grade fever 24 hours after birth, and her abdominal pain has developed over the past 12 hours. She is febrile to 39°C and is tachycardic. Abdominal examination is notable for marked tenderness in the lower abdomen. A pelvic examination shows a purulent material emanating from her cervix with marked adnexal tenderness. A Gram stain shows extensive neutrophils and gram-positive cocci in chains. Which of the following organisms is the most likely cause of her disease?

A. *Chlamydia trachomatis*
B. *Gardnerella vaginalis*
C. *Neisseria gonorrhea*
D. *Streptococcus agalactiae*
E. *Trichomonas vaginalis*

IV-63. All of the following statements regarding enterococci are true EXCEPT:

A. Enterococci are the second most common cause of hospital-acquired infections.
B. Infection with vancomycin-resistant strains of enterococci (VRE) does not increase the patient's risk of death compared with infection with vancomycin-sensitive strains of enterococci.
C. Patients with GI colonization by VRE are more likely to develop bacteremia than patients with GI colonization by vancomycin-sensitive strains of enterococci.
D. Physical proximity to a room colonized with VRE is a risk factor for patients developing gut colonization with VRE.
E. Strains of *E. faecium* are more likely to be resistant to vancomycin than strains of *E. faecalis*.

IV-64. A 74-year-old man with a recent history of diverticulitis is admitted to the hospital with 1 week of fever, malaise, and generalized weakness. His physical examination is notable for a temperature of 38.5°C, a new mitral heart murmur, and splinter hemorrhages. Three blood cultures grow *Enterococcus faecalis*, and an echocardiogram shows a small vegetation on the mitral valve. The organism is reported as being sensitive to ampicillin with no high-level resistance to aminoglycosides. Based on this information, which of the following is recommended therapy?

A. Ampicillin
B. Ampicillin plus gentamicin
C. Daptomycin
D. Linezolid
E. Tigecycline

IV-65. Which of the following drugs is bactericidal and approved by the FDA for some infections caused by vancomycin-resistant *E. faecium*?

A. Ceftriaxone
B. Cefoxitin
C. Linezolid
D. Quinupristin/dalfopristin
E. Vancomycin

IV-66. A 42-year-old man with HIV has been developing worsening disease because of HAART resistance and worsening viremia. Over the past 6 months, his CD4 T-cell count has fallen below 100/μL. He has not been compliant with prophylactic medication because he is tired of taking pills. He comes to clinic reporting 3 weeks of productive cough and low-grade fever. A chest radiograph shows multiple small necrotizing nodules in the bilateral lower lobes. A percutaneous needle biopsy reveals some neutrophils and small gram-positive coccobacilli that the laboratory says looks like corynebacterium. A culture grows *Rhodococcus equi*. All of the following are effective therapy EXCEPT:

A. Azithromycin
B. Cefotaxime
C. Linezolid
D. Tigecycline
E. Vancomycin

IV-67. An 87-year-old nursing home resident is brought by ambulance to a local emergency department. He is obtunded and ill-appearing. Per nursing home staff, the patient has experienced low-grade temperatures, poor appetite, and lethargy over several days. A lumbar puncture is performed, and the Gram stain returns gram-positive rods and many white blood cells. *Listeria* meningitis is diagnosed and appropriate antibiotics are begun. Which of the following statements regarding *Listeria* meningitis distinguishes it from other causes of bacterial meningitis?

A. There is more frequent nuchal rigidity.
B. More neutrophils are present on the cerebrospinal fluid (CSF) differential.
C. Photophobia is more common.
D. Presentation is often more subacute.
E. White blood cell (WBC) count is often more elevated in the CSF.

IV-68. Several family members present to a local emergency department 2 days after a large family summer picnic at which deli meats and salads were served. They all complain of profuse diarrhea, headaches, fevers, and myalgias. Their symptoms began about 24 hours after the picnic. It appears that everyone who ate Uncle Sandy's Salami Surprise was affected. Routine cultures of blood and stool are negative to date. Which of the following is true regarding *Listeria* gastroenteritis?

A. Antibiotic treatment is not necessary for uncomplicated cases.
B. Carriers are asymptomatic but can easily spread infection via the fecal–oral route.
C. Gastrointestinal illness can result from ingestion of a single organism.
D. Illness is toxin mediated, and organisms are not present at the time of infection.
E. Person-to-person spread is a common cause of outbreaks.

IV-69. A 26-year-old woman presents late in the third trimester of her pregnancy with high fevers, myalgias, backache, and malaise. She is admitted and started on empirical broad-spectrum antibiotics. Blood cultures return positive for *Listeria monocytogenes*. She delivers a 5-lb infant 24 hours after admission. Which of the following statements regarding antibiotic treatment for this infection is true?

A. Clindamycin should be used in patients with penicillin allergy.
B. Neonates should receive weight-based ampicillin and gentamicin.
C. Penicillin plus gentamicin is first-line therapy for the mother.
D. Quinolones should be used for *Listeria* bacteremia in late-stage pregnancy.
E. Trimethoprim–sulfamethoxazole has no efficacy against *Listeria* spp.

IV-70. A 64-year-old man with a long history of heroin abuse is brought to the hospital because of fever and worsening muscle spasms and pain over the past day. Because of long-standing venous sclerosis, he no longer injects intravenously but "skin pops," often with dirty needles. On examination, he is extremely sweaty and febrile to 101.4°F. There are widespread muscle spasms, including the face. He is unable to open his jaw because of muscle spasm and has severe back pain because of diffuse spasm. On his leg, there is a skin wound that is tender and erythematous. All of the following statements regarding this patient are true EXCEPT:

A. Culture of the wound may reveal *Clostridium tetani*.
B. Intrathecal antitoxin administration is recommended therapy.
C. Metronidazole is the recommended therapy.
D. Permanent muscle dysfunction is likely after recovery.
E. Strychnine poisoning and antidopaminergic drug toxicity should be ruled out.

IV-71. A 34-year-old injection drug user presents with a 2-day history of slurred speech, blurry vision that is worse with bilateral gaze deviation, dry mouth, and difficulty swallowing both liquids and solids. He states that his arms feel weak as well but denies any sensory deficits. He has had no recent illness but does describe a chronic ulcer on his left lower leg that has felt slightly warm and tender of late. He frequently injects heroin into the edges of the ulcer. On review of systems, he reports mild shortness of breath but denies any gastrointestinal symptoms, urinary retention, or loss of bowel or bladder continence. Physical examination reveals a frustrated, nontoxic appearing man who is alert and oriented but noticeably dysarthric. He is afebrile with stable vital signs. Cranial nerve examination reveals bilateral cranial nerve VI deficits and an inability to maintain medial gaze in both eyes. He has mild bilateral ptosis, and both pupils are reactive but sluggish. His strength is 5/5 in all extremities except for his shoulder shrug, which is 4/5. Sensory examination and deep tendon reflexes are within normal limits in all four extremities. His oropharynx is dry. Cardiopulmonary and abdominal examination findings are normal. He has a 4 cm × 5 cm well-granulated lower extremity ulcer with redness, warmth, and erythema noted on the upper margin of the ulcer. What is the treatment of choice?

A. Glucocorticoids
B. Equine antitoxin to *Clostridium botulinum* neurotoxin
C. Intravenous heparin
D. Naltrexone
E. Plasmapheresis

IV-72. A 19-year-old man presents to the emergency department with 4 days of watery diarrhea, nausea, vomiting, and low-grade fever. He recalls no unusual meals, sick contacts, or travel. He is hydrated with IV fluid, given antiemetics, and discharged home after feeling much better. Three days later, two of three blood cultures are positive for *Clostridium perfringens*. He is called at home and says that he feels fine and is back at work. What should your next instruction to the patient be?

A. Return for IV penicillin therapy.
B. Return for IV penicillin therapy plus echocardiography.
C. Return for IV penicillin therapy plus colonoscopy.
D. Return for surveillance blood culture.
E. Reassurance

IV-73. Which of the following is the most common clinical manifestation of *Neisseria meningitidis* infection?

A. Asymptomatic nasopharyngeal colonization
B. Chronic meningitis
C. Meningitis
D. Petechial or purpuric rash
E. Septicemia

IV-74. A 21-year-old college student is admitted to the hospital with meningitis. CSF cultures reveal *N. meningitides* type B. The patient lives in a dormitory suite with five other students. Which of the following is recommended for the close household contacts?

A. Culture all close contacts and offer prophylaxis to those with positive culture results
B. Immediate administration of ceftriaxone to all close contacts
C. Immediate administration of rifampin to all close contacts
D. Immediate vaccination with conjugate vaccine
E. No therapy necessary

IV-75. A 19-year-old man comes to clinic complaining of 2 days of severe dysuria and urethral discharge. Urine analysis shows pyuria. He reports unprotected sexual contact with a new partner within the past week. DNA probe is positive for *N. gonorrhea*. Which of the following is the most effective therapy?

A. Intravenous ceftriaxone
B. Intramuscular penicillin
C. Oral azithromycin
D. Oral cefixime
E. Oral levofloxacin

IV-76. A 44-year-old man presents to the emergency department for evaluation of a severe sore throat. His symptoms began this morning with mild irritation on swallowing and have gotten progressively severe over the course of 12 hours. He has been experiencing a fever to as high as 39°C at home and reports progressive shortness of breath. He denies antecedent rhinorrhea and tooth and jaw pain. He has had no ill contacts. On physical examination, the patient appears flushed and in respiratory distress with use of accessory muscles of respiration. Inspiratory stridor is present. He is sitting leaning forward and is drooling with his neck extended. His vital signs are as follows: temperature of 39.5°C, blood pressure of 116/60 mmHg, heart rate of 118 beats/min, respiratory rate of 24 breaths/min, and oxygen saturation of 95% on room air. Examination of his oropharynx shows erythema of the posterior oropharynx without exudates or tonsillar enlargement. The uvula is midline. There is no sinus tenderness and no cervical lymphadenopathy. His lung fields are clear to auscultation, and cardiovascular examination reveals a regular tachycardia with a II/VI systolic ejection murmur heard at the upper right sternal border. Abdominal, extremity, and neurologic examinations are normal. Laboratory studies reveal a white blood cell count of 17,000/μL with a differential of 87% neutrophils, 8% band forms, 4% lymphocytes, and 1% monocytes. Hemoglobin is 13.4 g/dL with a hematocrit of 44.2%. An arterial blood gas on room air has a pH of 7.32, a PCO_2 of 48 mmHg, and a PO_2 of 92 mmHg. A lateral neck radiograph shows an edematous epiglottis. What is the next most appropriate step in evaluation and treatment of this individual?

A. Ampicillin, 500 mg IV q6h
B. Ceftriaxone, 1 g IV q24h
C. Endotracheal intubation and ampicillin, 500 mg IV q6h
D. Endotracheal intubation, 1 g IV q24h of ceftriaxone, and 600 mg IV q6h of clindamycin
E. Laryngoscopy and close observation

IV-77. All of the following statements regarding *Moraxella catarrhalis* as an upper respiratory pathogen are true EXCEPT:

A. Clinical features allow distinction between COPD exacerbations caused by *M. catarrhalis* and *H. influenzae*.
B. It causes otitis media in children.
C. It is the second most common bacterial cause of COPD exacerbations.
D. Most strains are susceptible to azithromycin.
E. Most strains express β-lactamase activity.

IV-78. A 75-year-old patient presents with fevers and wasting. He describes fatigue and malaise over the past several months and is concerned that he has been losing weight. On examination, he is noted to have a low-grade fever, and a soft diastolic heart murmur is appreciated. Laboratory tests reveal a normocytic, normochromic anemia. Three separate blood cultures grow *Cardiobacterium hominis*. Which of the following statements is true about this patient's clinical condition?

A. Antibiotics are not likely to improve his condition.
B. Echocardiography findings will likely be normal.
C. He has a form of endocarditis with a high risk of emboli.
D. He will likely need surgery.
E. The positive blood culture results are likely because of a skin contaminant.

IV-79. A 38-year-old woman with frequent hospital admissions related to alcoholism comes to the emergency department after being bitten by a dog. There are open wounds on her arms and right hand that are purulent and have necrotic borders. She is hypotensive and is admitted to the intensive care unit. She is found to have disseminated intravascular coagulation and soon develops multiorgan failure. Which of the following is the most likely organism to have caused her rapid decline?

A. *Aeromonas* spp.
B. *Capnocytophaga* spp.
C. *Eikenella* spp.
D. *Haemophilus* spp.
E. *Staphylococcus* spp.

IV-80. A 56-year-old man with a history of hypertension and cigarette smoking is admitted to the intensive care unit after 1 week of fever and nonproductive cough. Imaging shows a new pulmonary infiltrate, and urine antigen test result for *Legionella* is positive. Each of the following is likely to be an effective antibiotic EXCEPT:

A. Azithromycin
B. Aztreonam
C. Levofloxacin
D. Tigecycline
E. Trimethoprim/sulfamethoxazole

IV-81. All of the following are risk factors for the development of *Legionella* pneumonia EXCEPT:

A. Glucocorticoid use
B. HIV infection
C. Neutropenia
D. Recent surgery
E. Tobacco use

IV-82. A 72-year-old woman is admitted to the intensive care unit with respiratory failure. She has fever, obtundation, and bilateral parenchymal consolidation on chest imaging. Which of the following is true regarding the diagnosis of *Legionella* pneumonia?

A. Acute and convalescent antibodies are not helpful because of the presence of multiple serotypes.
B. *Legionella* can never be seen on a Gram stain.
C. *Legionella* cultures grow rapidly on the proper media.
D. *Legionella* urinary antigen maintains utility after antibiotic use.
E. Polymerase chain reaction for *Legionella* DNA is the "gold standard" diagnostic test.

IV-83. An 18-year-old man seeks attention for a severe cough. He reports no past medical history and excellent health. Approximately 7 days ago, he developed an upper respiratory syndrome with low-grade fever, coryza, some cough, and malaise. The fever and coryza has improved, but over the past 2 days, he has had an episodic cough that often is severe enough to result in vomiting. He reports receiving all infant vaccinations but only tetanus in the past 12 years. He is afebrile, and while not coughing, his chest examination is normal. During a coughing episode, there is an occasional inspiratory whoop. Chest radiography findings are unremarkable. Which of the following is true regarding his likely illness?

A. A fluoroquinolone is recommended therapy.
B. Cold agglutinin results may be positive.
C. Nasopharyngeal aspirate for DNA testing is likely to be diagnostic.
D. Pneumonia is a common complication.
E. Urinary antigen testing results remain positive for up to 3 months.

IV-84. Which of the following is the most common cause of traveler's diarrhea in Latin America?

A. *Campylobacter jejuni*
B. *Entamoeba histolytica*
C. Enterotoxigenic *Escherichia coli*
D. *Giardia lamblia*
E. *Vibrio cholerae*

IV-85. In the inpatient setting, extended-spectrum β-lactamase (ESBL)–producing gram-negative infections are most likely to occur after frequent use of which of the following classes of antibiotics?

A. Carbapenems
B. Macrolides
C. Quinolones
D. Third-generation cephalosporins

IV-86. A 25-year-old woman presents to the clinic complaining of several days of worsening burning and pain with urination. She describes an increase in urinary frequency and suprapubic tenderness but no fever or back pain. She has no past medical history with the exception of two prior episodes similar to this in the past 2 years. Urinalysis shows moderate white blood cells. Which of the following is the most likely causative agent of her current symptoms?

A. *Candida* spp.
B. *Escherichia coli*
C. *Enterobacter* spp.
D. *Klebsiella* spp.
E. *Proteus* spp.

IV-87. All of the following statements regarding intestinal disease caused by strains of Shiga toxin–producing and enterohemorrhagic *E. coli* are true EXCEPT:

A. Antibiotic therapy lessens the risk of developing hemolytic uremic syndrome.
B. Ground beef is the most common source of contamination.
C. Gross bloody diarrhea without fever is the most common clinical manifestation.
D. Infection is more common in industrialized than developing countries.
E. O157:H7 is the most common serotype.

IV-88. A 63-year-old man has been in the ICU for 3 weeks with slowly resolving ARDS after an episode of acute pancreatitis. He remains on mechanical ventilation through a tracheostomy. Over the past week, he has had gradual lessening of his mechanical ventilator needs and slight improvement of his radiograph. He has been afebrile with a normal WBC for the past 10 days. Over the past 24 hours, his FiO_2 has been increased from 0.60 to 0.80 to maintain adequate oxygenation. In addition, he has developed newly purulent sputum with a right lower lobe infiltrate, fever to 101.5°C, and a rising WBC. Sputum gram stain shows gram-negative plump coccobacilli that are identified as *Acinetobacter baumannii*. All of the following are true about this organism EXCEPT:

A. Mortality from bloodstream infection approaches 40%.
B. Multidrug resistance is characteristic.
C. They are a growing cause of hospital-acquired pneumonia and bloodstream infections in the United States.
D. They are not yet a significant problem in Asia or Australia.
E. Tigecycline is treatment of choice for bloodstream infection.

IV-89. *Helicobacter pylori* colonization increases the odds ratio of developing all of the following conditions EXCEPT:

A. Duodenal ulcer disease
B. Esophageal adenocarcinoma
C. Gastric adenocarcinoma
D. Gastric mucosa-associated lymphoid tissue (MALT) lymphoma
E. Peptic ulcer disease

IV-90. One month after receiving a 14-day course of omeprazole, clarithromycin, and amoxicillin for *Helicobacter pylori*–associated gastric ulcer disease, a 44-year-old woman still has mild dyspepsia and pain after meals. What is the appropriate next step in management?

A. Empirical long-term proton pump inhibitor therapy
B. Endoscopy with biopsy to rule out gastric adenocarcinoma
C. *H. pylori* serology testing
D. Second-line therapy for *H. pylori* with omeprazole, bismuth subsalicylate, tetracycline, and metronidazole
E. Urea breath test

IV-91. In the developed world, seroprevalence of *Helicobacter pylori* infection is currently

A. Decreasing
B. Increasing
C. Staying the same
D. Unknown

IV-92. A 42-year-old man with heme-positive stools and a history of epigastric pain is found to have a duodenal ulcer that is biopsy-proven positive for *H. pylori*. All of the following are effective eradication regimens EXCEPT:

A. Amoxicillin and levofloxacin for 10 days
B. Omeprazole, clarithromycin, and metronidazole for 14 days
C. Omeprazole, clarithromycin, and amoxicillin for 14 days
D. Omeprazole, bismuth, tetracycline, and metronidazole for 14 days
E. Omeprazole and amoxicillin for 5 days followed by omeprazole, clarithromycin, and tinidazole for 5 days

IV-93. A sputum culture from a patient with cystic fibrosis showing which of the following organisms has been associated with a rapid decline in pulmonary function and a poor clinical prognosis?

A. *Burkholderia cepacia*
B. *Pseudomonas aeruginosa*
C. *Staphylococcus aureus*
D. *Staphylococcus epidermidis*
E. *Stenotrophomonas maltophilia*

IV-94. Which single clinical feature has the most specificity in differentiating *Pseudomonas aeruginosa* sepsis from other causes of severe sepsis in a hospitalized patient?

A. Ecthyma gangrenosum
B. Hospitalization for severe burn
C. Profound bandemia
D. Recent antibiotic exposure
E. Recent mechanical ventilation for >14 days

IV-95. All of the following agents may be effective when used as monotherapy in a nonneutropenic patient with *Pseudomonas aeruginosa* bacteremia EXCEPT:

A. Amikacin
B. Cefepime
C. Ceftazidime
D. Meropenem
E. Piperacillin/tazobactam

IV-96. Five healthy college roommates develop a rapid (<8 hours) onset of abdominal pain, cramping, fever to 38.5°C, vomiting, and copious nonbloody diarrhea while camping. They immediately return for hydration and diagnosis. A stool culture grows *Salmonella enteritidis*. All of the statements regarding their clinical syndrome are true EXCEPT:

A. Antibiotic therapy is not indicated.
B. Bacteremia occurs in fewer than 10% of cases.
C. The most likely source was undercooked eggs.
D. There is no vaccine available for this illness.
E. They have enteric (typhoid) fever.

IV-97. Two days after returning from a trip to Thailand, a 36-year-old woman develops severe crampy abdominal pain, fever to 40°C, nausea, and malaise. The next day, she begins having bloody mucopurulent diarrhea with worsening abdominal pain and continued fever. She reports she was in Bangkok during monsoonal flooding and ate fresh food from stalls. A stool examination shows many neutrophils, and culture grows *Shigella flexneri*. Which of the following statements regarding her clinical syndrome is true?

A. An effective vaccine for travelers is available.
B. Antibiotic therapy prolongs the carrier state and should not be administered unless she develops bacteremia.
C. Antimotility agents are effective in reducing the risk of dehydration.
D. Ciprofloxacin is recommended therapy.
E. Her disease can be distinguished from illness caused by *Campylobacter jejuni* on clinical grounds by the presence of fever.

IV-98. A previously healthy 32-year-old graduate student at the University of Wisconsin describes 1 to 2 days of fever, myalgia, and headache followed by abdominal pain and diarrhea. He has experienced up to 10 bowel movements over the past day. He has noted mucus and blood in the stool. The patient notes that 3 days ago, he was at a church barbecue, where several people contracted a diarrheal illness. He has not traveled in more than 6 months and has no history of GI illness. Physical examination is unremarkable except for a temperature of 38.8°C and diffuse abdominal tenderness. Laboratory findings are notable only for a slightly elevated leukocyte count and an elevated erythrocyte sedimentation rate. Wright's stain of a fecal sample reveals the presence of neutrophils. Colonoscopy reveals inflamed mucosa. Biopsy of an affected area discloses mucosal infiltration with neutrophils, monocytes, and eosinophils; epithelial damage, including loss of mucus; glandular degeneration; and crypt abscesses. Which of the following microbial pathogens is most likely to be responsible for his illness?

A. *Campylobacter*
B. *Escherichia coli*
C. Norwalk agent
D. Rotavirus
E. *Staphylococcus aureus*

IV-99. In the patient described in question IV-98, which of the following is recommended therapy?

A. Azithromycin
B. Ceftriaxone
C. Lomotil only for symptoms
D. Metronidazole
E. Tinidazole

IV-100. While working for a relief mission in Haiti, you are asked to see a 19-year-old patient with profuse watery diarrhea as shown in Figure IV-100. The patient is mildly hypotensive and tachycardic and is afebrile. There is no abdominal tenderness. All of the statements regarding this patient's illness are true EXCEPT:

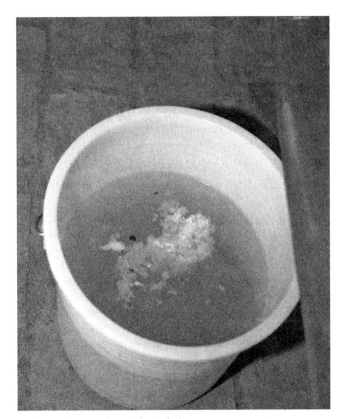

FIGURE IV-100 (see Color Atlas)

A. Antibiotic therapy shortens the duration of disease and hastens clearance of the organism from stool.
B. Morbidity or death is mediated by bacteremia and multiorgan failure.
C. Point of care antigen testing is available.
D. The diarrhea is toxin mediated.
E. Vaccines with moderate efficacy are available outside the United States.

IV-101. A 45-year-old man from western Kentucky presents to the emergency department in September complaining of fevers, headaches, and muscle pains. He recently had been on a camping trip with several friends during which they hunted for their food, including fish, squirrels, and rabbits. He did not recall any tick bites during the trip but does recall having several mosquito bites. For the past week, he has had an ulceration on his right hand with redness and pain surrounding it. He also has noticed some pain and swelling near his right elbow. None of the friends he camped with have been similarly ill. His vital signs are blood pressure of 106/65 mmHg, heart rate of 116 beats/min, respiratory rate of 24 breaths/min, and temperature of 38.7°C. His oxygen saturation is 93% on room air. He appears mildly tachypneic and flushed. His conjunctiva are not injected, and his mucous membranes are dry. The chest examination reveals crackles in the right mid-lung field and left base. His heart rate is tachycardic but regular. There is a II/VI systolic ejection murmur heard best at the lower left sternal border. His abdominal examination is unremarkable. On the right hand, there is an erythematous ulcer with a punched-out center covered by a black eschar. He has no cervical lymphadenopathy, but there are markedly enlarged and tender lymph nodes in the right axillae and epitrochlear regions. The epitrochlear node has some fluctuance with palpation. A chest radiograph shows fluffy bilateral alveolar infiltrates. Over the first 12 hours of his hospitalization, the patient becomes progressively hypotensive and hypoxic, requiring intubation and mechanical ventilation. What is the most appropriate therapy for this patient?

A. Ampicillin, 2 g IV q6h
B. Ceftriaxone, 1 g IV daily
C. Ciprofloxacin, 400 mg IV twice daily
D. Doxycycline, 100 mg IV twice daily
E. Gentamicin, 5 mg/kg twice daily

IV-102. A 35-year-old man comes to the emergency department complaining of an acute-onset high fever, malaise, and a tender lymph node. The patient returned from a camping trip in the Four Corners region of the United States (junction area of New Mexico, Arizona, Colorado, and Utah) 4 days ago and reports being bitten by fleas. He has no past medical history and works as a university professor. He denies illicit drug use. On physical examination, he is lethargic but oriented and has a temperature 39.4°C, heart rate of 105 beats/min, and blood pressure of 100/65 mmHg. There are numerous crusted flea bites on the upper legs. In the right inguinal region, there is an exquisitely tender 3- to 4-cm tense lymph node with surrounding edema but no lymphangitis. An aspirate of the node reveals small gram-negative coccobacilli that appear bipolar on Wright's stain. Which of the following is the most likely causative organism?

A. *Bartonella henselae*
B. Epstein-Barr virus
C. *Rickettsia rickettsia*
D. *Staphylococcus aureus*
E. *Yersinia pestis*

IV-103. In the patient in question IV-102, which of the following therapeutic options is recommended?

A. Azithromycin
B. Gentamicin
C. No therapy; it is a self-limited disease
D. Vancomycin
E. Voriconazole

IV-104. A 24-year-old man with advanced HIV infection presents to the emergency department with a tan painless nodule on the lower extremity (see Figure IV-104). He is afebrile and has no other lesions. He does not take antiretroviral therapy, and his last CD4+ T-cell count was 20/μL. He lives with a friend who has cats and kittens. A biopsy shows lobular proliferation of blood vessels lined by enlarged endothelial cells and a mixed acute and chronic inflammatory infiltrate. Tissue stains show gram-negative bacilli. Which of the following is most likely to be effective therapy for the lesion?

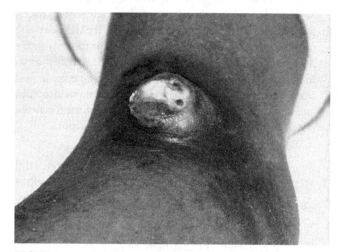

FIGURE IV-104 (see Color Atlas)

A. Azithromycin
B. Cefazolin
C. Interferon-α
D. Penicillin
E. Vancomycin

IV-105. A 38-year-old homeless man presents to the emergency department with a transient ischemic attack characterized by a facial droop and left arm weakness lasting 20 minutes and left upper quadrant pain. He reports intermittent subjective fevers, diaphoresis, and chills for the past 2 weeks. He has had no recent travel or contact with animals. He has taken no recent antibiotics. Physical examination reveals a slightly distressed man with disheveled appearance. His temperature is 38.2°C, heart rate is 90 beats/min, and blood pressure is 127/74 mmHg. He has poor dentition. Cardiac examination reveals an early diastolic murmur over the left third intercostal space. His spleen is tender and 2 cm descended below the costal margin. He has tender painful red nodules on the tips of the third finger of his right hand and on the fourth finger of his left hand that are new. He has nits evident on his clothes consistent with body louse infection. White blood cell count is 14,500/μL, with 5% band forms and 93% polymorphonuclear cells. Blood cultures are drawn followed by empirical vancomycin therapy. These culture results remain negative for growth 5 days later. He remains febrile but hemodynamically stable but does develop a new lesion on his toe similar to those on his fingers on hospital day 3. A transthoracic echocardiogram reveals a 1-cm mobile vegetation on the cusp of his aortic valve and moderate aortic regurgitation. A CT scan of the abdomen shows an enlarged spleen with wedge-shaped splenic and renal infarctions. What test should be sent to confirm the most likely diagnosis?

A. *Bartonella* serology
B. Epstein-Barr virus heterophile antibody
C. HIV polymerase chain reaction
D. Peripheral blood smear
E. Q fever serology

IV-106. A 26-year-old female college student presents with tender epitrochlear and axillary tender, firm, 3-cm lymph nodes on her left side. She has a 0.5-cm painless nodule on her left second finger. She reports low-grade fever and malaise over 2 weeks. She enjoys gardening and exotic fish collecting and owns several pets, including fish, kittens, and a puppy. She is sexually active with one partner. She traveled extensively throughout rural Southeast Asia 2 years before her current illness. The differential diagnosis includes all of the following EXCEPT:

A. *Bartonella henselae* infection
B. Lymphoma
C. *Sporothrix schenckii* infection
D. Staphylococcal infection

IV-107. A 24-year-old man seeks evaluation for painless penile ulcerations. He noted the first lesion about 2 weeks ago, and since that time, two adjacent areas have also developed ulceration. He states that there has been blood staining his underwear from slight oozing of the ulcers. He has no past medical history and takes no medication. He returned 5 weeks ago from a vacation in Brazil, where he did have unprotected sexual intercourse with a local woman. He denies other high-risk sexual behaviors and has never had sex with prostitutes. He was last tested for HIV 2 years ago. He has never had a chlamydial or gonococcal infection. On examination, there are three well-defined red, friable lesions measuring 5 mm or less on the penile shaft. They bleed easily with any manipulation. There is no pain with palpation. There is shotty inguinal lymphadenopathy. On biopsy of one lesion, there is a prominent intracytoplasmic inclusion of bipolar organisms in an enlarged mononuclear cell. Additionally, there

is epithelial cell proliferation with an increased number of plasma cells and few neutrophils. A rapid plasma reagin test result is negative. Cultures grow no organisms. What is the most likely causative organism?

A. *Calymmatobacterium granulomatis* (donovanosis)
B. *Chlamydia trachomatis* (lymphogranuloma venereum)
C. *Haemophilus ducreyi* (chancroid)
D. *Leishmania amazonensis* (cutaneous leishmaniasis)
E. *Treponema pallidum* (secondary syphilis)

IV-108. A 35-year-old man is seen 6 months after a cadaveric renal allograft. The patient has been on azathioprine and prednisone since that procedure. He has felt poorly for the past week with fever to 38.6°C (101.5°F), anorexia, and a cough productive of thick sputum. Chest radiography reveals a left lower lobe (5-cm) mass with central cavitation. Examination of the sputum reveals long, crooked, branching, beaded gram-positive filaments. The most appropriate initial therapy would include the administration of which of the following antibiotics?

A. Ceftazidime
B. Erythromycin
C. Penicillin
D. Sulfisoxazole
E. Tobramycin

IV-109. A 67-year-old woman with a history of systemic hypertension presents to her local emergency department with 2 weeks of right jaw pain that now has developed an area of purulent drainage into her mouth. She reports an accompanying fever. She denies recent dental work. Aside from osteoporosis, she is healthy. Her only medications are alendronate and lisinopril. Physical examination is notable for a temperature of 101.1°F, right-sided facial swelling, diffuse mandibular tenderness, and an area of yellow purulent drainage through the buccal mucosa on the right side. Microscopic examination of the purulent secretions is likely to show which of the following?

A. Auer rods
B. Sialolith
C. Squamous cell carcinoma
D. Sulfur granules
E. Weakly acid-fast branching, beaded filaments

IV-110. In the patient described above, what is the most appropriate therapy?

A. Amphotericin B
B. Itraconazole
C. Penicillin
D. Surgical debridement
E. Tobramycin

IV-111. A 68-year-old homeless man with a long history of alcohol abuse presents to his primary care physician with several weeks of fever, night sweats, and sputum production. He denies nausea, vomiting, and other gastrointestinal symptoms. Examination is notable for a low-grade temperature, weight loss of 15 lb since the previous visit, and foul breath but is otherwise normal. Blood work, including complete blood count and serum chemistries, is unremarkable. A PPD is placed, and the result is negative. His chest radiograph is shown in Figure IV-111. Which of the following is appropriate as initial therapy?

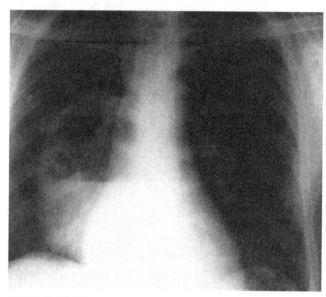

FIGURE IV-111

A. Bronchoscopy with biopsy of the cavity to diagnose squamous cell lung cancer
B. Esophagogastroduodenoscopy to diagnose hiatal hernia with aspiration
C. Immediate hospitalization and isolation to prevent spread of mycobacterium tuberculosis
D. Intravenous ceftriaxone and azithromycin for aspiration pneumonia
E. Oral clindamycin for lung abscess

IV-112. Which of the following is a major reservoir for anaerobic organisms in the human body?

A. Duodenum
B. Female genital tract
C. Gallbladder
D. Lung
E. Prostate

IV-113. All of the following factors influence the likelihood of transmitting active tuberculosis EXCEPT:

A. Duration of contact with an infected person
B. Environment in which contact occurs
C. Presence of extrapulmonary tuberculosis
D. Presence of laryngeal tuberculosis
E. Probability of contact with an infectious person

IV-114. Which of the following individuals with a known history of prior latent tuberculosis infection (without therapy) has the *lowest* likelihood of developing reactivation tuberculosis?

A. A 28-year-old woman with anorexia nervosa, a body mass index of 16 kg/m^2, and a serum albumin of 2.3 g/dL
B. A 36-year-old intravenous drug user who does not have HIV but is homeless
C. A 42-year-old man who is HIV-positive with a CD4 count of 350/μL on highly active antiretroviral therapy
D. A 52-year-old man who works as a coal miner
E. An 83-year-old man who was infected while stationed in Korea in 1958

IV-115. A 42-year-old Nigerian man comes to the emergency department because of fevers, fatigue, weight loss, and cough for 3 weeks. He complains of fevers and a 4.5-kg weight loss. He describes his sputum as yellow in color. It has rarely been blood streaked. He emigrated to the United States 1 year ago and is an undocumented alien. He has never been treated for tuberculosis, has never had a purified protein derivative (PPD) skin test placed, and does not recall receiving BCG vaccination. He denies HIV risk factors. He is married and reports no ill contacts. He smokes 1 pack of cigarettes daily and drinks 1 pint of vodka on a daily basis. On physical examination, he appears chronically ill with temporal wasting. His body mass index is 21 kg/m^2. Vital signs are blood pressure of 122/68 mmHg, heart rate of 89 beats/min, respiratory rate of 22 breaths/min, SaO$_2$ of 95% on room air, and temperature of 37.9°C. There are amphoric breath sounds posteriorly in the right upper lung field with a few scattered crackles in this area. No clubbing is present. The examination is otherwise unremarkable. His chest radiograph is shown in Figure IV-115. A stain for acid-fast bacilli is negative. What is the most appropriate approach to the ongoing care of this patient?

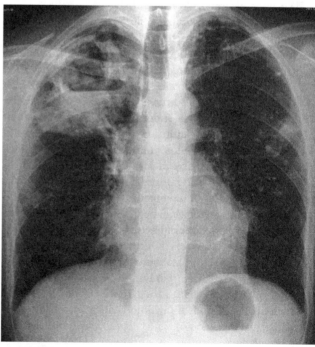

FIGURE IV-115

A. Admit the patient on airborne isolation until three expectorated sputums show no evidence of acid-fast bacilli.

B. Admit the patient without isolation as he is unlikely to be infectious with a negative acid-fast smear.

C. Perform a biopsy of the lesion and consult oncology.

D. Place a PPD test on his forearm and have him return for evaluation in 3 days.

E. Start a 6-week course of antibiotic treatment for anaerobic bacterial abscess.

IV-116. A 50-year-old man is admitted to the hospital for active pulmonary tuberculosis with a positive sputum acid-fast bacilli smear. He is HIV positive with a CD4 count of 85/μL and is not on highly active antiretroviral therapy. In addition to pulmonary disease, he is found to have disease in the L4 vertebral body. What is the most appropriate initial therapy?

A. Isoniazid, rifampin, ethambutol, and pyrazinamide

B. Isoniazid, rifampin, ethambutol, and pyrazinamide; initiate antiretroviral therapy

C. Isoniazid, rifampin, ethambutol, pyrazinamide, and streptomycin

D. Isoniazid, rifampin, and ethambutol

E. Withhold therapy until sensitivities are available.

IV-117. All of the following individuals receiving tuberculin skin purified protein derivative (PPD) reactions should be treated for latent tuberculosis EXCEPT:

A. A 23-year-old injection drug user who is HIV negative has a 12-mm PPD reaction.

B. A 38-year-old fourth grade teacher has a 7-mm PPD reaction and no known exposures to active tuberculosis. She has never been tested with a PPD previously.

C. A 43-year-old individual in the Peace Corps working in sub-Saharan Africa has a 10-mm PPD reaction. Eighteen months ago, the PPD reaction was 3 mm.

D. A 55-year-old man who is HIV positive has a negative PPD result. His partner was recently diagnosed with cavitary tuberculosis.

E. A 72-year-old man who is receiving chemotherapy for non-Hodgkin's lymphoma has a 16-mm PPD reaction.

IV-118. All of the following statements regarding interferon-gamma release assays for the diagnosis of latent tuberculosis are true EXCEPT:

A. There is no booster phenomenon.

B. They are more specific than tuberculin skin testing.

C. They have a higher sensitivity than tuberculin skin testing in high HIV-burden areas.

D. They have less cross reactivity with BCG and non-tuberculous mycobacteria than tuberculin skin testing.

E. They may be used to screen for latent tuberculosis in adults working in low prevalence U.S. settings.

IV-119. All of the following statements regarding BCG vaccination are true EXCEPT:

A. BCG dissemination may occur in severely immune-suppressed patients.

B. BCG vaccination is recommended at birth in countries with high TB prevalence.

C. BCG vaccination may cause a false-positive tuberculin skin test result.

D. BCG vaccine provides protection for infants and children from TB meningitis and miliary disease.

E. BCG vaccine provides protection from TB in HIV-infected patients.

IV-120. A 76-year-old woman is brought into the clinic by her son. She complains of a chronic nonproductive cough and fatigue. Her son adds that she has had low-grade fevers, progressive weight loss over months, and "just doesn't seem like herself." A representative slice from her chest CT is shown in Figure IV-120. She was treated for tuberculosis when she was in her 20s. A sputum sample is obtained, as are blood cultures. Two weeks later, both culture sets grow acid-fast bacilli consistent with *Mycobacterium avium* complex. Which of the following is the best treatment option?

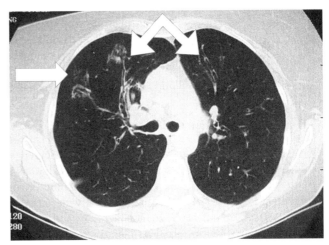

FIGURE IV-120

A. Bronchodilators and pulmonary toilet

B. Clarithromycin, ethambutol, and rifampin

C. Clarithromycin and rifampin

D. Moxifloxacin and rifampin

E. Pyrazinamide, isoniazid, rifampin, and ethambutol

IV-121. All of the following statements regarding anti-tuberculosis therapeutic agents are true EXCEPT:

A. In the United States, *M. tuberculosis* resistance to isoniazid remains below 10%.

B. Optic neuritis is the most severe adverse effect of ethambutol.

C. Pyrazinamide has utility in the therapy of *M. avium* complex and *M. kansasii* infections.

D. Rifabutin should be used instead of rifampin in patients receiving concurrent treatment with protease inhibitors or nevirapine.

E. Rifampin can decrease the half-life of warfarin, cyclosporine, prednisone, oral contraceptives, clarithromycin, and other important drugs.

IV-122. Which of the following patients with latent syphilis should undergo lumbar puncture for assessment of possible neurosyphilis?

A. A 24-year-old woman with an RPR titer of 1:128
B. A 38-year-old man with an RPR titer of 1:32 who was treated with benzathine G penicillin 2.4 million units intramuscularly. Repeat RPR titer 12 months after treatment is 1:16.
C. A 46-year-old man with HIV and a CD4 count of 150/μL
D. A 62-year-old woman with Bell's palsy and a recent change in mental status
E. All of the above

IV-123. An 18-year-old man presents with a firm, nontender lesion around his anal orifice. The lesion is about 1.5 cm in diameter and has a cartilaginous feel on clinical examination. The patient reports that it has progressed to this stage from a small papule. It is not tender. He reports recent unprotected anal intercourse. Bacterial culture result of the lesion is negative. A rapid plasmin reagin (RPR) test result is also negative. Therapeutic interventions should include:

A. Acyclovir 200 mg orally 5 times per day
B. Ceftriaxone 1 g intramuscularly
C. Observation
D. Penicillin G benzathine 2.4 million U intramuscularly
E. Surgical resection with biopsy

IV-124. A 46-year-old man presents to the emergency department in Honolulu, Hawaii, with myalgias, malaise, and fevers. He is homeless and has alcoholism and frequently sleeps in alleys that are infested with rats. He recalls blacking out from alcohol ingestion and waking with his legs in a fetid pool. He noted scratches and bites around his ankles about 2 weeks ago. Since that time, he has felt increasingly more ill. For the past day, he has also noted that his skin is increasingly yellow. In addition to alcohol abuse, he has a medical history of schizophrenia and smokes 1 to 2 packs of cigarettes daily. He currently receives olanzapine as an intramuscular injection at a dose of 300 mg monthly. On initial evaluation, his temperature is 38.6°C, pulse is 105 beats/min, respiratory rate is 24/min, and blood pressure is 98/59 mmHg with O₂ saturations of 92% on room air. He appears acutely ill and markedly jaundiced. His conjunctivae are injected bilaterally without discharge. Bibasilar crackles are present. His liver is enlarged and tender, but no splenomegaly is present. Laboratory results are notable for a BUN of 64 mg/dL, creatinine of 3.6 mg/dL, total bilirubin of 32.4 mg/dL, direct bilirubin of 29.8 mg/dL, AST of 80 U/L, ALT of 184 U/L, and alkaline phosphatase of 168 U/L. His complete blood count shows a white blood cell count of 12,500/μL with 13% bands and 80% polymorphonuclear forms, hematocrit of 33%, and platelets of 82,000/μL. Urinalysis reveals 20 white blood cells per high-power field, 3+ protein, and no casts. Coagulation study results are within normal limits. CT scan of the

chest shows diffuse flame-like infiltrates consistent with pulmonary hemorrhage. What is the likely diagnosis?

A. Acute alcoholic hepatitis
B. Disseminated intravascular coagulation due to *Streptococcus pneumoniae* infection
C. Microscopic polyangiitis
D. Rat bite fever (*Streptobacillus moniliformis* infection)
E. Weil's syndrome (*Leptospira interrogans* infection)

IV-125. A 26-year-old man presents to your office complaining of recurrent episodes of fever and malaise. He returned from a camping trip in the northwestern part of Montana about 3 weeks ago. While he was hiking, he denies eating or drinking any unpasteurized milk products. He sterilized all of his water before drinking. He had multiple insect bites, but did not identify any ticks. He primarily slept in cabins or tents and did not notice any rodent droppings in the areas where he camped. Two friends that accompanied him on the trip have not been ill. He initially experienced fevers as high as 104.7°F (40.4°C) with myalgias, headache, nausea, vomiting, and diarrhea beginning 5 days after his return home. These symptoms lasted for about 3 days and resolved spontaneously. He attributed his symptoms to the "flu" and returned to his normal functioning. Seven days later, the fevers returned with temperatures to 105.1°F (40.6°C). With these episodes, his family noted him to have intermittent confusion. Today is day 4 of his current illness, and the patient feels that his fevers have again subsided. What is the most likely cause of the patient's recurrent fevers?

A. Brucellosis
B. Colorado tick fever
C. Leptospirosis
D. Lymphocytic choriomeningitis
E. Tickborne relapsing fever

IV-126. A 36-year-old man presents to the emergency department in Pennsylvania complaining of lightheadedness and dizziness. On physical examination, the patient is found to have a heart rate of 38 beats/min, and the ECG demonstrates acute heart block. On further questioning, he reports that he lives in a wooded area. He has two dogs that often roam in the woods and have been found with ticks on many occasions. He takes no medications and is otherwise healthy. He is an avid hiker and is also training for a triathlon. He denies any significant childhood illness. His family history is positive for an acute myocardial infarction in his father at age 42 years. His physical examination is normal with the exception of a slow but regular heartbeat. His chemistry panel shows no abnormalities. His chest radiograph is normal. What is the most likely cause of complete heart block in this individual?

A. Acute myocardial infarction
B. Chagas disease
C. Lyme disease
D. Sarcoidosis
E. Subacute bacterial endocarditis

IV-127. *Borrelia burgdorferi* serology testing is indicated for which of the following patients, all of whom reside in Lyme-endemic regions?

A. 19-year-old female camp counselor who presents with her second episode of an inflamed, red, and tender left knee and right ankle

B. A 23-year-old male house painter who presents with a primary erythema migrans lesion at the site of a witnessed tick bite

C. A 36-year-old female state park ranger who presents with a malar rash; diffuse arthralgias or arthritis of her shoulders, knees, and metacarpophalangeal and proximal interphalangeal joints; pericarditis; and acute glomerulonephritis

D. A 42-year-old woman with chronic fatigue, myalgias, and arthralgias

E. A 46-year-old male gardener who presents with fevers, malaise, migratory arthralgias or myalgias, and three erythema migrans lesions

IV-128. A previously healthy 17-year-old woman presents in early October with profound fatigue and malaise, as well as fevers, headache, nuchal rigidity, diffuse arthralgias, and a rash. She lives in a small town in Massachusetts and spent her summer as a camp counselor at a local day camp. She participated in daily hikes in the woods but did not travel outside of the area during the course of the summer. Physical examination reveals a well-developed young woman who appears extremely fatigued but not in extremis. Her temperature is 37.4°C, pulse is 86 beats/min, blood pressure is 96/54 mmHg, and respiratory rate is 12 breaths/min. Physical examination documents clear breath sounds, no cardiac rub or murmur, normal bowel sounds, a nontender abdomen, no organomegaly, and no evidence of synovitis. Several erythema migrans lesions are noted on her lower extremities, bilateral axillae, right thigh, and left groin. All of the following are possible complications of her current disease state EXCEPT:

A. Bell's palsy
B. Large joint oligoarticular arthritis
C. Meningitis
D. Progressive dementia
E. Third-degree heart block

IV-129. In the patient described above, which of the following is appropriate therapy?

A. Azithromycin, 500 mg PO daily
B. Ceftriaxone, 2 g IV daily
C. Cephalexin, 500 mg PO bid
D. Doxycycline, 100 mg PO bid
E. Vancomycin, 1 g IV bid

IV-130. A 48-year-old man is admitted to the intensive care unit in July with hypotension and fever. He lives in a suburban area of Arkansas. He became ill yesterday with a fever as high as 104.0°F (40.0°C). Today, his wife noted increasing confusion and lethargy. Over this same time, he has complained of headaches and myalgias. He has had nausea with two episodes of vomiting. Before the acute onset of illness, he had no medical complaints. He has no other medical history and takes no medications. He works as a landscape architect. The history is obtained from the patient's wife, and she does not know if he has had any recent insect or tick bites. No one else in the family is ill, nor are the patient's coworkers. On presentation, the vital signs are blood pressure of 88/52 mmHg, heart rate of 135 beats/min, respiratory rate of 22 breaths/min, temperature 101.9°F (38.8°C), and oxygen saturation of 94% on room air. His physical examination reveals an ill-appearing man, moaning quietly. He is oriented to person only. No meningismus is present. His cardiac examination reveals regular tachycardia. His chest and abdominal examinations are normal. He has no rash. His laboratory values are as follows:

WBC count	4200/μL	Sodium	132 meq/L
PMNs	88%	Potassium	4.6 meq/L
Lymphocytes	10%	Chloride	98 meq/L
Monocytes	2%	Bicarbonate	22 meq/L
Eosinophils	0%	BUN	38 g/dL
Hemoglobin	12.3 g/dL	Creatinine	1.6 mg/dL
Hematocrit	37%	Glucose	102 mg/dL
Platelets	82,000/μL		

AST	215 U/L
ALT	199 U/L
Bilirubin	1.2 mg/dL
Alkaline phosphatase	98 U/L

He is fluid resuscitated and treated with intravenous ceftriaxone and vancomycin. A lumbar puncture shows no pleocytosis with normal protein and glucose. Despite this treatment, the patient develops worsening thrombocytopenia, neutropenia, and lymphopenia over the next 2 days. A bone marrow biopsy shows a hypercellular marrow with noncaseating granulomas. Which test is most likely to suggest the cause of the patient's illness?

A. Antibodies to double-stranded DNA and Smith antigens
B. Chest radiography
C. Levels of IgM and IgG on cerebrospinal fluid
D. Peripheral blood smear
E. Polymerase chain reaction on peripheral blood

IV-131. A 27-year-old woman who lives in North Carolina presents to her primary care physician complaining of fever, headache, myalgias, nausea, and anorexia 7 days after returning from hiking on the Appalachian Trail. Physical examination is remarkable for a temperature of 101.5°F (38.6°C). She appears generally fatigued but not toxic. She does not have a rash. She is reassured by her primary care physician that this likely represents a viral illness. She returns to clinic 3 days later with a progressive rash and ongoing fevers. She states that small red spots began to appear on her wrists and ankles within 24 hours of her previous visit and have now progressed up her extremities and onto her trunk. She also is noting increasing headache, and her husband thinks she has had some confusion. On physical examination, the patient is noted to be lethargic and answers questions slowly. What would be a reasonable course of action?

A. Admit the patient to the hospital for treatment with intravenous ceftriaxone 1 g twice daily and vancomycin 1 g twice daily.
B. Admit the patient to the hospital for treatment with doxycycline 100 mg twice daily.
C. Initiate treatment with doxycycline 100 mg orally twice daily as an outpatient.
D. Initiate treatment with trimethoprim–sulfamethoxazole DS twice daily.
E. Order rickettsial serologies and withhold treatment until a firm diagnosis is made.

IV-132. A previously healthy 20-year-old college student presents in September with several days of headache, extensive cough with scant sputum, and fever of 101.5°F (38.6°C). Several individuals in his dormitory have also been ill with a similar illness. On examination, pharyngeal erythema is noted, and lung examination reveals bilateral expiratory wheezing and scattered crackles in the lower lung zones. He coughs frequently during the examination. Chest radiography reveals bilateral peribronchial pneumonia with increased interstitial markings. No lobar consolidation is seen. Which organism is most likely to cause the patient's presentation?

A. Adenovirus
B. *Chlamydia pneumoniae*
C. *Legionella pneumophila*
D. *Mycoplasma pneumoniae*
E. *Streptococcus pneumoniae*

IV-133. A previously healthy 19-year-old man presents with several days of headache, cough with scant sputum, dyspnea, and fever of 38.6°C. On examination, pharyngeal erythema is noted, and lung fields show scattered wheezes and some crackles. Chest radiography reveals focal bronchopneumonia in the lower lobes. His hematocrit is

24.7%, down from a baseline measure of 46%. The only other laboratory abnormality is an indirect bilirubin of 3.4. A peripheral smear reveals no abnormalities. A cold agglutinin titer is measured at 1:64. What is the most likely infectious agent?

A. *Coxiella burnetii*
B. *Legionella pneumophila*
C. Methicillin-resistant *Staphylococcus aureus*
D. *Mycoplasma pneumoniae*
E. *Streptococcus pneumoniae*

IV-134. A 42-year-old woman is admitted to the intensive care unit with hypoxemic respiratory failure and pneumonia in August. She was well until 2 days before admission, when she developed fevers, myalgias, and headache. She works in a poultry processing plant and is originally from El Salvador. She has been in the United States for 15 years. She has no major health problems. Her PPD result was negative upon arrival to the United States. Several other workers have been ill with a similar illness, although no one else has developed respiratory failure. She is currently intubated and sedated. Her oxygen saturation is 93% on an FiO$_2$ of 0.80 and positive end-expiratory pressure of 12 cm H$_2$O. On physical examination, crackles are present in both lung fields. There is no cardiac murmur. Hepatosplenomegaly is present. Laboratory studies reveal a mild transaminitis. The influenza nasal swab result is negative for the presence of influenza A. Which of the following test results is most likely to be positive in this patient?

A. Acid-fast bacilli stain and mycobacterial culture for *Mycobacterium tuberculosis*
B. Blood cultures growing *Staphylococcus aureus*
C. Microimmunofluorescence testing for *Chlamydia psittaci*
D. Urine *Legionella* antigen
E. Viral cultures of bronchoscopic samples for influenza A

IV-135. A 20-year-old woman is 36 weeks pregnant and presents for her first evaluation. She is diagnosed with *Chlamydia trachomatis* infection of the cervix. Upon delivery, for what complication is her infant most at risk?

A. Jaundice
B. Hydrocephalus
C. Hutchinson triad
D. Conjunctivitis
E. Sensorineural deafness

IV-136. A 19-year-old man presents to an urgent care clinic with urethral discharge. He reports three new female sexual partners over the past 2 months. What should his management be?

A. Nucleic acid amplification test for *Neisseria gonor-rhoeae* and *Chlamydia trachomatis* and return to clinic in 2 days

B. Ceftriaxone 250 mg IM × 1 and azithromycin 1 g PO × 1 for the patient and his recent partners

C. Nucleic acid amplification test for *N. gonorrhoeae* and *C. trachomatis* plus ceftriaxone 250 mg IM × 1 and azithromycin 1 g PO × 1 for the patient

D. Nucleic acid amplification test for *N. gonorrhoeae* and *C. trachomatis* plus ceftriaxone 250 mg IM × 1 and azithromycin 1 g PO × 1 for the patient and his recent partners

E. Nucleic acid amplification test for *N. gonorrhoeae* and *C. trachomatis* plus ceftriaxone 250 mg IM × 1, azithromycin 1 g PO × 1, and Flagyl 2 g PO × 1 for the patient and his partners

IV-137. All of the following viruses have been implicated as a cause of human cancer EXCEPT:

A. Dengue fever virus
B. Epstein-Barr virus
C. Hepatitis B virus
D. Hepatitis C virus
E. Human papillomavirus

IV-138. All of the following antiviral medications are correctly matched with a significant side effect EXCEPT:

A. Acyclovir—thrombotic thrombocytopenic purpura
B. Amantadine—anxiety and insomnia
C. Foscarnet—acute renal failure
D. Ganciclovir—bone marrow suppression
E. Interferon—fevers and myalgias

IV-139. All of the following regarding herpes simplex virus-2 (HSV-2) infection are true EXCEPT:

A. Approximately one in five Americans harbors HSV-2 antibodies.
B. Asymptomatic shedding of HSV-2 in the genital tract occurs nearly as frequently in those with no symptoms as in those with ulcerative disease.
C. Asymptomatic shedding of HSV-2 is associated with transmission of virus.
D. HSV-2 seropositivity is an independent risk factor for HIV transmission.
E. Seroprevalence rates of HSV-2 are lower in Africa than in the United States.

IV-140. A 23-year-old woman is newly diagnosed with genital herpes simplex virus-2 (HSV-2) infection. What can you tell her that the chance of reactivation disease will be during the first year after infection?

A. 5%
B. 25%
C. 50%
D. 75%
E. 90%

IV-141. A 65-year-old man is brought to the hospital by his wife because of new onset of fever and confusion. He was well until 3 days ago but then developed a high fever, somnolence, and progressive confusion. His current medical history is unremarkable except for an elevated cholesterol level, and his only medication is atorvastatin. He is a civil engineer at an international construction company. His wife reports that he obtains regular health screening and has always been PPD negative. On admission, his temperature is 40°C, and his vital signs are otherwise normal. He is confused and hallucinating. Soon after admission, he develops a tonic-clonic seizure that requires lorazepam to terminate. His head CT shows no acute bleeding or elevated ICP. An EEG shows an epileptiform focus in the left temporal lobe, and diffusion-weighted MRI shows bilateral temporal lobe inflammation. Which of the following is most likely to be diagnostic?

A. CSF acid-fast staining
B. CSF India ink stain
C. CSF PCR for herpes virus
D. CSF oligoclonal band testing
E. Serum cryptococcal antigen testing

IV-142. Which of the following statements regarding administration of varicella-zoster vaccine to patients above the age of 60 is true?

A. It is a killed virus vaccine, so it is safe in immunocompromised patients.
B. It is not recommended for patients in this age group.
C. It will decrease the risk of developing postherpetic neuralgia.
D. It will not decrease the risk of developing shingles.
E. It will not decrease the burden of disease.

IV-143. A 19-year-old college student comes to clinic reporting that he has been ill for 2 weeks. About 2 weeks ago, he developed notable fatigue and malaise that prevented him from his usual exercise regimen and caused him to miss some classes. Last week, he developed low-grade fevers, sore throat, and swollen lymph nodes in his neck. He has a history of strep pharyngitis, so 3 days ago, he took some ampicillin that he had in his possession. Over the past 2 days, he has developed a worsening slightly itchy rash as shown in Figure IV-143. His physical examination is notable for a temperature of 38.1°C, pharyngeal erythema, bilateral tonsillar enlargement without exudates, bilateral tender cervical adenopathy, and a palpable spleen. All of the following statements regarding his illness are true EXCEPT:

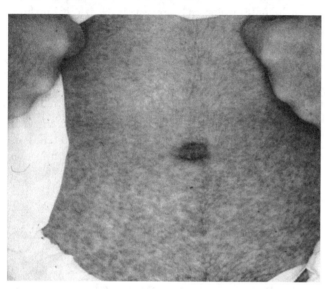

FIGURE IV-143 (see Color Atas)

A. Greater than 10% atypical lymphocytosis is likely.
B. Heterophile antibody testing will likely be diagnostic.
C. If the heterophile antibody test result is negative, testing for IgG antibodies against viral capsid antigen will likely be diagnostic.
D. It is spread via contaminated saliva.
E. The patient can receive ampicillin in the future if indicated.

IV-144. In the patient described above, which of the following is indicated treatment?

A. Acyclovir
B. Acyclovir plus prednisone
C. Ganciclovir
D. Prednisone
E. Rest, supportive measures, and reassurance

IV-145. Which of the following manifestations of cytomegalovirus (CMV) infection is *least* likely to occur after lung transplantation?

A. Bronchiolitis obliterans
B. CMV esophagitis
C. CMV pneumonia
D. CMV retinitis
E. CMV syndrome (fever, malaise, cytopenias, transaminitis, and CMV viremia)

IV-146. Which of the following serology patterns places a transplant recipient at the lowest risk of developing cytomegalovirus (CMV) infection after renal transplantation?

A. Donor CMV IgG negative; recipient CMV IgG negative.
B. Donor CMV IgG negative; recipient CMV IgG positive.
C. Donor CMV IgG positive; recipient CMV IgG negative.
D. Donor CMV IgG positive; recipient CMV IgG positive.
E. The risk is equal regardless of serology results.

IV-147. All of the following statements regarding human herpes virus-8 (HHV-8) are true EXCEPT:

A. It has been implicated causally in invasive cervical carcinoma.
B. It has been implicated causally in Kaposi's sarcoma.
C. It has been implicated causally in multicentric Castleman's disease.
D. It has been implicated causally in primary pleural lymphoma.
E. Primary infection may manifest with fever and maculopapular rash.

IV-148. All of the following clinical findings are consistent with the diagnosis of molluscum contagiosum EXCEPT:

A. Involvement of the genitals
B. Involvement of the soles of the feet
C. Lack of inflammation or necrosis at the site of the rash
D. Rash associated with an eczematous eruption
E. Rash spontaneously resolving over 3 to 4 months

IV-149. A 42-year-old man with AIDS and a CD4+ lymphocyte count of 23 cells/mm^3 presents with shortness of breath and fatigue in the absence of fevers. On examination, he appears chronically ill with pale conjunctiva. Hematocrit is 16%. Mean corpuscular volume is 84/fl. Red blood cell distribution width is normal. Bilirubin, lactose dehydrogenase, and haptoglobin are all within normal limits. Reticulocyte count is zero. White blood cell count is 4300/μL with an absolute neutrophil count of 2500. Platelet count is 105,000/ul. Which of the following tests is most likely to produce a diagnosis?

A. Bone marrow aspirate and biopsy
B. Parvovirus B19 IgG
C. Parvovirus B19 polymerase chain reaction
D. Parvovirus B19 IgM
E. Peripheral blood smear

IV-150. A 22-year-old woman presents with diffuse arthralgias and morning stiffness in her hands, knees, and wrists. Two weeks earlier, she had a self-limited febrile illness notable for a red facial rash and lacy reticular rash on her extremities. On examination, her bilateral wrists, metacarpophalangeal joints, and proximal interphalangeal joints are warm and slightly boggy. Which of the following tests is most likely to reveal her diagnosis?

A. Antinuclear antibody
B. *Chlamydia trachomatis* ligase chain reaction of the urine
C. Joint aspiration for crystals and culture
D. Parvovirus B19 IgM
E. Rheumatoid factor

IV-151. Which of the following statements regarding the currently licensed human papillomavirus (HPV) vaccines is true?

A. Both protect against genital warts.
B. After becoming sexually active, women will derive little protective benefit from vaccination.
C. They are inactivated live virus vaccines.
D. They are targeted toward all oncogenic strains of HPV but are only 70% effective at decreasing infection in an individual.
E. Vaccinees should continue to receive standard Pap smear testing.

IV-152. A 32-year-old woman experiences an upper respiratory illness that began with rhinorrhea and nasal congestion. She also is complaining of a sore throat but has no fever. Her illness lasts for about 5 days and resolves. Just before her illness, her 4-year-old child who attends daycare also experienced a similar illness. All of the following statements regarding the most common etiologic agent causing this illness are true EXCEPT:

A. After the primary illness in a household, a secondary case of illness will occur in 25% to 70% of cases.
B. The seasonal peak of the infection is in early fall and spring in temperate climates.
C. The virus can be isolated from plastic surfaces up to 3 hours after exposure.
D. The virus grows best at a temperature of 37°C, the temperature within the nasal passages.
E. The virus is a single-stranded RNA virus of the Picornaviridae family.

IV-153. All of the following respiratory viruses is a cause of the common cold syndrome in children or adults EXCEPT:

A. Adenoviruses
B. Coronaviruses
C. Enteroviruses
D. Human respiratory syncytial viruses
E. Rhinoviruses

IV-154. All of the following viruses are correctly matched with their primary clinical manifestations EXCEPT:

A. Adenovirus—Gingivostomatitis
B. Coronavirus—Severe acute respiratory syndrome
C. Human respiratory syncytial virus—Bronchiolitis in infants and young children
D. Parainfluenza—Croup
E. Rhinovirus—Common cold

IV-155. A 9-month-old infant is admitted to the hospital with a febrile respiratory illness with wheezing and cough. Upon admission to the hospital, the baby is tachypneic and tachycardic with an oxygen saturation of 75% on room air. Rapid viral diagnostic testing confirms the presence of human respiratory syncytial virus. All of the following treatments should be used as part of the treatment plan for this child EXCEPT:

A. Aerosolized ribavirin
B. Hydration
C. Immunoglobulin with high titers of antibody directed against human respiratory syncytial virus
D. Nebulized albuterol
E. Oxygen therapy to maintain oxygen saturation greater than 90%

IV-156. In March 2009, the H1N1 strain of the influenza A virus emerged in Mexico and quickly spread worldwide over the next several months. Ultimately, more than 18,000 people died from the pandemic. This virus had genetic components of swine influenza viruses, an avian virus, and a human influenza virus. The genetic process by which this pandemic strain of influenza A emerged is an example of:

A. Antigenic drift
B. Antigenic shift
C. Genetic reassortment
D. Point mutation
E. B and C

IV-157. A 65-year-old woman is admitted to the hospital in January with a 2-day history of fevers, myalgias, headache, and cough. She has a history of end-stage kidney disease, diabetes mellitus, and hypertension. Her medications include darbepoetin, selamaver, calcitriol, lisinopril, aspirin, amlodipine, and insulin. She receives hemodialysis three times weekly. Upon admission, her blood pressure is 138/65 mmHg, heart rate is 122 beats/min, temperature is 39.4°C, respiratory rate is 24 breaths/min, and oxygen saturation is 85% on room air. On physical examination, diffuse crackles are heard, and a chest radiograph confirms the presence of bilateral lung infiltrates concerning for pneumonia. It is known that the most common cause of seasonal influenza in this area is an H3N2 strain of influenza A. All of the following should be included in the initial management of this patient EXCEPT:

A. Amantadine
B. Assessment of the need for close household contacts to receive chemoprophylaxis if influenza swab result is positive
C. Droplet precautions
D. Nasal swab for influenza
E. Oxygen therapy

IV-158. In which of the following individuals has the intranasal influenza vaccine been determined to be safe and effective?

A. A 3-year-old child who was hospitalized on one occasion for wheezing in association with human respiratory syncytial virus infection at 9 months of age

B. A 32-year-old woman who is currently 32 weeks pregnant

C. A 42-year-old registered nurse who had a known exposure to an individual with pandemic H1N1 who is currently receiving chemoprophylaxis with oseltamivir. He does not have contact with transplant, oncology, or HIV-positive patients.

D. A 48-year-old hematologist whose primary specialty is bone marrow transplant

E. A 69-year-old man with hypertension

IV-159. A 17-year-old woman with a medical history of mild intermittent asthma presents to your clinic in February with several days of cough, fever, malaise, and myalgias. She notes that her symptoms started 3 days earlier with a headache and fatigue and that several students and teachers at her high school have been diagnosed recently with "the flu." She did not receive a flu shot this year. Which of the following medication treatment plans is the best option for this patient?

A. Aspirin and a cough suppressant with codeine

B. Oseltamivir, 75 mg PO bid for 5 days

C. Rimantadine, 100 mg PO bid for 1 week

D. Symptom-based therapy with over-the-counter agents

E. Zanamivir, 10 mg inhaled bid for 5 days

IV-160. All of the following statements regarding human T-cell lymphotropic virus-I (HTLV-I) infection are true EXCEPT:

A. Acute T-cell leukemia is associated with HTLV-I infection.

B. HTLV-I endemic regions include southern Japan, the Caribbean, and South America.

C. HTLV-I infection is associated with a gradual decline in T-cell function and immunosuppression.

D. HTLV-I is transmitted parenterally, sexually, and from mother to child.

E. Tropical spastic paraparesis is associated with HTLV-I infection.

IV-161. A 28-year-old man is diagnosed with HIV infection during a clinic visit. He has no symptoms of opportunistic infection. His CD4+ lymphocyte count is 150/μL. All of the following are approved regimens for primary prophylaxis against *Pneumocystis jiroveci* infection EXCEPT:

A. Aerosolized pentamidine, 300 mg monthly

B. Atovaquone, 1500 mg PO daily

C. Clindamycin, 900 mg PO q8h, plus primaquine, 30 mg PO daily

D. Dapsone, 100 mg PO daily

E. Trimethoprim–sulfamethoxazole, 1 single-strength tablet PO daily

IV-162. All of the following statements regarding HIV epidemiology in the United States as of 2010 are true EXCEPT:

A. Most patients in the United States with HIV infection are nonwhite.

B. The annual number of AIDS-related deaths has fallen since 1995.

C. The percentage of AIDS cases attributed to male-to-male transmission has fallen steadily since 1985.

D. The proportion of prevalent HIV cases caused by injection drug use is currently decreasing.

E. Up to 20% of patients in the United States are unaware of being infected with HIV.

IV-163. Which of the following scenarios is most likely associated with the lowest risk of HIV transmission to a health care provider after an accidental needle stick from a patient with HIV?

A. The needle is visibly contaminated with the patient's blood.

B. The needle stick injury is a deep tissue injury to the health care provider.

C. The patient whose blood is on the contaminated needle has been on antiretroviral therapy for many years with a history of resistance to many available agents but most recently has had successful viral suppression on current therapy.

D. The patient whose blood is on the contaminated needle was diagnosed with acute HIV infection 2 weeks ago.

IV-164. Abacavir is a nucleoside transcription inhibitor that carries which side effect unique for HIV antiretroviral agents?

A. Fanconi's anemia

B. Granulocytopenia

C. Lactic acidosis

D. Lipoatrophy

E. Severe hypersensitivity reaction

IV-165. A 38-year-old man with HIV/AIDS presents with 4 weeks of diarrhea, fever, and weight loss. Which of the following tests makes the diagnosis of cytomegalovirus (CMV) colitis?

A. CMV IgG

B. Colonoscopy with biopsy

C. Serum CMV polymerase chain reaction

D. Stool CMV antigen

E. Stool CMV culture

IV-166. A 40-year-old man is admitted to the hospital with 2 to 3 weeks of fever, tender lymph nodes, and right upper quadrant abdominal pain. He reports progressive weight loss and malaise over 1 year. On examination, he is found to be febrile and frail with temporal wasting and oral thrush. Matted, tender anterior cervical lymphadenopathy smaller than 1 cm and tender hepatomegaly are noted. He is diagnosed with AIDS (CD4+ lymphocyte count = 12/μL and HIV RNA = 650,000 copies/mL). Blood cultures grow *Mycobacterium avium*. He is started on rifabutin and clarithromycin, as well as dapsone for *Pneumocystis* prophylaxis, and discharged home 2 weeks later after his fevers subside. He follows up with an HIV provider 4 weeks later and is started on tenofovir, emtricitabine, and efavirenz. Two weeks later, he returns to clinic with fevers, neck pain, and abdominal pain. His temperature is 39.2°C, heart rate is 110 beats/min, blood pressure is 110/64 mmHg, and oxygen saturations are normal. His cervical nodes are now 2 cm in size and extremely tender, and one has fistulized to his skin and is draining yellow pus that is acid-fast bacillus stain positive. His hepatomegaly is pronounced and tender. What is the *most likely* explanation for his presentation?

A. Cryptococcal meningitis
B. HIV treatment failure
C. Immune reconstitution syndrome to *Mycobacterium avium*
D. Kaposi's sarcoma
E. *Mycobacterium avium* treatment failure caused by drug resistance

IV-167. Per-coital rate of HIV acquisition in a man who has unprotected sexual intercourse with an HIV-infected female partner is likely to increase under which of the following circumstances?

A. Acute HIV infection in the female partner
B. Female herpes simplex virus (HSV-2)–positive serostatus
C. Male nongonococcal urethritis at the time of intercourse
D. Uncircumcised male status
E. All of the above

IV-168. Current Centers for Disease Control and Prevention recommendations are that screening for HIV be performed in which of the following?

A. All high-risk groups (injection drug users, men who have sex with men, and high-risk heterosexual women)
B. All U.S. adults
C. Injection drug users
D. Men who have sex with men
E. Women who have sex with more than two men per year

IV-169. A 38-year-old woman is seen in the clinic for a decrease in cognitive and executive function. Her husband is concerned because she is no longer able to pay bills, keep appointments, or remember important dates. She also seems to derive considerably less pleasure from caring for her children and her hobbies. She is unable to concentrate for long enough to enjoy movies. This is a clear change from her functional status 6 months prior. A workup reveals a positive HIV antibody by enzyme immunoassay and Western blot. Her CD4+ lymphocyte count is 378/μL with a viral load of 78,000/mL. She is afebrile with normal vital signs. Her affect is blunted, and she seems disinterested in the medical interview. Neurologic examination for strength, sensation, cerebellar function, and

cranial nerve function is nonfocal. Funduscopic examination is normal. Mini-Mental Status Examination score is 22 of 30. A serum rapid plasmin reagin (RPR) test result is negative. MRI of the brain shows only cerebral atrophy disproportionate to her age but no focal lesions. What is the next step in her management?

A. Antiretroviral therapy
B. Cerebrospinal fluid (CSF) JV virus polymerase chain reaction (PCR)
C. CSF mycobacterial PCR
D. CSF VDRL test
E. Serum cryptococcal antigen
F. *Toxoplasma* IgG

IV-170. Indinavir is a protease inhibitor that carries which side effect unique for HIV antiretroviral agents?

A. Abnormal dreams
B. Benign hyperbilirubinemia
C. Hepatic necrosis in pregnant women
D. Nephrolithiasis
E. Pancreatitis

IV-171. In an HIV-infected patient, *Isospora belli* infection is different from *Cryptosporidium* infection in which of the following ways?

A. *Isospora* causes a more fulminant diarrheal syndrome, leading to rapid dehydration and even death in the absence of rapid rehydration.
B. *Isospora* infection may cause biliary tract disease, but cryptosporidiosis is strictly limited to the lumen of the small and large bowel.
C. *Isospora* spp. are more likely to infect immunocompetent hosts than *Cryptosporidium* spp.
D. *Isospora* spp. are less challenging to treat and generally respond well to trimethoprim–sulfamethoxazole treatment.
E. *Isospora* spp. occasionally cause large outbreaks among the general population.

IV-172. A 27-year-old man presents to your clinic with 2 weeks of sore throat, malaise, myalgias, night sweats, fevers, and chills. He visited an urgent care center and was told that he likely had the flu. He was told that he had a "negative test for mono." The patient is homosexual and states that he is in a monogamous relationship and has unprotected receptive and insertive anal and oral intercourse with one partner. He had several partners before his current partner 4 years ago but none recently. He reports a negative HIV-1 test 2 years ago and recalls being diagnosed with *Chlamydia* infection 4 years ago. He is otherwise healthy with no medical problems. You wish to rule out the diagnosis of acute HIV. Which blood test should you order?

A. CD4+ lymphocyte count
B. HIV enzyme immunoassay (EIA)/Western blot combination testing
C. HIV resistance panel
D. HIV RNA by polymerase chain reaction (PCR)
E. HIV RNA by ultrasensitive PCR

IV-173. A 47-year-old woman with known HIV/AIDS (CD4+ lymphocyte, 106/μL and viral load, 35,000/mL) presents with painful growths on the side of her tongue as shown in Figure IV-173. What is the most likely diagnosis?

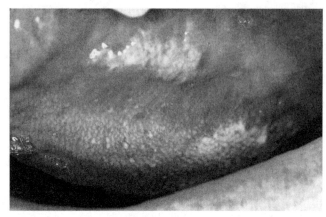

FIGURE IV-173 (see Color Atas)

A. Aphthous ulcers
B. Hairy leukoplakia
C. Herpes stomatitis
D. Oral candidiasis
E. Oral Kaposi's sarcoma

IV-174. Which of the following patients should receive HIV antiretroviral therapy?

A. A 24-year-old man with newly diagnosed acute HIV infection by viral PCR
B. A 44-year-old man who reports having unprotected anal intercourse with another man who has active HIV infection
C. A 26-year-old pregnant women found at screening to have HIV infection of unknown duration and a CD4 lymphocyte count of 700/μL
D. A 51-year-old man found to at screening to have HIV infection of unknown duration and a CD4 lymphocyte count of 150/μL
E. All of the patients should receive antiretroviral therapy

IV-175. All of the following statements regarding antiretroviral therapy for HIV are true EXCEPT:

A. CD4+ lymphocyte count should rise by more than 100 cells/mm^3 within 2 months of initiation of therapy.
B. Intermittent administration regimens have equivalent efficacy to constant administration regimens.
C. Plasma HIV RNA should fall by 1 log order within 2 months of initiation of therapy.
D. Recommended initial regimens include three drugs.
E. Viral genotype should be checked before initiation of therapy.

176. All of the following statements regarding Norwalk virus gastroenteritis are true EXCEPT:

A. Fever is common.
B. Incubation period is typically 5 to 7 days.
C. Infection is common worldwide.
D. It is a major cause of nonbacterial diarrhea outbreaks in the United States.
E. Transmission is typically fecal–oral.

IV-177. All of the following statements regarding rotavirus gastroenteritis are true EXCEPT:

A. Fever occurs in more than 25% of cases.
B. Inflammatory diarrhea distinguishes rotaviral illness from Norwalk agent gastroenteritis.
C. It is a major cause of diarrheal death among children in the developing world.
D. Nausea is common.
E. Vaccination is recommended for all children in the United States.

IV-178. A 9-year-old boy is brought to a pediatric emergency department by his father. He has had 2 days of headache, neck stiffness, and photophobia and this morning had a temperature of 38.9°C (102°F). He has also had several episodes of vomiting and diarrhea overnight. A lumbar puncture is performed, which reveals pleocytosis in the cerebrospinal fluid (CSF). Which of the following is true regarding enteroviruses as a cause of aseptic meningitis?

A. An elevated CSF protein level rules out enteroviruses as a cause of meningitis.
B. Enteroviruses are responsible for up to 90% of aseptic meningitis in children.
C. Lymphocytes will predominate in the CSF early on, with a shift to neutrophils at 24 hours.
D. Symptoms are more severe in children than in adults.
E. They occur more commonly in the winter and spring.

IV-179. A 25-year-old woman presents with 1 day of fever to 38.3°C (101°F); sore throat; dysphagia; and a number of grayish-white papulovesicular lesions on the soft palate, uvula, and anterior pillars of the tonsils (see Figure IV-179). The patient is most likely infected with which of the following?

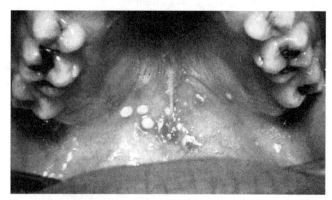

FIGURE IV-179 (see Color Atas)

A. *Candida albicans*
B. Coxsackievirus
C. Herpesvirus
D. HIV
E. *Staphylococcus lugdunensis*

IV-180. The human enterovirus family includes poliovirus, coxsackieviruses, enteroviruses, and echovirus. Which of the following statements regarding viral infection with one of the members of this group is true?

A. Among children infected with poliovirus, paralysis is common.

B. Enteroviruses are not transmitted via blood transfusions and insect bites.

C. In utero exposure to maternal enteroviral antibodies is not protective.

D. Infections are most common in adolescents and adults, although serious illness is most common in young children.

E. Paralysis from poliovirus infection was more commonly seen in developing countries.

IV-181. A 23-year-old previously healthy female letter carrier works in a suburb in which the presence of rabid foxes and skunks has been documented. She is bitten by a bat, which then flies away. Initial examination reveals a clean break in the skin in the right upper forearm. She has no history of receiving treatment for rabies and is unsure about vaccination against tetanus. The physician should:

A. Clean the wound with a 20% soap solution.

B. Clean the wound with a 20% soap solution and administer tetanus toxoid.

C. Clean the wound with a 20% soap solution, administer tetanus toxoid, and administer human rabies immune globulin intramuscularly.

D. Clean the wound with a 20% soap solution, administer tetanus toxoid, administer human rabies immune globulin IM, and administer human diploid cell vaccine.

E. Clean the wound with a 20% soap solution and administer human diploid cell vaccine.

IV-182. While working at a new medical school in Kuala Lumpur, Malaysia, a 35-year-old previously healthy man from Baltimore develops a sudden onset of malaise, fever, headache, retro-orbital pain, backache, and myalgias. On examination, his temperature is 39.6°C with normal blood pressure and slight tachycardia. He has some vesicular lesions on his palate and scleral injection. Laboratory studies are notable for a platelet count of 100,000/μL. All of the following are true regarding his illness EXCEPT:

A. A second infection could result in hemorrhagic fever.

B. After resolution, he has lifelong immunity.

C. IgM ELISA may be diagnostic.

D. In equatorial areas, year-round transmission occurs.

E. The disease is transmitted by mosquitoes.

IV-183. Which of the following fungi is considered dimorphic?

A. *Aspergillus fumigatus*

B. *Candida glabrata*

C. *Cryptococcus neoformans*

D. *Histoplasma capsulatum*

E. *Rhizopus* spp.

IV-184. All of the following antifungal medications are available in an oral form EXCEPT:

A. Caspofungin

B. Fluconazole

C. Griseofulvin

D. Itraconazole

E. Posaconazole

F. Terbinafine

IV-185. All of the following antifungal medications are approved for the treatment of *Candida albicans* fungemia EXCEPT:

A. Caspofungin

B. Fluconazole

C. Micafungin

D. Posaconazole

E. Voriconazole

IV-186. Clinically useful serum or urine diagnostic tests exist for all of the following invasive fungal infections EXCEPT:

A. Aspergillus

B. Blastomycosis

B. Coccidioidomycosis

C. Cryptococcosis

D. Histoplasmosis

IV-187. A 24-year-old female student at the Ohio State University is seen in the emergency department for shortness of breath and chest pain. She has no significant past medical history. Her only medication is an oral contraceptive. As a component of her evaluation, she receives a contrast-enhanced CT scan of the chest. Fortunately, there is no pulmonary embolism (she is diagnosed with viral pleuritis), but there are numerous lung, mediastinal, and splenic calcifications. Based on these findings, which of the following remote infections was most likely?

A. Blastomycosis

B. Coccidioidomycosis

C. Cryptococcosis

D. Histoplasmosis

E. Tuberculosis

IV-188. A 43-year-old woman with a history of rheumatoid arthritis is admitted to the hospital with respiratory failure. She was started on infliximab 2 months ago because of refractory disease. Before initiation of the medication, her physician found no evidence of latent tuberculosis infection. She reports 2 days of fever and worsening shortness of breath. On admission, she is hypotensive and hypoxemic with a chest radiograph showing bilateral interstitial and reticulonodular infiltrates. After administration of fluids, broad-spectrum antibiotics, intubation, and initiation of mechanical ventilation, a bronchoalveolar lavage is performed. A silver stain of the BAL fluid shows the organisms shown in Figure IV-188. Which of the following is the most likely causative organism?

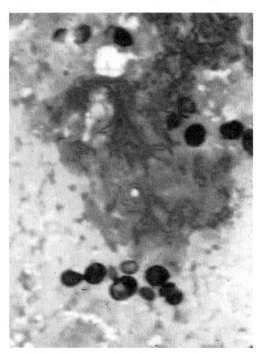

FIGURE IV-188 (see Color Atas)

A. *Aspergillus fumigatus*
B. Cytomegalovirus
C. *Histoplasma capsulatum*
D. *Mycobacteria avium* complex
E. Mycobacterial tuberculosis

IV-189. In the patient described above, which of the following therapies should be continued?

A. Caspofungin
B. Clarithromycin, rifampin, and ethambutol
C. Ganciclovir
D. INH, rifampin, PZA, and ethambutol
E. Liposomal amphotericin B

IV-190. A 24-year-old man is brought to the emergency department by his friends because of worsening mental status, confusion, and lethargy. He has been complaining of a severe headache for more than 1 week. The patient works as a migrant farm worker, most recently in the Fresno, California, area. He is originally from the Philippines and has been in the United States for 4 years with no medical

therapy. Vital signs include blood pressure of 95/45 mmHg, heart rate of 110 beats/min, respiratory rate of 22 breaths/min, oxygen saturation of 98%, and temperature of 101.1°F. He appears cachectic and is confused. There is minimal nuchal rigidity but notable photophobia. His CBC is notable for a WBC of 2000/μL (95% neutrophils) and a hemoglobin of 9 g/dL. An LP reveals a WBC count of 300/μL (90% lymphocytes), glucose of 10 mg/dL, and protein of 130 mg/dL. Silver stain of the CSF reveals large (30–100 μm) round structures measuring with thick walls containing small round spores and internal septations. Which of the following is the most appropriate therapy?

A. Caspofungin
B. Ceftriaxone plus vancomycin
C. Fluconazole
D. INH, rifampin, ethambutol, and pyrazinamide (PZA)
E. Penicillin G

IV-191. You are a physician for an undergraduate university health clinic in Arizona. You have evaluated three students with similar complaints of fever, malaise, diffuse arthralgias, cough without hemoptysis, and chest discomfort, and one of the patients has a skin rash on her upper neck consistent with erythema multiforme. Chest radiography is similar in all three, with hilar adenopathy and small pleural effusions. Her CBC is notable for eosinophilia. Upon further questioning, you learn that all three students are in the same archaeology class and participated in an excavation 1 week ago. Your leading diagnosis is:

A. Mononucleosis
B. Primary pulmonary aspergillosis
C. Primary pulmonary coccidioidomycosis
D. Primary pulmonary histoplasmosis
E. Streptococcal pneumonia

IV-192. A 62-year-old man returns from a vacation to Arizona with fever, pleurisy, and a nonproductive cough. All of the following factors on history and laboratory examination favor a diagnosis of pulmonary coccidioidomycosis rather than community-acquired pneumonia EXCEPT:

A. Eosinophilia
B. Erythema nodosum
C. Mediastinal lymphadenopathy on chest radiography
D. Positive *Coccidioides* complement fixation titer result
E. Travel limited to Northern Arizona (Grand Canyon area)

IV-193. In a patient with lung and skin lesions, a travel history to which of the following regions would be most compatible with the potential diagnosis of blastomycosis?

A. Brazil (Amazon River basin)
B. Malaysia
C. Northern Wisconsin
D. Southern Arizona
E. Western Washington state

IV-194. A 43-year-old man comes to the physician complaining of 1 month of low-grade fever, malaise, shortness of breath, and a growing skin lesion. He resides in the upper peninsula of Michigan and works as a landscaper. He avoids medical care as much as possible. He is on no medications and smokes 2 packs per day of cigarettes. Over the past month, he notices that his daily productive cough has worsened and the phlegm in dark yellow. He also reports that he has developed a number of skin lesions that start as a painful nodule and then over 1 week ulcerate and discharge pus (see Figure IV-194). His physical examination is notable for egophony and bronchial breath sounds in the right lower lobe, and approximately five to 10 ulcerating 4- to 8-cm skin lesions on the lower extremities consistent with the one shown in the figure. His chest radiograph shows right lower lobe consolidation with no pleural effusion and no evidence of hilar or mediastinal adenopathy. After obtaining sputum for cytology and culture and a biopsy of the skin lesion, which is the next most likely diagnostic or therapeutic intervention?

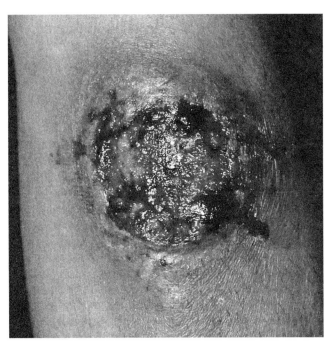

FIGURE IV-194 (see Color Atas) *(Used with permission from Elizabeth M. Spiers, MD.)*

A. Colonoscopy to evaluate for inflammatory bowel disease
B. INH, rifampin, PZA, and ethambutol
C. Itraconazole
D. PET scan to evaluate for metastatic malignant disease
E. Vancomycin

IV-195. A 34-year-old female aviary worker who has no significant past medical history, is taking no medications, has no allergies, and is HIV negative presents to the emergency department with fever, headache, and fatigue. She reports that her headache has been present for at least 2 weeks, is bilateral, and is worsened by bright lights and loud noises. She is typically an active person who has recently been fatigued and has lost 8 lb because of anorexia. Her work involves caring for birds and maintaining their habitat. Her vital signs are notable for a temperature of 101.8°F. The neurologic examination findings are normal except for notable photophobia. Head CT examination is normal. Lumbar puncture is significant for an opening pressure of 20 cmH$_2$O, white blood cell count of 15 cells/μL (90% monocytes), protein of 0.5 g/L (50 mg/mL), glucose of 2.8 mmol/L (50 mg/dL), and positive India ink stain. What is the appropriate therapy for this patient?

A. Amphotericin B for 2 weeks followed by lifelong fluconazole
B. Amphotericin B plus flucytosine for 2 weeks followed by oral fluconazole for 10 weeks
C. Caspofungin for 3 months
D. Ceftriaxone and vancomycin for 2 weeks
E. Voriconazole for 3 months

IV-196. An HIV-positive patient with a CD4 count of 110/μL who is not taking any medications presents to an urgent care center with complaints of a headache for the past week. He also notes nausea and intermittently blurred vision. Examination is notable for normal vital signs without fever but mild papilledema. Head CT does not show dilated ventricles. The definitive diagnostic test for this patient is:

A. Cerebrospinal fluid culture
B. MRI with gadolinium imaging
C. Ophthalmologic examination, including visual field testing
D. Serum cryptococcal antigen testing
E. Urine culture

IV-197. All of the following have been identified as a predisposing factor or condition associated with the development of hematogenously disseminated candidiasis EXCEPT:

A. Abdominal surgery
B. Indwelling vascular catheters
C. Hyperalimentation
D. Pulmonary alveolar proteinosis
E. Severe burns

IV-198. A 19-year-old young man is undergoing intensive chemotherapy for acute myelogenous leukemia. He has been neutropenic for more than 5 days and has been taking prophylactic meropenem and vancomycin for 3 days in addition to parenteral alimentation. His absolute neutrophil count yesterday was 50 cells/mm³, and today it is 200 cells/mm³. He had a fever spike to 101°F yesterday. A chest and abdomen CT at that time was unremarkable. You are asked to see him because over the past 3 hours, he has developed fever greater than 102°F, severe myalgias and joint pains, and new skin lesions (see Figure IV-198). New skin lesions are appearing in all body areas. Initially, they are red areas that become macronodular and are mildly painful. Vital signs are otherwise notable for a blood pressure of 100/60 mmHg and heart rate of 105 beats/min. An urgent biopsy of the skin lesion is most likely to show:

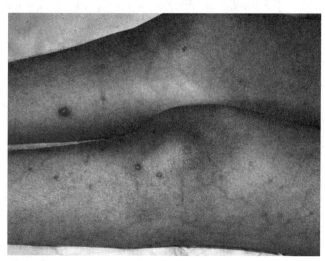

FIGURE IV-198 (see Color Atas)

A. Branching (45°) septated hyphae on methenamine silver stain
B. Budding yeast on methenamine silver stain
C. Encapsulated yeast on India ink stain
D. Pseudohyphae and hyphae on tissue Gram stain
E. Rounded internally septated spherules on methenamine silver stain

IV-199. In the patient described above, all of the following medications are appropriate additions to the current antibiotic regimen EXCEPT:

A. Amphotericin
B. Caspofungin
C. Fluconazole
D. Flucytosine
E. Voriconazole

IV-200. Which of the following statements regarding the use of antifungal agents to prevent *Candida* infections is true?

A. HIV-infected patients should receive prophylaxis for oropharyngeal candidiasis when CD4 count is below 200 cells/mm³.
B. Most centers administer fluconazole to recipients of allogeneic stem cell transplants.
C. Most centers administer fluconazole to recipients of living related renal transplants.
D. Voriconazole has been shown to be superior to other agents as prophylaxis in liver transplant recipients.
E. Widespread candida prophylaxis in postoperative patients in the SICU has been shown to be cost effective.

IV-201. *Candida albicans* is isolated from the following patients. Rate the likelihood in order from greatest to least that the positive culture represents true infection rather than contaminant or noninfectious colonization.

Patient X: A 63-year-old man admitted to the intensive care unit (ICU) with pneumonia who has recurrent fevers after receiving 5 days of levofloxacin for pneumonia. A urinalysis drawn from a Foley catheter shows positive leukocyte esterase, negative nitrite, 15 white blood cells/hpf, 10 red blood cells/hpf, and 10 epithelial cells/hpf. Urine culture grows *Candida albicans*.

Patient Y: A 38-year-old woman on hemodialysis presents with low-grade fevers and malaise. Peripheral blood cultures grow *C. albicans* in one of a total of three sets of blood cultures in the aerobic bottle only.

Patient Z: A 68-year-old man presents with a 2-day history of fever, productive cough, and malaise. Chest radiography reveals a left lower lobe infiltrate. A sputum Gram stain shows many PMNs, few epithelial cells, moderate gram-positive cocci in chains, and yeast consistent with *Candida* spp.

A. Patient X > patient Z > patient Y
B. Patient Y > patient Z > patient X
C. Patient Y > patient X > patient Z
D. Patient X > patient Y > patient Z
E. Patient Z > patient X > patient Y

IV-202. A 72-year-old man is admitted to the hospital with bacteremia and pyelonephritis. He is HIV-negative and has no other significant past medical history. Two weeks into his treatment with antibiotics, a fever evaluation reveals a blood culture positive for *Candida albicans*. Examination is unremarkable. White blood cell count is normal. The central venous catheter is removed, and systemic antifungal agents are initiated. What further evaluation is recommended?

A. Abdominal CT scan to evaluate for abscess
B. Chest radiography
C. Funduscopic examination
D. Repeat blood cultures
E. Transthoracic echocardiography

IV-203. A local oncology center is concerned about the occurrence of an outbreak of cases of invasive *Aspergillus* in patients receiving bone marrow transplants. Which of the following is the most likely source of *Aspergillus* infection?

A. Contaminated air source
B. Contaminated water source
C. Patient-to-patient spread in outpatient clinic waiting rooms
D. Provider-to-patient spread because of poor hand washing technique
E. Provider-to-patient spread because of poor utilization of alcohol disinfectant

IV-204. A 23-year-old man receiving chemotherapy for relapsed acute myelogenous leukemia has had persistent neutropenia for the past 4 weeks. Over the past 5 days, his absolute neutrophil count has risen from zero to 200 cells/mm^3, and he has had persistent fevers despite receiving cefepime and vancomycin empiric therapy. Other than fever, tachycardia, and malaise, he has no focal findings, and his vital signs are otherwise unremarkable, including a normal oxygen saturation on room air. A chest and abdomen CT performed because of the fever shows a few scattered 1- to 2-cm nodules with surrounding ground glass infiltrates in the lower lobes. Which of the following test results will most likely be positive in this patient?

A. Serum cryptococcal antigen
B. Serum galactomannan assay
C. Sputum fungal culture
D. Urine *Histoplasma* antigen
E. Urine *Legionella* antigen

IV-205. In the patient described above, which of the following medications should be initiated immediately?

A. Amphotericin B
B. Caspofungin
C. Fluconazole
D. Trimethoprim–sulfamethoxazole
E. Voriconazole

IV-206. A 40-year-old male smoker with a history of asthma is admitted to the inpatient medical service with fever, cough, brownish-green sputum, and malaise. Physical examination shows a respiratory rate of 15 breaths/min, no use of accessory muscles of breathing, and bilateral polyphonic wheezes throughout the lung fields. There is no clubbing or skin lesions. You consider a diagnosis of allergic bronchopulmonary aspergillosis. All the following clinical features are consistent with allergic bronchopulmonary aspergillosis EXCEPT:

A. Bilateral peripheral cavitary lung infiltrates
B. Elevated serum IgE
C. Peripheral eosinophilia
D. Positive serum antibodies to *Aspergillus* spp.
E. Positive skin testing for *Aspergillus* spp.

IV-207. A 26-year-old patient with asthma continues to have coughing fits and dyspnea despite numerous steroid tapers and frequent use of albuterol over the past few months. Persistent infiltrates are seen on chest radiography. A pulmonary consultation suggests an evaluation for allergic bronchopulmonary aspergillosis. Which of the following is the best diagnostic test for this diagnosis?

A. Bronchoalveolar lavage (BAL) with fungal culture
B. Galactomannan enzyme immunoassay (EIA)
C. High-resolution CT
D. Pulmonary function tests
E. Serum IgE level

IV-208. Patients with which of the following have the lowest risk of invasive pulmonary *Aspergillus* infection?

A. Allogeneic stem cell transplant with graft-versus-host disease
B. HIV infection
C. Long-standing high-dose glucocorticoids
D. Post-solid organ transplant with multiple episodes of rejection
E. Relapsed or uncontrolled leukemia

IV-209. Patients with all of the following conditions have increased risk of developing mucormycosis EXCEPT:

A. Deferoxamine therapy
B. Factitious hypoglycemia
C. Glucocorticoid therapy
D. Metabolic acidosis
E. Neutropenia

IV-210. A 36-year-old woman with a history of diabetes mellitus, hypertension, and chronic renal insufficiency reports comes to the emergency department complaining of double vision for 1 day. She is on chronic hemodialysis and missed her last appointment. She also notes 12 hours of facial swelling and difficulty speaking. Her vital signs are notable for a temperature of 39.0°C and blood pressure 155/95 mmHg. Her facial examination is shown in Figure IV-210. Laboratory examination reveals a white blood cell count of 15,000/μL, serum glucose of 205 mg/dL, serum creatinine of 6.3 mg/dL, and hemoglobin A1c of 9.7%. Arterial blood gas on room air is pH of 7.24, PCO_2 of 20 mmHg, and PO_2 of 100 mmHg. Needle biopsy of a retro-orbital mass reveals wide, thick–walled, ribbon-shaped nonseptate hyphal organisms that branch at 90 degrees with tissue and vascular invasion on PAS stain. All of the following are components of the initial therapy EXCEPT:

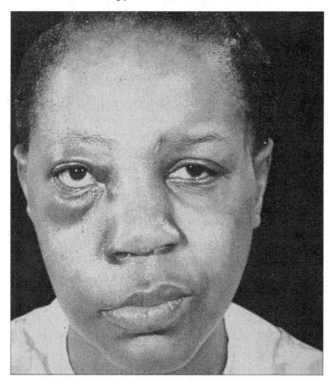

FIGURE IV-210 (see Color Atas)

A. Hemodialysis
B. Insulin
C. Liposomal amphotericin B
D. Surgical debridement
E. Voriconazole

IV-211. Which of the following is the most common form of infection in patients with mucormycosis?

A. Cutaneous
B. Gastrointestinal
C. Hematogenous dissemination
D. Pulmonary
E. Rhinocerebral

IV-212. A 21-year-old college student seeks your opinion because of a lesion on his head. He has no significant medical history and reports a solitary lesion on the crown of his head for more than month that has been growing slowly. He has had no fever and reports that although the area is itchy, he feels well. On examination, you note a 3-cm round area of alopecia without redness, pain, or inflammation. It is well demarcated with central clearing, scaling, and broken hair shafts at the edges. There is no redness or pain. Which of the following should you recommend?

A. Caspofungin
B. Clindamycin
C. Doxycycline
D. Minoxidil
E. Terbinafine

IV-213. A 68-year-old woman seeks evaluation for an ulcerative lesion on her right hand. She reports that the area on the back of her right hand was initially red and not painful. There appeared to be a puncture wound in the center of the area, and she thought she had a simple scratch acquired while gardening. Over the next several days, the lesion became verrucous and ulcerated. Now the patient has noticed several nodular areas along the arm, one of which ulcerated and began draining a serous fluid today. She is also noted to have an enlarged and tender epitrochlear lymph node on the right arm. A biopsy of the edge of the lesion shows ovoid and cigar-shaped yeasts. Sporotrichosis is diagnosed. What is the most appropriate therapy for this patient?

A. Amphotericin B intravenously
B. Caspofungin intravenously
C. Clotrimazole topically
D. Itraconazole orally
E. Selenium sulfide topically

IV-214. A 35-year-old woman with long-standing rheumatoid arthritis has been treated with infliximab for the past 6 months with improvement of her joint disease. She has a history of positive PPD and takes INH prophylaxis. For the past week, she reports worsening dyspnea on exertion with low-grade fevers and a nonproductive cough. On examination, her vital signs are notable for normal blood pressure, temperature of 38.0°C, heart rate of 105 beats/min, respiratory rate of 22 breaths/min, and SaO_2 of 91% on room air. Her lungs are clear. Within one flight of steps, she becomes dyspneic, and her SaO_2 falls to 80%. A chest CT scan is shown in Figure IV-214. Which of the following is the most likely diagnosis?

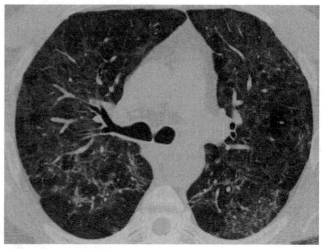

FIGURE IV-214

A. *Aspergillus fumigatus* pneumonia
B. *Nocardia asteroides* pneumonia
C. *Pneumocystis jiroveci* pneumonia
D. Rheumatoid nodules
E. Staphylococcal bacteremia and septic pulmonary emboli

IV-215. Which of the following patients should receive prophylaxis against *Pneumocystis jiroveci* pneumonia?

A. A 19-year-old woman with acute myelogenous leukemia initiating induction chemotherapy
B. A 24-year-old man with HIV initiated on HAART therapy 9 months ago when his CD4 count was 100/μL and now has a CD4 count of 500/μL for the past 4 months
C. A 36-year-old man with newly diagnosed HIV and a CD4 count of 300/μL
D. A 42-year-old woman with rheumatoid arthritis who recovered from an episode of *Pneumocystis* pneumonia while taking infliximab who is now initiating therapy with abatacept
E. A 56-year-old man with COPD receiving prednisone for an acute exacerbation

IV-216. A 45-year-old woman with known HIV infection and medical nonadherence to therapy is admitted to the hospital with 2 to 3 weeks of increasing dyspnea on exertion and malaise. A chest radiograph shows bilateral alveolar infiltrates, and induced sputum is positive for *Pneumocystis jiroveci*. Which of the following clinical conditions is an indication for administration of adjunct glucocorticoids?

A. Acute respiratory distress syndrome
B. CD4+ lymphocyte count <100/μL
C. No clinical improvement 5 days into therapy
D. Pneumothorax
E. Room air PaO_2 <70 mmHg

IV-217. All of the following statements regarding the drug mefloquine are true EXCEPT:

A. Dose adjustment is necessary in patients with renal insufficiency.
B. It is only available in oral form.
C. It is the preferred drug for prophylaxis of chloroquine-resistant malaria.
D. It should not be administered concurrently with halofantrine.
E. Psychiatric side effects limit it use in certain patients.

IV-218. A 45-year-old migrant worker originally from Mexico is evaluated for right upper quadrant pain, fever, and hepatic tenderness. He reports no diarrhea or bloody stool. He is found to have a large hepatic abscess on CT scan of the abdomen. Of note, he has been in the United States for approximately 10 years and was well until approximately 10 days ago. Which of the following tests can be used to confirm the diagnosis?

A. Examination of stool for trophozoites
B. Liver biopsy
C. PCR of stool for *Campylobacter* spp.
D. Response to empiric trial of iodoquinol
E. Serologic test for antibody to *E. histolytica*

IV-219. A 23-year-old woman is seen in the emergency department for fever and altered mental status. She is from Tanzania and arrived in the United States earlier that day. She reported 3 days of episodic fever before leaving home. Over the course of the day, her family describes deteriorating mental status. Now she is confused and lethargic. Her physical examination is notable for a temperature of 40°C, heart rate of 145 beats/min, and systemic blood pressure of 105/62 mmHg. She has a clearly gravid uterus, approximately 24 weeks of gestational age, and a neurologic examination shows confusion but no focal findings. A thick and thin smear are shown in Figure IV-219. Treatment with IV quinidine is started immediately. Which of the followings are potential complications of this therapy?

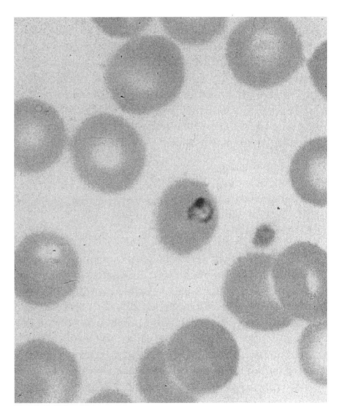

FIGURE IV-219 (see Color Atas)

A. Hyperthyroidism
B. Hypoglycemia
C. Nightmares
D. Retinopathy
E. Seizures

IV-220. A 20-year-old man is seen in the university walk-in health clinic for evaluation of recurrent fever. He reports fever greater than 101°F lasting less than a day occurring approximately weekly for the past 3 weeks. He feels otherwise relatively poorly with diffuse myalgias and headache that are much worse during the febrile episodes. Of note, he returned recently from a mission trip to Central America and reports not taking malaria prophylaxis. Examination of the peripheral smear confirms the diagnosis of *Plasmodium vivax*. If present, which of the following findings indicates that the patient has severe malaria and is not a candidate for outpatient therapy?

A. Fever >40°C
B. One seizure last week
C. Parasitemia of >5% affected erythrocytes on peripheral smear
D. Serum bilirubin level of >2 mg/dL
E. The presence of headache

IV-221. A 51-year-old woman is diagnosed with *Plasmodium falciparum* malaria after returning from a safari in Tanzania. Her parasitemia is 6%, hematocrit is 21%, bilirubin is 7.8 mg/dL, and creatinine is 2.7 mg/dL. She is still making 60 mL/hr of urine. She rapidly becomes obtunded. Intensive care is initiated with frequent creatinine checks, close monitoring for hypoglycemia, infusion of phenobarbital for seizure prevention, mechanical ventilation for airway protection, and exchange transfusion to address her high parasitemia. Which of the following regimens is recommended as first-line treatment for her malarial infection?

A. Chloroquine
B. Intravenous artesunate
C. Intravenous quinine
D. Intravenous quinidine
E. Mefloquine

IV-222. A 28-year-old woman presents with fevers, headache, diaphoresis, and abdominal pain 2 days after returning from an aid mission to the coast of Papua New Guinea. Several of her fellow aid workers developed malaria while abroad, and she stopped her doxycycline prophylaxis because of a photosensitivity reaction 5 days earlier. You send blood cultures, routine labs, and a thick and thin smear to evaluate the source of her fevers. Which of the following statements is accurate in reference to diagnosis of malaria?

A. A thick smear is performed to increase sensitivity compared with a thin smear but can only be performed in centers with experienced laboratory personnel and has a longer processing time.
B. Careful analysis of the thin blood film allows for prognostication based on estimation of parasitemia and morphology of the erythrocytes.
C. In the absence of rapid diagnostic information, empirical treatment for malaria should be strongly considered.
D. Morphology on blood smear is the current criterion used to differentiate the four species of *Plasmodium* that infect humans.
E. All of the above are true.

IV-223. A 19-year-old college student is employed during the summer months on Nantucket Island in Massachusetts. She is evaluated in the local emergency department with 5 days of fever, malaise, and generalized weakness. Although she does recall a tick bite approximately 6 weeks ago, she denies rash around that time or presently. Physical examination is unremarkable with the exception of a temperature of 39.3°C. Which of the following statements is true regarding her most likely illness?

A. *B. duncani* is the most likely organism to be found in her peripheral blood smear.
B. First-line therapy for severe disease in this patient is immediate complete RBC exchange transfusion in addition to clindamycin and quinine.
C. If babesiosis is not demonstrated on thick or thin preparations of peripheral blood, PCR amplification of babesial 18S rRNA is recommended.
D. The ring form of *B. microti* seen in red blood cells on microscopy is indistinguishable from *Plasmodium falciparum*.
E. Without a current or historical rash, she is unlikely to have babesiosis.

IV-224. A 35-year-old man from India is seen for evaluation of several weeks of fever that has decreased in intensity, but he now has developed abdominal swelling. He has no significant past medical history. Physical examination shows palpable splenomegaly and hepatomegaly and diffuse lymphadenopathy. Diffuse hyperpigmentation is present in his skin. Visceral leishmaniasis is suspected. Which of the following diagnostic techniques is most commonly used?

A. Culture of peripheral blood for *Leishmania* spp.
B. PCR for *L. infantum* nucleic acid in peripheral blood
C. Rapid immunochromatographic test for recombinant antigen rK39 from *L. infantum*
D. Smear of stool for amastigotes
E. Splenic aspiration to demonstrate amastigotes

IV-225. All of the following statements regarding infection with *Trypanosoma cruzi* are true EXCEPT:

A. It is found only in the Americas.
B. It is the causative agent of Chagas disease.
C. It is transmitted to humans by the bite of deer flies.
D. It may be transmitted to humans by blood transfusion.
E. It may cause acute and chronic disease.

IV-226. A 36-year-old man is admitted to the hospital with 3 months of worsening dyspnea on exertion and orthopnea. Over the past 2 weeks, he has been sleeping upright. He denies any chest pain with exertion or syncope. There is no history of hypertension, hyperlipidemia, or diabetes. He is a lifelong nonsmoker and since arriving to the United States from rural Mexico 16 years ago works as an electrician. His physical examination is notable for being afebrile with a heart rate 105 beats/min, blood pressure of 100/80 mmHg, respiratory rate of 22 breaths/min, and oxygen saturation of 88% on room air. He has notable jugular venous distension upright with no Kussmaul sign,

3+ pitting edema to the knees, and bilateral crackles two-thirds up the lung fields. Cardiac examination shows a laterally displaced PMI, a 2/6 systolic murmur at the apex and axilla, an S3, and no friction rub or pericardial knock. Which of the following is likely to reveal the most likely diagnosis?

A. Coronary angiography
B. Right heart catheterization
C. Serum PCR for *T. cruzi* DNA
D. Serum *T. cruzi* IgG antibodies
E. Serum troponin

IV-227. A 36-year-old medical missionary recently returned from a 2-week trip to rural Honduras. During the trip, she lived in the jungle, where she received multiple bug bites and developed open sores. One week after her return, she comes to the clinic reporting 2 days of malaise, fever to 38.5°C, and anorexia. There is an indurated swollen area of erythema on her calf and femoral adenopathy. Because of her exposure history, you obtain a thin and thick blood smear that demonstrates organisms consistent with *T. cruzi*. Which of the following is the best next intervention?

A. Immediate therapy with benznidazole
B. Immediate therapy with primaquine
C. Immediate therapy with voriconazole
D. Observation only
E. Serologic confirmation with specific *T. cruzi* IgG testing

IV-228. A 44-year-old man who recently returned from a safari trip to Uganda seeks attention for a painful lesion on the leg and new fevers. He was on a safari tour, where he stayed in the animal park that was populated extensively with antelope, lions, giraffes, and hippos. They often toured savannah and jungle settings. He returned within the past week and noticed a painful lesion on his neck at the site of some bug bites. He reports fever over 38°C, and you find palpable cervical lymphadenopathy. Review of systems is notable for malaise and anorexia for 2 days. A thick and thin smear of the blood reveals protozoa consistent with trypanosomes. All of the following are true about his disease EXCEPT:

A. Humans are the primary reservoir.
B. If untreated, death is likely.
C. It was transmitted by the bite of a tsetse fly.
D. Lumbar puncture should be performed.
E. Suramin is effective treatment.

IV-229. A 36-year-old man with HIV/AIDS is brought to the hospital after a grand mal seizure at home. He has a history of ongoing IV drug use and is not taking HAART. His last CD4 T-cell count was below 50/μL more than 1 month ago. Further medical history is unavailable. Vital signs are normal. On examination, he is barely arousable and disoriented. He is cachectic. There is no nuchal rigidity or focal motor deficits. Serum creatinine is normal. An urgent head MRI with gadolinium is performed, and the results of the T1-gated images are shown in Figure IV-229. Which of the following will be the most effective therapy?

A. Caspofungin
B. INH, rifampin, PZA, and ethambutol
C. Pyrimethamine plus sulfadiazine
D. Streptokinase
E. Voriconazole

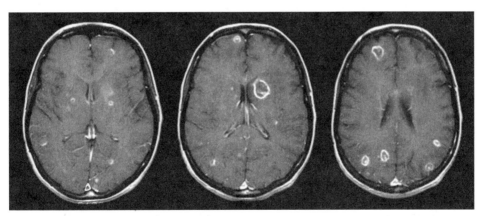

FIGURE IV-229

IV-230. Which of the following intestinal protozoal infections can be diagnosed with stool ova and parasite examination?

A. *Cryptosporidium* spp.
B. *Cyclospora* spp.
C. *Giardia* spp.
D. *Isospora* spp.
E. *Microsporidia* spp.
F. All of the above

IV-231. A 17-year-old woman presents to the clinic complaining of vaginal itchiness and malodorous discharge. She is sexually active with multiple partners, and she is interested in getting tested for sexually transmitted diseases. A wet-mount microscopic examination is performed, and trichomonal parasites are identified. Which of the following statements regarding trichomoniasis is true?

A. A majority of women are asymptomatic.
B. No treatment is necessary because the disease is self-limited.
C. The patient's sexual partner need not be treated.
D. Trichomoniasis can only be spread sexually.
E. Trichomoniasis is 100% sensitive to metronidazole

IV-232. A 19-year-old college student presents to the emergency department with crampy abdominal pain and watery diarrhea that has worsened over 3 days. He recently returned from a volunteer trip to Mexico. He has no past medical history and felt well throughout the trip. Stool examination shows small cysts containing four nuclei, and stool antigen immunoassay is positive for *Giardia* spp. Which of the following is a recommend treatment regimen for this patient?

A. Albendazole
B. Clindamycin
C. Giardiasis is self-limited and requires no antibiotic therapy
D. Paromomycin
E. Tinidazole

IV-233. A 28-year-old woman is brought to the hospital because of abdominal pain, weight loss, and dehydration. She has been diagnosed with HIV/AIDS for the past 2 years with a history of oral candidiasis and pneumocystis pneumonia. She reports voluminous watery diarrhea over the past 2 weeks. Because of medical nonadherance, she has not taken any antiretroviral therapy. Routine stool ova and parasite examination is normal, but stool antigen testing reveals *Cryptosporidium* spp. Which of the following is the recommended therapy?

A. Metronidazole
B. Nitazoxanide
C. No therapy recommended because the diarrhea is self-limited.
D. No effective specific therapy is available.
E. Tinidazole

IV-234. Which of the following has resulted in a significant decrease in the incidence of trichinellosis in the United States?

A. Adequate therapy that allows for eradication of infection in index cases before person-to-person spread can occur
B. Earlier diagnosis because of a new culture assay
C. Federal laws limiting the import of foreign cattle
D. Laws prohibiting the feeding of uncooked garbage to pigs
E. Requirements for handwashing by commercial kitchen staff who handle raw meat

IV-235. A patient comes into the clinic and describes progressive muscle weakness over several weeks. He has also experienced nausea, vomiting, and diarrhea. One month ago, he had been completely healthy and describes a bear hunting trip in Alaska, where they ate some of the game they killed. Soon after he returned, his gastrointestinal symptoms began followed by muscle weakness in his jaw and neck that has now spread to his arms and lower back. Examination confirms decreased muscle strength in the upper extremities and neck. He also has slowed extraocular movements. Laboratory examination shows panic values for elevated eosinophils and serum creatine phosphokinase. Which of the following organisms is most likely the cause of his symptoms?

A. *Campylobacter* spp.
B. Cytomegalovirus
C. *Giardia* spp.
D. *Taenia solium*
E. *Trichinella* spp.

IV-236. A 3-year-old boy is brought by his parents to the clinic. They state that he has experienced fevers, anorexia, weight loss, and most recently has started wheezing at night. He had been completely healthy until these symptoms started 2 months ago. The family had travelled through Europe several months earlier and reported no unusual exposures or exotic foods. They have a puppy at home. On examination, the child is ill-appearing and is noted to have hepatosplenomegaly. Laboratory results show a panic value of 82% eosinophils. Total white blood cells are elevated. A complete blood count is repeated to rule out a laboratory error, and eosinophils are 78%. Which of the following is the most likely organism or process?

A. *Cysticercus* spp.
B. Giardiasis
C. *Staphylococcus lugdunensis*
D. Toxocariasis
E. Trichinellosis

IV-237. The patient described above continues to decline over the next 2 to 3 days, developing worsening respiratory status, orthopnea, and cough. On physical examination, his heart rate is 120 beats/min, blood pressure is 95/80 mmHg, respiratory rate is 24 breaths/min, and oxygen saturation is 88% on room air. His neck veins are elevated, there is an apical S3, and his lungs have bilateral crackles halfway up the lung fields. An echocardiogram shows an ejection fraction of 25%. Which of the following therapies should be initiated?

A. Albendazole
B. Methylprednisolone
C. Metronidazole
D. Praziquantel
E. Vancomycin

IV-238. A 28-year-old man is brought to the emergency department by his wife for altered mental status, fevers, vomiting, and headache. He developed a bilateral headache began about 1 day ago that has progressively worsened. He and his wife returned from a trip to Thailand and Vietnam, where they spent a lot of time in rural settings eating local mollusks, seafood, and vegetables. His physical examination is notable for fever, nuchal rigidity, confusion, and lethargy. Lumbar puncture reveals elevated opening pressure; elevated protein; normal glucose; and white blood cell count of 200/μL with 50% eosinophils, 25% neutrophils, and 25% lymphocytes. Which of the following is the most likely etiology of his meningitis?

A. *Angiostrongylus cantonensis*
B. *Gnathostoma spinigerum*
C. *Trichinella murrelli*
D. *Trichinella nativa*
E. *Toxocara canis*

IV-239. While attending the University of Georgia, a group of friends go on a 5-day canoeing and camping trip in rural southern Georgia. A few weeks later, one of the campers develops a serpiginous, raised, pruritic, erythematous eruption on the buttocks. *Strongyloides* larvae are found in his stool. Three of his companions, who are asymptomatic, are also found to have *Strongyloides* larvae in their stool. Which of the following is indicated in the asymptomatic carriers?

A. Fluconazole
B. Ivermectin
C. Mebendazole
D. Mefloquine
E. Treatment only for symptomatic illness

IV-240. All of the following are clinical manifestations of *Ascaris lumbricoides* infection EXCEPT:

A. Asymptomatic carriage
B. Fever, headache, photophobia, nuchal rigidity, and eosinophilia
C. Nonproductive cough and pleurisy with eosinophilia
D. Right upper quadrant pain and fever
E. Small bowel obstruction

IV-241. A 21-year-old college student in Mississippi comes to student health to ask advice about treatment for ascaris infection. He is an education major and works 1 day a week in an elementary school, where a number of the students were recently diagnosed with ascariasis over the past 3 months. He feels well and reports being asymptomatic. A stool O&P reveals characteristic ascaris eggs. Which of the following should you recommend?

A. Albendazole
B. Diethylcarbamazine (DEC)
C. Fluconazole
D. Metronidazole
E. Vancomycin

IV-242. A 38-year-old woman presents to the emergency department with severe abdominal pain. She has no past medical or surgical history. She recalls no recent history of abdominal discomfort, diarrhea, melena, bright red blood per rectum, nausea, or vomiting before this acute episode. She ate ceviche (lime-marinated raw fish) at a Peruvian restaurant 3 hours before presentation. On examination, she is in terrible distress and has dry heaves. Her temperature is 37.6°C, heart rate is 128 beats/min, and blood pressure is 174/92 mmHg. Examination is notable for an extremely tender abdomen with guarding and rebound tenderness. Bowel sounds are present and hyperactive. Rectal examination findings are normal, and Guaiac test result is negative. The pelvic examination is unremarkable. The white blood cell count is 6738/μL and hematocrit is 42%. A complete metabolic panel and lipase and amylase levels are all within normal limits. CT of the abdomen shows no abnormality. What is the next step in her management?

A. CT angiogram of the abdomen
B. Pelvic ultrasonography
C. Proton pump inhibitor therapy and observation
D. Right upper quadrant ultrasonography
E. Upper endoscopy

IV-243. While participating in a medical missionary visit to Indonesia, you are asked to see a 22-year-old man with new onset of high fever, groin pain, and a swollen scrotum. His symptoms have been present for about 1 week and worsening steadily. His temperature is 38.8°C, and his examination is notable for tender inguinal lymphadenopathy, scrotal swelling with a hydrocele, and lymphatic streaking. All of the following may be useful in diagnosing his condition EXCEPT:

A. Examination of blood
B. Examination of hydrocele fluid
C. Scrotal ultrasonography
D. Serum ELISA
E. Stool O&P

IV-244. The patient described above should be treated with which of the following medications?

A. Albendazole
B. Diethylcarbamazine (DEC)
C. Doxycycline
D. Ivermectin
E. Praziquantel

IV-245. A 45-year-old woman is brought to the Emergency department by her daughter because she saw something moving in her mother's eye. The patient is visiting from Zaire, where she lives in the rain forest. The patient reports some occasional eye swelling and redness. On examination, you find a worm in the subconjunctiva (Figure IV-245). Which of the following medications is indicated for therapy?

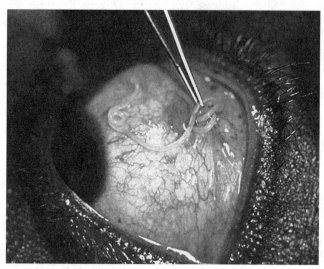

FIGURE IV-245 (see Color Atlas)

A. Albendazole
B. Diethylcarbazine (DEC)
C. Ivermectin
D. Terbinafine
E. Voriconazole

IV-246. All of the following statements regarding the epidemiology of schistosomal infection are true EXCEPT:

A. *S. haematobium* infection is seen mostly in South America.
B. *S. japonicum* infection is seen mostly in China, Philippines, and Indonesia.
C. *S. mansoni* infection is seen in Africa, South America, and the Middle East.
D. Schistosomal infection causes acute and chronic manifestations.
E. Transmission of all human schistosomal infections is from snails.

IV-247. A 48-year-old female presents to her physician with a 2-day history of fever, arthralgias, diarrhea, and headache. She recently returned from an ecotour in tropical sub-Saharan Africa, where she went swimming in inland rivers. Notable findings on physical examination include a temperature of 38.7°C (101.7°F); 2-cm tender mobile lymph nodes in the axilla, cervical, and femoral regions; and a palpable spleen. Her white blood cell count is 15,000/μL with 50% eosinophils. She should receive treatments with which of the following medications?

A. Chloroquine
B. Mebendazole
C. Metronidazole
D. Praziquantel
E. Thiabendazole

IV-248. A person with liver disease caused by *Schistosoma mansoni* would be most likely to have what condition?

A. Ascites
B. Esophageal varices
C. Gynecomastia
D. Jaundice
E. Spider nevi

IV-249. A 26-year-old man is brought to the emergency department after the onset of a grand mal seizure. On arrival to the hospital, the seizure had terminated, and he was somnolent without focal findings. Vital signs were normal except for tachycardia. The patient has no known medical history and no history of illicit drug or alcohol use. He takes no medications. At a routine clinic visit 3 months earlier, he was documented to be HIV antibody and PPD negative. He is originally from rural Guatemala and has been in the United States working as a laborer for the past 3 years. A contrast CT shows multiple parenchymal lesions in both hemispheres that are identical to the one shown in the posterior right brain (Figure IV-249). After acute stabilization, including anticonvulsant therapy, which of the following is the most appropriate next step in this patient's management?

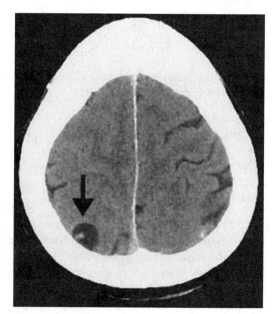

FIGURE IV-249

A. Echocardiogram with Doppler examination of aortic and mitral valves
B. Initiation of praziquantel therapy
C. Initiation of pyrimethamine and sulfadiazine therapy
D. Measurement of HIV viral load
E. Neurosurgical consultation for brain biopsy

IV-250. A 44-year-old woman presents to the emergency department with recurrent episodes of right upper quadrant pain, typically soon after meals. These episodes have been present for at least 1 month and seem to be worsening. The patient emigrated from Lebanon more than 20 years ago and works as an attorney. She takes no medications and is physically active. On examination, she is jaundiced and in obvious discomfort because of right upper quadrant pain. She is afebrile and tachycardic. Her physical examination is notable for an enlarged liver. Ultrasound examination confirms the large liver and demonstrates a complex 14-cm cyst with daughter cysts extending to the liver edge with associated biliary tract dilation. Which of the following is the most appropriate management approach to this patient?

A. Albendazole medical therapy
B. Albendazole followed by surgical resection
C. Needle biopsy of the cystic lesion
D. PAIR (percutaneous aspiration, infusion of scolicidal agent, and reaspiration)
E. Serologic testing for *E. granulosus*

ANSWERS

IV-1. **The answer is B.** *(Chap. 119)* Deficiencies in the complement system predispose patients to a variety of infections. Most of these deficits are congenital. Patients with sickle cell disease have acquired functional defects in the alternative complement pathway. They are at risk of infection from *Streptococcus pneumoniae* and *Salmonella* spp. Patients with liver disease, nephrotic syndrome, and systemic lupus erythematosus may have defects in C3. They are at particular risk for infections with *Staphylococcus aureus, S. pneumoniae, Pseudomonas* spp., and *Proteus* spp. Patients with congenital or acquired (usually systemic lupus erythematosus) deficiencies in the terminal complement cascade (C5-8) are at particular risk of infection from *Neisseria* spp. such as *N. meningitis* or *N. gonorrhoeae*.

IV-2. **The answer is A.** *(Chap. 121)* Choosing the appropriate empiric coverage for patients with severe sepsis is important for improving outcomes. This patient has undergone splenectomy in the distant past and is at 58 times greater risk for overwhelming bacterial sepsis than the normal population. The risk is greatest in the first 2 years after splenectomy but persists across the entire lifetime. The most common organisms causing severe sepsis in asplenic patients are encapsulated bacteria, especially *Streptococcus pneumoniae, Neisseria meningitidis*, and *Haemophilus influenzae*. *S. pneumoniae* causes 50% to 70% of severe sepsis in asplenic patients. The recommended empiric antibiotics in asplenic patients with sepsis are ceftriaxone 2 g IV every 12 hours and vancomycin 1 g IV every 12 hours.

IV-3. **The answer is C.** *(Chap. 121)* Necrotizing fasciitis is a life-threatening infection that leads to extensive necrosis of the subcutaneous tissue and fascia. It is most commonly caused by group A streptococci and a mixed facultative and anaerobic flora. Recently, there have been an increasing number of cases of necrotizing fasciitis caused by community-acquired methicillin-resistant *Staphylococcus aureus*. Risk factors include diabetes mellitus, intravenous drug use, and peripheral vascular disease. The infection often arises at a site of minimal trauma, and the physical findings initially are minimal compared with the severity of pain and fever. The mortality rate for necrotizing fasciitis is between 15% and 34% but rises to as high as 70% if toxic shock syndrome is present. Wide surgical debridement of the affected tissue is necessary, and without surgery, the mortality rate is near 100%. A high index of clinical suspicion is important for selecting the appropriate antibiotic therapy and early consultation of surgery. The initial antibiotics should cover the typical organisms and include vancomycin 1 g IV every 12 hours, clindamycin 600 mg IV every 6–8 hours, and gentamicin 5 mg/kg/day intravenously.

IV-4. **The answer is B.** *(Chap. 121)* Cat bites are the most likely animal bites to lead to cellulitis because of deep inoculation and the frequent presence of *Pasteurella multicoda*. In an immunocompetent host, only cat bites warrant empirical antibiotics. Often the first dose is given parenterally. Ampicillin–sulbactam followed by oral amoxicillin–clavulanate is effective empirical therapy for cat bites. However, in an asplenic patient, a dog bite can lead to rapid overwhelming sepsis as a result of *Capnocytophaga canimorsus* bacteremia. These patients should be followed closely and given third-generation cephalosporins early in the course of infection. Empirical therapy should also be considered for dog bites in elderly adults, for deep bites, and for bites on the hand.

IV-5. **The answer is A.** *(Chap. 122)* Immunization programs have the goals to control, eliminate, and eradicate disease. *Disease control* refers to decreases the impact of a specific illness on both health-related and societal outcomes. Examples of vaccinations that have lead to improved control of disease include the pneumococcal and influenza vaccines. Elimination can have two meanings. The first definition is to have zero cases in a defined geographic area. A second meaning is to reduce or eliminate the indigenous sustained transmission of an infection in a specific geographic area. In 2010, vaccine programs had eliminated measles, rubella, poliomyelitis, and diphtheria in the United States, although increasing numbers of cases of measles have been reported is some parts of the United States because of incomplete vaccination in children. Disease eradication is the most difficult goal to achieve. A disease can be considered eradicated when its elimination can be sustained without ongoing interventions. The only disease that has been globally eradicated at this point is smallpox. Poliomyelitis has been eradicated in most of the world although Afghanistan, Pakistan, India, and Nigeria continue to have ongoing transmission of the disease.

IV-6. **The answer is B.** *(Chap. 122)* Pneumococcal vaccination has been recommended for all individuals at any age with a variety of chronic medical conditions, including chronic respiratory disease, chronic heart disease, chronic liver failure, diabetes mellitus, asplenia, and chronic kidney disease. Determining when to revaccinate individuals has been somewhat controversial. The current recommendations are to revaccinate individuals ages 19 to 64 5 years after the initial vaccine if they have chronic renal failure or nephrotic syndrome, asplenia, or other immunocompromising conditions. All other individuals should receive a one-time revaccination at age 65 years and older if they were vaccinated 5 or more years previously and younger than 65 years old at the time of original vaccination.

IV-7. **The answer is C.** *(Chap. 122)* The varicella-zoster vaccine is a live virus vaccine that was recently introduced for prevention of shingles in older adults. The current recommendation is all adults older than 60 years be offered the zoster vaccine regardless of whether they report a childhood history of chickenpox. As this is a live virus vaccine, it cannot be administered to anyone who has severe immunodeficiency. Specific recommendations for whom the zoster vaccine is contraindicated include:

1. Pregnancy

2. Anyone younger than 60 years

3. Patients with leukemia, lymphoma, or other malignant neoplasms affecting the bone marrow. If a patient is in remission and has not received chemotherapy or radiation therapy within 3 months, the vaccine can be given.

4. Individuals with AIDS or HIV with a CD4+ count <200/μL or ≤15% peripheral lymphocytes

5. Individuals taking immunosuppressive therapy equivalent to prednisone ≥20 mg/day, methotrexate 0.4 mg/kg/wk, or azathioprine <3 mg/kg/day

6. Anyone with suspected cellular immunodeficiency (e.g., hypogammaglobulinemia)

7. Individuals receiving a hematopoietic stem cell transplant

8. Individuals receiving recombinant human immune mediators or modulators, especially antitumor necrosis factor agents

IV-8. **The answer is E.** *(Chap. 122)* Live-attenuated viruses are generally contraindicated as vaccines for immunocompromised hosts for fear of vaccine-induced disease. The most cited example of this is smallpox vaccine resulting in disseminated vaccinia infection. However, yellow fever vaccine is another example of a live virus vaccine. The other examples listed in this example are inactivated organisms (rabies, IM typhoid) or polysaccharide (meningococcal) and are therefore noninfectious. Oral typhoid vaccine is a live-attenuated strain, so the IM form is likely preferable in this host. Malaria prophylaxis currently involves chemoprophylaxis rather than vaccination. Although safe from an infectious standpoint, potential interactions with cyclosporine should be monitored.

IV-9. **The answer is E.** *(Chap. 122)* In recent years, rabies virus has been most frequently transmitted by bats in the United States. Usually a bite is noted but not always. Therefore, patients who have unexpected, unmonitored (i.e., while they are asleep) close contact with bats should be told to seek medical attention and likely vaccination. A bite is a clear indication for the most effective immunization strategy involving both active (inactivated virus vaccine) and passive (human rabies immunoglobulins) immune activation unless the offending bat is captured and found to be rabies negative with further testing. The vaccination schedule for nonimmunes is intensive, with doses at 0, 3, 7, 14, and 28 days. Although there has been at least one report of successful antiviral treatment of rabies, there is no indication for prophylactic antiviral therapy.

IV-10. **The answer is E.** *(Chap. 123)* When traveling abroad, it is important to plan ahead and consider the potential infectious agents to which one might be exposed. The Centers for Disease Control and Prevention and the World Health Organization publish guidelines for recommended vaccinations before travel to countries around the world. Before travel, it is certainly recommended that an individual be up to date on all routine vaccinations, including measles, diphtheria, and polio. Influenza is perhaps the most common preventable illness in travelers, and the influenza vaccine should be administered per routine guidelines. There are, however, very few required vaccinations in most countries. Yellow fever is one exception, and proof of vaccination is required by many countries in sub-Saharan Africa and equatorial South America. This is especially important for individuals traveling from areas where yellow fever is endemic or epidemic. The only other required vaccinations are meningococcal meningitis and influenza vaccination to travel in Saudi Arabia during the Hajj.

IV-11. **The answer is E.** *(Chap. 123,* http://wwwnc.cdc.gov/travel/destinations/haiti.htm). Malaria remains endemic in many parts of the world, and an estimated 30,000 travelers from the United States and Europe are infected with malaria during travel yearly. The areas of highest risk are in sub-Saharan Africa and Oceania with the lowest risk in South and Central America, including Haiti and the Dominican Republic. Chloroquine resistance is growing throughout the world and is especially notable in parts of South America, Africa, and Southeast Asia. However, in Haiti, the incidence of chloroquine resistant malaria is low. For a traveler to Haiti, the Centers for Disease Control and Prevention states that travelers have a choice of chloroquine, doxycycline, atovaquone–proguanil, or mefloquine. In addition, travelers should be cautioned to use appropriate techniques for malarial prevention, including protective clothing, DEET-containing insect repellants, permethrin-impregnated bednets, and screened sleeping accommodations, if possible.

IV-12. **The answer is E.** *(Chap. 123)* Individuals with HIV are generally considered at high risk of infectious complications when traveling abroad. However, individuals who have no symptoms and a CD4+ count greater than 500/μL appear to be at no greater risk than individuals without HIV infection. Before travel, it is important to research the travel requirements for the specific country of travel. Many countries routinely deny entry for HIV-positive individuals for prolonged stays, and proof of HIV testing is required in many countries for stays longer than 3 months. Consular offices should be contacted before travel to determine if any special documentation is required. HIV-infected travelers should have all routine immunizations before travel, including influenza and pneumococcal vaccinations. The response rate to influenza in an asymptomatic HIV-positive person is greater than 80%. Generally, live-attenuated viruses are not given to HIV-infected individuals. However, because measles can be lethal in those with HIV, this vaccine is recommended unless the CD4+ count is less than 200/μL, and the expected response rate would be between 50% and 100%. In contrast, the live yellow fever vaccine is not given to HIV-infected travelers, and individuals with CD4+ counts below 200/μL should be discouraged from traveling to countries with endemic yellow fever. Some countries in sub-Saharan Africa require yellow fever vaccination. However, because this patient is traveling from a low-risk area, a medical waiver would likely be issued.

IV-13. **The answer is E.** *(Chap. 124)* The etiologic agents of infective endocarditis vary by host (see Figure IV-13). Community-acquired native valve endocarditis remains an important clinical problem, particularly in elderly people. In those patients, streptococci (*Viridans* spp., *S. gallolyticus*, other non–group A and other group streptococci, and *Abiotrophia* spp.) account for approximately 40% of cases. *Staphylococcus aureus* (30%) is next most common. Enterococci, HACEK group, coagulase-negative, and culture-negative cases each account for less than 10% of community-acquired native valve cases. In health care–associated, injection drug use–associated, and greater than 12-month-old prosthetic valve endocarditis, *S. aureus* is most common. Coagulase-negative staphylococcus is the most common organism in prosthetic valve endocarditis less than 12 months. Enterococci cause endocarditis in approximately 10% to 15% of cases in health care–associated, 2- to 12-month prosthetic valve, and injection drug use cases. Culture-negative endocarditis accounts for 5% to 10% of cases in all of the aforementioned clinical scenarios.

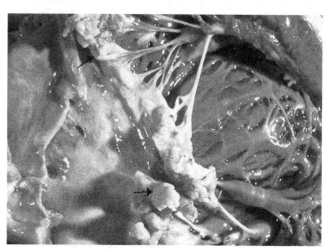

FIGURE IV-13 (see Color Atlas)

IV-14. **The answer is B.** *(Chap. 124)* The Duke criteria for diagnosis of infective endocarditis are a set of major and minor clinical, laboratory, and echocardiographic criteria that are highly sensitive and specific. The presence of two major criteria, one major criterion and three minor criteria, or five minor criteria allows a clinical diagnosis of definite endocarditis (see Table IV-14). Evidence of echocardiographic involvement as evidenced by an oscillating mass (vegetation) on a valve, supporting structure, or implanted material; an intracardiac abscess or partial dehiscence of a prosthetic valve; or a new valvular regurgitation are major criteria in the Duke classification. An increase or change in preexisting murmur by clinical examination is not sufficient. Transthoracic echocardiography is specific for infective endocarditis but only finds vegetations in about 65% of patients with definite endocarditis. It is not adequate for evaluation of prosthetic valves or for intracardiac complications. Transesophageal echocardiography is more sensitive, detecting abnormalities in more than 90% of cases of definite endocarditis.

IV-15. **The answer is C.** *(Chap. 124)* The recommendations for prophylaxis to prevent infective endocarditis have undergone change recently with a change to recommending it for fewer

TABLE IV-14 The Duke Criteria for the Clinical Diagnosis of Infective Endocarditis [a]

Major Criteria

1. Positive blood culture

   Typical microorganism for infective endocarditis from two separate blood cultures

       Viridans streptococci, *Streptococcus gallolyticus*, HACEK group, *Staphylococcus aureus, or*

       Community-acquired enterococci in the absence of a primary focus, *or*

   Persistently positive blood culture, defined as recovery of a microorganism consistent with infective endocarditis from:

       Blood cultures drawn >12 h apart; *or*

       All of 3 or a majority of ≥4 separate blood cultures, with first and last drawn at least 1 h apart

   Single positive blood culture for *Coxiella burnetii* or phase I IgG antibody titer of >1:800

2. Evidence of endocardial involvement

   Positive echocardiogram[b]

       Oscillating intracardiac mass on valve or supporting structures or in the path of regurgitant jets or in implanted material in the absence of an alternative anatomic explanation, *or*

       Abscess, *or*

       New partial dehiscence of prosthetic valve, *or*

   New valvular regurgitation (increase or change in preexisting murmur not sufficient)

Minor Criteria

1. Predisposition: predisposing heart condition or injection drug use

2. Fever ≥38.0°C (≥100.4°F)

3. Vascular phenomena: major arterial emboli, septic pulmonary infarcts, mycotic aneurysm, intracranial hemorrhage, conjunctival hemorrhages, Janeway lesions

4. Immunologic phenomena: glomerulonephritis, Osler's nodes, Roth's spots, rheumatoid factor

5. Microbiologic evidence: positive blood culture but not meeting major criterion as noted previously[c] or serologic evidence of active infection with organism consistent with infective endocarditis

[a]Definite endocarditis is defined by documentation of two major criteria, of one major criterion and three minor criteria, or of five minor criteria. See text for further details.
[b]Transesophageal echocardiography is recommended for assessing possible prosthetic valve endocarditis or complicated endocarditis.
[c]Excluding single positive cultures for coagulase-negative staphylococci and diphtheroids, which are common culture contaminants, and organisms that do not cause endocarditis frequently, such as gram-negative bacilli.
Abbreviation: HACEK, *Haemophilus* spp., *Aggregatibacter actinomycetemcomitans, Cardiobacterium hominis, Eikenella corrodens, Kingella* spp.
Source: Adapted from Li JS et al: Proposed modifications to the Duke criteria for the diagnosis of infective endocarditis. *Clin Infect Dis* 30:633, 2000, with permission from the University of Chicago Press.

patients. The most recent American Heart Association guidelines (*Circulation* 116:1736, 2007) reverse many of the former recommendations based on indirect evidence suggesting that benefit is minimal and is not supported by cost-benefit or cost-effectiveness studies. Current recommendations advise prophylactic antibiotics only for those at highest risk for severe morbidity or mortality from endocarditis undergoing manipulation of gingival tissue or periapical region of the teeth, perforation of the oral mucosa, or a procedure on an infected site. Prophylaxis is not advised for routine gastrointestinal or genitourinary procedures. High-risk patients include those with prior endocarditis, prosthetic heart valves, unrepaired cyanotic congenital heart disease lesions, recently (<6 months) repaired congenital heart lesions, incompletely repaired congenital heart disease lesions, and valvulopathy after cardiac transplant. The British Society for Antimicrobial Chemotherapy does recommend prophylaxis for at-risk patients undergoing selected gastrointestinal or genitourinary procedures; however, the National Institute for Health and Clinical Excellence in the United Kingdom advised discontinuation of the practice (*http://www.nice.org.uk/guidance/cg64*).

IV-16. **The answer is A.** *(Chap. 124)* This patient has culture-negative endocarditis, a rare entity defined as clinical evidence of infectious endocarditis in the absence of positive blood cultures. In this case, evidence for subacute bacterial endocarditis includes valvular regurgitation; an aortic valve vegetation; and embolic phenomena on the extremities, spleen, and kidneys. A common reason for negative blood cultures is prior antibiotics. In the absence of this, the two most common pathogens (both of which are technically difficult to isolate in blood culture bottles) are Q fever, *Coxiella burnetii* (typically associated with close contact with livestock), and *Bartonella* spp. In this case, the patient's homelessness and body louse infestation are clues for *Bartonella quintana* infection. Diagnosis is made by blood culture about 25% of the time. Otherwise, direct polymerase chain reaction of valvular tissue, if available, or acute and convalescent serologies are diagnostic options. Empirical therapy for culture-negative endocarditis usually includes ceftriaxone and gentamicin with or without doxycycline. For confirmed *Bartonella* endocarditis, optimal therapy is gentamicin plus doxycycline. EBV and HIV do not cause endocarditis. A peripheral blood smear would not be diagnostic.

IV-17. **The answer is D.** *(Chap. 124)* Although any valvular vegetation can embolize, vegetations located on the mitral valve and vegetations larger than 10 mm are greatest risk of embolizing. Of the answer choices, C, D, and E are large enough to increase the risk of embolization. However, only choice D demonstrates the risks of both size and location. Hematogenously seeded infection from an embolized vegetation may involve any organ but particularly affects those organs with the highest blood flow. They are seen in up to 50% of patients with endocarditis. Tricuspid lesions lead to pulmonary septic emboli, which are common in injection drug users. Mitral and aortic lesions can lead to embolic infections in the skin, spleen, kidneys, meninges, and skeletal system. A dreaded neurologic complication is mycotic aneurysm, focal dilations of arteries at points in the arterial wall that have been weakened by infection in the vasa vasorum or septic emboli, leading to hemorrhage.

IV-18. **The answer is A.** *(Chap. 124)* Patients with infective endocarditis on antibiotic therapy can be expected to demonstrate clinical improvement within 5 to 7 days. Blood cultures frequently remain positive for 3 to 5 days for *Staphylococcus aureus* treated with β-lactam antibiotics and 7 to 9 days with vancomycin. Neither rifampin nor gentamicin has been shown to provide clinical benefit in the scenario described in this question. Vancomycin peak and trough levels have not been shown to improve drug efficacy in infective endocarditis. It is too early in therapy to consider this case representative of vancomycin failure. The efficacy of daptomycin or linezolid because an alternative to vancomycin for left-sided MRSA endocarditis has not been established.

IV-19. **The answer is B.** *(Chap. 125)* Bullae (Latin for bubbles) are skin lesions that are greater than 5 mm and fluid filled. They may be regular or irregularly shaped and filled with serous or seropurulent fluid. *Clostridium* spp., including *perfringens*, may cause bullae through myonecrosis. Staphylococcus causes scalded skin syndrome through elaboration of the exfoliatin toxin from phage group II, particularly in neonates. *Streptococcus pyogenes*, the causative agent of impetigo, may cause bullae initially that progress to crusted lesions. MRSA may also cause impetigo. The halophilic *Vibrio*, including *V. vulnificus*, may cause an aggressive fasciitis with bullae formation. Patients with cirrhosis exposed to Gulf of Mexico or Atlantic waters (or ingestion of raw seafood from those waters) are at greatest risk. Infection with the dimorphic fungus, *Sporothrix schenckii*, presents with discrete crusted lesions resembling ringworm. Lesions may progress to ulcerate. Patients often have a history of working with soil or roses.

IV-20. **The answer is D.** *(Chap. 125)* This patient has necrotizing fasciitis and myonecrosis. His computed tomography scan shows edema and inflammation of the left chest wall. Necrotizing fasciitis and myonecrosis may also be caused by infection with mixed aerobes and anaerobes, *Staphylococcus aureus* including, methicillin-resistant *S. aureus*, and *Clostridium* spp. Treatment involves prompt surgical evaluation and empiric therapy for the causative agents. *Mycobacterium tuberculosis* would most commonly cause cavitary lung lesions.

Coxsackie virus causes vesicular lesions during acute infection. There may be myalgias and elevated muscle enzymes but not frank myonecrosis. *Rickettsia akari* is the causative agent of rickettsialpox. It occurs after a mite bite with a papule with central vesicle that evolves to form a painless black eschar. Rickettsialpox has been recently described in Ohio, Arizona, and Utah. Varicella-zoster virus causes chickenpox with acute infection and zoster with reactivation. The lesions are crusting vesicles, not fasciitis or myonecrosis.

IV-21. **The answer is C.** *(Chap. 126)* Although *Staphylococcus aureus* (methicillin-resistant *S. aureus* and methicillin-sensitive *S. aureus*) is the most common bacteria causing osteomyelitis, the infection may also be caused by gram-negative organisms (*Pseudomonas aeruginosa, Escherichia coli*), coagulase-negative staphylococci, enterococci, and propionibacteria. *Mycobacterium tuberculosis* is an important cause of vertebral osteomyelitis in countries with fewer medical resources and high prevalence (along with brucellosis). Prosthetic joint implants and stabilization devices are commonly sources of osteomyelitis, often seeded from bacteremia or after trauma. MRSA osteomyelitis is a growing problem in hospitals throughout the developed world, particularly after surgery. The reason for the higher morbidity and cost may be related to virulence factors or less effective or timely treatment. Patients with diabetes are at very high risk of osteomyelitis of the foot and require a high index of suspicion.

IV-22. **The answer is A.** *(Chap. 126)* The therapy for osteomyelitis is challenging because of the multiplicity of potential causative organisms, the diagnostic difficulty, and the prolonged necessary therapy. Early surgical intervention may be beneficial diagnostically and therapeutically. In this case, the Gram stain is polymicrobial, and the putrid smell is very specific for anaerobic organisms. The diagnosis of acute osteomyelitis is also very likely based on the positive probe to bone test and wide ulcer. Broad-spectrum antibiotics are indicated. Vancomycin and linezolid cover methicillin-resistant *Staphylococcus aureus* (MRSA) and streptococcal isolates but would miss gram-negative rods and anaerobic bacteria. Metronidazole covers only anaerobes, missing gram-positive organisms that are key in the initiation of diabetic foot infections. Clindamycin covers gram-positive organisms and anaerobes but misses gram-negative rods. Ampicillin–sulbactam is broad-spectrum antibiotic and covers all three classes of organism except MRSA. If the patient has a history of MRSA or MRSA risk factors, then the addition of vancomycin or linezolid is a strong consideration. Recent studies have also suggested that daptomycin may be a promising therapy for MRSA osteomyelitis.

IV-23. **The answer is A.** *(Chap. 127)* Primary (spontaneous) bacterial peritonitis (PBP) occurs when the peritoneal cavity becomes infected without an apparent source of contamination. PBP occurs most often in patients with cirrhosis, usually with preexisting ascites. The bacterial likely invade the peritoneal fluid because of poor hepatic filtration in cirrhosis. Although fever is present in up to 80% of cases, abdominal pain, acute onset, and peritoneal signs are often absent. Patients may present with nonspecific findings such as malaise or worsening encephalopathy. A neutrophil count in peritoneal fluid of greater than 250/μL is diagnostic; there is no % neutrophil differential threshold. Diagnosis is often difficult because peritoneal culture findings are often negative. Blood cultures may reveal the causative organism. The most common organisms are enteric gram-negative bacilli, but gram-positive cocci are often found. Anaerobes are not common (in contrast to secondary bacterial peritonitis), and empiric antibiotics targeting them are not necessary if PBP is suspected. Third-generation cephalosporins or piperacillin–tazobactam are reasonable initial empiric therapy. Diagnosis requires exclusion of a primary intraabdominal source of peritonitis.

IV-24. **The answer is D.** *(Chap. 127)* This patient has continuous ambulatory peritoneal dialysis (CAPD)–associated peritonitis. Unlike primary or secondary bacterial peritonitis, this infection is usually caused by skin organisms, most commonly *Staphylococcus* spp. The organisms migrate into the peritoneal fluid via the device. There may not be a tunnel or exit-site infection. Peritonitis is the most common reason for discontinuing CAPD. Y-connectors and diligent technique decrease the risk of CAPD. In contrast to PBP and similar to spontaneous bacterial peritonitis (SBP), the onset of symptoms is usually acute with diffuse pain and peritoneal signs. The dialysate will be cloudy with greater than 100 WBC/μL and greater than 50% neutrophils. Dialysate should be placed in blood culture media and often is often positive with one organism. Finding more than one organism in culture should prompt an evaluation for SBP. Empirical intraperitoneal coverage for CAPD peritonitis should be directed against staphylococcal species based on local epidemiology. If the patient is severely ill, intravenous antibiotics should be added. If the patient does not respond within 4 days, catheter removal should be considered.

IV-25.   **The answer is D.** *(Chap. 127)* The computed tomography scan shows a large complex liver abscess in the right lobe. Liver abscesses may arise from hematogenous spread, biliary disease (most common currently), pylephlebitis, or contiguous infection in the peritoneal cavity. Fever is the only common physical finding in liver abscess. Up to 50% of patients may not have symptoms or signs to direct attention to the liver. Nonspecific symptoms are common, and liver abscess is an important cause of fever of unexplained origin in elderly patients. The only reliably abnormal serum studies are elevated alkaline phosphatase or WBC in 70% of patients. Liver abscess may be suggested by an elevated hemidiaphragm on chest radiograph. The most common causative organisms in presumed biliary disease are gram-negative bacilli. Anaerobes are not common unless pelvic or other enteric sources are suspected. Fungal liver abscesses occur after fungemia in immunocompromised patients receiving chemotherapy, often presenting symptomatically with neutrophil reconstitution. Drainage, usually percutaneous, is the mainstay of therapy and is useful initially diagnostically (Figure IV-25B).

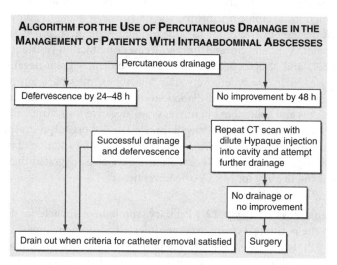

FIGURE IV-25B

IV-26.   **The answer is C.** *(Chap. 127)* It is important to distinguish between primary (spontaneous) and secondary peritonitis. Primary peritonitis is a result of long-standing ascites, usually as a result of cirrhosis. The pathogenesis is poorly understood but may involve bacteremic spread or translocation across the gut wall of usually only a single species of pathogenic bacteria. Secondary peritonitis is caused by rupture of a hollow viscous or irritation of the peritoneum caused by a contiguous abscess or pyogenic infection. It typically presents with peritoneal signs and in most cases represents a surgical emergency. Secondary peritonitis in a patient with cirrhosis is difficult to distinguish on clinical grounds from primary (spontaneous) peritonitis. It is often overlooked because classic peritoneal signs are almost always lacking, and it is uniformly fatal in the absence of surgery. Suspicion for this diagnosis should occur when ascites shows a protein greater than 1 g/dL, lactate dehydrogenase (LDH) greater than serum LDH, glucose level below 50 mg/dL, or a polymicrobial Gram stain. When this diagnosis is suspected, abdominal radiography is indicated to rule out free air, and prompt surgical consultation is warranted. Unlike with primary (spontaneous) bacterial peritonitis, in cases of secondary peritonitis, antibiotics should include anaerobic coverage and often antifungal agents. This patient requires intravenous fluid because he has hypotension and tachycardia caused by sepsis. Drotrecogin alfa has been shown to reduce mortality in patients with sepsis, but it is not indicated in patients with thrombocytopenia, cirrhosis, and ascites.

IV-27. **The answer is B.** *(Chap. 128)* Acute infectious diarrhea remains a leading cause of death worldwide, especially among children younger than 5 years of age. The major categories of acute diarrheal illness include noninflammatory, inflammatory, and penetrating diarrhea. *Vibrio cholerae* causes diarrhea through production of an enterotoxin, which is characteristic of noninflammatory diarrhea. After ingestion of a large volume ($10^5–10^6$) of organisms, *V. cholerae* attaches to the brush border of the small intestinal enterocytes and produces cholera toxin. The primary clinical characteristic of diarrheal illness caused by toxin production is profuse watery diarrhea that is not bloody. Fecal leukocytes are typically not present in noninflammatory diarrhea. However, a mild increase in fecal lactoferrin can be seen because this test is more sensitive for the presence of mild inflammation. Other pathogens that are common causes of noninflammatory diarrhea are enterotoxigenic *Escherichia coli*, *Bacillus cereus*, *Staphylococcus aureus*, and viral diarrhea, among others.

The site of inflammation in inflammatory diarrhea is typically the colon or distal small bowel. In inflammatory diarrhea, there is invasion of leukocytes into the wall of the intestines. The prototypical pathogen of inflammatory diarrhea is *Shigella dysenteriae*. Bloody stools are common, and the stool contains large quantities of fecal leukocytes and fecal lactoferrin. Other pathogens that cause inflammatory diarrhea are most *Salmonella* species, *Campylobacter jejuni*, enterohemorrhagic *Escherichia coli*, and *Clostridium difficile*.

Penetrating diarrhea is caused by either *Salmonella typhi* or *Yersinia enterocolitica*. The site of inflammation in penetrating diarrhea is the distal small bowel. In penetrating diarrhea, these organisms penetrate the intestinal wall and multiply within Peyer's patches and intestinal lymph nodes before disseminating into the bloodstream. Clinically, penetrating diarrhea presents as enteric fever with fever, relative bradycardia, abdominal pain, leukopenia, and splenomegaly.

IV-28 and IV-29. **The answers are B and D, respectively.** *(Chap. 128)* Traveler's diarrhea is common among individuals traveling to Asia, Africa, and Central and South America, affecting 25% to 50% of travelers to these areas. Most traveler's diarrhea begins within 3 to 5 days after arrival and is self-limited, lasting 1 to 5 days. Most individuals acquire traveler's diarrhea after consuming contaminated food or water. Although some organisms have a geographic association, enterotoxigenic and enteroaggregative *Escherichia coli* are found worldwide and are the most common causes of traveler's diarrhea. In Asia, *Campylobacter jejuni* is also common. This presentation would be uncommon for *Shigella* spp. because it most frequently causes bloody diarrhea. Norovirus is associated with a more profuse diarrhea. It has been the causative organism in large outbreaks on cruise ships. *Giardia lamblia* is a parasite that is responsible for 5% or less of traveler's diarrhea.

The approach to treatment of traveler's diarrhea should be tailored to the severity of the patient's symptoms. In general, most cases are self-limited. As long as an individual is able to maintain adequate fluid intake, no specific therapy may be required if there are no more than one or two unformed stools daily without distressing abdominal symptoms, bloody stools, or fever. In this scenario, the patient is not having a large number of stools, but in the presence of distressing abdominal symptoms, use of bismuth subsalicylate or loperamide is recommended. If loperamide is used, an initial dose of 4 mg is given followed by 2 mg after passage of each unformed stool. Antibacterial therapy is only recommended if there is evidence of inflammatory diarrhea (bloody stools or fever) or there are more than two unformed stools daily. The antibacterial agent of choice is usually a fluoroquinolone. Ciprofloxacin given as a single dose of 750 mg or 500 mg three times daily for 3 days is typically effective. In Thailand, *Campylobacter jejuni* is a common agent and has a high degree of fluoroquinolone resistance. For travelers to Thailand who require antibiotics, azithromycin is recommended with an initial dose of 10 mg/kg on the first day followed by 5 mg/kg on days 2 and 3 if diarrhea persists.

IV-30. **The answer is C.** *(Chap. 128)* Acute bacterial food poisoning occurring 1 to 6 hours after ingestion of contaminated food is most commonly caused by infection with *Staphylococcus aureus* or *Bacillus cereus*. *S. aureus* is associated with ingestion of ham, poultry, potato or egg salad, mayonnaise, or cream pastries that have been allowed to remain at room temperature after cooking. *B. cereus* is classically associated with contaminated fried rice. The symptoms of bacterial food poisoning begin abruptly with nausea, vomiting, abdominal cramping, and diarrhea. However, fever is not a common finding and should cause one to consider other etiologies of vomiting and diarrhea.

IV-31. **The answer is C.** *(Chap. 128)* The patient most likely has food poisoning caused by contamination of the fried rice with *Bacillus cereus*. This toxin-mediated disease occurs when heat-resistant spores germinate after boiling. Frying before serving may not destroy the preformed toxin. The emetic form of illness occurs within 6 hours of eating and is self-limited. No therapy is necessary unless the patient develops severe dehydration. This patient currently has no symptoms consistent with volume depletion; therefore, she does not need intravenous fluids at present. Sarcoidosis does not predispose patients to infectious diseases.

IV-32. **The answer is E.** *(Chap. 129)* Although frequent nonbloody diarrheal illness is commonly associated with *Clostridium difficile* infection, other presentations are well described, including fever in 28% of cases, abdominal pain, and leukocytosis. Adynamic ileus is often seen with *C. difficile* infection, and leukocytosis in this condition should be a clue that *C. difficile* is at play. Recurrent infection after therapy has been described in 15% to 30% of cases.

IV-33. **The answer is D**. *(Chap. 129)* *Clostridium difficile* infection is diagnosed by the following means: diarrhea of three or more stools per day for 2 or more days with no other cause plus (1) demonstration of toxin A or B in the stool, (2) polymerase chain reaction for toxin-producing *C. difficile* of the stool, or (3) demonstration of pseudomembranes on colonoscopy. Although many tests are available, none has adequate sensitivity to definitively rule out *C. difficile* infection. Thus, empiric therapy is appropriate in a patient (such as patient C) with a high likelihood of *C. difficile* infection.

IV-34. **The answer is C.** *(Chap. 129)* The patient has evidence of recurrent *Clostridium difficile* infection, which occurs in up to 30% of treated patients. Because there is no evidence that she has severe infection and this is her first recurrence, the recommended therapy is to retreat with oral metronidazole. Vancomycin is reserved for patients with severe infection either initially or with recurrence. Fecal transplantation, intravenous immunoglobulin, and oral nitazoxanide are all potential therapies for patients with multiple recurrences.

IV-35. **The answer is E.** *(Chap. 129)* Clindamycin, ampicillin, and cephalosporins (including ceftriaxone) were the first antibiotics associated with *Clostridium difficile*–associated disease and still are. More recently, broad-spectrum fluoroquinolones, including moxifloxacin and ciprofloxacin, have been associated with outbreaks of *C. difficile*, including outbreaks in some locations of a more virulent strain that has caused severe disease among elderly outpatients. For unclear reasons, β-lactams other than the later generation cephalosporins appear to carry a lesser risk of disease. Penicillin–β-lactamase combination antibiotics appear to have lower risk of *C. difficile*–associated disease than the other agents mentioned. Cases have even been reported associated with metronidazole and vancomycin administration. Nevertheless, all patients initiating antibiotics should be warned to seek care if they develop diarrhea that is severe or persists for more than 1 day because all antibiotics carry some risk for *C. difficile*–associated disease.

IV-36. **The answer is A.** *(Chap. 130)* Common causes of urethral discomfort and discharge in men include *Chlamydia trachomatis*, *Neisseria gonorrhoeae*, *Mycoplasma genitalium*, *Ureaplasma urealyticum*, *Trichomonas vaginalis*, and herpes simplex virus. *Gardnerella* spp. is the usual cause of bacterial vaginosis in women and is not a pathogen in men.

IV-37. **The answer is C.** *(Chap. 130)* The patient has symptoms consistent with the urethral syndrome characterized by "internal" dysuria with urgency and frequency and pyuria but no uropathogens at counts of 10^2/mL or greater in urine. This is most commonly caused by infection with *Chlamydia trachomatis* or *Neisseria gonorrhoeae* and can be readily confirmed by nucleic acid amplification testing for these pathogens in the urine. "External" dysuria includes pain in the vulva during urination, often without frequency or urgency. This is found in vulvovaginal candidiasis and herpes simplex infection, which can be visualized on physical examination. Cervical culture would not be useful with her urinary symptoms. Elevated vaginal pH above 5.0 is commonly present in trichomonal vaginitis. Clue cells on vaginal secretion microscopy suggest bacterial vaginosis.

IV-38. **The answer is B.** *(Chap. 130)* Bacterial vaginosis is associated with *Gardnerella vaginalis* and various anaerobic or noncultured bacteria. It generally has malodorous discharge that is white or gray. There is no external irritation, and pH of vaginal fluid is usually above 4.5; a fishy odor is present with 10% KOH preparation; and microscopy shows clue cells, few leukocytes, and many mixed microbiota. Normal vaginal findings are described in patient D with pH below 4.5 and lactobacilli seen on microscopic examination. A high pH above 5 with external irritation is often found in vulvovaginal candidiasis, but the presence of motile trichomonads is diagnostic for trichomonal vaginitis.

IV-39. **The answer is E.** *(Chap. 130)* In a study of patients with mucopurulent cervicitis seen at a sexually transmitted disease clinic in the 1980s, more than one-third of cervical samples failed to reveal any etiology. In a recent similar study in Baltimore using nucleic acid amplification testing, more than half of the cases were not microbiologically identified. *Chlamydia trachomatis* is the most frequently diagnosed organism followed by *Neisseria gonorrhoeae*. Because of the difficulty in making a microbiologic diagnosis, empiric therapy for *C. trachomatis* and, in areas were *N. gonorrhoeae* is highly endemic, gonococcus is indicated.

IV-40. **The answer is C.** *(Chap. 130)* The presence of right upper quadrant tenderness in conjunction with classic findings of pelvic inflammatory disease is highly suggestive of Fitz-Hugh-Curtis syndrome or perihepatitis caused by inflammation of the liver capsule caused by either *Neisseria gonorrhoeae* or *Chlamydia trachomatis* infection. Although this condition may be easily visualized by laproscopic examination, the resolution of right upper quadrant symptoms with therapy of pelvic inflammatory disease is the more common proof of the diagnosis. The presence of normal liver function testing is reassuring that hepatitis is not present, making hepatitis C virus infection unlikely.

IV-41. **The answer is A.** *(Chap. 130)* The most common causes of genital ulceration are herpes simplex virus, syphilis, and chancroid. Gonorrhea typically manifests as a urethritis, not genital ulcers. Syphilitic ulcers (primary chancre) are firm, shallow single ulcers that are not pustular and are generally not painful. Despite these usual findings, rapid plasma reagin testing is indicated in all cases of genital ulceration given the disparate presentations of *Treponema pallidum*. Herpes simplex virus ulcers are quite painful but are vesicular rather than pustular. In primary infection, they may be bilateral, but with reactivation, they are generally unilateral. *Haemophilus ducreyi*, the agent responsible for chancroid, causes multiple ulcers, often starting as pustules, that are soft, friable, and exquisitely tender, as present in this case. Primary infection with HIV usually causes an acute febrile illness, not focal ulcers. The presence of genital ulcers increases the likelihood of acquisition and transmission of HIV.

IV-42. **The answer is F.** *(Chap. 130)* HIV is the leading cause of death in some developing countries. Efforts to decrease transmission include screening and treatment of sexually associated infections. All of the listed conditions have been linked with higher acquisition of HIV based on epidemiologic studies and high biologic plausibility. Up to 50% of women of reproductive age in developing countries have bacterial vaginosis. All of the bacterial infections are curable, and treatment can decrease the frequency of genital herpes recurrences. This highlights an additional reason that primary care doctors should screen for each of these infections in female patients with detailed historic questions, genitourinary and rectal examinations, and evidence-based routine screening for these infections based on age and risk category.

IV-43. **The answer is B.** *(Chap. 131)* Nosocomial infections have reservoirs and sources just as do community-acquired pathogens. In hospitalized patients, cross-contamination (i.e., indirect spread of organisms from one patient to the next) accounts for many nosocomial infections. Although hand hygiene is uniformly recommended for health care practitioners, adherence to hand washing is low often because of time pressure, inconvenience, and skin damage. Because of improved adherence, alcohol-based hand rubs are now recommended for all heath care workers except when hands are visibly soiled or after care of a patient with *Clostridium difficile* infection, whose spores may not be killed by alcohol and thus require thorough hand wash with soap and water.

IV-44. **The answer is E.** *(Chap. 132)* Ultimately, solid organ transplant patients are at highest risk for infection because of T-cell immunodeficiency from antirejection medicines. As a result, they are also at risk for reactivation of many of the viruses from the herpes virus family, most notably cytomegalovirus, varicella-zoster virus, and Epstein-Barr virus. However, immediately after transplant, these deficits have not yet developed in full. Neutropenia is not common after solid organ transplantation as in bone marrow transplantation. In fact, patients are most at risk of infections typical for all hospitalized patients, including wound infections, urinary tract infection, pneumonia, *Clostridium difficile* infection, and line-associated infection. Therefore, a standard evaluation of a febrile patient in the first weeks after a solid organ transplant should include a detailed physical examination, blood and urine cultures, urinalysis, chest radiography, and *C. difficile* stool antigen or toxin studies if warranted, in addition to a transplant-specific evaluation.

IV-45. **The answer is E.** *(Chap. 132)* The patient presents with symptoms suggestive of infection in the middle period after transplantation (1–4 months). In patients with prior cytomegalovirus (CMV) exposure or receipt of CMV-positive organ transplant, this is a period of time when CMV infection is most common. The patient presented here has classic signs of CMV disease with generalized symptoms in addition to dysfunction of her transplanted organ (kidney). Often bone marrow suppression is present, demonstrated here by lymphopenia. Because CMV infection is linked with graft dysfunction and rejection, prophylaxis is frequently used, including valganciclovir. Trimethoprim–sulfamethoxazole is used for *Pneumocystis jiroveci* prophylaxis, acyclovir generally is used for varicella-zoster virus prophylaxis, itraconazole may be considered in patients considered at risk for histoplasmosis reactivation, and isoniazid is used for individuals with recent purified protein derivative conversion or positive chest imaging and no prior treatment.

IV-46. **The answer is E.** *(Chap. 132)* *Toxoplasma gondii* commonly achieves latency in cysts during acute infection. Reactivation in the central nervous system in AIDS patients is well known. However, *Toxoplasma* cysts also reside in the heart. Thus, transplanting a *Toxoplasma*-positive heart into a *Toxoplasma*-negative recipient may cause reactivation in the months after transplant. Serologic screening of cardiac donors and recipients for *T. gondii* is important. To account for this possibility, prophylactic doses of trimethoprim–sulfamethoxazole, which is also effective prophylaxis against *Pneumocystis* and *Nocardia* spp., is standard after cardiac transplantation. Cardiac transplant recipients, similar to all other solid organ transplant recipients, are at risk of developing infections related to impaired cellular immunity, particularly more than 1 month to 1 year post-transplant. Wound infections or mediastinitis from skin organisms may complicate the early transplant (<1 month) period.

IV-47. **The answer is C.** *(Chaps. 132 and 204)* During the first week after hematopoietic stem cell transplantation, the highest risk of infection comes from aerobic nosocomially acquired bacteria. However, after about 7 days, the risk of fungal infection rises, particularly with prolonged neutropenia. The patient presented here presents with symptoms and signs of a respiratory illness after prolonged neutropenia; fungal infection is high on the differential diagnosis list. The computed tomography scan with nodules and associated halo sign is suggestive of *Aspergillus* infection. The halo sign often occurs in *Aspergillus* infection in the context of an increasing neutrophil count after a prolonged nadir. The serum galactomannan antigen test detects galactomannan, a major component of the *Aspergillus* cell wall that is released during growth of hyphae. The presence of this compound suggests invasion and growth of the mold. This noninvasive test is receiving wider acceptance in the diagnosis of invasive *Aspergillus* spp. in immunocompromised hosts. Additionally, galactomannan assays in bronchoalveolar lavage fluid may aid diagnosis of invasive *Aspergillus* in immunocompromised hosts (*American Journal of Respiratory and Critical Care Medicine* 177: 27-34, 2008). In the absence of purulent sputum, sputum cultures are unlikely to be helpful. *Aspergillus* is seldom cultured from the sputum in cases of invasive aspergillosis. Examination of buffy coat is useful for the diagnosis of histoplasmosis, but the focal nodules with halo sign and absence of other systemic symptoms makes histoplasmosis less likely. *Legionella* spp. and cytomegalovirus pneumonia are generally not associated with nodules and have either lobar infiltrates or diffuse infiltrates.

IV-48. **The answer is E.** *(Chap. 133)* All bacteria, both gram negative and gram positive, have rigid cell walls that protect bacterial intracellular hyperosmolarity from the host environment. Peptidoglycan is the present in both gram-negative and gram-positive bacteria, but only gram-negative bacteria have an additional outer membrane external to peptidoglycan. Many antibiotics target cell wall synthesis and thus lead to inhibition of growth or cell death. These antibiotics include bacitracin, glycopeptides such as vancomycin, and β-lactam antibiotics. Macrolides such as azithromycin, lincosamides (clindamycin), linezolid, chloramphenicol, aminoglycosides such as tobramycin, mupirocin, and tetracycline all inhibit protein synthesis. Sulfonamides and trimethoprim interrupt cell metabolism. Rifampin and metronidazole alter nucleic acid synthesis. The quinolones, such as ciprofloxacin, and novobiocin inhibit DNA synthesis. Finally, polymixins, gramicid, and daptomycin disrupt the cellular membrane.

IV-49. **The answer is B.** *(Chap. 133)* The patient presents with evidence of methicillin-resistant *Staphylococcus aureus*–associated soft tissue infection that has failed therapy with clindamycin. Linezolid is an appropriate choice for antibiotic coverage in this situation. Subsequent development of neurologic symptoms, including agitated delirium, evidence of autonomic instability coupled with tremor, muscular rigidity, hyperreflexia, and clonus, suggests serotonin syndrome. Because linezolid is a monoamine oxidase inhibitor, it interacts with selective serotonin reuptake inhibitors and can cause serotonin syndrome. Other potential triggers include tyramine-rich foods and sympathomimetics such as phenylpropanolamine. The other drug–drug combinations in the answer choices are not described to be associated with serotonin syndrome.

IV-50. **The answer is A.** *(Chap. 134)* Pneumococcal infections, particularly pneumonia, remain a worldwide public health problem. Intermittent colonization of the nasopharynx by pneumococcus transmitted by respiratory droplet is common and is the likely reservoir for invasive disease. Infants and elderly adults are at greatest risk of developing invasive pneumococcal disease (IPD) and death. In the developed world, children are the most common source of pneumococcal transmission. By 1 year of age, 50% of children have had at least one episode of colonization. Prevalence studies show carriage rates of 20% to 50% in children up to 5 years old and up to 15% for adults. These numbers approach 90% for children and 40% for adults in the developing world. Pneumococcal vaccination has dramatically impacted the epidemiology with reduced IPD in the United States attributable to reductions in serotypes included in the vaccine. Similar reductions have been observed in other countries implementing routine childhood vaccinations; however, in certain populations (Alaska native populations and United Kingdom), the reduction in vaccine covered serotype cases has been offset by increases in nonvaccine serotypes. Case fatality rates caused by pneumococcal pneumonia vary by host factors, age, and access to care. Interestingly, there appears to be no reduction in case fatality during the first 24 hours of hospitalization since the introduction of antibiotics. This is likely because of the development of severe multiorgan failure as a result of severe infection. Appropriate care in an intensive setting can reduce case fatality rate for severe infection. Outbreaks of disease are well recognized in crowded settings with susceptible individuals, such as infant daycare facilities, military barracks, and nursing homes. Furthermore, there is a clear association between preceding viral respiratory disease (especially but not exclusively influenza) and risk of secondary pneumococcal infections. The significant role of pneumococcal pneumonia in the morbidity and mortality associated with seasonal and pandemic influenza is increasingly recognized.

IV-51.   **The answer is C.** *(Chap. 134)* This elderly man presents with a typical story of pneumococcal pneumonia. His age, chronic conditions, and nursing home residence put him a high risk of invasive disease acquisition. Outbreaks commonly occur in crowded environments or nursing homes often after preceding upper respiratory or influenza viral infections and are spread through respiratory droplets. Although the differential diagnosis includes viral pathogens, mycoplasmas, *Haemophilus influenzae*, *Klebsiella pneumoniae*, *Staphylococcus aureus*, and *Legionella* spp., pneumococcal disease remains most common in this demographic. Blood cultures, even in severe disease are positive in fewer than 30% of cases. Diagnosis relies on a positive culture from blood or sputum or a positive urinary antigen test result. Urinary antigen testing has a high positive predictive value in adults because the intermittent colonization rate is low. The urinary antigen test is less specific for invasive disease in children who may be colonized. The radiograph in this case is typical for consolidation (with air bronchograms) of the right lower lobe. The clear right heart border and confinement below the major fissure suggests unilobar disease. With time and hydration, further radiologic extension may be apparent. Parapneumonic (noninfected) pleural effusions are common. The most common focal complication of pneumococcal disease is empyema, occurring in approximately 5% of cases. It should be suspected in cases of new or enlarging pleural effusion or persistent fever particularly after initiation of therapy. Meningitis may occur from hematogenous spread in conjunction with pneumonia or may be the sole presenting syndrome of pneumococcal infection. Pneumococcal resistance to penicillin has increased dramatically since the 1990s, and it is not recommended for empiric therapy of acute pneumonia. However, in culture-proven cases with minimal inhibitory concentration below 2 µg/mL, penicillin may remain an appropriate therapeutic choice for severe disease or meningitis.

IV-52 and IV-53.   **The answers are E and A, respectively.** *(Chaps. 134 and 143)* In a previously healthy student, particularly one living in a dormitory, *Streptococcus pneumoniae* and *Neisseria meningitides* are the pathogens most likely to be causing community-acquired bacterial meningitis. As a result of the increasing prevalence of penicillin- and cephalosporin-resistant streptococci, initial empirical therapy should include a third- or fourth-generation cephalosporin plus vancomycin. Dexamethasone has been shown in children and adults to decrease meningeal inflammation and unfavorable outcomes in acute bacterial meningitis. In a recent study of adults, the effect on outcome was most notable in patients with *S. pneumoniae* infection. The first dose (10 mg IV) should be administered 15 to 20 minutes before or with the first dose of antibiotics and is unlikely to be of benefit unless it is begun 6 hours after the initiation of antibiotics. Dexamethasone may decrease the penetration of vancomycin into the cerebrospinal fluid.

IV-54.   **The answer is B.** *(Chap. 135)* Although new genetic diagnostic kits for distinguishing microbes are becoming more common, basic biochemical characterization of bacterial pathogens is still widely used in microbiology laboratories. Clinicians should be familiar with the most common of these techniques when interpreting laboratory results. Whereas all staphylococci are catalase positive, streptococci are catalase negative. Whereas *S. aureus* are coagulase positive, *Staphylococcus epidermidis* (as well as *S. hominis*, *S. saprophyticus*, and others) are coagulase negative. This is the initial result that can make this important clinical distinction. Lactose fermentation is used to distinguish many gram-negative bacteria. *Salmonella*, *Proteus*, and *Shigella* spp. *and Pseudomonas aeruginosa* are unable to ferment lactose. The oxidase test is commonly used to identify *P. aeruginosa*. The urease test is used to identify *Proteus* spp., *Helicobacter* spp., and other gram-negative organisms.

IV-55.   **The answer is D.** *(Chap. 135)* The major clinical concern in this patient is epidural abscess or vertebral osteomyelitis, as well as line infection caused by *Staphylococcus aureus*. These concerns plus her significant likelihood of clinical deterioration necessitate close inpatient monitoring. Empiric therapy for methicillin-resistant *S. aureus* and gram-negative bacteria is warranted after obtaining blood cultures pending further evaluation. Metastatic seeding during *S. aureus* bacteremia has been estimated to occur as often as 30% of the time. The bones, joints, kidneys, and lungs are the most common sites. Metastatic infection to the spine should be evaluated in an emergent fashion with magnetic resonance imaging. The dialysis catheter should be removed because it is infected based on clinical examination. Infective endocarditis is a major concern. This diagnosis is based on positive blood culture results and either a vegetation on echocardiogram, new pathologic murmur, or evidence of septic embolization on physical examination. A transthoracic echocardiogram is warranted in the evaluation for endocarditis (a disease that this patient is at risk for). However, it need not be ordered emergently because it will not impact management during the initial phase of hospitalization. Moreover, because the diagnosis can only be established in the presence of positive blood cultures (or in rare cases serology of a difficult-to-culture organism), a rational approach is to await positive blood cultures before ordering an echocardiogram.

IV-56. **The answer is C.** *(Chap. 135)* In the past 10 years, numerous outbreaks of community-based infection caused by methicillin-resistant *Staphylococcus aureus* (MRSA) in individuals with no prior medical exposure have been reported. These outbreaks have taken place in both rural and urban settings in widely separated regions throughout the world. The reports document a dramatic change in the epidemiology of MRSA infections. The outbreaks have occurred among such diverse groups as children, prisoners, athletes, Native Americans, and drug users. Risk factors common to these outbreaks include poor hygienic conditions, close contact, contaminated material, and damaged skin. The community-associated infections have been caused by a limited number of MRSA strains. In the United States, strain USA300 (defined by pulsed-field gel electrophoresis) has been the predominant clone. Although the majority of infections caused by this community-based clone of MRSA have involved the skin and soft tissue, 5% to 10% have been invasive, including severe necrotizing lung infections, necrotizing fasciitis, infectious pyomyositis, endocarditis, and osteomyelitis. The most feared complication is a necrotizing pneumonia that often follows influenza upper respiratory infection and can affect previously healthy people. This pathogen produces the Panton-Valentine leukocidin protein that forms holes in the membranes of neutrophils as they arrive at the site of infection and serves as marker for this pathogen. An easy way to identify this strain of MRSA is its sensitivity profile. Unlike MRSA isolates of the past, which were sensitive only to vancomycin, daptomycin, quinupristin–dalfopristin, and linezolid, CA-MRSA are almost uniformly susceptible to trimethoprim–sulfamethoxazole and doxycycline as well. The organism is also usually sensitive to clindamycin. The term *community acquired* has probably outlived its usefulness because this isolate has become the most common *S. aureus* isolate causing infection in many hospitals around the world.

IV-57. **The answer is A.** *(Chap. 135)* Vancomycin remains the drug of choice for methicillin-resistant *Staphylococcus aureus* (MRSA). New patterns of staphylococcal resistance are developing including a strain (VISA, first reported in Japan) that shows vancomycin intermediate resistance. Of the drugs listed all have activity against MRSA. Telavancin is a derivative of vancomycin that is approved by the U.S. Food and Drug Administration for complicated skin and soft tissue infections. VISA strains appear to be susceptible. Linezolid is bacteriostatic against staphylococci and has oral and parenteral formulations. Quinupristin–dalfopristin is bactericidal against all staphylococcal strains, including VISA. It has been used in severe MRSA infections. Daptomycin is not effective for respiratory infections. It can be used for bacteremia and right-sided endocarditis.

IV-58. **The answer is E.** *(Chap. 135)* Probably because of its ubiquity and ability to stick to foreign surfaces, *Staphylococcus epidermidis* is the most common cause of infections of central nervous system shunts as well as an important cause of infections on artificial heart valves and orthopedic prostheses. *Corynebacterium* spp. (diphtheroids), similar to *S. epidermidis*, colonize the skin. When these organisms are isolated from cultures of shunts, it is often difficult to be sure if they are the cause of disease or simply contaminants. Leukocytosis in cerebrospinal fluid, consistent isolation of the same organism, and the character of a patient's symptoms are all helpful in deciding whether treatment for infection is indicated.

IV-59. The answer is D. *(Chap. 135)* This patient has infectious pyomyositis, a disease of the tropics and of immunocompromised hosts such as patients with poorly controlled diabetes mellitus or AIDS. The pathogen is usually *Staphylococcus aureus*. Management includes aggressive debridement, antibiotics, and attempts to reverse the patient's immunocompromised status. *Clostridium perfringens* may cause gas gangrene, particularly in devitalized tissues. Streptococcal infections may cause cellulitis or an aggressive fasciitis, but the presence of abscesses in a patient with poorly controlled diabetes makes staphylococcal infection more likely. Polymicrobial infections are common in diabetic ulcers, but in this case, the imaging and physical examination show intramuscular abscesses.

IV-60. The answer is D. *(Chap. 136)* Recurrent episodes of rheumatic fever are most common in the first 5 years after the initial diagnosis. Penicillin prophylaxis is recommended for at least this period. After the first 5 years, secondary prophylaxis is determined on an individual basis. Ongoing prophylaxis is currently recommended for patients who have had recurrent disease, have rheumatic heart disease, or work in occupations that have a high risk for reexposure to group A streptococcal infection. Prophylactic regimens are penicillin V, PO 250 mg bid; benzathine penicillin, 1.2 million units IM every 4 weeks; and sulfadiazine, 1 g PO daily. Polyvalent pneumococcal vaccine has no cross-reactivity with group A streptococcus.

IV-61. The answer is E. *(Chap. 136)* Necrotizing fasciitis involves the superficial or deep fascia (or both) investing the muscles of an extremity or the trunk. The source of the infection is either the skin, with organisms introduced into tissue through trauma (sometimes trivial), or the bowel flora, with organisms released during abdominal surgery or from an occult enteric source, such as a diverticular or appendiceal abscess. The inoculation site may be unapparent and is often some distance from the site of clinical involvement; for example, the introduction of organisms via minor trauma to the hand may be associated with clinical infection of the tissues overlying the shoulder or chest. Cases originating from the skin are most commonly caused by infection with *Streptococcus pyogenes* (group A streptococcus), sometimes with *Staphylococcus aureus* coinfection. In this case, the presence of fasciitis without myositis (which is more commonly caused by staphylococci) makes *S. pyogenes* the most likely organism. The onset of disease is often acute and the course fulminant. Although pain and tenderness may be severe, physical findings may be subtle initially. Local anesthesia (caused by cutaneous nerve infarction) and skin mottling are late findings. Cases associated with the bowel flora are usually polymicrobial, involving a mixture of anaerobic bacteria (e.g., *Bacteroides fragilis* or anaerobic streptococci) and facultative organisms (usually gram-negative bacilli). Necrotizing fasciitis is a surgical emergency with extensive debridement potentially life saving. At surgery, the extent of disease is typically more extensive than clinically or radiologically indicated. Antibiotic therapy is adjunctive. Patients with necrotizing fasciitis may develop streptococcal toxic shock syndrome. *Streptococcus pneumoniae* and *Staphylococcus epidermidis* are not causes of necrotizing fasciitis. *Clostridium difficile* causes antibiotic-associated colitis.

IV-62. The answer is D. *(Chap. 136)* *Streptococcus agalactiae* is the only species of group B streptococci (GBS) and is a major cause of sepsis and meningitis in neonates. The infection in neonates is acquired by passage through a maternally colonized birth canal. Although 40% to 50% of neonates born of colonized mothers will themselves become colonized, only 1% to 2% develop infection. GBS is also a cause of peripartum fever and can cause significant endometritis or chorioamnionitis. Vaginal swab culture results are typically positive. Risk factors for infection of the mother and child include premature labor and prolonged rupture of membranes. Treatment is with penicillin. The Centers for Disease Control and Prevention recommends screening pregnant women for anogenital colonization at 35 to 37 weeks of pregnancy by a swab culture of the lower vagina and anorectum. Intrapartum chemoprophylaxis is recommended for culture-positive women.

IV-63. **The answer is B.** *(Chap. 137)* Enterococci are the second most common organisms (after staphylococci) isolated from hospital-associated infections in the United States. Although *Enterococcus faecalis* remains the predominant species recovered from nosocomial infections, the isolation of *E. faecium* has increased substantially in the past 10 to 15 years. More than 80% of *E. faecium* isolates recovered in U.S. hospitals are resistant to vancomycin and more than 90% are resistant to ampicillin. The most important factors associated with vancomycin-resistant enterococci (VRE) colonization and persistence in the gut include prolonged hospitalization; long courses of antibiotic therapy; hospitalization in long-term-care facilities, surgical units, or intensive care units; organ transplantation; renal failure (particularly in patients undergoing hemodialysis) or diabetes; high APACHE scores; and physical proximity to patients infected or colonized with VRE or to these patients' rooms. VRE infection increases the risk of death, independent of the patient's clinical status, over that among individuals infected with a glycopeptide-susceptible enterococcal strain.

IV-64. **The answer is B.** *(Chap. 137)* This patient has enterococcal endocarditis, which often occurs in patients with underlying gastrointestinal or genitourinary pathology. *Enterococcus faecalis* is a more common causative organism than *E. faecium* in community-acquired endocarditis. Patients tend to more commonly be men with underlying chronic disease. The typical presentation is one of subacute bacterial endocarditis and with involvement of the mitral or aortic valves. Prolonged therapy beyond 4 to 6 weeks is often necessary for organisms with drug resistance. Complications requiring valve replacement are common. Enterococci are intrinsically resistant or tolerant to several antimicrobial agents (with *tolerance* defined as lack of killing by drug concentrations 16 times higher than the minimal inhibitory concentration). Monotherapy for endocarditis with a β-lactam antibiotic (to which many enterococci are tolerant) has produced disappointing results with low cure rates at the end of therapy. However, the addition of an aminoglycoside to a cell wall–active agent (a β-lactam or a glycopeptide) increases cure rates and eradicates the organisms; moreover, this combination is synergistic and bactericidal in vitro. Therefore, combination therapy with a cell wall–active agent and an aminoglycoside is the standard of care for endovascular infections caused by enterococci. This synergistic effect can be explained, at least in part, by the increased penetration of the aminoglycoside into the bacterial cell, presumably as a result of cell wall alterations attributable to the β-lactam or glycopeptide.

IV-65. **The answer is D.** *(Chap. 137)* Resistance to ampicillin and vancomycin is far more common in strains of *Enterococcus faecium* than *E. faecalis*. Linezolid and quinupristin–dalfopristin are approved by the U.S. Food and Drug Administration for the treatment of some vancomycin-resistant enterococci (VRE) infections. Linezolid is not bactericidal, and its use in severe endovascular infections has produced mixed results; therefore, it is recommended only as an alternative to other agents. Quinupristin–dalfopristin is not active against most *E. faecalis* isolates. Resistance to VRE strains of *E. faecium* is also emerging with increasing usage. Cephalosporins are generally inactive against enterococcal infections.

IV-66. **The answer is B.** *(Chap. 138)* *Rhodococcus* spp., including *R. equi*, are phylogenetically related to the corynebacteria. They predominantly cause necrotizing lung infections in immunocompromised hosts. The differential diagnosis of the cavitating lung lesions includes tuberculosis, *Nocardia* infection, and septic emboli. The organisms can initially be mistaken for corynebacteria, but they should not be misconstrued as skin contaminants. The organism is routinely susceptible to vancomycin, which is considered the drug of choice. Infection caused by *R. equi* has also been treated successfully with antibiotics that penetrate intracellularly, including macrolides, clindamycin, trimethoprim–sulfamethoxazole, rifampin, tigecycline, and linezolid. β-Lactam antibiotics are not effective.

IV-67. **The answer is D.** *(Chap. 139) Listeria* meningitis typically affects elderly and the chronically ill individuals. It is frequently a more subacute (developing over days) illness than other etiologies of bacterial meningitis. It may be mistaken for aseptic meningitis. Meningeal signs, including nuchal rigidity, are less common, as is photophobia, than in other more acute causes of bacterial meningitis. Typically, white blood cell (WBC) counts in the cerebrospinal fluid range from 100 to 5000/μL with a less pronounced neutrophilia. About 75% of patients will have a WBC count below 1000/μL. Gram stain is only positive in 30% to 40% of cases. Case fatality rates are approximately 20%.

IV-68. **The answer is A.** *(Chap. 139)* *Listeria monocytogenes* causes gastrointestinal (GI) illness via ingestion of food that has been contaminated with high concentrations of bacteria. The bacteria may survive and multiply at refrigeration temperatures; therefore, deli meats, soft cheeses, hot dogs, and milk are common sources. The attack rate is very high, with close to 100% of exposed patients experiencing symptoms. Symptoms develop within 48 hours of exposure, and there is no prolonged asymptomatic carrier state. Person-to-person spread (other than vertically from mother to fetus) does not appear to occur during outbreaks. Although the bacteria have several virulence factors that lead to clinical symptoms, the organism, and not a specific toxin, mediates infection. A large inoculum is necessary to produce symptoms. Surveillance studies show that fewer than 5% of asymptomatic adults have positive stool cultures, and fecal–oral spread is not common. Typical symptoms, including fever, are as described in the case above. Patients with isolated GI illness do not require antibiotics.

IV-69. **The answer is B.** *(Chap. 139)* *Listeria* bacteremia in pregnancy is a relatively rare but serious infection both for the mother and fetus. Vertical transmission may occur, with 70% to 90% of fetuses developing infection from their mothers. Preterm labor is common. Prepartum treatment of the mother increases the chances of a healthy delivery. Mortality among fetuses approaches 50% and is much lower in neonates receiving appropriate antibiotics. First-line therapy is with ampicillin, with gentamicin often added for synergy. This recommendation is the same for the mother and child. In patients with true penicillin allergy, the therapy of choice is trimethoprim–sulfamethoxazole. There are case reports of successful therapy with vancomycin, imipenem, linezolid, and macrolides, but there is not enough clinical evidence, and there have been some reports of failure that maintain ampicillin as recommended therapy.

IV-70. **The answer is D.** *(Chap. 140)* Tetanus is an acute disease manifested by skeletal muscle spasm and autonomic nervous system disturbance. It is caused by a powerful neurotoxin produced by the bacterium *Clostridium tetani* and is now a rare disease because of widespread vaccination. There were fewer than 50 cases reported recently in the United States, but there is a rising frequency in drug users. Older patients may be at higher risk because of waning immunity. The differential diagnosis of a patient presenting with tetanus includes strychnine poisoning and drug-related dystonic reactions. The diagnosis is clinical. Cardiovascular instability is common because of autonomic dysfunction and is manifest by rapid fluctuation in heart rate and blood pressure. Wound culture results are positive in approximately 20% of cases. Metronidazole or penicillin should be administered to clear infection. Tetanus immune globulin is recommended over equine antiserum because of a lower risk of anaphylactic reactions. Recent evidence suggests that intrathecal administration is efficacious in inhibiting disease progression and improving outcomes. Muscle spasms may be treated with sedative drugs. With effective supportive care and often respiratory support, muscle function recovers after clearing the toxin with no residual damage.

IV-71. **The answer is B.** *(Chap. 141)* This patient most likely has wound botulism. The use of "black-tar" heroin has been identified as a risk factor for this form of botulism. Typically, the wound appears benign, and unlike in other forms of botulism, gastrointestinal symptoms are absent. Symmetric *descending* paralysis suggests botulism, as does cranial nerve involvement. This patient's ptosis, diplopia, dysarthria, dysphagia, lack of fevers, normal reflexes, and lack of sensory deficits are all suggestive. Botulism can be easily confused with Guillain-Barré syndrome (GBS), which is often characterized by an antecedent infection and rapid, symmetric *ascending* paralysis and treated with plasmapheresis. The Miller

Fischer variant of GBS is known for cranial nerve involvement with ophthalmoplegia, ataxia, and areflexia being the most prominent features. Elevated protein in the cerebrospinal fluid also favors GBS over botulism. Both botulism and GBS can progress to respiratory failure, so making a diagnosis by physical examination is critical. Other diagnostic modalities that may be helpful are wound culture, serum assay for toxin, and examination for decreased compound muscle action potentials on routine nerve stimulation studies. Patients with botulism are at risk of respiratory failure caused by respiratory muscle weakness or aspiration. They should be followed closely with oxygen saturation monitoring and serial measurement of forced vital capacity.

IV-72. **The answer is E.** *(Chap. 142)* Clostridia are gram-positive, spore-forming obligate anaerobes that reside normally in the gastrointestinal (GI) tract. Several clostridial species can cause severe disease. *Clostridium perfringens,* which is the second most common clostridial species to normally colonize the GI tract, is associated with food poisoning, gas gangrene, and myonecrosis. *C. septicum* is seen often in conjunction with GI tumors. *C. sordellii* is associated with septic abortions. All can cause a fulminant overwhelming bacteremia, but this condition is rare. The fact that this patient is well several days after his acute complaints rules out this fulminant course. A more common scenario is transient, self-limited bacteremia caused by transient gut translocation during an episode of gastroenteritis. There is no need to treat when this occurs, and no further workup is necessary. *Clostridium* spp. sepsis rarely causes endocarditis because overwhelming disseminated intravascular coagulation and death occur so rapidly. Screening for GI tumor is warranted when *C. septicum* is cultured from the blood or a deep wound infection.

IV-73. **The answer is A.** *(Chap. 143)* *Neisseria meningitidis* is an effective colonizer of the human nasopharynx, with asymptomatic infection rates of greater than 25% described in some series of adolescents and young adults and among residents of crowded communities. Despite the high rates of carriage among adolescents and young adults, only 10% of adults carry meningococci, and colonization is very rare in early childhood. Colonization should be considered the normal state of meningococcal infection. Meningeal pharyngitis rarely occurs. Meningococcal disease occurs when a virulent form of the organism invades a susceptible host. The most important bacterial virulence factor relates to the presence of the capsule. Unencapsulated forms of *N. meningitides* rarely cause disease. A nonblanching petechial or purpuric rash occurs in more than 80% of cases of meningococcal disease. Of patients with meningococcal disease, 30% to 50% present with meningitis, approximately 40% with meningitis plus septicemia, and 20% with septicemia alone. Patients with complement deficiency, who are at highest risk of developing meningococcal disease, may develop chronic meningitis.

IV-74. **The answer is B.** *(Chap. 143)* Close contacts of individuals with meningococcal disease are at increased risk of developing secondary disease with reports of secondary cases in up to 3% of primary cases. The rate of secondary cases is highest during the week after presentation of the index case with most cases presenting within 6 weeks. Increased risk remains for up to 1 year. Prophylaxis is recommended for persons who are intimate or household contacts of the index case and health care workers who have been directly exposed to respiratory secretions. Mass prophylaxis is not usually offered. The aim of prophylaxis is to eradicate colonization of close contacts with the strain that has caused invasive disease. Prophylaxis should be given as soon as possible to all contacts at the same time to avoid recolonization. Waiting for culture is not recommended. Ceftriaxone as a single dose is currently the most effective option in reducing carriage. Rifampin is no longer the optimal agent because it requires multiple doses and fails to eliminate carriage in up to 20% of cases. In some countries, ciprofloxacin or ofloxacin is used, but resistance has been reported in some areas. Current conjugated vaccines do not include *N. meningitides* serotype B. Most sporadic cases in the United States are now caused by this serotype. Vaccination should be offered in cases of meningococcal disease caused by documented infection by a serotype included in the current vaccine.

IV-75. **The answer is D.** *(Chap. 144)* Because of emerging resistance, treatment recommendations for gonorrhea require frequent updating. Fluoroquinolones and penicillin are no longer generally recommended in the United States because of resistance. Current effective therapies use single-dose therapies to maximize adherence. Oral cefixime or intramuscular ceftriaxone are effective for urethritis, cervicitis, and proctitis. Azithromycin is no longer effective for gonorrhea because of resistance, but it should be administered because of the presumption of chlamydial co-infection. Doxycycline also an option for co-treatment in nonpregnant women. Patients with uncomplicated infection who receive therapy do not require a test of cure. Patients should be instructed to contact sexual partners for screening and therapy. Recent studies have demonstrated that the provision of medications or prescriptions to treat gonorrhea and chlamydia in sexual partners diminishes the risk of reinfection in the affected patient.

IV-76. **The answer is D.** *(Chap. 145)* Generally thought of as a disease of children, epiglottitis is also a disease of adults since the wide use of *Haemophilus influenzae* type B vaccination. Epiglottitis can cause life-threatening airway obstruction caused by cellulitis of the epiglottis and supraglottic tissues, classically caused by *H. influenzae* type B infection. However, other organisms are also common causes, including nontypeable *H. influenzae, Streptococcus pneumoniae, H. parainfluenzae, Staphylococcus aureus*, and viral infection. The initial evaluation and treatment for epiglottitis in adults includes airway management and intravenous antibiotics. The patient presented here is demonstrating signs of impending airway obstruction with stridor, inability to swallow secretions, and use of accessory muscles of inspiration. A lateral neck radiograph shows the typical thumb sign indicative of a swollen epiglottis. In addition, the patient has evidence of hypoventilation with carbon dioxide retention. Thus, in addition to antibiotics, this patient should also be intubated and mechanically ventilated electively under a controlled setting because he is at high risk for mechanical airway obstruction. Antibiotic therapy should cover the typical organisms outlined above and include coverage for oral anaerobes.

In adults presenting without overt impending airway obstruction, laryngoscopy would be indicated to assess airway patency. Endotracheal intubation would be recommended for those with more than 50% airway obstruction. In children, endotracheal intubation is often recommended because laryngoscopy in children has provoked airway obstruction to a much greater degree than adults, and increased risk of mortality has been demonstrated in some series in children when the airway is managed expectantly.

IV-77. **The answer is A.** *(Chap. 145)* *Moraxella catarrhalis* is an unencapsulated gram-negative diplococcus that causes upper respiratory tract disease in children and adults. Some studies suggest that the widespread implementation of pneumococcal vaccination has increased the prevalence of *M. catarrhalis* and related organisms as a cause of disease. *M. catarrhalis* causes approximately 10% to 20% of cases of otitis media in children, often after a preceding viral infection. It is the second most common proven bacterial cause of chronic obstructive pulmonary disease (COPD) exacerbations after *Haemophilus influenzae*. Clinical features do not distinguish among the various bacterial and viral causes of COPD exacerbations. In most cases, a proven cause is not found. Currently, most strains of *M. catarrhalis* demonstrate β-lactamase activity. Recommended therapy includes agents effective for upper respiratory, sinus, and otic infections presumed to be caused by *M. catarrhalis, H. influenzae*, and *S. pneumoniae*, including amoxicillin–clavulanic acid, extended-spectrum cephalosporins, azithromycin, clarithromycin, and flouroquinolones.

IV-78. **The answer is C.** *(Chap. 146)* This patient has subacute bacterial endocarditis caused by infection with one of the HACEK organisms. The HACEK organisms (*Haemophilus, Actinobacillus, Cardiobacterium, Eikenella*, and *Kingella* spp.) are gram-negative rods that reside in the oral cavity. They are responsible for about 3% of cases of infective endocarditis in most series. They are the most common cause of gram-negative endocarditis in nondrug abusers. Most patients have a history of poor dentition or a recent dental procedure. Often, patients are initially diagnosed with culture-negative endocarditis because these organisms may be slow growing and fastidious. Cultures must be specified for prolonged culture of fastidious organisms. HACEK endocarditis is typically subacute, and the risk of embolic phenomena to the bone, skin, kidneys, and vasculature is high. Vegetations are seen on approximately 85% of transthoracic echocardiograms. Cure rates are excellent with antibiotics alone; native valves require 4 weeks, and prosthetic valves require 6 weeks of treatment. Ceftriaxone is the treatment of choice, with ampicillin–gentamicin as an alternative. Sensitivities may be delayed because of the organisms' slow growth.

IV-79. **The answer is B.** *(Chap. 146) Capnocytophaga canimorsus* is the most likely organism to have caused fulminant disease in this patient with alcoholism after a dog bite. Patients with a history of alcoholism, asplenia, and glucocorticoid therapy are at risk of developing disseminated infection, sepsis, and disseminated intravascular coagulation. Because of increasing β-lactamase expression, recommended treatment is with ampicillin–sulbactam or clindamycin. One of these therapies should be administered to asplenic patients with a dog bite. Other species of *Capnocytophaga* cause oropharyngeal disease and can cause sepsis in neutropenic patients, particularly in the presence of oral ulcers. *Eikenella* and *Haemophilus* spp. are common mouth flora in humans but not in dogs. *Staphylococcus* spp. can cause sepsis but is less likely in this scenario.

IV-80. **The answer is B.** *(Chap. 147)* Despite antibiotic treatment, pneumonia from all causes remains a major source of mortality in the United States. Mortality from *Legionella* pneumonia varies from 0% to 11% in treated immunocompetent patients to about 30% if not treated effectively. Because *Legionella* spp. is an intracellular pathogen, antibiotics that reach intracellular MICs are most likely to be effective. Newer macrolides and quinolones are antibiotics of choice and are effective as monotherapy. Doxycycline and tigecycline are active in vitro. Anecdotal reports have described successes and failures with trimethoprim–sulfamethoxazole and clindamycin. Aztreonam, most β-lactams, and cephalosporins cannot be considered effective therapy for *Legionella* pneumonia. For severe cases, rifampin may be initially added to azithromycin or a fluoroquinolone.

IV-81. **The answer is C.** *(Chap. 147) Legionella* is an intracellular pathogen that enters the body through aspiration or direct inhalation. Numerous prospective studies have found it is one of the four most common causes of community-acquired pneumonia with *Streptococcus pneumoniae*, *Haemophilus influenzae*, and *Chlamydia pneumoniae* accounting for 2% to 9% of cases. Postoperative patients are at risk because of an increased risk of aspiration. Cell-mediated immunity is the primary host defense against *Legionella* spp., and patients with HIV or those who take glucocorticoids are at risk based on their depressed cell-mediated immune function. Alveolar macrophages phagocytose *Legionella* spp. Smokers and those with chronic lung disease are at risk given their poor local immune responses and decreased ability for widespread phagocytosis. Neutrophils play a comparatively small role in the host defense against *Legionella* spp., and those with neutropenia are not predisposed to *Legionella* infection.

IV-82. **The answer is D.** *(Chap. 147) Legionella* urine antigen is detectable within 3 days of symptoms and will remain positive for 2 months. It is not affected by antibiotic use. The urinary antigen test is formulated to detect only *L. pneumophila* (which causes 80% of *Legionella* infections) but cross-reactivity with other *Legionella* spp. has been reported. The urinary test result is sensitive and highly specific. Typically, Gram staining of specimens from sterile sites such as pleural fluid show numerous white blood cells but no organisms. However, *Legionella* spp. may appear as faint, pleomorphic gram-negative bacilli. *Legionella* spp. may be cultured from sputum even when epithelial cells are present. Cultures, grown on selective media, take 3 to 5 days to show visible growth. Antibody detection using acute and convalescent serum is an accurate means of diagnosis. A fourfold rise is diagnostic, but this takes up to 12 weeks, so it is most useful for epidemiologic investigation. *Legionella* polymerase chain reaction has not been shown to be adequately sensitive and specific for clinical use. It is used for environmental sampling.

IV-83. **The answer is C.** (*Chap. 148*) Pertussis caused by the gram-negative bacteria *Bordetella pertussis*, is an upper respiratory infection characterized by a violent cough. Its prevalence has been dramatically reduced, but not eliminated, by widespread infant vaccination. It causes an extremely morbid and often mortal disease in infants younger than 6 months old, particularly in the developing world. The prevalence appears to be increasing in young adults and adolescents because of waning immunity. Some are recommending booster vaccination after 10 years. *B. pertussis* is also a growing pathogen in patients with chronic obstructive pulmonary disease. The clinical manifestations typically include a persistent, episodic cough developing a few days after a cold-like upper respiratory infection. The cough may become persistent. It often wakes the patient from sleep and results in posttussive vomiting. An audible whoop is only present in fewer than half of cases. Diagnosis is with nasopharyngeal culture or DNA probe testing. There is no urinary antigen testing available. The goal of antibiotic therapy is to eradicate the organism from the nasopharynx. It does not alter the clinical course. Macrolide antibiotics are the treatment of choice. Pneumonia is uncommon with *B. pertussis*. Cold agglutinins may be positive in infection with *Mycoplasma pneumoniae*, which is on the differential diagnosis of *B. pertussis*.

IV-84. **The answer is C.** (*Chap. 149*) Enterotoxigenic *Escherichia coli* is the most common cause of traveler's diarrhea, accounting for 50% of cases in Latin America and 15% in Asia. Enterotoxigenic and enteroaggregative *E. coli* are the most common isolates from persons with classic secretory traveler's diarrhea. Bloody stools, fecal leukocytes, and fever are typically absent. Symptoms typically last less than 3 days. The spectrum of disease can range from mild to severe with life-threatening volume loss. Treatment of frequent watery stools caused by presumed *E. coli* infection with ciprofloxacin, or because of concerns regarding increasing ciprofloxacin resistance, azithromycin may shorten the duration of symptoms. *Entamoeba histolytica* and *Vibrio cholerae* account for smaller percentages of traveler's diarrhea in Mexico. *Campylobacter* infection is more common in Asia and during the winter in subtropical areas. *Giardia* infection is associated with contaminated water supplies and in campers who drink from freshwater streams.

IV-85. **The answer is D.** (*Chap. 149*) β-lactamases are a major source of antibiotic resistance in gram-negative bacilli. Many gram-negative bacteria produce broad-spectrum β-lactamases that confer resistance to penicillins and first-generation cephalosporins. The addition of clavulanate, a β-lactamase inhibitor, to an antibiotic regimen is often enough to overcome this resistance. Extended-spectrum β-lactamases (ESBLs), however, lead to resistance to all β-lactam drugs, including third- and fourth-generation cephalosporins. ESBL-producing genes can be acquired by gram-negative bacteria via plasmids and are becoming increasingly prevalent in hospitals worldwide. *Klebsiella* and *Escherichia coli* are the most common bacteria that acquire ESBLs, although it can be seen in many other gram-negatives, including *Serratia, Proteus, Enterobacter*, and *Citrobacter* spp. The most common scenario for the development of ESBL-gram negative organisms in the hospital is prevalent use of third-generation cephalosporins. Carbapenems should be considered first-line antibiotics for these bacteria. Macrolides and quinolones have different mechanisms of action than β-lactam antibiotics and do not apply selective pressure to generate ESBL-producing bacteria.

IV-86. **The answer is B.** (*Chap. 149*) *E. coli* is the etiologic agent in 85% to 95% of uncomplicated urinary tract infections (UTIs) that occur in premenopausal women. Uncomplicated cystitis is the most common UTI syndrome. About 20% of women will develop a recurrence in 1 year after their initial UTI. Pregnant women are at high risk of cystitis developing into pyelonephritis. *Proteus* infection represents only 1% to 2% of uncomplicated UTIs. *Proteus* infection causes 20% to 45% of UTIs in patients with long-term bladder catheterization. *Klebsiella* spp. also accounts for only 1% to 2% of uncomplicated UTIs; however, it is responsible for 5% to 17% of complicated UTIs. *Enterobacter* spp. is a rare cause of infection outside of the hospital. *Candida* spp. is most often a genitourinary colonizer in healthy patients and is rarely the cause of infection.

IV-87. **The answer is A.** *(Chap. 149) Shiga* toxic and enterohemorrhagic strains of *Escherichia coli* (STEC/EHEC) cause hemorrhagic colitis and hemolytic uremic syndrome (HUS). Several large outbreaks resulting from the consumption of fresh produce (e.g., lettuce, spinach, sprouts) and of undercooked ground beef have received significant attention in the media. O157:H7 is the most prominent serotype, but others have been reported to cause similar disease. The ability of STEC/EHEC to produce Shiga toxin (Stx2 and/or Stx1) or related toxins is a critical factor in the expression of clinical disease. Manure from domesticated ruminant animals in industrialized countries serves as the major reservoir for STEC/EHEC. Ground beef—the most common food source of STEC/EHEC strains—is often contaminated during processing. Low bacterial numbers can transmit disease in humans, accounting for widespread infection from environmental sources and person-to-person spread. O157:H7 strains are the fourth most commonly reported cause of bacterial diarrhea in the United States (after *Campylobacter*, *Salmonella*, and *Shigella* spp.). STEC/EHEC characteristically causes grossly bloody diarrhea in more than 90% of cases. Significant abdominal pain and fecal leukocytes are common (70% of cases), but fever is not; absence of fever can incorrectly lead to consideration of noninfectious conditions (e.g., intussusception and inflammatory or ischemic bowel disease). STEC/EHEC disease is usually self-limited, lasting 5 to 10 days. HUS may develop in very young or elderly patients within 2 weeks of diarrhea. It is estimated that it occurs in 2% to 8% of cases of STEC/EHEC and that more than 50% of all cases of HUS in the United States and 90% of cases in children are caused by STEC/EHEC. Antibiotic therapy of STEC/EHEC cases of diarrhea should be avoided because antibiotics may increase the likelihood of developing HUS.

IV-88. **The answer is E.** *(Chap. 150)* Infections with *Acinetobacter* spp. are a growing cause of hospital-acquired infections worldwide. Surveillance data from Australia and Asia suggest that infections are common, and there are reports of community-acquired *Acinetobacter* infection. They typically infect patients receiving long-term care in intensive care units by causing ventilator-associated pneumonia, bloodstream infections, or urinary tract infections. They are particularly of concern because of their propensity to develop multidrug (or pan-drug) resistance and their ability to colonize units because of health care worker transmission. *A. baumannii* is the most common isolate and develops drug resistance avidly. Many strains are currently resistant to carbapenems (imipenem, meropenem). Last-line agents such as colistin, polymyxin A, and tigecycline are often the only available therapeutic options. Tigecycline has been used for pneumonia caused by carbapenem-resistant strains but is not thought to be efficacious in bloodstream infection because usual dosing does not achieve therapeutic levels against *Acinetobacter* spp.

IV-89. **The answer is B.** *(Chap. 151) Helicobacter pylori* is thought to colonize about 50% (30% in developed countries and >80% in developing countries) of the world's population. The organism induces a direct tissue response in the stomach, with evidence of mononuclear and polymorphonuclear infiltrates in all of those with colonization regardless of whether or not symptoms are present. Gastric ulceration and adenocarcinoma of the stomach arise in association with this gastritis. MALT is specific to *H. pylori* infection and because of prolonged B-cell activation in the stomach. Although *H. pylori* does not directly infect the intestine, it does diminish somatostatin production, indirectly contributing to the development of duodenal ulcers. Gastroesophageal reflux disease is not caused by *H. pylori* colonization. Recent studies have demonstrated that colonization by some strains of *H. pylori* may be protective for the development of adenocarcinoma of the esophagus and premalignant lesions such as Barrett's esophagus (odds ratio, 0.2–0.6).

IV-90. **The answer is E.** *(Chap. 151)* It is impossible to know whether the patient's continued dyspepsia is attributable to persistent *Helicobacter pylori* as a result of treatment failure or to some other cause. A quick noninvasive test to look for the presence of *H. pylori* is a urea breath test. This test can be done as an outpatient and gives a rapid, accurate response. Patients should not have received any proton pump inhibitors or antimicrobials in the meantime. Stool antigen test is another good option if urea breath testing is not available. If the urea breath test is positive more than 1 month after completion of first-line therapy, second-line therapy with a proton pump inhibitor, bismuth subsalicylate, tetracycline, and metronidazole may be indicated. If the urea breath test result is negative, the remaining symptoms are unlikely attributable to persistent *H. pylori* infection. Serology is useful only for diagnosing infection initially, but it can remain positive and therefore misleading in those who have cleared *H. pylori*. Endoscopy is a consideration to rule out ulcer or upper gastrointestinal malignancy but is generally preferred after two failed attempts to eradicate *H. pylori*. Figure IV-90 outlines the algorithm for management of *H. pylori* infection.

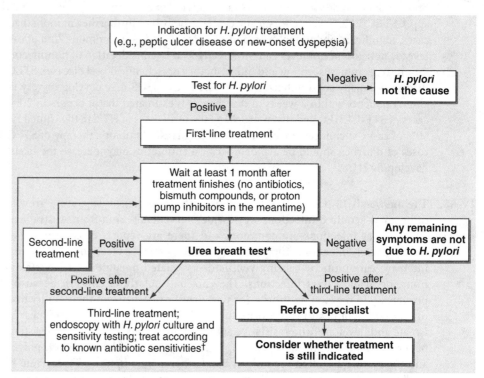

FIGURE IV-90

IV-91. **The answer is A.** *(Chap. 151)* Helicobacter pylori is a disease of overcrowding. Transmission has therefore decreased in the United States as the standard of living has increased. It is predicated that the percentage of duodenal ulcers caused by factors other than *H. pylori* (e.g., use of nonsteroidal anti-inflammatory drugs) will increase over the upcoming decades. Controversial but increasing evidence suggests that *H. pylori* colonization may provide some protection from recent emerging gastrointestinal disorders, such as gastroesophageal reflux disease (and its complication, esophageal carcinoma). Therefore, the health implications of *H. pylori* eradication may not be simple.

IV-92. **The answer is A.** *(Chap. 151)* In vitro, *Helicobacter pylori* is susceptible to a wide variety of antibiotics. However, monotherapy is no longer recommended because of inadequate antibiotic delivery to the colonization niche and the development of resistance. All current regimens include a proton pump inhibitor (omeprazole or equivalent), H2 blocker (ranitidine or equivalent), and/or bismuth. Regimens including quinolones may not be advisable because of common resistance and the risk of developing *Clostridium difficile* colitis. Current regimens have an eradication rate of 75% to 80%. (See Table IV-92.)

TABLE IV-92 Recommended Treatment Regimens for *Helicobacter pylori* Infection

Regimen (Duration)	Drug 1	Drug 2	Drug 3	Drug 4
Regimen 1: OCM (7–14 days)[a]	Omeprazole[b] (20 mg bid)	Clarithromycin (500 mg bid)	Metronidazole (500 mg bid)	—
Regimen 2: OCA (7–14 days)[a]	Omeprazole[b] (20 mg bid)	Clarithromycin (500 mg bid)	Amoxicillin (1 g bid)	—
Regimen 3: OBTM (14 days)[c]	Omeprazole[b] (20 mg bid)	Bismuth subsalicylate (2 tabs qid)	Tetracycline HCl (500 mg qid)	Metronidazole (500 mg tid)
Regimen 4[d]: sequential (5 days + 5 days)	Omeprazole[b] (20 mg bid)	Amoxicillin 1 g bid		
	Omeprazole[b] (20 mg bid)	Clarithromycin (500 mg bid)	Tinidazole (500 mg bid)	
Regimen 5[e]: OAL (10 days)	Omeprazole[b] (20 mg bid)	Amoxicillin (1 g bid)	Levofloxacin (500 mg qid)	

[a]Meta-analyses show that a 14-day course of therapy is slightly superior to a 7-day course. However, in populations in which 7-day treatment is known to have very high success rates, this shorter course is still often used.
[b]Omeprazole may be replaced with any proton pump inhibitor at an equivalent dosage or, in regimens 1 and 2, with ranitidine bismuth citrate (400 mg).
[c]Data supporting this regimen come mainly from Europe and are based on the use of bismuth subcitrate and metronidazole (400 mg tid). This is the most commonly used second-line regimen.
[d]Data supporting this regimen come from Europe. Although the two 5-day courses of different drugs have usually been given sequentially, recent evidence suggests no added benefit from this approach. Thus 10 days of the four drugs combined may be as good and may aid compliance.
[e]Data supporting this second- or third-line regimen come from Europe. This regimen may be less effective where rates of quinolone use are high. Theoretically, it may also be wise to avoid it in populations where *Clostridium difficile* infection is common after broad-spectrum antibiotic use.
Abbreviations: bid, twice a day; qid, four times a day; tid, three times a day.

IV-93. **The answer is A.** *(Chap. 152) Burkholderia cepacia* is an opportunistic pathogen that has been responsible for nosocomial outbreaks. It also colonizes and infects the lower respiratory tract of patients with cystic fibrosis, chronic granulomatous disease, and sickle cell disease. In patients with cystic fibrosis, it portends a rapid decline in pulmonary function and a poor clinical prognosis. It also may cause a resistant necrotizing pneumonia. *B. cepacia* is often intrinsically resistant to a variety of antimicrobials, including many β-lactams and aminoglycosides. Trimethoprim–sulfamethoxazole (TMP/SMX) is usually the first-line treatment. *Pseudomonas aeruginosa* and *Staphylococcus aureus* are common colonizers and pathogens in patients with cystic fibrosis. *Stenotrophomonas maltophilia* is an opportunistic pathogen, particularly in patients with cancer, transplants, and critical illness. *S. maltophilia* is a cause of pneumonia, urinary tract infection, wound infection, and bacteremia. TMP/SMX is usually the treatment of choice for *Stenotrophomonas* infections.

IV-94. **The answer is A.** *(Chap. 152)* Ecthyma gangrenosum is a disseminated collection of geographic, painful, reddish, maculopapular lesions that rapidly progress from pink to purple and finally to a black, dry necrosis. They are teeming with causative bacteria. In reviews on ecthyma, *Pseudomonas aeruginosa* is the most common isolate from blood and skin lesions. However, many organisms can cause this foreboding rash. Neutropenic patients and AIDS patients are at highest risk, but diabetics and intensive care unit (ICU) patients are also affected. Pseudomonal sepsis is severe with a high mortality rate. Its presentation is otherwise difficult to discern from other severe sepsis syndromes, with hypothermia, fever, hypotension, organ damage, encephalopathy, bandemia, and shock being common findings. Although antibiotic use, severe burns, and long ICU stays increase the risk for *Pseudomonas* infection, these exposures are also risk factors for other bacterial infections, many of which also carry daunting resistant profiles. Because of *P. aeruginosa*'s propensity for multidrug resistance, two agents (usually an antipseudomonal β-lactam plus an aminoglycoside or ciprofloxacin) are warranted until culture data return confirming sensitivity to one or both agents. At this point, the choice to narrow to one antibiotic or not is still debated and is largely physician preference.

IV-95. **The answer is A.** *(Chap. 152)* Antibiotic therapy against *Pseudomonas aeruginosa* is often controversial, and the practitioner must interpret recommendations in light of local resistance patterns. Traditionally, many recommended two-drug therapy for *Pseudomonas* bacteremia because of synergy between aminoglycosides and β-lactam agents. Since the introduction of newer antipseudomonal antibiotics, most studies conclude that monotherapy with one of those drugs to which the isolate is sensitive is as effective as combination therapy. That conclusion holds for bacteremic patients with or without neutropenia. However, monotherapy with an aminoglycoside for *P. aeruginosa* bacteremia is not recommended. Many recommend adding an aminoglycoside to an antipseudomonal drug in cases of shock or where the prevalence of resistance to the primary drug is high. The Infectious Diseases Society of America recommends adding an aminoglycoside or ciprofloxacin for *Pseudomonas* pneumonia.

IV-96. **The answer is E.** *(Chap. 153)* *Salmonella enteritidis* is one of the causes of nontyphoidal salmonellosis (NTS) along with *Salmonella typhimurium* and other strains. Enteric (typhoid) fever is caused by *Salmonella typhi* or *Salmonella paratyphi*. Recent cases of gastroenteritis caused by NTS have been associated with undercooked or raw eggs. In contrast to *S. typhi* and *S. paratyphi*, which only have human reservoirs, the NTS can colonize livestock accounting for outbreaks related to contaminated water (fresh produce, undercooked ground meat, dairy products). The gastroenteritis caused by NTS is indistinguishable clinically for other enteric pathogens. The diarrhea is nonbloody and may be copious. The disease is typically self-limited in healthy hosts, and antibiotic therapy is not recommended because it does not change the course of disease and promotes resistance. Therapy may be necessary for neonates or debilitated elderly patients who are more likely to develop bacteremia. Bacteremia occurs in fewer than 10% of cases. Metastatic infections of bone, joint, and endovascular devices may occur. There is no vaccine for NTS. Oral and parenteral vaccines for *S. typhi* are available.

IV-97. **The answer is D.** *(Chap. 154)* Shigellosis remains a cause of dysentery in the developing world and sporadic cases caused by fecal–oral contamination occur in the developing and developed world. The human intestinal tract is the most prevalent reservoir for the bacteria. Clinical illness from *Shigella* infection can be caused by a very small inoculum. Shigellosis typically evolves through four phases: incubation, watery diarrhea, dysentery, and the postinfectious phase. The incubation period is usually 1 to 4 days, and the dysentery follows within hours to days. The dysentery syndrome is indistinguishable from other invasive enteropathogens (including *Campylobacter* spp.), and inflammatory bowel disease is also in the differential diagnosis. Because the organism is enteroinvasive, antibiotic therapy is indicated. Ciprofloxacin is generally recommended unless there is no or proven resistance. Ceftriaxone, azithromycin, pivmecillinam, and some recent quinolones are also effective. *Shigella* infection typically does not cause life-threatening dehydration. Antimotility agents are not recommended because they are thought to prolong the systemic symptoms and may increase the risk of toxic mega-colon and hemolytic uremic syndrome. There is currently no commercially available vaccine for *Shigella* infection.

IV-98. **The answer is A.** *(Chap. 155)* *Campylobacter* spp. are motile, curved gram-negative rods. The principal diarrheal pathogen is *Campylobacter jejuni*. This organism is found in the gastrointestinal tract of many animals used for food production and is usually transmitted to humans in raw or undercooked food products or through direct contact with infected animals. More than half of cases are caused by insufficiently cooked contaminated poultry. *Campylobacter* infection a common cause of diarrheal disease in the United States. The illness usually occurs within 2 to 4 days after exposure to the organism in food or water. Biopsy of an affected patient's jejunum, ileum, or colon reveals findings indistinguishable from those of Crohn's disease and ulcerative colitis. Although the diarrheal illness is usually self-limited, it may be associated with constitutional symptoms, lasts more than 1 week, and recurs in 5% to 10% of untreated patients. Complications include pancreatitis, cystitis, arthritis, meningitis, and Guillain-Barré syndrome. The symptoms of *Campylobacter* enteritis are similar to those resulting from infection with *Salmonella typhi, Shigella* spp., and *Yersinia* spp.; all of these agents cause fever and the presence of fecal leukocytes. The diagnosis is made by isolating *Campylobacter* organisms from the stool, which requires selective media. *Escherichia coli* (enterotoxigenic), Norwalk agent, and rotavirus are generally not associated with the finding of fecal leukocytes. About 5% to 10% of untreated patients with *Campylobacter* enteritis develop recurrences that may be clinically and pathologically confused with inflammatory bowel disease.

IV-99. **The answer is A.** *(Chap. 155)* As is true with all acute diarrheal diseases, adequate volume resuscitation is central to treatment. Many patients with mild *Campylobacter* enteritis will resolve spontaneously, and not all patients clearly benefit from therapy. In the presence of high or persistent fever, bloody diarrhea, severe diarrhea, worsening symptoms, or symptoms persisting for more than 1 week, antibiotics are recommended. A 5- to 7-day course of erythromycin, azithromycin (and other macrolides), or ciprofloxacin is effective. Drug resistance to flouroquinolones and tetracycline is increasing. Antimotility agents are not recommended because they have been associated with the development of serious complications, including toxic megacolon and hemolytic uremic syndrome. Tinidazole and metronidazole are used to treat a variety of nonbacterial diarrhea syndromes, including giardiasis and amoebiasis. Metronidazole is also used for *Clostridium difficile*–associated colitis.

IV-100. **The answer is B.** *(Chap. 156)* Cholera remains a worldwide problem with sporadic cases usually related to contact with fecally contaminated water or seafood. Humans are the only known reservoir of *Vibrio cholera*. Most cases are reported in Africa or Asia. After a century, cholera returned to Haiti after recent natural disasters and breakdown of public health measures. The watery diarrhea of cholera is mediated by a specific cholera toxin that binds to small intestine epithelium to cause profuse fluid secretion. The diarrhea of cholera is painless, nonbloody, and watery with mucus and few inflammatory cells. The term "rice-water" diarrhea refers to the appearance of water after soaking rice. Morbidity and mortality from cholera are from profound volume depletion. Rehydration is essential to therapy. Major improvements in care came from the development of oral rehydration solutions that take advantage of glucose–sodium co-transport in the small intestine. These solutions allowed effective rehydration in resource limited settings where intravenous rehydration was not practical. Diagnosis is by culture or point-of-care antigen detection dipstick assay. Antibiotics are not necessary for cure, but they diminish the duration and volume of fluid loss and hasten the clearance of the organism from stool. A single dose of doxycycline is effective in adults in areas where there is not resistance. Ciprofloxacin or azithromycin may be alternatives.

IV-101. **The answer is E.** *(Chap. 158)* The most likely infecting organism in this patient is *Francisella tularensis*. Gentamicin is the antibiotic of choice for the treatment of tularemia. Fluoroquinolones have shown in vitro activity against *F. tularensis* and have successfully been used in a few cases of tularemia. Currently, however, it cannot be recommended as first-line therapy because data are limited regarding its efficacy relative to gentamicin, but it can be considered if an individual is unable to tolerate gentamicin. To date, there have been no clinical trials of fluoroquinolones to definitively demonstrate equivalency with gentamicin. Third-generation cephalosporins have in vitro activity against *F. tularensis*. However, use of ceftriaxone in children with tularemia resulted in almost universal failure. Likewise, tetracycline and chloramphenicol also have limited usefulness with a higher relapse rate (up to 20%) compared with gentamicin. *F. tularensis* is a small gram-negative, pleomorphic bacillus that is found both intra- and extracellularly. It is found in mud, water, and decaying animal carcasses, and ticks and wild rabbits are the sources for most human infections in the southeast United States and Rocky Mountains. In western states, tabanid flies are the most common vectors. The organisms usually enter the skin through the bite of a tick or through an abrasion. On further questioning, the patient above reported that during the camping trip, he was primarily responsible for skinning the animals and preparing dinner. He did sustain a small cut on his right hand at the site where the ulceration is apparent. The most common clinical manifestations of *F. tularensis* are ulceroglandular and glandular disease, accounting for 75% to 85% of cases. The ulcer appears at the site of entry of the bacteria and lasts for 1 to 3 weeks and may develop a black eschar at the base. The draining lymph nodes become enlarged and fluctuant. They may drain spontaneously. In a small percentage of patients, the disease becomes systemically spread, as is apparent in this case, with pneumonia, fevers, and sepsis syndrome. When this occurs, the mortality rate approaches 30% if untreated. However, with appropriate antibiotic therapy, the prognosis is very good. Diagnosis requires a high clinical suspicion because demonstration of the organism is difficult. It rarely seen on Gram stain because the organisms stain weakly and are so small that they are difficult to distinguish from background material. On polychromatically stained tissue, they may be seen both intra- and extracellularly, singly or in clumps. Moreover, *F. tularensis* is a difficult organism to culture and requires cysteine-glucose–blood agar. However, most laboratories do not attempt to culture the organism because of the risk of infection in laboratory workers, requiring biosafety level 2 practices. Usually the diagnosis is confirmed by agglutination testing with titers above 1:160 confirming diagnosis.

IV-102 and IV-103. The answers are E and B, respectively. *(Chap. 159)* This patient has a classic presentation of bubonic plague caused by *Yersinia pestis*. Plague is transmitted to humans from rodents via flea bites. The clinical manifestations include bubonic (most common, 80%–95% of cases), septicemic (bacteremia without a bubo), primary pneumonic, and secondary pneumonic. The untreated mortality is up to 20% with higher rates for septicemic and pneumonic presentations. Most cases in the United States occur in the Four Corners region or in the border zone of northern California, southern Oregon, and western Nevada. The presenting bubo in bubonic plague is usually near the inciting flea bite. The differential diagnosis includes streptococcal or staphylococcal infection, tularemia, cat-scratch disease, tick typhus, infectious mononucleosis, and lymphatic filariasis. These infections do not progress as rapidly as plague, are not as painful, and are associated with visible cellulitis or ascending lymphangitis, which are absent in plague. The organisms may be visualized on bubo aspirate. The gram-negative coccobacillus *Y. pestis* is characteristically bipolar on Wright's stain. Bartonella and rickettsia are generally not visible on Gram staining. Traditionally, streptomycin was the first-line treatment, but because of fewer side effects, gentamicin is currently recommended. Fluoroquinolones have in vitro activity and have been reported effective in case reports. They would likely be administered in the event of pneumonic plague as a bioterrorism event.

IV-104. The answer is A. *(Chap. 160)* This patient has bacillary angiomatosis caused by cutaneous infection with *Bartonella quintana* or *Bartonella henselae*. Kittens are the likely source of the infection in this case. Bacillary angiomatosis occurs in HIV-infected patients with CD4+ T-cell counts below 100/μL. The cutaneous lesions of bacillary angiomatosis are typically painless cutaneous lesions but may appear as subcutaneous nodules, ulcerated plaques, or verrucous growths. They may be single or multiple. The differential diagnosis includes Kaposi's sarcoma, pyogenic granuloma, and tumors. Biopsy findings are as described in this case, and the diagnosis is best made with histology. Treatment is with azithromycin or doxycycline. Oxacillin or vancomycin is the treatment for staphylococcal or streptococcal skin infections. Treatment with antiretrovirals to restore CD4+ T-cell count will prevent further episodes.

IV-105. The answer is A. *(Chap. 160)* This patient has culture-negative endocarditis, a rare entity defined as clinical evidence of infectious endocarditis in the absence of positive blood cultures. In this case, evidence for subacute bacterial endocarditis includes valvular regurgitation; an aortic valve vegetation; and embolic phenomena on the extremities, spleen, and kidneys. A common reason for negative blood culture results is prior antibiotics. In the absence of this, the two most common pathogens (both of which are technically difficult to isolate in blood culture bottles) are Q fever, or *Coxiella burnetii* (typically associated with close contact with livestock), and *Bartonella* spp. In this case, the patient's homelessness and body louse infestation are clues for *Bartonella quintana* infection. Diagnosis is made by blood culture about 25% of the time. Otherwise, direct polymerase chain reaction of valvular tissue, if available, or acute and convalescent serologies are diagnostic options. Empirical therapy for culture-negative endocarditis usually includes ceftriaxone and gentamicin with or without doxycycline. For confirmed *Bartonella* endocarditis, optimal therapy is gentamicin plus doxycycline. Epstein-Barr virus and HIV do not cause endocarditis. A peripheral blood smear would not be diagnostic.

IV-106. **The answer is C.** *(Chap. 160)* Although the patient's gardening puts her at risk for *Sporothrix* infection, this infection typically causes a more localized streaking nodular lymphadenitis affecting the forearm. The differential diagnosis for nodular adenitis includes *Sporothrix schenckii, Nocardia brasiliensis, Mycobacterium marinum, Leishmania braziliensis,* and *Francisella tularensis* and is based on direct inoculation of organism caused by contact with soil, a marine environment, or an insect or animal bite. This patient has regional lymphadenitis involving larger lymph nodes that drain the site of inoculation. Most likely in her case is cat-scratch disease caused by infection with *Bartonella henselae*, based on the kittens in her home, but lymphoma and staphylococcal infection must also be considered, and often a lymph node biopsy is required to make this distinction. Most cases of cat-scratch disease resolve without therapy. In immunocompetent patients, antibiotic therapy has minimal benefit but may expedite resolution of lymphadenopathy. Antimicrobial therapy, usually with azithromycin, is indicated in immunosuppressed patients.

IV-107. **The answer is A.** *(Chap. 161)* Donovanosis is caused by the intracellular organism *Calymmatobacterium granulomatis* and most often presents as a painless erythematous genital ulceration after a 1- to 4-week incubation period. However, incubation periods can be as long as 1 year. The infection is predominantly sexually transmitted, and autoinoculation can lead to formation of new lesions by contact with adjacent infected skin. Typically, the lesion is painless but bleeds easily. Complications include phimosis in men and pseudo-elephantiasis of the labia in women. If the infection is untreated, it can lead to progressive destruction of the penis or other organs. Diagnosis is made by demonstration of Donovan bodies within large mononuclear cells on smears from the lesion. *Donovan bodies* refers to the appearance of multiple intracellular organisms within the cytoplasm of mononuclear cells. These organisms are bipolar and have an appearance similar to a safety pin. On histologic examination, there is an increase in the number of plasma cells with few neutrophils; additionally, epithelial hyperplasia is present and can resemble neoplasia. A variety of antibiotics can be used to treat donovanosis, including macrolides, tetracyclines, trimethoprim–sulfamethoxazole, and chloramphenicol. Treatment should be continued until the lesion has healed, often requiring 5 or more weeks of treatment. All of the choices listed in the question are in the differential diagnosis of penile ulcerations. Lymphogranuloma venereum is endemic in the Caribbean. The ulcer of primary infection heals spontaneously, and the second phase of the infection results in markedly enlarged inguinal lymphadenopathy, which may drain spontaneously. *Haemophilus ducreyi* results in painful genital ulcerations, and the organism can be cultured from the lesion. The painless ulcerations of cutaneous leishmaniasis can appear similarly to those of donovanosis but usually occur on exposed skin. Histologic determination of intracellular parasites can distinguish leishmaniasis definitively from donovanosis. Finally, it is unlikely that the patient has syphilis in the setting of a negative rapid plasma reagin test result, and the histology is inconsistent with this diagnosis.

IV-108. **The answer is D.** *(Chaps. 16 and 155)* This patient is chronically immunosuppressed from his antirejection prophylactic regimen, which includes both glucocorticoids and azathioprine. However, the finding of a cavitary lesion on chest radiography considerably narrows the possibilities and increases the likelihood of nocardial infection. The other clinical findings, including production of profuse thick sputum, fever, and constitutional symptoms, are also quite common in patients who have pulmonary nocardiosis. The Gram stain, which demonstrates filamentous branching gram-positive organisms, is characteristic. Most species of *Nocardia* are acid fast if a weak acid is used for decolorization (e.g., modified Kinyoun method). These organisms can also be visualized by silver staining. They grow slowly in culture, and the laboratory must be alerted to the possibility of their presence on submitted specimens. After the diagnosis, which may require an invasive approach, is made, sulfonamides are the drugs of choice. Sulfadiazine or sulfisoxazole from 6 to 8 g/day in four divided doses generally is administered, but doses up to 12 g/day have been given.

The combination of sulfamethoxazole and trimethoprim has also been used, as have the oral alternatives minocycline and ampicillin and intravenous amikacin. There is little experience with the newer β-lactam antibiotics, including the third-generation cephalosporins and imipenem. Erythromycin alone is not effective, although it has been given successfully along with ampicillin. In addition to appropriate antibiotic therapy, the possibility of disseminated nocardiosis must be considered; common sites include brain, skin, kidneys, bone, and muscle.

IV-109. The answer is D. *(Chap. 163)* The patient presents with symptoms suggestive of osteonecrosis of her jaw possibly caused by bisphosphonate use. Additionally, her jaw pain has progressed and now appears to be infected. *Actinomyces* is a classic oral organism with a propensity to infect the jaw, particularly when the bone is abnormal, usually because of radiation or osteonecrosis. Osteonecrosis of the jaw caused by bisphosphonates is an increasingly recognized risk factor for actinomyces infection. Frequently, the soft tissue swelling is confused for either parotitis or a cancerous lesion. *Actinomyces* spp. frequently form fistulous tracts, which provide an opportunity to examine the secretions and identify either the organism itself (less common) or sulfur granules. Sulfur granules are an in vivo concretion of *Actinomyces* bacteria, calcium phosphate, and host material. Gram stain of *Actinomyces* infection shows intensely positive staining at the center with branching rods at the periphery. Auer rods are found in acute promyelocytic leukemia. Although head and neck cancer is in the differential diagnosis, the acuity of the presentation and fever make this less likely. Weakly acid-fast branching filaments are found in nocardial infection, which is unlikely to involve the head and neck, although both organisms frequently cause pulmonary infiltrates. Although parotitis with obstruction caused by sialolith is possible, the symptoms are in the jaw and diffuse, not specifically involving the parotid gland, thus making sialolith less likely.

IV-110. The answer is C. *(Chap. 163)* Therapy for actinomyces requires a long course of antibiotics even though the organism is very sensitive to penicillin therapy. This is presumed to be attributable to the difficulty of using antibiotics to penetrate the thick-walled masses and sulfur granules. Current recommendations are for penicillin IV for 2 to 6 weeks followed by oral therapy for a total of 6 to 12 months. Surgery should be reserved for patients who are not responsive to medical therapy.

IV-111. The answer is E. *(Chap. 164)* The patient presents with symptoms suggestive of lung infection, his demographics suggest that an abscess might be present, and the foul-smelling breath supports this diagnosis. His chest radiograph shows a cavity with air-fluid level, thus confirming the diagnosis of lung abscess. Lung abscess generally presents in the dependent lobes, as it did in this patient, and often involves oral anaerobic bacteria that are normally found in the crevices of teeth. Although infections are frequently polymicrobial, clindamycin is usually adequate to treat the infection. In this case, if there is no response to therapy targeted at lung abscess for several weeks, then further testing would be warranted, generally including bronchoscopy to evaluate possible malignancy. The negative purified protein derivative result makes tuberculosis very unlikely, and chest radiography did not show upper lobe infiltrates or cavities.

IV-112. The answer is B. *(Chap. 164)* The major reservoirs in the human body for anaerobic bacteria are the mouth, lower gastrointestinal tract, skin, and female genital tract. Generally, anaerobic infections occur proximal to these sites after the normal barrier (i.e., skin or mucous membrane) is disrupted. Thus, common infections resulting from these organisms are abdominal or lung abscess, periodontal infection, gynecologic infections such as bacterial vaginosis, and deep tissue infection. Properly obtained cultures in these circumstances generally grow a mixed population of anaerobes typical of the microenvironment of the original reservoir.

IV-113. The answer is C. *(Chap. 165)* Tuberculosis is most commonly transmitted from person to person by airborne droplets. Factors that affect the likelihood of developing tuberculosis infection include the probability of contact with an infectious person, the intimacy and duration of contact, the degree of infectiousness of the contact, and the environment in which the contact takes place. The most infectious patients are those with cavitary pulmonary or laryngeal tuberculosis with about 10^5 to 10^7 tuberculous bacteria per milliliter of sputum. Individuals who have a negative acid-fast bacillus smear with a positive culture for tuberculosis are less infectious but may transmit the disease. However, individuals with only extrapulmonary (e.g., renal, skeletal) tuberculosis are considered noninfectious.

IV-114. The answer is D. *(Chap. 165)* Aging, chronic disease, and suppression of cellular immunity are risk factors for developing active tuberculosis in patients with latent infection. (See Table IV-114.) The greatest absolute risk factor for development of active tuberculosis is HIV positivity. The risk of developing active infection is greatest in those with the lowest CD4 counts; however, having a CD4 count above a threshold value does not negate the risk of developing an active infection. The reported incidence of developing active tuberculosis in HIV-positive individuals with a positive purified protein derivative result is 10% per year compared with a lifetime risk of 10% in immunocompetent individuals. Whereas malnutrition and severe underweight confer a twofold greater risk of developing active tuberculosis, IV drug use increases the risk 10 to 30 times. Silicosis also increases the risk of developing active tuberculosis 30 times. Although the risk of developing active tuberculosis is greatest in the first year after exposure, the risk also increases in elderly adults. Coal mining has not been associated with increased risk independent of other factors, such as tobacco smoking.

TABLE IV-114   **Risk Factors for Active Tuberculosis Among Persons Who Have Been Infected With Tubercle Bacilli**

Factor	Relative Risk/Odds[a]
Recent infection (<1 year)	12.9
Fibrotic lesions (spontaneously healed)	2–20
Comorbidity	
HIV infection	21–>30
Silicosis	30
Chronic renal failure/hemodialysis	10–25
Diabetes	2–4
IV drug use	10–30
Immunosuppressive treatment	10
Gastrectomy	2–5
Jejunoileal bypass	30–60
Posttransplantation period (renal, cardiac)	20–70
Tobacco smoking	2–3
Malnutrition and severe underweight	2

[a]Old infection = 1.
Abbreviation: IV, intravenous.

IV-115. The answer is A. *(Chap. 165)* The chest radiograph shows a right upper lobe infiltrate with a large cavitary lesion. In this man from an endemic area for tuberculosis, this finding should be treated as active pulmonary tuberculosis until proven otherwise. In addition, this patient's symptoms suggest a chronic illness with low-grade fevers, weight loss, and temporal wasting that would be consistent with active pulmonary tuberculosis. If a patient is suspected of having active pulmonary tuberculosis, the initial management should include documentation of disease while protecting health care workers and the population in general. This patient should be hospitalized in a negative-pressure room on airborne isolation until three expectorated sputum samples have been demonstrated to be negative. The samples should preferably be collected in the early morning because the burden of organisms is expected to be higher on a more concentrated sputum. The sensitivity of a single sputum for the detection of tuberculosis in confirmed cases is only 40% to 60%. Thus, a single sputum sample is inadequate to determine infectivity and the presence of active pulmonary tuberculosis. Skin testing with a purified protein derivative of the tuberculosis mycobacterium is used to detect latent infection with tuberculosis and has no role in determining whether active disease is present. The cavitary lung lesion shown on the chest imaging could represent malignancy or a bacterial lung abscess, but because the patient is from a high-risk area for tuberculosis, tuberculosis would be considered the most likely diagnosis until ruled out by sputum testing.

IV-116. The answer is A. *(Chap. 165)* Initial treatment of active tuberculosis associated with HIV disease does not differ from that of a non-HIV-infected person. The standard treatment regimen includes four drugs: isoniazid, rifampin, pyrazinamide, and ethambutol (RIPE). These drugs are given for a total of 2 months in combination with pyridoxine (vitamin B_6) to prevent neurotoxicity from isoniazid. After the initial 2 months, patients continue on isoniazid and rifampin to complete a total of 6 months of therapy. These recommendations are the same as those of non–HIV-infected individuals. If the sputum culture remains positive for tuberculosis after 2 months, the total course of antimycobacterial therapy is increased from 6 to 9 months. If an individual is already on antiretroviral therapy (ART) at the time of diagnosis of tuberculosis, it may be continued, but often rifabutin is substituted for rifampin because of drug interactions between rifampin and protease inhibitors. In individuals not on ART at the time of diagnosis of tuberculosis, it is not recommended to start ART concurrently because of the risk of immune reconstitution inflammatory syndrome (IRIS) and an increased risk of medication side effects. IRIS occurs as the immune system improves with ART and causes an intense inflammatory reaction directed against the infecting organism(s). There have been fatal cases of IRIS in association with tuberculosis and initiation of ART. In addition, both ART and antituberculosis drugs have many side effects. It can be difficult for a clinician to decide which medication is the cause of the side effects and may lead unnecessarily to alterations in the antituberculosis regimen. ART should be initiated as soon as possible and preferably within 2 months. Three-drug regimens are associated with a higher relapse rate if used as a standard 6-month course of therapy and, if used, require a total of 9 months of therapy. Situations in which three-drug therapy may be used are pregnancy, intolerance to a specific drug, and in the setting of resistance. A five-drug regimen using Rifampin, isoniazide, pyrazinamide, ethambutol (RIPE) plus streptomycin is recommended as the standard retreatment regimen. Streptomycin and pyrazinamide are discontinued after 2 months if susceptibility testing is unavailable. If susceptibility testing is available, the treatment should be based on the susceptibility pattern. In no instance is it appropriate to withhold treatment in the setting of active tuberculosis to await susceptibility testing.

IV-117. The answer is B. *(Chap. 165)* The aim of treatment of latent tuberculosis is to prevent development of active disease, and the tuberculin skin test (purified protein derivative [PPD]) is the most common means of identifying cases of latent tuberculosis in high-risk groups. To perform a tuberculin skin test, 5 tuberculin units of PPD are placed subcutaneously in the forearm. The degree of induration is determined after 48 to 72 hours. Erythema only does not count as a positive reaction to the PPD. The size of the reaction to the tuberculin skin test determines whether individuals should receive treatment for latent tuberculosis. In general, individuals in low-risk groups should not be tested. However, if tested, a reaction larger than 15 mm is required to be considered as positive. School teachers are considered low-risk individuals. Thus, the reaction of 7 mm is not a positive result, and treatment is not required. A size of 10 mm or larger is considered positive in individuals who have been infected within 2 years or those with high-risk medical conditions. The individual working in an area where tuberculosis is endemic has tested newly positive by skin testing and should be treated as a newly infected individual. High-risk medical conditions for which treatment of latent tuberculosis is recommended include diabetes mellitus, injection drug use, end-stage renal disease, rapid weight loss, and hematologic disorders. PPD reactions 5 mm or larger are considered positive for latent tuberculosis in individuals with fibrotic lesions on chest radiographs, those with close contact with an infected person, and those with HIV or who are otherwise immunosuppressed. There are two situations in which treatment for latent tuberculosis is recommended regardless of the results on skin testing. First, infants and children who have had close contact with an actively infected person should be treated. After 2 months of therapy, a skin test should be performed. Treatment can be discontinued if the skin test result remains negative at that time. Also, individuals who are HIV positive and have had close contact with an infected person should be treated regardless of their skin test results.

IV-118. **The answer is C.** *(Chap. 165)* T-lymphocyte release of interferon-gamma in response to highly specific tuberculosis antigen stimulation is the basis for the commercially available interferon-gamma release assays (IGRAs). IGRAs are more specific than tuberculin skin testing caused by less cross-reactivity with non-mTB organisms, including Bacillus Calmette-Guérin and nontuberculous mycobacteria. The absolute sensitivity of IGRAs is not clearly known because of the difficulty in establishing a gold standard, but most studies demonstrate superior performance in detecting latent tuberculosis in low-incidence settings. They also are more user friendly because there is no administration expertise, interpretation is less subjective, and results do not require a second visit. The results are far less clear in settings of high tuberculosis or HIV burden. The tuberculin skin testing booster phenomenon, a spurious conversion caused by serial testing, does not occur with IGRAs; however, a tuberculin skin test may cause a false-positive IGRA result. In the United States, IGRA is preferred for most persons older than 5 years of age being screened for latent tuberculosis.

IV-119. **The answer is E.** *(Chap. 165)* Bacillus Calmette-Guérin (BCG) is derived from an attenuated strain of *Mycobacterium bovis*. It has been available since 1921. Many vaccines are available, but they vary in efficacy from 0% to 80% in clinical trials. The vaccine protects infants and young children from serous forms of tuberculosis, including meningitis and miliary disease. Side effects from the vaccine are rare, but BCG dissemination (BCGitis) may occur in patients with severe combined immunodeficiency or advanced HIV-induced immune suppression. BCG cross-reacts with tuberculin skin testing, but the size of the response wanes with time. BCG vaccination is currently recommended in countries with a high TB prevalence. It is not recommended in the United States because of the low prevalence of disease and cross-reactivity with tuberculin skin testing. Infants with unknown HIV infection status, infants of mothers with known HIV infection, and HIV-infected individuals should not receive BCG vaccination.

IV-120. **The answer is B.** *(Chap. 167)* The chest computed tomography shows a "tree-in-bud" pattern in the peripheral right lung and bilateral bronchiectasis. This pattern is consistent with bronchiolar inflammation and is typical of nontuberculous mycobacterial infection. Nontuberculous mycobacteria, such as *Mycobacterium avium* complex (MAC), may cause chronic pulmonary infections in normal hosts and those with underlying pulmonary disease immunosuppression. In normal hosts, bronchiectasis is the most common underlying condition. In immunocompetent patients without underlying disease, treatment of pulmonary infection with MAC is considered on an individual basis based on symptoms, radiographic findings, and bacteriology. Treatment should be initiated in the presence of progressive pulmonary disease or symptoms. In patients without any prior lung disease, no structural lung disease, and who do not demonstrate progressive clinical decline, *M. avium* pulmonary infection can be managed conservatively. Patients with underlying lung disease, such as chronic obstructive pulmonary disease, bronchiectasis, or cystic fibrosis, or those with a history of pulmonary tuberculosis should receive antibiotics. This patient has both clinical and historic reasons for antibiotic treatment. The appropriate regimen in this case is clarithromycin (or azithromycin), ethambutol, and rifampin (or rifabutin) for 12 months after culture sterilization (typically 18 months). The combination of pyrazinamide, isoniazid, rifampin, and ethambutol is effective treatment for *M. tuberculosis* infection, which is not present here. Other drugs with activity against MAC include intravenous and aerosolized aminoglycosides, fluoroquinolones, and clofazimine.

IV-121. **The answer is C.** *(Chap. 168)* Pyrazinamide (PZA) is the first-line treatment for *Mycobacterium tuberculosis*. Addition of PZA for 2 months to isoniazid and rifampin allows the total duration of treatment to be shortened from 9 months to 6 months. PZA has no utility in the treatment of nontuberculous mycobacteria. Ethambutol has no serious drug interactions, but patients must be closely monitored for optic neuritis, which may manifest with decreased visual acuity, central scotoma, or difficulty seeing green (or red). All patients initiating therapy with ethambutol should have a visual and ophthalmologic examination at baseline. In the United States overall, isoniazid resistance remains uncommon. Primary isoniazid resistance is more common in patients with tuberculosis born outside the United States. Rifampin is a potent inducer of cytochrome P450 system and has numerous drug interactions. The Centers for Disease Control and Prevention has guidelines for managing antituberculosis drug interactions including rifampin. Rifabutin is a less potent inducer of hepatic cytochromes. Rifabutin is recommended for HIV-infected patients who are on antiretroviral therapy with protease inhibitors or non-nucleoside reverse transcriptase inhibitors (particularly nevirapine) in place of rifampin.

IV-122. The answer is E. *(Chap. 169)* Neurosyphilis has generally been thought to be a late complication of syphilis infection, but this is now known to be inaccurate. Within weeks after infection, the central nervous system is invaded with treponemal organisms. The vast majority of cases are asymptomatic. Abnormal protein levels within the cerebrospinal fluid (CSF) or positive CSF Venereal Disease Research Laboratory (VDRL) test can be seen in up to 40% of individuals with primary or secondary syphilis and 25% of cases of latent syphilis. In symptomatic cases, neurosyphilis can have a variety of manifestations that are typically considered in three broad categories: meningeal, meningovascular, and parenchymal syphilis. Meningeal syphilis is dominated by headache, neck stiffness, and cranial nerve abnormalities. Meningovascular syphilis has signs of meningitis but also can include a vasculitis complicated by stroke. Parenchymal syphilis does indeed represent a late manifestation of disease. Changes in personality, dementia, Argyll Robertson pupils, and paresis are typical findings.

It can be difficult to determine which patients with syphilis required a lumbar puncture to assess for central nervous system involvement of the disease. However, it is quite important because the treatment of neurosyphilis requires 14 days of treatment with intravenous penicillin. Clearly, any patient with a positive test result for syphilis with concerning neurologic symptoms should undergo a lumbar puncture. Some experts also recommend lumbar puncture in all patients with syphilis who are HIV positive. However, this is controversial with others recommending lumbar puncture only if the CD4 count is less than 350/μL. Other instances in which a lumbar puncture is recommended is in the setting of a very high titer rapid plasma reagin (RPR) or VDRL (>1:32) or failure of the RPR or VDRL to fall by a factor of 4 after appropriate treatment. Thus, all of the patients presented would be recommended to undergo a lumbar puncture.

IV-123. The answer is D. *(Chap. 169)* The patient's clinical examination is consistent with primary syphilis and he should receive appropriate therapy. In primary syphilis, 25% of patients will have negative nontreponemal tests for syphilis (rapid plasma reagin or Venereal Disease Research Laboratory). A single dose of long-acting benzathine penicillin is the recommended treatment for primary, secondary, and early latent syphilis. Ceftriaxone is the treatment of choice for gonorrhea, but this lesion is not consistent with that diagnosis. Ceftriaxone given daily for 7 to 10 days is an alternative treatment for primary and secondary syphilis. Acyclovir is the drug of choice for genital herpes. Herpetic lesions are classically multiple and painful. Observation is not an option because the chancre will resolve spontaneously without treatment and the patient will remain infected and infectious. Given the appearance and clinical history, there is no indication for tissue biopsy or surgical resection.

IV-124. The answer is E. *(Chap. 171)* The patient has Weil's syndrome caused by infection with *Leptospira interrogans*. *L. interrogans* is a spirochete that is acquired through contact with an infected animal. Species that commonly transmit the organism to human include rats, dogs, cattle, and pigs. The organism is excreted in urine and can survive in water for months. For a human to become infected, susceptible individuals typically have indirect contact with infected animal urine through contaminated water sources and other wet environments. Tropical human environments, rodent infestations, and large populations of infected dogs are also important for transmission. Leptospirosis occurs only sporadically in the United States with most cases occurring in Hawaii.

Clinically, leptospirosis can take many manifestations, including subclinical infection, a self-limited febrile illness, and Weil's disease. Leptospirosis is classically a biphasic disease. After the acute exposure, fevers last for 3 to 10 days. During this time, the patient will complain of malaise and myalgias. Conjunctival suffusion (dilated conjunctival blood vessels without drainage) is common as are pharyngeal edema, muscle tenderness, and crackles on lung examination. Weil's disease is the most serious form of leptospirosis and occurs during the immune phase of the disease. Clinically, severe jaundice in the absence of hepatocellular injury is a striking feature of the disease. In addition, acute kidney injury, hypotension, and diffuse hemorrhage are common. The lungs are the most common site of hemorrhage, but the gastrointestinal tract, retroperitoneum, pericardium, and brain can also be affected. The diagnosis is most often made by serologic assays because culture of the organism takes several weeks. Treatment of leptospirosis is typically intravenous penicillin, ceftriaxone, or cefotaxime.

Acute alcoholic hepatitis can produce fevers and malaise, but a more marked increase in liver enzymes would be expected with the aspartate aminotransferase elevated out of proportion to alanine aminotransferase. Disseminated intravascular coagulation in the setting of an infection would demonstrate abnormalities of coagulation, which were not present here. Microscopic polyangiitis is a small to medium vessel vasculitis that could cause pulmonary hemorrhage and acute renal failure. Rarely, the liver can be affected as well. However, the urinalysis does not suggest acute glomerulonephritis because no casts or red blood cells are present. Rat-bite fever causes intermittent fevers, polyarthritis, and a nonspecific rash.

IV-125. **The answer is E.** (*Chap. 172*) Tickborne relapsing fever (TBRF) is a spirochetal infection caused by any one of several species of *Borrelia*. The Borrelia are small spirochetes that are transmitted to humans through the bite of an infected tick. The tick that transmits TBRF is *Ornithodoros* spp., which feeds on a variety of squirrels and chipmunks that live near freshwater lakes. TBRF is endemic in several areas of the western United States, southern British Columbia, the Mediterranean, Africa, and the plateau regions of Mexico and South and Central America. In the United States, TBRF is rarely reported east of Montana, Colorado, New Mexico, and Texas. The general areas where TBRF is contracted is in the forested and mountainous regions of these states, although it can be contracted in the limestone caves of central Texas. Only 13 counties in the entire United States have had 50% of all cases reported in the United States.

After an incubation period of about 7 days, an individual infected with TBRF will begin to experience fevers that can reach as high as 106.7°F (41.5°C). Symptoms that accompany the fevers include myalgias, chills, nausea, vomiting, abdominal pain, confusion, and arthralgias. The average duration of a first episode is 3 days. If the disease is not recognized and treated, the fever will recur after a period of about 7 days. The duration of fevers is typically shorter with repeated episodes but will continue to relapse about every 7 days until the disease is treated. Diagnosis of TBRF requires detection of the spirochetes in the blood during a febrile episode or serologic conversion. TBRF is typically treated with doxycycline or erythromycin for 7 to 10 days.

The other options should be on the differential diagnosis for an individual with recurrent and relapsing fevers. In addition, this list would also include yellow fever, dengue fever, malaria, rat-bite fever, and infection with echovirus 9 or *Bartonella* spp. Brucellosis is a bacterial infection most commonly transmitted by ingestion of contaminated milk or cheese, which this patient did not report. Colorado tick fever is a viral infection transmitted by the bite of a *Dermacentor andersoni* tick that is endemic in the western areas of the United States. The pattern of fever is slightly different from TBRF because the cycle is 2 to 3 days of fever followed by 2 to 3 days of normal temperature. Leptospirosis often has two phases of fever. The first occurs during the acute infection, lasting 7 to 10 days. In some individuals, the fever recurs 3 to 10 days later during the immune phase. The typical route of infection is prolonged contact with infected rodent droppings in wet environments. Lymphocytic choriomeningitis is a viral infection that is most commonly transmitted via contact with urine or droppings from common house mice. This illness usually has two phases as well. During the first phase that occurs 8 to 13 days after exposure, an individual will experience fevers, malaise, and myalgias. In the second phase of illness, symptoms more typical of meningitis occur.

IV-126. The answer is C. *(Chap. 174)* About 8% of individuals affected by Lyme disease have cardiac involvement during the second stage of disease. Caused by *Borrelia burgdorferi*, Lyme disease is transmitted by the bite of an infected *Ixodes* tick. The first phase of the disease represents localized infection and is characterized by the presence of the erythema migrans rash. The second stage of the disease represents disseminated infection. The most common manifestations of this stage are new annular skin lesions, headache, fever, and migratory arthralgias. When cardiac involvement is present, the most common presentation is related to conduction abnormalities, including all categories of heart block. Diffuse cardiac involvement can occur with acute myopericarditis and left ventricular dysfunction. The cardiac involvement typically resolves within a few weeks even without treatment.

Acute myocardial infarction (MI) can cause complete heart block, particularly in the event of an inferior MI. However, this patient has minimal risk factors for cardiac disease, is otherwise healthy, and has no symptoms to suggest this as a cause. Chagas disease is caused *Trypanosoma cruzi*, an parasite endemic to Mexico and Central and South America. Sarcoidosis is a systemic disease that pathologically demonstrates the diffuse presence of noncaseating granulomas in a variety of tissues. Conduction abnormalities, including complete heart block and ventricular tachycardia, can be the presenting symptoms of the disease. More commonly, sarcoidosis would have pulmonary manifestations. Although sarcoidosis is certainly possible in this patient, it would be a diagnosis of exclusion because his risk factors make Lyme disease more likely. Subacute bacterial endocarditis can also result in complete heart block if the endocarditis progresses to develop a valve ring abscess. The patient with subacute bacterial endocarditis would present with a more acute illness than this patient with fevers, weight loss, and most likely secondary signs of endocarditis such as Osler nodes, splinter hemorrhages, and Janeway lesions.

IV-127. The answer is A. *(Chap. 173)* Lyme serology tests should be done only in patients with an intermediate pretest probability of having Lyme disease. The presence of erythema migrans in both patient B and patient E is diagnostic of Lyme disease in the correct epidemiologic context. The diagnosis is entirely clinical. Patient C's clinical course sounds more consistent with systemic lupus erythematosus, and initial laboratory evaluation should focus on this diagnosis. Patients with chronic fatigue, myalgias, and cognitive change are occasionally concerned about Lyme disease as a potential etiology for their symptoms. However, the pretest probability of Lyme is low in these patients, assuming the absence of antecedent erythema migrans, and a positive serology is unlikely to be a true positive test result. Lyme arthritis typically occurs months after the initial infection and occurs in about 60% of untreated patients. The typical attack is large joint, oligoarticular, and intermittent, lasting weeks at a time. Oligoarticular arthritis carries a broad differential diagnosis, including sarcoidosis, spondyloarthropathy, rheumatoid arthritis, psoriatic arthritis, and Lyme disease. Lyme serology is appropriate in this situation. Patients with Lyme arthritis usually have the highest IgG antibody responses seen in the infection.

IV-128 and IV-129. The answers are D and D, respectively. *(Chap. 173)* This patient's rash is a classic erythema migrans lesion and is diagnostic for Lyme disease in her geographic region. In the United States, Lyme disease is caused by infection with *Borrelia burgdorferi*. Partial central clearing, a bright red border, and a target center are very suggestive of this lesion. The fact that multiple lesions exist implies disseminated infection rather than a primary tick bite inoculation in which only one lesion is present. Potential complications of secondary Lyme disease in the United States include migratory arthritis, meningitis, cranial neuritis, mononeuritis multiplex, myelitis, varying degrees of atrioventricular block, and (less commonly) myopericarditis, splenomegaly, and hepatitis. Third-degree or persistent Lyme disease is associated with oligoarticular arthritis of large joints and subtle encephalopathy but not frank dementia. *Borrelia garinii* infection is seen only in Europe and can cause a more pronounced encephalomyelitis.

Acute Lyme disease involving the skin or joints (or both) is treated with oral doxycycline unless the patient is pregnant or younger than 9 years old. Amoxicillin and macrolides (azithromycin) are less effective therapies. Ceftriaxone is indicated for acute disease in the presence of nervous system involvement (meningitis, facial palsy, encephalopathy, radiculoneuritis) or third-degree heart block. It may also be used for treatment of patients with arthritis who do not respond to oral therapy. First-generation cephalosporins are not active against *B. burgdorferi*. Although the rash of erythema migrans may look like cellulitis caused by staphylococci or streptococci, there is no proven efficacy of vancomycin for Lyme disease.

IV-130. The answer is E. *(Chap. 174)* This clinical vignette describes an individual infected with *Ehrlichia chaffeensis*, the causative agent of human monocytic ehrlichiosis (HME). This rickettsial infection is transmitted through the bite of an infected deer tick and is most common in the southeast, south-central, and mid-Atlantic states. In 2008, the incidence was highest in Arkansas, Oklahoma, and Missouri. This patient is at risk given his occupation, which requires him to spend a significant amount of time outdoors. The time from incubation to symptoms of infection is about 8 days. The most prominent symptoms of HME are nonspecific and include fevers, malaise, headaches, and myalgias. Nausea, vomiting, diarrhea, cough, confusion, and rash are less common. HME can be quite severe with 62% of all individuals requiring hospitalization and a mortality rate of about 3%. In severe cases, septic shock, adult respiratory distress syndrome, and meningoencephalitis can occur. Laboratory findings are helpful in suggesting possible HME. Common findings are lymphopenia, neutropenia, thrombocytopenia, and elevations in aminotransferases. If a bone marrow biopsy is done, the marrow is hypercellular, and noncaseating granulomas can be observed. Diagnosis of HME relies on polymerase chain reaction detection of *E. chaffeensis* nucleic acids in peripheral blood. Morulae are seen only rarely (<10%) in the cytoplasm of monocytes on peripheral blood smears. Paired sera demonstrating a rise in antibody titers to above 1:64 over a course of about 3 weeks can also be confirmatory. Treatment of HME is oral or intravenous doxycycline that is continued for 3 to 5 days after fever has resolved.

In rare instances, systemic lupus erythematosus could present with a fulminant illness that could include pancytopenia and liver function abnormalities. However, it would be more likely to have a rash and renal involvement, which this patient did not exhibit. Antibody testing for double-stranded DNA and Smith antigens would not be helpful in this case. Because the patient had a normal lumbar puncture result, further testing of the cerebrospinal fluid is unlikely to yield the diagnosis. This testing is most common used to diagnose viral encephalitides or meningitis such as West Nile virus and herpes simplex virus. The presence of noncaseating granulomas on bone marrow biopsy is a nondiagnostic finding. In the appropriate clinical setting, this could be suggestive of sarcoidosis. However, sarcoidosis does not present with a fulminant febrile illness over a matter of days. Moreover, although a chest radiograph may demonstrate hilar adenopathy or lung infiltrate, this, too, is a nondiagnostic finding.

IV-131. The answer is B. *(Chap. 174)* This patient demonstrates evidence of Rocky Mountain spotted fever (RMSF), which has progressed over the course of several days because of a lack of initial recognition and treatment. RMSF is caused by infection with *Rickettsia rickettsii* and is transmitted through the bite of an infected dog tick. RMSF has been diagnosed in 47 states and is most commonly diagnosed in the south-central and southeastern states. Symptoms typically begin about 1 week after inoculation. The initial symptoms are vague and are easily misdiagnosed as a viral infection with fever, myalgias, malaise, and headache predominating. Although almost all patients with RMSF develop a rash during the course of the illness, rash is present in only 14% on the first day, and the lack of rash in a patient who is at risk for RMSF should not delay treatment. By day 3, 49% of individuals develop a rash. The rash initially is a macular rash that begins on the wrists and ankles and progresses to involve the extremities and trunk. Over time, hemorrhaging into the macules occurs and has a petechial appearance. As the illness progresses, respiratory failure and central nervous system (CNS) manifestations can develop. Encephalitis, presenting as confusion and lethargy, is present about 25% of the time. Other manifestations can include renal failure, hepatic injury, and anemia. Treatment for RMSF is doxycycline 100 mg twice daily. It can be administered orally or intravenously. Because this patient shows progressive disease with CNS involvement, hospital admission for treatment is warranted to monitor for further decompensation in the patient's condition. If the patient were more clinically stable, outpatient therapy would be appropriate. Treatment should not be delayed while awaiting confirmatory serologic testing because untreated cases of RMSF are fatal, usually within

8 to 15 days. Treatment with any sulfa drugs should be avoided because these drugs are ineffective and can worsen the disease course. Intravenous ceftriaxone and vancomycin are appropriate agents for bacterial meningitis. Although this could be a consideration in this patient with fever, confusion, and a rash, meningococcemia would present with a more fulminant course, and the patient's risk factor (hiking in an endemic area) would make RMSF more likely.

IV-132. **The answer is D.** *(Chap. 175)* This patient presents with symptoms of atypical pneumonia, and the most common causative organism for atypical pneumonia is *Mycoplasma pneumoniae*. Pneumonia caused by *Mycoplasma* occurs worldwide without a specific seasonal preference. *M. pneumoniae* is a highly infectious organism and is spread by respiratory droplets. It is estimated that about 80% of individuals within the same family will experience the infection after one person becomes infected. Outbreaks of *M. pneumoniae* also occur in institutional settings, including boarding schools and military bases. Clinical manifestations of *M. pneumoniae* typically are pharyngitis, tracheobronchitis, wheezing, or nonspecific upper respiratory syndrome. Although many commonly believe the organism is associated with otitis media and bullous myringitis, there are little clinical data to support this assertion. Atypical pneumonia occurs in fewer than 15% of individuals infected with *M. pneumoniae*. The onset of pneumonia typically is gradual with preceding symptoms of upper respiratory infection. Cough is present, and often extensive, but nonproductive. Examination typically demonstrates wheezing or rales in about 80% of patients. The most common radiographic findings are bilateral peribronchial pneumonia with increased interstitial markings. Lobar consolidation is uncommon. Definitive diagnosis requires demonstration of *M. pneumoniae* nucleic acids on polymerase chain reaction of respiratory secretions or performance of serologic testing. Often, however, the patients are treating empirically without obtaining definitive diagnosis.

Other causes of atypical pneumonia are *Chlamydia pneumoniae* and *Legionella pneumophila*. *C. pneumoniae* more commonly causes pneumonia in school-aged children, although adults can become re-infected. *Legionella* pneumonia is often associated with outbreaks of disease caused by contaminated water supplies. Individuals with *Legionella* pneumonia can become quite sick and develop respiratory failure. Adenovirus is a common viral cause of upper respiratory tract infection and has been associated with outbreaks of pneumonia among military recruits.

Streptococcus pneumoniae is the most common cause of community-acquired pneumonia, but it typically presents with lobar or segmental consolidation.

IV-133. **The answer is D.** *(Chap. 175)* *Mycoplasma pneumoniae* is a common cause of pneumonia that is often underdiagnosed based on difficult and time-consuming culture techniques, because it likely causes mild respiratory symptoms, and because it is adequately treated with standard antibiotic regimens for community-acquired pneumonia. It is spread easily person to person, and outbreaks in crowded conditions, such as schools or barracks, are common. Most patients develop a cough without radiographic abnormalities. When radiographic abnormalities are present, there is usually a diffuse bronchopneumonia pattern without any lobar consolidation. Pharyngitis and rhinitis are also common. *M. pneumoniae* commonly induces the production of cold agglutinins, which in turn can cause an IgM- and complement-mediated intravascular hemolytic anemia. The presence of cold agglutinins is specific for *M. pneumoniae* infection only in the context of a consistent clinical picture for infection, as in this patient. Cold agglutinins are more common in children. Blood smear shows no abnormality, which is in contrast to IgG or warm-type hemolytic anemia in which spherocytes are seen. Because there is no easy diagnostic test, empirical therapy is often administered.

IV-134. **The answer is C.** *(Chap. 176)* This patient likely has pneumonia caused by infection with *Chlamydia psittaci*. This organisms is a relatively rare cause of pneumonia with only about 50 confirmed cases yearly in the United States. Contrary to common belief, the organism is not limited to psittacine birds (parrots, parakeets, cockatiels, macaws), but any bird can be infected, including poultry. Most infections are seen in owners of pet birds, poultry farmers, or poultry processing workers, and outbreaks of pneumonia have been seen in poultry processing factories. Untreated psittacosis has a mortality rate of as high as 10%. The illness presents with nonspecific symptoms of fevers, chills, myalgias, and severe headache. Gastrointestinal symptoms with hepatosplenomegaly are also common. Severe pneumonia requiring ventilatory support can occur, and other rare manifestations include endocarditis, myocarditis, and neurologic complications. The current diagnostic tool of choice is the microimmunofluorescence test, which is a serologic test. Any titer greater than 1:16 is considered evidence of exposure to psittacosis, and paired acute and convalescent titers showing a fourfold rise in titer are consistent with psittacosis. Complement fixation tests are also used. Treatment of choice for psittacosis is tetracycline 250 mg four times daily for a minimum of 4 weeks. Public health officials should be notified to assess other workers in the factory for disease and limit exposure.

Although this patient has immigrated from an area endemic for tuberculosis, she had a previous negative purified protein derivative result and no known tuberculosis exposures. Her chest radiograph shows diffuse consolidation, which would not be typical for reactivation of tuberculosis. Systemic infection with *Staphylococcus aureus* from an abscess or endocarditis could present with respiratory failure related to septic emboli. However, her chest imaging is not consistent with this, and she has no risk factors (i.e., intravenous drug use, indwelling intravenous catheter) for development of *S. aureus* bloodstream infection. *Legionella pneumophila* is associated with outbreaks of disease related to contaminated water supplies or air conditioning. It should be considered in this patient in light of her ill coworkers. However, hepatosplenomegaly is not consistent with this diagnosis. Influenza A is also a consideration for this patient, but the time of year is not consistent for seasonal influenza. In outbreaks of pandemic influenza, this would be more likely.

IV-135. **The answer is D.** *(Chap. 176)* Congenital infection from maternal transmission can lead to severe consequences for the neonate; thus, prenatal care and screening for infection are very important. *Chlamydia trachomatis* is associated with up to 25% of exposed neonates who develop inclusion conjunctivitis. It can also be associated with pneumonia and otitis media in the newborn. Pneumonia in the newborn has been associated with later development of bronchitis and asthma. Hydrocephalus can be associated with toxoplasmosis. Hutchinson triad, which is Hutchinson teeth (blunted upper incisors), interstitial keratitis, and eighth nerve deafness, is caused by congenital syphilis. Sensorineural deafness can be associated with congenital rubella exposure. Treatment of *C. trachomatis* infection in infants consists of oral erythromycin.

IV-136. **The answer is D.** *(Chap. 176)* Urethritis in men causes dysuria with or without discharge, usually without frequency. The most common causes of urethritis in men include *Neisseria gonorrhoeae, Chlamydia* trachomatis, *Mycoplasma genitalium, Ureaplasma urealyticum, Trichomonas vaginalis*, herpes simplex virus, and possibly adenovirus. Until recently, *C. trachomatis* accounted for 30% to 40% of cases; however, this number may be decreasing. Recent studies suggest that *M. genitalium* is a common cause of nonchlamydial cases. Currently, the initial diagnosis of urethritis in men includes specific tests only for *N. gonorrhoeae* and *C. trachomatis*. Tenets of urethral discharge treatment include providing treatment for the most common causes of urethritis with the assumption that the patient may be lost to follow-up. Therefore, prompt empirical treatment for gonorrhea and Chlamydia infections with ceftriaxone and azithromycin should be given on the day of presentation to the clinic to the patient, and recent partners should be contacted for treatment. Azithromycin will also be effective for *M. genitalium*. If pus can be milked from the urethra, cultures should be sent for definitive diagnosis and to allow for contact tracing by the health department because both of these are reportable diseases. Urine nucleic acid amplification tests are an acceptable substitute in the absence of pus. It is also critical to provide empirical treatment for at-risk sexual contacts. If symptoms do not respond to the initial empirical therapy, patients should be reevaluated for compliance with therapy, reexposure, and *T. vaginalis* infection.

IV-137. **The answer is A.** *(Chap. 177)* Persistent viral infection is speculated to be pathogenically important in up to 20% of human malignancies. Strong associations based on epidemiology, the presence of viral nucleotides in tumor cells, the transformational ability of viruses on human cells, and animal models have been established. Most hepatocellular carcinoma is thought to be related to chronic infection with hepatitis B or C virus. Most cervical cancer is caused by persistent infection with human papilloma virus type 16 or 18. Epstein-Barr virus plays a role in the development of many B-lymphocyte and epithelial cell malignancies such as Hodgkin's lymphoma, Burkitt's lymphoma, and nasopharyngeal carcinoma. HTLV-1 is associated with a number of T-cell lymphomas and leukemias. KSHV (Kaposi's sarcoma associated herpes virus, HHV-8) is associated with Kaposi's sarcoma, pleural effusion lymphoma, and multicentric Castleman's disease. Dengue fever virus, a flavovirus, is the cause of dengue fever and has not been associated with human malignancy.

IV-138. The answer is A. *(Chap. 178)* Compared with the large number of antimicrobials directed against bacterial, antiviral therapies have been fewer, and advances in antiviral therapy have come more slowly. However, in recent years, a large number of antiviral medications have been introduced, and it is generally important to be familiar with the common side effects of these medications. Acyclovir and valacyclovir are most commonly used for the treatment of herpes simplex viruses I and II as well as varicella-zoster virus. Acyclovir is generally a well-tolerated drug, but it can crystallize in the kidneys, leading to acute renal failure if the patient is not properly hydrated. Valacyclovir is an ester of acyclovir that significantly improves the bioavailability of the drug. It is also well tolerated but has been associated with thrombotic thrombocytopenic purpura or hemolytic uremic syndrome when used at high doses. Ganciclovir and foscarnet are medications used to treat cytomegalovirus (CMV) infection. Ganciclovir is primarily given intravenously because the oral bioavailability is less than 10%. Ganciclovir is associated with bone marrow suppression and can cause renal dysfunction. Foscarnet is used for ganciclovir-resistant CMV infections. Renal impairment commonly occurs with its use and causes hypokalemia, hypocalcemia, and hypomagnesemia. Thus, careful monitoring of electrolytes and renal function is warranted with foscarnet use. Amantadine is an antiviral medication used for the treatment of influenza A. It has been demonstrated to have a variety of central nervous system (CNS) side effects, including dizziness, anxiety, insomnia, and difficulty concentrating. Although initially used as an antiviral drug, the CNS effects of amantadine have led to its use in Parkinson's disease. Interferons are a group of cytokines produced endogenously in response to a variety of pathogens, including viruses and bacteria. Therapeutically, interferons have been studied extensively in the treatment of patients with chronic hepatitis B and C. Interferons lead to a host of systemic effects, including symptoms of a viral syndrome (fevers, chills, fatigue, and myalgias) as well as leukopenia.

IV-139. The answer is E. *(Chap. 179)* Antibodies to herpes simplex virus-2 (HSV-2) are not routinely detected until puberty, consistent with the typical sexual transmission of the virus. Serosurveys suggest that 15% to 20% of American adults have HSV-2 infection; however, only 10% report a history of genital lesions. Seroprevalence is similar or higher in Central America, South America, and Africa. Recent studies in African obstetric clinics have found seroprevalence rates as high as 70%. HSV-2 infection is believed to be so pervasive in the general population based on ease of transmission, both in symptomatic and asymptomatic states. Therefore, this sexually transmitted disease (STD) is significantly more common in individuals who less frequently engage in high-risk behavior than other STDs. HSV-2 is an independent risk factor for HIV acquisition and transmission. HIV virion is shed from herpetic lesions, thus promoting transmission.

IV-140. The answer is E. *(Chap. 179)* Primary genital herpes caused by herpes simplex virus-2 (HSV-2) is characterized by fever, headache, malaise, inguinal lymphadenopathy, and diffuse genital lesions of varying stage. The cervix and urethra are usually involved in women. Although both HSV-2 and HSV-1 can involve the genitals, the recurrence rate of HSV-2 is much higher (90% in the first year) than with HSV-1 (55% in the first year). The rate of reactivation for HSV-2 is very high. Acyclovir, valacyclovir, and famciclovir are effective in shortening the duration of symptoms and lesions in genital herpes. Chronic daily therapy can reduce the frequency of recurrences in those with frequent reactivation. Valacyclovir has been shown to reduce transmission of HSV-2 between sexual partners.

IV-141. **The answer is C.** *(Chap. 179)* Herpes encephalitis accounts for 10% to 20% of sporadic cases of viral encephalitis in the United States. It most commonly occurs in patients 5 to 30 years and older than 50 years old. HSV-1 accounts for more than 95% of cases, and most adults have clinical or serologic evidence of HSV-1 mucocutaneous infection before onset of central nervous system symptoms. Herpes simplex virus (HSV) encephalitis is characterized by the acute onset of fever and focal neurologic signs, particularly in the temporal lobe. Electroencephalographic (EEG) abnormalities in the temporal lobe are common. The cerebrospinal fluid (CSF) will show elevated protein, lymphocyte leukocytosis with red blood cells, and normal glucose. HSV polymerase chain reaction testing of CSF is highly sensitive and specific for diagnosis. Treatment with acyclovir reduces mortality; however, neurologic sequelae are common, particularly in older patients. Differentiation of HSV encephalitis from other viral forms is difficult. Most experts recommend initiation of empiric acyclovir in any patient with suspected encephalitis pending a confirmed or alternative diagnosis. Tuberculosis meningitis presents typically as a basilar meningitis and not encephalitis. The history, clinical findings, EEG abnormalities, and radiologic findings make fungal meningitis unlikely. CSF oligoclonal bands are typically seen in patient with multiple sclerosis.

IV-142. **The answer is C.** *(Chap. 180)* Recently, a varicella-zoster virus vaccine that has 18 times the viral content of the live-attenuated virus vaccine used in children was shown efficacious for shingles in patients older than 60 years of age. The vaccine decreased the incidence of shingles by 51%, the burden of illness by 61%, and the incidence of postherpetic neuralgia by 66%. The Advisory Committee on Immunization Practices has therefore recommended that persons in this age group be offered this vaccine to reduce the frequency of shingles and the severity of postherpetic neuralgia. Because is it a live virus vaccine, it should not be used in immunocompromised patients.

IV-143 and IV-144. **The answers are C and E, respectively.** *(Chap. 181)* Epstein-Barr virus (EBV) is the cause of heterophile-positive infectious mononucleosis (IM), which is characterized by fever, sore throat, lymphadenopathy, and atypical lymphocytosis. EBV is also associated with several human tumors, including nasopharyngeal carcinoma, Burkitt's lymphoma, Hodgkin's disease, and (in patients with immunodeficiencies) B-cell lymphoma. EBV infection occurs worldwide with more than 90% of adults seropositive. In the developing world, most are infected as young children, and IM is uncommon; in the more developed world, most are infected as adolescents or young adults, and IM is more common. The virus is spread by contaminated saliva. Asymptomatic seropositive individuals shed the virus in saliva. In young children, the EBV infection causes mild disease with sore throat. Adolescents and young adults develop IM as described above plus often splenomegaly in the second to third week of disease. The white blood cell count is usually elevated and peaks at 10,000 to 20,000/μL during the second or third week of illness. Lymphocytosis is usually demonstrable, with greater than 10% atypical lymphocytes. A morbilliform rash may occur in about 5% of patients as part of the acute illness. Most patients treated with ampicillin develop a macular rash as pictured; this rash is not predictive of future adverse reactions to penicillins. Heterophile antibody testing results will be positive in up to 40% of cases of IM in the first week of illness and up to 90% by the third week. If heterophile antibody testing results are negative, the more expensive testing for immunoglobulin M (IgM) antibodies to viral capsid antigen is more sensitive and specific. IgG antibodies to viral capsid antigen will stay present indefinitely after initial infection and are not useful for diagnosing acute disease. Treatment of uncomplicated IM is with rest, supportive measures, and reassurance. Excessive physical activity should be avoided in the first month to avoid splenic trauma. Prednisone is not indicated and may predispose to secondary infection. It has been used at high dose when IM is complicated by airway compromise caused by pharyngeal swelling, autoimmune hemolytic anemia, severe thrombocytopenia, hemophagocytic syndrome, or other severe complications. Controlled trials have shown that acyclovir has no significant impact on the course of uncomplicated IM. One study showed no benefit for combined prednisone plus acyclovir.

IV-145. **The answer is D.** *(Chap. 182)* Cytomegalovirus (CMV) retinitis, a common CMV infection in HIV patients, occurs less commonly in solid organ transplant patients. CMV does affect the lung in a majority of transplant patients if either the donor or recipient is CMV-seropositive pretransplant. CMV disease in transplant recipients typically develops 30 to 90 days after transplant. It rarely occurs within 2 weeks of transplantation. CMV very commonly causes a pneumonitis that clinically is difficult to distinguish from acute rejection. Prior CMV infection has been associated with bronchiolitis obliterans syndrome (chronic rejection) in lung transplant recipients. As with HIV, the gastrointestinal tract is commonly involved with CMV infection. Endoscopy with biopsy showing characteristic giant cells, not serum polymerase chain reaction (PCR), is necessary to make this diagnosis. The CMV syndrome is also common in lung transplant patients. Serum CMV PCR should be sent as part of the workup for all nonspecific fevers, worsening lung function, liver function abnormalities, or falling leukocyte counts occurring more than a couple of weeks after transplant.

IV-146. **The answer is A.** *(Chap. 182)* When the transplant donor is cytomegalovirus (CMV) immunoglobulin G (IgG) positive and the recipient is negative, there is a very high risk of primary CMV infection in the recipient. However, if the recipient is IgG positive, CMV occurs as a reactivation infection. When both the donor and recipient are seronegative, then the risk of any CMV infection is lowest, but not zero, because contact with an infected host could prompt primary CMV infection. Unlike nearly all other transplant patients, many donor and recipient seronegative patients do not receive chemoprophylaxis with ganciclovir. In patients who are CMV IgG negative and received a CMV IgG negative transplant, transfusions should be from CMV IgG negative donors or white blood cell filtered products administered to reduce the risk of primary CMV infection. It is not clear whether universal prophylaxis or preemptive therapy is the preferable approach in CMV-seropositive immunocompromised hosts. Both ganciclovir and valganciclovir have been used successfully for prophylaxis and preemptive therapy in transplant recipients. A CMV glycoprotein B vaccine reduced infections in a placebo-controlled trial among 464 CMV-seronegative women; this outcome raises the possibility that this experimental vaccine will reduce congenital infections, but further studies must validate this approach.

IV-147. **The answer is A.** *(Chap. 182)* Human herpes virus-8 (HHV-8) or Kaposi's sarcoma–associated herpes virus (KSHV infects B lymphocytes, macrophages, and both endothelial and epithelial cells) appears to be causally related to Kaposi's sarcoma and a subgroup of AIDS-related B-cell body cavity–based lymphomas (primary effusion lymphomas) and to multicentric Castleman's disease. HHV-8 infection is more common in parts of Africa than in the United States. Primary HHV-8 infection in immunocompetent children may manifest as fever and maculopapular rash. Among individuals with intact immunity, chronic asymptomatic infection is the rule, and neoplastic disorders generally develop only after subsequent immunocompromise. In patients with AIDS, effective antiretroviral therapy has caused improvement in HHV-8–related disease. The virus is sensitive to ganciclovir, foscarnet, and cidofovir, but clinical benefit has not been demonstrated in trials. Invasive cervical carcinoma has been causally implicated with human papilloma virus infection.

IV-148. **The answer is B.** *(Chap. 183)* Molluscum contagiosum is a cutaneous poxvirus infection with a distinctive cutaneous appearance. The rash typically consists of collections of 2- to 5-mm umbilicated papules that can occur anywhere on the body except the palms and soles. It can be accompanied by an eczematous reaction. Molluscum contagiosum is transmitted through close contact, including sexual contact, which causes genital involvement. Unlike other poxvirus lesions, molluscum contagiosum is not associated with inflammation or necrosis. In immunocompetent patients, the disease is usually self-limited; rash will subside within several months. Systemic involvement does not occur.

IV-149. **The answer is C.** *(Chap. 184)* Immunocompromised patients occasionally cannot clear parvovirus infection because of a lack of T-cell function. Because parvovirus B19 selectively infects red cell precursors, persistent infection can lead to a prolonged red blood cell aplasia and a persistent drop in hematocrit, with low or absent reticulocytes. Pure red blood cell aplasia has been reported in HIV infection, lymphoproliferative diseases, and after transplantation. Iron studies show adequate iron but decreased utilization. The peripheral smear usually shows no abnormalities other than normocytic anemia and the absence of reticulocytes. Antibody tests are not useful in this setting because immunocompromised patients do not produce adequate antibodies against the virus. Therefore, polymerase chain reaction (PCR) is the most useful diagnostic test. Bone marrow biopsy may be suggestive because it will show no red blood cell precursors, but usually a less invasive PCR test is adequate. Immediate therapy is with red blood cell transfusion followed by intravenous immunoglobulins, which contain adequate titers of antibody against parvovirus B19.

IV-150. **The answer is D.** *(Chap. 184)* The most likely diagnosis based on the patient's antecedent illness with a facial rash is parvovirus infection. Arthropathy is uncommon in childhood parvovirus infection but may cause a diffuse symmetric arthritis in up to 50% of adults. This corresponds to the immune phase of illness when immunoglobulin M antibodies are developed. The arthropathy syndrome is more common in women than men. The distribution of affected joints is typically symmetric, most commonly in the small joints of the hands and less commonly the ankles, knees, and wrists. Occasionally the arthritis persists over months and can mimic rheumatoid arthritis. Rheumatoid factor can be detected in serum. Parvovirus B19V infection may trigger rheumatoid disease in some patients and has been associated with juvenile idiopathic arthritis. Reactive arthritis caused by *Chlamydia* spp. or a list of other bacterial pathogens tends to affect large joints such as the sacroiliac joints and spine. It is also sometimes accompanied by uveitis and urethritis. The large number of joints involved with a symmetric distribution argues against crystal or septic arthropathy.

IV-151. **The answer is E.** *(Chap. 185)* The currently available human papillomavirus (HPV) vaccines dramatically reduce rates of infection and disease produced by the HPV types in the vaccines. These products are directed against virus types that cause anogenital tract disease. Both vaccines consist of virus-like particles without any viral nucleic acid and therefore are not active. To date, one quadrivalent product (Gardasil, Merck) containing HPV types 6, 11, 16, and 18 and one bivalent product (Cervarix, GlaxoSmithKline) containing HPV types 16 and 18 have been licensed in the United States. HPV types 6 and 11 cause 90% of anogenital warts, and types 16 and 18 are responsible for 70% of cervical cancers. Efficacy has varied according to the immunologic and virologic characteristics of study populations at baseline and according to the endpoints evaluated. Among study participants who are shown at baseline not to be infected with a specific virus type contained in the vaccine and who adhere to the study protocol, rates of vaccine efficacy regularly exceed 90%, as measured by both infection and disease caused by that specific virus type. Study participants who are already infected at baseline with a specific virus type contained in the vaccine do not benefit from vaccination against that type but may benefit from vaccination against other virus types contained in the vaccine preparation. Thus, the available HPV vaccines have potent prophylactic effects but no therapeutic effects. The Advisory Committee on Immunization Practices (ACIP) of the Centers for Disease Control and Prevention has recommended that HPV vaccination be routinely offered to girls and young women 9 to 26 years of age. The quadrivalent vaccine has also been licensed in the United States for use in boys and young men; the ACIP has stated that this product may be used to prevent anogenital warts in boys and young men 9 to 26 years of age. Because 30% of cervical cancers are caused by HPV types not contained in the vaccines, no changes in cervical cancer screening programs are currently recommended. Ongoing studies are examining self-testing for HPV to replace many Pap studies in patients with no evidence of cervical infection. Recent studies implicate HPV in some forms of squamous cell carcinoma of the oropharynx. The utility of the current vaccines in preventing these cancers in not yet known.

IV-152. **The answer is D.** *(Chap. 186)* This patient presents with symptoms of the common cold with a self-limited illness characterized by rhinorrhea and sore throat. The most common viruses causing the common cold are rhinoviruses, which are implicated in as many as 50% of common colds. Rhinoviruses are small single-stranded RNA viruses of the Picornaviridae family. There are three genetic species of rhinoviruses with 102 serotypes identified. Rhinoviruses grow preferentially at the temperature of the

235

nasal passages (33° to 34°C) rather than the temperature of the lower airways (37°C). Although rhinovirus infections occur year round, there are seasonal peaks of the infection in the early fall and spring in temperate climates. Overall, the rates of rhinovirus infection are highest in infants and young children and decrease with age. The virus is most often introduced into families through young children in preschool or grade school. After the index infection, secondary infections occur in other family members 25% to 70% of the time. Rhinovirus spreads through direct contact with infected secretions, which can occur through respiratory droplets or hand-to-hand contact. It can also be transmitted through large or small particle aerosols. Finally, the virus can be isolated from plastic surfaces from 1 to 3 hours after inoculation, raising the possibility that the virus can also be transmitted through environmental contact.

IV-153. **The answer is C.** *(Chap. 186)* Acute viral respiratory illnesses are the most common illness worldwide, and a wide variety of viruses have been implicated as causes. Rhinoviruses are the most common virus causing the common cold and are found in about 50% of cases. The second most commonly isolated viruses are coronaviruses. These viruses are more common in the late fall, winter, and early spring, primarily at times when rhinoviruses are less active. Other causes of common cold in children are adenoviruses, whereas these viruses are uncommon in adults with the exception of outbreaks in individuals living in close quarters such as military recruits. Although human respiratory syncytial virus characteristically causes pneumonia and bronchiolitis in young children, the virus can cause common cold and pharyngitis in adults. Parainfluenza virus is another virus classically associated with croup in children, but it causes common cold in adults. Enteroviruses most often cause an undifferentiated febrile illness.

IV-154. **The answer is A.** *(Chap. 186)* The common viruses causing respiratory infections often have specific associated clinical syndromes. Rhinoviruses are primarily responsible for the common cold. Coronaviruses are also commonly associated with colds. However, in 2002 to 2003, there was an outbreak of a coronavirus-associated illness that originated in China and spread to 28 countries in Asia, Europe, and North and South America. This illness was named severe acute respiratory syndrome (SARS) and caused severe lower respiratory illness and acute respiratory distress syndrome. Overall, the case-fatality rate was 9.5%. Human respiratory syncytial virus is the primary agent responsible for lower respiratory disease and bronchiolitis in infants and young children. Another virus primarily associated with childhood illness is parainfluenza virus. This virus is a frequent cause of croup in young children characterized by a febrile illness with a barking cough and stridor. Adenovirus often causes a febrile illness with the common cold and pharyngitis in children. In adults, it is associated with outbreaks of respiratory illness in military recruits. Herpes simplex virus is associated gingivostomatitis in children and pharyngotonsillitis in adults.

IV-155. **The answer is C.** *(Chap. 186)* In infants, human respiratory syncytial virus (HRSV) is frequently associated with lower respiratory infections in 25% to 40% of infections. This can present as pneumonia, tracheobronchitis, or bronchiolitis. In cases of lower respiratory infections, tachypnea, wheezing, and hypoxemia are common and can progress to respiratory failure. Treatment is primarily supportive with hydration, suctioning of secretions, and administration of humidified oxygen. Bronchodilators are also used to treat wheezing and bronchospasm. In more severe cases, aerosolized ribavirin has been demonstrated to modestly improve the time to resolution of respiratory illness. The American Academy of Pediatrics states that aerosolized ribavirin may be considered in infants who are seriously ill or who are at high risk of complications, including bronchopulmonary dysplasia and congenital heart disease and those who are immunosuppressed. However, no benefit has been demonstrated with use of standard intravenous immunoglobulin or HRSV-specific immunoglobulin.

IV-156. **The answer is E.** *(Chap. 187)* Pandemic strains of influenza emerge through genetic reassortment of RNA segments between viruses that affect different species, including humans, swine, and birds. This process is also called antigenic shift during which a new strain of influenza emerges to which very few people have immunity. Antigenic shift only occurs with influenza A because it is the only influenza that crosses between species. Antigenic drift is the result of point mutations in the hemagglutinin or neuraminidase proteins. Antigenic drift occurs frequently and is responsible for the interpandemic influenza outbreaks.

IV-157. The answer is A. *(Chap. 187, www.cdc.gov/flu)* This patient is presenting with an influenza-like illness during the typical flu season. Hospital infection control practices in this setting are to treat all patients presenting with an influenza-like illness as if they have influenza until proven otherwise. This includes institution of droplet precautions to prevent spread to other individuals as well as performing testing to confirm influenza diagnosis. This is most commonly done via a nasopharyngeal swab but can also be done on throat swab, sputum, nasotracheal aspirates, or bronchoscopic specimens if available. If influenza diagnosis is confirmed, assessment of close household contacts for individuals who may be candidates for chemoprophylaxis against influenza is important, particularly individuals who would be high risk of complications from influenza infection. This group includes children younger than 4 years old, pregnant women, individuals age 65 years or older, individuals with heart or lung disease, individuals with abnormal immune systems, and individuals with chronic metabolic diseases or renal disease.

As far as treatment is concerned, clearly, oxygen should be given to individuals who are hypoxemic. Other appropriate supportive care should also be administered, including intravenous fluids and respiratory therapy support to manage secretions. In general, treatment with antiviral medications has been demonstrated to decrease the duration of symptoms by 1 to 1.5 days when initiated within the first 48 hours after the onset of symptoms. However, the Centers for Disease Control and Prevention (CDC) recommends treatment with antiviral medications as early as possible in patients hospitalized with severe pneumonia. Some evidence indicates that use of antiviral therapy might be effective in decreasing morbidity and mortality in individuals who are hospitalized with severe pneumonia even when given more than 48 hours after the onset of symptoms. The preferred class of antiviral therapy is the neuraminidase inhibitors, which have efficacy against both influenza A and B. In addition, resistance is much lower among this class of medications. This class includes the drugs zanamivir, oseltamivir, and peramivir. Of these, oseltamivir is most commonly used because it is an oral medication with limited side effects. Zanamivir is given by inhalation and can cause bronchoconstriction in individuals with asthma. Peramivir is currently an investigational medication that is administered intravenously.

The adamantine agents include amantadine and rimantadine. These medications have no efficacy against influenza B and also have a high degree of antiviral resistance (>90%) in North America to H3N2 strains of influenza A. It is important to know the resistance patterns to antiviral agents during the local flu season. The CDC currently does not recommend amantadine as first-line therapy for severe influenza. Antibacterial therapy should be reserved for individuals with suspected bacterial complications of influenza.

IV-158. The answer is A. *(Chap. 187, www.cdc.gov/flu)* The intranasal influenza vaccine contains a cold-adapted, live-attenuated influenza virus. Because of this, its use is more limited than intramuscular inactivated influenza vaccine. It is currently only recommended for healthy individuals between the ages of 2 and 49 years. Contraindications to the use of the live-attenuated intranasal influenza vaccine include pregnancy, chronic pulmonary or cardiovascular conditions, immunosuppressed patients, individuals with a history of Guillain-Barré syndrome, and individuals with a history of severe egg allergy. In addition, individuals who regularly are in contact with immunosuppressed people should not receive the intranasal vaccine, or if it is given, they should avoid contact with severely immunosuppressed patients for 7 days after receipt of the vaccine. In young children, a history of asthma precludes the use of intranasal influenza vaccination because the vaccine can precipitate episodes of wheezing. The Centers for Disease Control and Prevention recommends avoiding the use of the live-attenuated vaccine in individuals whose parents report an episode of wheezing within the past 12 months regardless of whether asthma is a chronic diagnosis. A final caveat in the use of the live-attenuated intranasal influenza vaccine is its use in individuals who are actively taking antiviral medications as chemoprophylaxis against influenza because antiviral medications interfere with the immune response to the live-attenuated influenza vaccine. The current recommendations are that live-attenuated influenza vaccination not be administered for 48 hours after antiviral medications have been stopped and that antiviral medications not be given for 2 weeks after receipt of the live-attenuated influenza vaccine. However, the immune response to the intramuscular inactivated vaccine is not affected by coadministration with antiviral drugs.

IV-159. The answer is D. *(Chap. 187)* The majority of influenza infections are clinically mild and self-limited. Treatment with over-the-counter cough suppressants and analgesics such as acetaminophen is often adequate. Patients who are younger than the age of 18 years are at risk of developing Reye's syndrome if they are exposed to salicylates such as aspirin. The neuraminidase inhibitors oseltamivir and zanamivir have activity against influenza A and B. They can be used within 2 days of symptom onset and have been shown to reduce the duration of symptoms by 1 or 2 days. This patient has had symptoms for more than 48 hours, so neither drug is likely to be effective. The patient's history of asthma is an additional contraindication to zanamivir because this drug can precipitate bronchospasm. The M2 inhibitors amantadine and rimantadine have activity against influenza A only. However, since 2005, more than 90% of A/H3N2 viral isolates demonstrated resistance to amantadine, and these drugs are no longer recommended for use in influenza A.

IV-160. The answer is C. *(Chap. 188)* Human T-cell lymphotropic virus-I (HTLV-I) is a retrovirus that is a chronic infection like HIV, but it does not cause similar sequelae. It was the first identified human retrovirus. Gradual decline of CD4+ lymphocyte number and function is a feature of HIV but not of HTLV-I. Although many people in endemic areas have sero-logic evidence of infection, most do not develop disease. The two major complications of HTLV-I are tropical spastic paraparesis and acute T-cell leukemia. Tropical spastic paraparesis is an upper motor neuron disease of insidious onset leading to weakness, lower extremity stiffness, urinary incontinence, and eventually a thoracic myelopathy, leading to a bedridden state in about one-third of patients after 10 years. It is more common in women than men. It can easily be confused with multiple sclerosis; this is why it is important to be able to recall the geographic regions where HTLV-I is endemic when evaluating a myelopathy. Acute T-cell leukemia is a difficult-to-treat leukemia that is specific to chronic HTLV-I infection. HTLV-I is thought to be transmitted in a similar fashion to HIV.

IV-161. The answer is C. *(Chap. 189)* Clindamycin plus primaquine is a therapeutic, not prophylactic, regimen for mild to moderate disease caused by *Pneumocystis* infection. Trimethoprim–sulfamethoxazole is usually given as a first-line agent but carries a significant side effect profile that includes hyperkalemia; renal insufficiency; elevation of serum creatinine; granulocytopenia; hemolysis in persons with G6PD insufficiency; and frequent allergic reactions, particularly in those with severe T-cell deficiency. Atovaquone is a common alternative that is given at the same dose for *Pneumocystis* prophylaxis as for therapy. Gastrointestinal symptoms are common with atovaquone. Aerosolized pentamidine can be given on a monthly basis with a risk of bronchospasm and pancreatitis. Patients who develop *Pneumocystis* pneumonia while receiving aerosolized pentamidine often have upper lobe–predominant disease. Dapsone is commonly used for *Pneumocystis* prophylaxis; however, the physician must be aware of the possibility of methemoglobinemia, G6PD-mediated hemolysis, rare hepatotoxicity, and rare hypersensitivity reaction when using this medicine.

IV-162. The answer is C. *(Chap. 189)* HIV/AIDS continues to have an extraordinary public health impact in the United States. As of January 1, 2010, an estimated 1,108,611 cases of AIDS had been diagnosed in the United States. Approximately 1.1 million individuals in the United States were living with HIV infection, approximately 20% of whom are unaware of their infection. Approximately two-thirds of those living with HIV/AIDS were nonwhite, and nearly half (48%) were men who have sex with men. The annual death rate from HIV/AIDS has fallen steadily in the past 15 years. This trend is attributable to several factors, including improved prophylaxis and treatment of opportunistic infections, the growing experience among health professions in caring for HIV-infected individuals, improved access to health care, and a decrease in new infections because of saturational effects and prevention efforts. However, the most influential factor clearly has been the increased use of potent antiretroviral drugs, generally administered in a combination of three or four agents. After a decrease in the percentage of new HIV infections attributed to male-to-male sexual contact from 1985 to 1999, this percentage has increased. In 2009, this transmission category accounted for 48% of all AIDS diagnoses. The estimated percentage of AIDS diagnoses attributed to injection drug use increased from 20% to 31% from 1985 to 1994 and decreased since that time, accounting for 15% of diagnoses in 2009. The estimated percentage of AIDS diagnoses attributed to heterosexual contact increased from 3% in 1985 to 31% in 2009. HIV infection and AIDS have disproportionately affected minority populations in the United States. Among those diagnosed with HIV (regardless of AIDS status) in 2009, 52% percent were blacks, a group that constitutes only 12% of the U.S. population.

IV-163. **The answer is C.** *(Chap. 189)* The quoted risk for HIV transmission via a needle stick is 0.3%. This risk can be reduced to less than 0.1% if the at-risk health care worker is treated with antiretroviral therapy within 24 hours. The risk of transmission is likely highly variable according to a number of factors. Large-bore needle sticks where infected patient blood is visible are higher risk, as are deep tissue puncture to the health care provider. The patient's degree of virologic control is generally inferred to be critical as well. Patients with viral loads below 1500/mL are considerably less likely to transmit via a needle stick than those with high viral loads. An extension of this point is that during acute and end-stage HIV infection, viral loads are extremely high, and contagion by needle stick is likely to be much higher. In addition, during end-stage disease, virulent viral forms predominate, which may increase the risk to an even greater extent. Each of these variables must be assessed rapidly after an accidental high-risk needle stick. Antiretroviral therapy (ART) is effective at preventing HIV transmission via needle stick if given before viral RNA incorporates into the host genome as proviral DNA. This is thought to occur within about 48 hours, but under the best scenario, ART should be given within 1 hour of a needle stick. Circumstances are often murky, with key information such as viral load, viral resistance history, and even HIV serostatus of the patient variably available; therefore, urgent consultation with an HIV or occupational health specialist is imperative after a needle stick. (Hepatitis B and C transmission must also be considered.)

IV-164. **The answer is E.** *(Chap. 189)* Abacavir use is associated with a potentially severe hypersensitivity reaction in about 5% of patients. There is likely a genetic component, with HLA-B*5701 being a significant risk factor for hypersensitivity syndrome. Symptoms, which usually occur within 2 weeks of therapy but can take more than 6 weeks to emerge, include fever, maculopapular rash, fatigue, malaise, gastrointestinal symptoms, and dyspnea. When a diagnosis is suspected, the drug should be stopped and never given again because rechallenge can be fatal. For this reason, both the diagnosis and patient education after the diagnosis is made must be performed thoroughly and carefully. It is important to note that two available combination pills contain abacavir (Epzicom, Trizivir), so patients must know to avoid these as well. Fanconi's anemia is a rare disorder associated with tenofovir. Zidovudine causes anemia and sometimes granulocytopenia. Stavudine and other nucleoside reverse transcriptase inhibitors are associated with lipoatrophy of the face and legs.

IV-165. **The answer is B.** *(Chap. 189)* Cytomegalovirus (CMV) colitis should be considered in AIDS patients with CD4+ lymphocyte counts below 50/μL, fevers, and diarrhea. Diarrhea is often bloody but can be watery. Initial evaluation often involves stool studies to rule out other parasitic or bacterial causes of diarrhea in AIDS patients. A standard panel includes some or all of the following depending on epidemiologic and historical data: *Clostridium difficile* stool antigen; stool culture; stool *Mycobacterium avium intracellulare* culture; stool ova and parasite examination; and special stains for *Cryptosporidium, Isospora, Cyclospora,* and *Microsporidium* spp. There is no stool or serum test that is useful for the evaluation of CMV colitis in an HIV-infected patient. A positive CMV immunoglobulin G result is merely a marker of past infection. If this test result is negative, then the pretest probability of developing active CMV decreases substantially. Serum CMV polymerase chain reaction (PCR) has gained utility in solid organ and bone marrow transplant patients for following treatment response for invasive CMV infection. However, in HIV-infected patients, CMV viremia correlates imprecisely with colitis. Furthermore, because CMV is a latent-lytic herpesvirus, a positive serum PCR does not imply disease unless drawn in the right clinical context, for which there is none in HIV infection. Colonic histology is sensitive and specific for the diagnosis of CMV colitis, with large-cell inclusion bodies being diagnostic.

IV-166. The answer is C. *(Chap. 189)* Immune reconstitution syndrome (IRIS) is commonly seen after the initiation of antiretroviral therapy (ART) in patients with AIDS and a concomitant opportunistic infection (OI). It is a syndrome in which either a previously recognized OI worsens after ART despite an initial period of improvement after standard therapy for that particular infection or in which an OI that was not previously recognized is unmasked after ART therapy. The latter scenario occurs presumably as immune cells become reactivated and recognize the presence of a pathogen that disseminated in the absence of adequate T-cell response with the patient remaining subclinical before ART. Many opportunistic pathogens are known to behave this way, but *Cryptococcus* spp., *Mycobacterium tuberculosis*, and *Mycobacterium avium* complex (MAI/MAC) are the most likely to be associated with IRIS. Risk factors for IRIS are a CD4+ lymphocyte count below 50/μL at ART initiation, initiation of ART within 2 months of treatment initiation for the OI, adequate virologic response to ART, and increase in CD4+ lymphocyte count as a result of ART. IRIS can be diagnostically challenging and is very diverse in terms of clinical presentation and severity. Depending on the organ system and pathogen involved, drug-resistant OI and new OI must be considered, sometimes necessitating invasive biopsies and cultures. In this case, the overlap of organ system with the original presentation, low likelihood of MAI drug resistance, and timing of the syndrome favor IRIS. Therapy is with nonsteroidal anti-inflammatory drugs and sometimes glucocorticoids. OI treatment is continued, and all efforts are made to continue ART as well except under the most dire of clinical circumstances.

IV-167. The answer is E. *(Chap. 189)* The biologic determinants of HIV transmission and acquisition are complex and have been difficult to study. However, several key factors are now known to increase the per-coital rate of HIV transmission, at least for heterosexual couples. In discordant couples, there is a dose-dependent relationship between serum viral load and HIV transmission. In fact, in carefully done studies, there was virtually no transmission between discordant couples when serum viral load was low (<400/mL). It is likely that this is attributable to a fairly tight correlation between serum and genital viral load. A corollary is that during acute HIV or AIDS, the viral load and therefore transmissibility are high. Strong clinical data from randomized trials indicate that circumcised men are less likely to acquire HIV because the interior surface of the foreskin is replete with cellular targets for HIV infection. Nonulcerative sexually transmitted infections cause mucosal breakdown that has been shown to allow for greater acquisition of HIV infection. Herpes simplex virus-2 (HSV-2) carriage (not necessarily requiring active genital ulcer disease) leads to increases in HIV genital shedding as well as HIV-1 target cell migration to the genital mucosa, making both transmission and acquisition of HIV higher in HSV-2–positive persons.

IV-168. The answer is B. *(Chap. 189)* Centers for Disease Control and Prevention guidelines now state that all adults should receive HIV testing, with the availability of a patient opt-out mechanism rather than informed consent. The basis for this is that about 25% of the 1 million Americans infected with HIV are unaware of their status, there is good available treatment for HIV that serves to extend the lifespan and decrease HIV transmission, and HIV testing is shown to correlate with a decrease in risk-taking behaviors. Cost-benefit analysis has suggested this approach has advantages to current approaches focusing on screening high-risk populations. Pretest counseling is desirable but not always built into the testing process, so physicians should provide some degree of preparation for a positive test result. If the diagnosis is made, support systems should be activated that may include trained nurses, social workers, or community support centers.

IV-169. **The answer is A.** *(Chap. 189)* This patient most likely has HIV encephalopathy of moderate severity. Other neurologic conditions associated with HIV may be considered with a broad initial workup, but her reasonably high CD4+ count, lack of focal deficits, and lack of mass lesions on high-resolution brain imaging makes toxoplasmosis, central nervous system (CNS) tuberculoma, progressive multifocal leukoencephalopathy (PML), and CNS lymphoma all less unlikely. Immediate highly active antiretroviral therapy is the treatment of choice for HIV encephalopathy, and she warrants this despite her CD4+ lymphocyte count, placing her in a gray zone according to current guidelines in regards to starting therapy. A lumbar puncture for the Venereal Disease Research Laboratory test is unnecessary because a serum rapid plasma reagin test is a very good screening test for any type of syphilis; JC virus detected in the cerebrospinal fluid would suggest PML, but her pretest probability for this is low because it usually affects patients with low CD4+ T-cell counts. Serum cryptococcal antigen has excellent performance characteristics, but there is little reason to suspect cryptococcal meningitis in the absence of headache or elevated intracerebral pressure.

IV-170. **The answer is D.** *(Chap. 189)* Indinavir is the only agent to cause nephrolithiasis. Nucleoside reverse transcriptase inhibitors, particularly stavudine and didanosine (d4T and ddI), are associated with mitochondrial toxicity and pancreatitis. Nevirapine can cause hepatic necrosis in women, particularly with CD4+ lymphocyte counts above 350/μL. Efavirenz, a very commonly used agent, causes dream disturbances that usually, but not always, subside after the first month of therapy. Both indinavir and atazanavir cause a benign indirect hyperbilirubinemia reminiscent of Gilbert's syndrome.

IV-171. **The answer is D.** *(Chap. 189)* *Isospora* and *Cryptosporidium* spp. cause very similar clinical disease in AIDS patients that ranges from intermittent, self-resolved watery diarrhea with abdominal cramping and sometimes nausea to a potentially fatal cholera-like presentation in the most immunocompromised hosts. *Cryptosporidium* spp. may cause biliary disease and can lead to cholangitis. *Isospora* spp. is limited to the gut lumen. *Cryptosporidium* spp. is not always an opportunistic infection and has led to widespread community outbreaks. *Isospora* spp. is not seen in immunocompetent hosts. Finally, treatment for *Isospora* infection is usually successful. In fact, this infection is rarely seen in the developed world because trimethoprim–sulfamethoxazole, which is commonly used for *Pneumocystis* prophylaxis, tends to eradicate *Isospora* spp. Cryptosporidiosis, on the other hand, is very difficult to cure, and interventions are controversial. Some clinicians favor nitazoxanide, but cure rates are mediocre, and immune reconstitution with antiretroviral therapy is ultimately critical to cure the gastrointestinal disease.

IV-172. **The answer is D.** *(Chap. 189)* Acute HIV should be suspected in any at-risk person who presents with a mono-like illness; it is diagnosed by positive plasma RNA polymerase chain reaction (PCR). Patients typically have not developed sufficient antibodies to the virus yet to develop a positive enzyme immunoassay result, and the diagnosis of HIV is usually missed if this test is sent within the first 2 months of HIV acquisition. It is tempting for clinicians to send an ultrasensitive PCR, but this only decreases specificity (false-positive tests with detection of very low levels of HIV are possible because of cross-contamination in the laboratory) with no other benefit. There is typically a massive amount of HIV virus in the plasma during acute infection, and the ultrasensitive assay is never required for detection at this stage of disease. Ultrasensitive assays are helpful in the context of therapy to ensure that there is not persistence of low-level viremia. CD4+ lymphocyte count decreases during many acute infections, including HIV, and is therefore not diagnostically appropriate. CD4+ lymphocyte counts are useful to risk stratify for opportunistic infection in stable patients with known HIV infection. Resistance tests are sent only when the diagnosis is confirmed.

IV-173. **The answer is B.** *(Chap. 189)* Oral hairy leukoplakia is caused by a severe overgrowth of Epstein-Barr virus infection in T-cell–deficient patients. It is not premalignant and is often unrecognized by the patient but is sometimes a cosmetic, symptomatic, and therapeutic nuisance. The white, thickened folds on the side of the tongue can be pruritic or painful and sometimes resolve with acyclovir derivatives or topical podophyllin resin. Ultimate resolution occurs after immune reconstitution with antiretroviral therapy. Oral candidiasis or thrush is a very common, relatively easy-to-treat condition in HIV patients and takes on an appearance of white plaques on the tongue, palate, and buccal mucosa that bleed with blunt removal. Herpes simplex virus (HSV) recurrences or aphthous ulcers present as painful ulcerating lesions. The latter should be considered when oral ulcers persist, do not respond to acyclovir, and do not culture HSV. Kaposi's sarcoma is uncommon in the oropharynx and takes on a violet hue, suggesting its highly vascularized content.

IV-174. The answer is E. *(Chap. 189)* Current recommendations are to initiate antiretroviral therapy in patients with the acute HIV syndrome, all pregnant women, patients with an AIDS-defining illness, patients with HIV-associated nephropathy, and patients with asymptomatic disease with CD4+ T-cell counts below 500/μL. Clinical trials are under way to determine the value of even earlier intervention, and some experts would place everyone with HIV infection on antiretroviral therapy. In addition, one may wish to administer a 6-week course of therapy to uninfected individuals immediately after a high-risk exposure to HIV. For patients diagnosed with an opportunistic infection and HIV infection at the same time, one may consider a 2- to 4-week delay in the initiation of antiretroviral therapy during which time treatment is focused on the opportunistic infection. Although not proven, it is postulated that this delay may decrease the severity of any subsequent immune reconstitution inflammatory syndrome by lowering the antigenic burden of the opportunistic infection.

TABLE IV-174 **Indications for the Initiation of Antiretroviral Therapy in Patients With HIV Infection**

I. Acute infection syndrome
II. Chronic infection
A. Symptomatic disease (including HIV-associated nephropathy)
B. Asymptomatic disease
1. CD4+ T-cell count <500/μL[a]
2. Pregnancy
III. Postexposure prophylaxis

[a]This is an area of controversy. Some experts would treat everyone regardless of CD4+ T-cell count.
Source: Guidelines for the Use of Antiretroviral Agents in HIV-Infected Adults and Adolescents, USPHS.

IV-175. The answer is B. *(Chap. 189)* Therapy of HIV infection does not lead to eradication or cure of HIV. Treatment decisions must take into account the fact that one is dealing with a chronic infection. Patients initiating antiretroviral therapy must be willing to commit to lifelong treatment and understand the importance of adherence to their prescribed regimen. Treatment interruption regimens are associated with rapid increases in HIV RNA levels, rapid declines in CD4+ T-cell counts, and an increased risk of clinical progression. In clinical trials, there has been an increase in serious adverse events in the patients randomized to intermittent therapy, suggesting that some "non–AIDS-associated" serious adverse events such as heart attack and stroke may be linked to HIV replication. Given that patients can be infected with viruses that harbor drug resistance mutations, it is recommended that a viral genotype be done before the initiation of therapy to optimize the selection of antiretroviral agents. The three options for initial therapy most commonly in use today are three different three-drug regimens. These include (1) tenofovir, emtricitabine, and efavirenz; (2) tenofovir, emtricitabine, and atazanavir (or darunavir); and (3) tenofovir, emtricitabine, and raltegravir. There are no clear data at present on which to base distinctions among these three regimens. After the initiation of therapy, one should expect a rapid, at least 1-log (10-fold) reduction in plasma HIV RNA levels within 1 to 2 months and then a slower decline in plasma HIV RNA levels to less than 50 copies per milliliter within 6 months. There should also be a rise in the CD4+ T-cell count of 100 to 150/μL that is also particularly brisk during the first month of therapy. Subsequently, one should anticipate a CD4+ T-cell count increase of 50 to 100 cells per year until numbers approach normal. Many clinicians believe that failure to achieve these endpoints is an indication for a change in therapy.

IV-176. The answer is B. *(Chap. 190)* The Norwalk virus is the prototype calicivirus that causes human disease. The calicivirus family, many of which cause gastroenteritis and diarrhea, particularly in children, includes norovirus and sapovirus. Most adults worldwide have antibodies to these viruses. However, they are a major cause of morbidity throughout the world and a frequent cause of nonbacterial diarrhea outbreaks in the United States. They spread via fecal–oral spread and have a low inoculum necessary for disease. In temperate regions, they tend to occur in cold weather months. The incubation period is less than 3 days, typically 24 hours. The onset of disease is rapid. Fever, myalgias, and headache are common. The diarrhea is nonbloody without fecal leukocytes. The disease is self-limited, and therapy is supportive.

IV-177. The answer is B. *(Chap. 190)* Nearly all children worldwide are infected with rotavirus by age 5 years. In the developing world, it remains a major cause of diarrheal death caused by volume depletion. Repeated infections occur with each subsequent episode of lesser severity. Therefore, severe disease is uncommon in adolescents and adults who may develop disease, particularly after contact with ill children. The disease typically has an abrupt onset with vomiting usually preceding diarrhea. Fever occurs in approximately one-third of cases. Stools usually do not contain blood, mucus, or inflammatory material. The disease is usually self-limited in 3 to 7 days. Because rotavirus is a major cause of childhood hospitalization and morbidity in the United States, vaccination is recommended for all U.S. children. Vaccination has less efficacy in the developing world because of a higher frequency of malnutrition, co-infection, and comorbidities, but is recommended by the World Health Organization for all children worldwide.

IV-178. The answer is B. *(Chap. 191)* Enteroviruses are responsible for up to 90% of aseptic meningitis in which an etiologic agent can be identified. Symptoms are typically more severe in adults than children. Illness is more frequent in the summer and fall in temperate climates, but other causes of viral meningitis are more common in winter and spring. Cerebrospinal fluid (CSF) analysis always shows an elevated (although usually <1000 cells/μL) white blood cell count. Early, there may be a neutrophil predominance; however, this typically shifts toward lymphocyte predominance by 24 hours. CSF glucose and protein are usually normal, although the latter can sometimes be elevated. The illness is typically self-limiting, and the prognosis is excellent.

IV-179. The answer is B. *(Chap. 191)* These lesions are diagnostic of herpangina, which is caused by coxsackievirus A. They are typically round and discrete, which helps differentiate them from thrush caused by *Candida* spp. Unlike herpes simplex virus stomatitis, herpangina lesions are not associated with gingivitis. Lesions are typically concentrated in the posterior portion of the mouth. Herpangina usually presents with dysphagia, odynophagia, and fever; these lesions can persist for several weeks. The lesions do not ulcerate.

IV-180. The answer is B. *(Chap. 191)* Enteroviruses are single-strand RNA viruses that multiply in the gastrointestinal (GI) tract but rarely cause GI illness. Typical person-to-person spread occurs via the fecal–oral route; enteroviruses are not known to spread via blood transfusions or insect vectors. Infection is most common among infants and small children; serious illness occurs in neonates, older children, and adults. Most infections with poliovirus are symptomatic or cause a minor illness. Before the implementation of polio vaccines, paralysis was a rare clinical presentation of poliovirus infection and was less frequent in developing countries, likely because of earlier exposure. Paralytic disease caused by polio infection is more common in older adults, pregnant women, and persons exercising strenuously or with trauma at the time of central nervous system symptoms. Exposure to maternal antibodies leads to a lower risk of symptomatic neonatal infection.

IV-181. The answer is D. *(Chap. 195)* The patient has been bitten by a member of a species known to carry rabies in an area in which rabies is endemic. Based on the animal vector and the facts that the skin was broken and that saliva possibly containing the rabies virus was present, postexposure rabies prophylaxis should be administered. If an animal involved in an unprovoked bite can be captured, it should be killed humanely, and the head should be sent immediately to an appropriate laboratory for rabies examination by the technique of fluorescent antibody staining for viral antigen. If a healthy dog or cat bites a person in an endemic area, the animal should be captured, confined, and observed for 10 days. If the animal remains healthy for this period, the bite is highly unlikely to have transmitted rabies. Postexposure prophylactic therapy includes vigorous cleaning of the wound with a 20% soap solution to remove any virus particles that may be present. Tetanus toxoid and antibiotics should also be administered. Passive immunization with anti-rabies antiserum in the form of human rabies immune globulin (rather than the corresponding equine antiserum because of the risk of serum sickness) is indicated at a dose of 10 units/kg into the wound and 10 units/kg IM into the gluteal region. Second, one should actively immunize with an antirabies vaccine (either human diploid cell vaccine or rabies vaccine absorbed) in five 1-mL doses given intramuscularly, preferably in the deltoid or anterior lateral thigh area. The five doses are given over a 28-day period. The administration of either passive or active immunization without the other modality results in a higher failure rate than does the combination therapy.

IV-182. The answer is B. *(Chap. 196)* This patient has a typical presentation of dengue fever. All four distinct dengue viruses (dengue 1–4) have the mosquito *Aedes aegypti* as their principal vector, and all cause a similar clinical syndrome. Thus, lifelong immunity cannot be presumed. In rare cases, second infection with a serotype of dengue virus different from that involved in the primary infection leads to dengue hemorrhagic fever with severe shock. Year-round transmission between latitudes 25°N and 25°S has been established, and seasonal forays of the viruses to points as far north as Philadelphia are thought to have taken place in the United States. Dengue fever is seen throughout Southeast Asia, including Malaysia, Thailand, Vietnam, and Singapore. the Western hemisphere, it may be found in the Caribbean region, including Puerto Rico. With increasing spread of the vector mosquito throughout the tropics and subtropics, large areas of the world have become vulnerable to the introduction of dengue viruses, particularly through air travel by infected humans, and both dengue fever and the related dengue hemorrhagic fever are becoming increasingly common. The *A. aegypti* mosquito, which is also an efficient vector of the yellow fever and chikungunya viruses, typically breeds near human habitation, using relatively fresh water from sources such as water jars, vases, discarded containers, coconut husks, and old tires. *A. aegypti* usually inhabits dwellings and bites during the day. After an incubation period of 2 to 7 days, the typical patient experiences the symptoms described above along with the severe myalgia that gave rise to the colloquial designation "break-bone fever." There is often a macular rash on the first day as well as adenopathy, palatal vesicles, and scleral injection. The illness may last 1 week, with additional symptoms usually including anorexia, nausea or vomiting, marked cutaneous hypersensitivity, and—near the time of defervescence—a maculopapular rash beginning on the trunk and spreading to the extremities and the face. Laboratory findings include leukopenia; thrombocytopenia; and, in many cases, serum aminotransferase elevations. The diagnosis is made by immunoglobulin G enzyme-linked immunosorbent assay (ELISA) or paired serology during recovery or by antigen-detection ELISA or reverse transcription polymerase chain reaction during the acute phase. In endemic regions where specific testing is not easily available, the diagnosis is presumed in cases of a typical clinical presentation and thrombocytopenia. Given the frequency of disease and the potential for hemorrhagic fever, active investigation is pursuing an effective vaccine.

IV-183. The answer is D. *(Chap. 198)* The classification of fungal infections is typically based on anatomic location of infection and epidemiology of the organism. Additionally, it is important to know the descriptive characteristics of fungi in culture because that information may be useful clinically. Endemic mycoses (e.g., coccidioidomycosis, blastomycosis) are infections that are caused by fungi that are not typically part of human microbial flora. Opportunistic mycoses (e.g., *Candida, Aspergillus*) are infections that are caused by fungi that are commonly part of the human microbial flora. Yeasts (*Candida, Cryptococcus*) are seen microscopically as single cells or rounded organisms. Molds (*Aspergillus, Rhizopus*) grow as filamentous forms (hyphae) at room temperature and in tissue. *Dimorphic* is the term to describe fungi that exist as yeasts or large spherical structures in tissue but in filamentous forms in the environment. Blastomycosis, histoplasmosis, paracoccidioidomycosis, coccidioidomycosis, and sporotrichosis are typically dimorphic. *Candida* may exist as a yeast or filamentous form in tissue infection, with the exception of *Candida glabrata*, which only exists as a yeast in tissue infection.

IV-184. The answer is A. *(Chap. 198)* The azole antifungals (fluconazole, itraconazole, voriconazole, and posaconazole) all have oral formulations. The azoles inhibit ergosterol synthesis in the fungal cell wall. Compared with amphotericin B, they are considered fungistatic but do not cause significant renal toxicity. Fluconazole is effective for *Candida albicans* and coccidioidomycosis. Voriconazole has broader spectrum against *Candida* spp., including *Candida glabrata* and *Candida krusei*. Itraconazole is the drug of choice for mild to moderate histoplasmosis and blastomycosis. Posaconazole is approved in immunocompromised patients as prophylaxis against *Candida* and *Aspergillus* infection. Studies of posaconazole have suggested efficacy for zygomycosis, *Aspergillus*, and cryptococcal infections. It also has activity against fluconazole-resistant *Candida*. The echinocandins (caspofungin, anidulafungin, micafungin) only have intravenous formulations at this time. They are considered fungicidal for *Candida* and fungistatic for *Aspergillus*. Griseofulvin is an oral medication used historically primarily for ringworm infection. Terbinafine is more effective than griseofulvin for ringworm and onychomycosis.

IV-185. The answer is D. *(Chap. 198)* All patients with *Candida* fungemia should be treated with systemic antifungals. Fluconazole has been shown to be an effective agent for candidemia with equivalence to amphotericin products and caspofungin. Voriconazole is also active against *Candida albicans* but has many drug interactions that make it less desirable against this pathogen. However, it has broader activity against *Candida* spp. including *Candida glabrata* and *Candida krusei*. No trials of posaconazole for candidemia have yet been reported. The echinocandins, including micafungin and caspofungin, have broad activity, are fungicidal against *Candida* spp., and have low toxicity. They are among the safest antifungal agents.

IV-186. The answer is B. *(Chap. 198)* The definitive diagnosis of an invasive fungal infection generally requires histologic demonstration of fungus invading tissue along with an inflammatory response. However, *Coccidioides* serum complement fixation, cryptococcal serum and cerebrospinal fluid antigen, and urine/serum *Histoplasma* antigen are all tests with good performance characteristics, occasionally allowing for presumptive diagnoses before pathologic tissue sections can be examined or cultures of blood or tissue turn positive. Serum testing for galactomannan is approved for the diagnosis of *Aspergillus* infection. However, false-negative test results may occur. Multiple serial tests may decrease the incidence of false-negative test results. There is no approved urine or serologic test for blastomycosis.

IV-187. The answer is D. *(Chap. 199)* All of these pathogens are typically inhaled and cause pulmonary infection, which may resolve spontaneously or progress to active disease. Resolved infection with blastomycosis, coccidioidomycosis, *Cryptococcus* spp., and tuberculosis will often leave a radiographic lesion that typically looks like a solitary nodule and may be confused with potential malignancy. Latent tuberculosis is often suggested by the radiographic finding of a calcified lymph node that is typically solitary. Of the listed infections, histoplasmosis is most likely to resolve spontaneously in an immunocompetent individual, leaving multiple mediastinal and splenic calcifications. These represent calcified granulomas formed after an appropriate cellular immunity response involving interleukin-12, tumor necrosis factor-α in combination with functional lymphocytes, macrophages, and epithelial cells. In endemic areas, 50% to 80% of adults have evidence of previous infection without clinical manifestations. In patients with impaired cellular immunity, the infection may disseminate to the bone marrow, spleen, liver, adrenal glands, and mucocutaneous membranes. Unlike tuberculosis, remote *Histoplasma* infection rarely reactivates.

IV-188. The answer is C. *(Chap. 199)* This silver stain shows the typical small (2–5 μm) budding yeast of *Histoplasma capsulatum* on bronchoalveolar lavage (BAL). Patients receiving infliximab and other anti–tumor necrosis factor therapies are at risk of developing opportunistic infection with tuberculosis, *Histoplasma*, other pathogenic fungi (including pneumocystis), *Legionella*, and viruses (including cytomegalovirus). These infections typically manifest after approximately 2 months of therapy, although shorter and longer durations are described. Patients with AIDS (CD4 <200 cells/mm^3), at extremes of age, and receiving prednisone therapy are also at risk of disseminated histoplasmosis. Disseminated histoplasmosis may present with shock, respiratory failure, pancytopenia, disseminated intravascular coagulation, and multiorgan failure or as a more indolent illness with focal organ dissemination, fever, and systemic symptoms. Culture results of BAL are positive in more than 50% of cases of acute respiratory histoplasmosis. Bone marrow and blood cultures have a high yield in disseminated cases. *Histoplasma* antigen testing of blood and BAL is also sensitive and specific. There is potential cross-reactivity with blastomycosis, coccidioidomycosis, and paracoccidioidomycosis.

IV-189. The answer is E. *(Chap. 199)* Patients with severe life-threatening *Histoplasma* infection should be treated with a lipid formulation of amphotericin B followed by itraconazole (see Table IV-189). In immunosuppressed patients, the degree of immunosuppression should be reduced if possible. Caspofungin (and other echinocandins) is not active against *Histoplasma* spp. but would be used for infection with *Candida* or *Aspergillus*. Ganciclovir is recommended for cytomegalovirus infection. The combination isoniazid, rifampin, pyrazinamide, and ethambutol is recommended therapy for *Mycobacterium tuberculosis*. Clarithromycin, rifampin, and ethambutol therapy is recommended therapy for *Mycobacterium avium* complex.

TABLE IV-189 Recommendations for the Treatment of Histoplasmosis

Type of Histoplasmosis	Treatment Recommendations	Comments
Acute pulmonary, moderate to severe illness with diffuse infiltrates or hypoxemia	Lipid AmB (3–5 mg/kg per day) ± glucocorticoids for 1–2 weeks; then itraconazole (200 mg bid) for 12 weeks. Monitor renal and hepatic function.	Patients with mild cases usually recover without therapy, but itraconazole should be considered if the patient's condition has not improved after 1 month.
Chronic cavitary pulmonary	Itraconazole (200 mg qd or bid) for at least 12 months. Monitor hepatic function.	Continue treatment until radiographic findings show no further improvement. Monitor for relapse after treatment is stopped.
Progressive disseminated	Lipid AmB (3–5 mg/kg per day) for 1–2 weeks; then itraconazole (200 mg bid) for at least 12 months. Monitor renal and hepatic function.	Liposomal AmB is preferred, but the AmB lipid complex may be used because of cost. Chronic maintenance therapy may be necessary if the degree of immunosuppression cannot be reduced.
Central nervous system	Liposomal AmB (5 mg/kg per day) for 4–6 weeks; then itraconazole (200 mg bid or tid) for at least 12 months. Monitor renal and hepatic function.	A longer course of lipid AmB is recommended because of the high risk of relapse. Itraconazole should be continued until cerebrospinal fluid or CT abnormalities clear.

Abbreviation: AmB, amphotericin B; bid, twice a day; CT, computed tomography; tid, three times a day.

IV-190. The answer is C. *(Chap. 200)* This patient likely has coccidioidomycosis with meningitis caused by HIV infection as evidenced by his history, physical examination, laboratory findings, and diagnostic microbes in the cerebrospinal fluid (CSF). Fresno is in the heart of the San Joaquin Valley, the highest endemic region for coccidioidomycosis. For reasons that are unclear, African American men and Filipino males are at highest risk of developing coccidioidal infection. Coccidioidomycosis becomes disseminated in fewer than 1% of cases, but the meninges as well as the skin, bone, and joints are the most common extrapulmonary sites. Defective cellular immunity and immunosuppression increase the likelihood of dissemination and meningitis. Nuchal rigidity is mild when present, but chronic headache and confusion are typical. Untreated infection may lead to hydrocephalus. Untreated meningitis is uniformly fatal. The CSF findings in this case are typical with lymphocyte predominance, markedly low glucose, and high protein. The findings on silver stain are characteristic of spherules with are unique to coccidioidal infection and are diagnostic when found in tissue (often in granulomas) or body fluids. Complement fixation antibodies in the CSF also indicate infection. Traditionally, amphotericin B was used for treatment of meningitis, but azole antifungals may now be used. Studies have shown itraconazole and fluconazole effective for coccidioidal infections. Fluconazole has excellent CSF penetration and is currently the recommended therapy. Itraconazole is likely preferred for bone and joint disease. Therapy should be lifelong because the relapse rate is greater than 80%. Although the clinical presentation and CSF findings are consistent with tuberculosis meningitis, the finding of spherules is diagnostic. Caspofungin is active against *Candida* and *Aspergillus* but not coccidioidomycosis. Penicillin G is the preferred therapy for tertiary syphilis.

IV-191. **The answer is C.** *(Chap. 200) Coccidioides immitis* is a mold that is found in the soil in the southwestern United States and Mexico. Case clusters of primary disease may appear 10 to 14 days after exposure, and the activities with the highest risk include archaeological excavation, rock hunting, military maneuvers, and construction work. Only 40% of primary pulmonary infections are symptomatic. Symptoms may include those of a hypersensitivity reaction such as erythema nodosum (typically on the lower extremities), erythema multiforme (typically in a necklace distribution), arthritis, or conjunctivitis. Blood eosinophilia is common during acute infection. Although pleurisy is common, significant pleural effusion only occurs in 10% of cases (typically mononuclear with negative culture). Diagnosis can be made by culture of sputum; however, when this organism is suspected, the laboratory needs to be notified because it is a biohazard level 3 fungus. Serologic tests of blood may also be helpful; however, seroconversion of primary disease may take up to 8 weeks. Skin testing is useful only for epidemiologic studies and is not done in clinical practice. Asymptomatic and most cases of focal uncomplicated pneumonia do not require therapy.

IV-192. **The answer is E.** *(Chap. 200)* Northern Arizona (i.e., the Grand Canyon region) is not a region of high incidence of coccidioidomycosis. The organism can be cultured from dry top soil in the high desert of Southern Arizona surrounding Phoenix and Tucson. In North America, the areas of greatest endemicity include the San Joaquin valley in California, south central Arizona, and northern Mexico. Endemic foci have also been described in the Texas Rio Grande Valley, some areas of Central America, Columbia, Venezuela, northeastern Brazil, Paraguay, Bolivia, and north central Argentina. Eosinophilia is a common laboratory finding in acute coccidioidomycosis, and erythema nodosum is a common cutaneous clinical feature (particularly on the lower extremities in women). Mediastinal lymphadenopathy is more commonly seen on radiographs for all acute pneumonias caused by endemic mycoses, including *Coccidioides* spp., rather than caused by bacterial pneumonia. A positive complement fixation test result is one method to definitively diagnose acute infection.

IV-193. **The answer is C.** *(Chap. 201)* Blastomycosis is caused by the dimorphic fungus *Blastomyces dermatides,* which commonly resides in soil and is acquired through inhalation. Pulmonary infection is most common and can be acute or indolent. Extrapulmonary extension via hematogenous spread from the lungs is common with skin lesions and osteomyelitis most common. In patients with AIDS, central nervous system involvement, usually as a brain abscess, has been reported in approximately 40% of cases of blastomycosis. Most cases of blastomycosis are reported from North America with the most common regions being bordering the Mississippi and Ohio River basins, the upper Midwest and Canada bordering the Great Lakes, and a small area of New York and Ontario bordering the St. Lawrence River. Outside of North American, most blastomycosis cases are in Africa. Coccidioidomycosis is endemic in Southern Arizona.

IV-194. **The answer is C.** *(Chap. 201)* The constellation of symptoms including chronic pneumonia with ulcerating skin lesions and soil exposure in the upper Midwest in the Great Lakes region is highly suggestive of disseminated blastomycosis infection. Sputum or skin biopsy may show broad-based budding yeast. The definitive diagnosis would be made by growth of the organism from sputum or skin biopsy. Serologic testing is of limited use because of cross-reactivity with other endemic fungi. There is a urine *Blastomyces* antigen test that appears more sensitive than serum testing. Therapy for blastomycosis in a non–life-threatening condition is with itraconazole. Lipid formulations of amphotericin are indicated in life-threatening disease or central nervous system (CNS) disease (fluconazole can also be used for CNS disease). Blastomycosis may present with solitary pulmonary lesions that may be suggestive of malignancy and should be evaluated as such. The chronic indolent form may also be confused with pulmonary tuberculosis. The differential diagnosis of blastomycosis skin lesions includes pyoderma gangrenosum that may be associated with inflammatory bowel disease. Methicillin-resistant *Staphylococcus aureus* skin lesions may be nodular then ulcerate but, when associated with hematologic dissemination from the lung, are usually more acute than this indolent presentation.

IV-195. **The answer is B.** *(Chap. 202)* The goal of therapy for cryptococcal meningoencephalitis in an HIV-negative patient is cure of the fungal infection, not simply control of symptoms. Thus, intravenous amphotericin plus flucytosine is recommended as induction followed by prolonged therapy with fluconazole. Amphotericin plus flucytosine for 6 to 10 weeks may also be used in non-immunocompromised patients. Patients with immunocompromising conditions may receive the same initial regimen with a more prolonged course of fluconazole to prevent relapse. Although not relevant in this case, isolated pulmonary cryptococcosis in an immunocompetent patient may be treated with fluconazole for 3 to 6 months after clear demonstration that the cerebrospinal fluid (CSF) is not affected. Cryptococcal meningitis often causes increased intracranial pressure (ICP), which is thought to contribute to irreversible brain and cranial nerve damage. ICP should be measured during lumbar puncture, and CSF should be removed as needed to avoid elevated ICP. Shunt placement may be indicated in refractory cases. Newer triazoles, such as voriconazole, are highly active against *Cryptococcus*, but clinical experience is limited at this time. Neither caspofungin nor micafungin have activity against *Cryptococcus*. Ceftriaxone and vancomycin are the recommended treatments for bacterial meningitis in an immunocompetent patient younger than 50 years of age and have no role in the therapy of *Cryptococcus* infection.

IV-196. **The answer is A.** *(Chap. 202)* Cryptococcal meningoencephalitis presents with early manifestations of headache, nausea, gait disturbance, confusion, and visual changes. Fever and nuchal rigidity are often mild or absent. Papilledema is present in more than 30% of cases. Asymmetric cranial nerve palsies occur in 25% of cases. Neuroimaging findings are often normal. If there are focal neurologic findings, magnetic resonance imaging may be used to diagnose cryptococcomas in the basal ganglia or caudate nucleus, although they are more common in immunocompetent patients with *Cryptococcus neoformans* var. *gattii*. Imaging does not make the diagnosis. The definitive diagnosis remains cerebrospinal fluid (CSF) culture. However, capsular antigen testing in both the serum and the CSF is very sensitive and can provide a presumptive diagnosis. Approximately 90% of patients, including all with a positive CSF smear, and the majority of AIDS patients have detectable cryptococcal antigen. The result is often negative in patients with isolated pulmonary disease. However, because of a very small false-positive rate in antigen testing, CSF culture remains the definitive diagnostic test. In this condition *C. neoformans* often can also be cultured from the urine; however, other testing methods are more rapid and useful.

IV-197. **The answer is D.** *(Chap. 203)* Reviews of cases reveal consistent conditions and risk factors associated with hematogenous dissemination of *Candida*. Many refer to the fact that innate immunity is the most important defense mechanism against hematogenous dissemination of the fungus and that neutrophils are the most important component of this defense. Many immunocompetent people have antibodies to *Candida* spp.; the role of these antibodies in the defense against hematogenous spread is not clear. Therefore, patients the conditions and risk factors listed in the question plus indwelling urinary catheters, parenteral glucocorticoids, neutropenia, cytotoxic chemotherapy, and immunosuppressive agents for organ transplantation all confer risk of disseminated candidiasis. Additionally, low birth weight infants, HIV-infected patients with low CD4 counts, and patients with diabetes are at great risk of local infection with *Candida* that may disseminate when other predisposing factors are present (e.g., catheters). Women receiving antibiotics are at risk of developing vaginal candidiasis. Patients with pulmonary alveolar proteinosis are at risk of infection with unusual organisms such as *Nocardia*, atypical mycobacteria, *Aspergillus*, and pneumocystis but are not at increased risk of disseminated candidiasis in the absence of other risk factors.

IV-198. The answer is D. *(Chaps. 198 and 203)* This patient presents with the classic skin presentation of disseminated candidiasis. The skin lesions, severe myalgias, joint pains, and fever are typical manifestations of hematogenous spread from either a gastrointestinal or skin source in a patient predisposed by neutropenia and indwelling catheters. The severe myalgias are a characteristic of this syndrome and should be taken seriously as a new complaint in a susceptible host. Blood culture results are likely be positive, but staining of the skin lesions is positive in virtually 100% of cases. *Candida* is the only fungus that can typically be visualized on tissue Gram stain in the form of pseudohyphae and hyphae. *Aspergillus* is seen in tissue as clumps of branching (45 degrees) septated hyphae often with angioinvasion and necrosis. *Aspergillus* may also disseminate in a prolonged neutropenic patient, usually from a lung infection, and cause rapidly progressive skin lesions, usually with a necrotic center. *Histoplasma* and *Blastomyces* can be visualized in tissue as budding yeast. Encapsulated yeasts on India ink are indicative of *Cryptococcus*. Spherules are specific to coccidioidomycosis.

IV-199. The answer is D. *(Chap. 203) Candida* spp. are susceptible to a number of systemic antifungal agents. Most institutions chose an agent based on their local epidemiology and resistance patterns. Fluconazole is the most commonly used agent for nonneutropenic hemodynamically stable patients unless azole resistance is considered an issue. In a hemodynamically unstable neutropenic patient, more broad-spectrum agents are typically used such as polyenes, echinocandins, or later-generation azoles such as voriconazole. (See Table IV-199.) Lipid formulations of amphotericin, although not approved by the U.S. Food and Drug Administration as primary therapy, are commonly used because they are less toxic than amphotericin B deoxycholate. At present, the vast majority of isolates of *Candida albicans* are sensitive to fluconazole. *Candida glabrata* and *Candida krusei* are more sensitive to polyenes and echinocandins. Flucytosine is not used as sole therapy for *Candida*. It may be combined with amphotericin for treatment of *Candida* endophthalmitis and meningitis.

TABLE IV-199   Agents for the Treatment of Disseminated Candidiasis

Agent	Route of Administration	Dose[a]	Comment
Amphotericin B deoxycholate	IV only	0.5–1.0 mg/kg daily	Being replaced by lipid formulations
Amphotericin B lipid formulations			Not FDA approved as primary therapy but used commonly because less toxic than amphotericin B deoxycholate
Liposomal (AmBi some, Abelcet)	IV only	3.0–5.0 mg/kg daily	
Lipid complex (ABLC)	IV only	3.0–5.0 mg/kg daily	
Colloidal dispersion (ABCD)	IV only	3.0–5.0 mg/kg daily	Associated with frequent infusion reactions
Azoles			
Fluconazole	IV and oral	400 mg/d	Most commonly used
Voriconazole	IV and oral	400 mg/d	Multiple drug interactions
			Approved for candidemia in nonneutropenic patients
Echinocandins			Broad spectrum against *Candida* spp.; approved for disseminated candidiasis
Caspofungin	IV only	50 mg/d	
Anidulafungin	IV only	100 mg/d	
Micafungin	IV only	100 mg/d	

[a]See Pappas et al. (2009) for loading doses and adjustments in renal failure. The recommended duration of therapy is 2 weeks beyond the last positive blood cultures and resolution of signs and symptoms of infection.
Note: Although ketoconazole is approved for the treatment of disseminated candidiasis, it has been replaced by the newer agents listed in this table. Posaconazole has been approved for prophylaxis in neutropenic patients and for oropharyngeal candidiasis.
Abbreviations: FDA, Food and Drug Administration; IV, intravenous.

IV-200. The answer is B. *(Chap. 203)* The use of antifungal agents to prevent *Candida* infections remains controversial, but some general principles have emerged in recent years. Most centers start prophylactic fluconazole to allogeneic stem cell transplant recipients. Many centers also administer them to high-risk liver transplant recipients but not routine living related renal transplant recipients. This prophylaxis should be differentiated from the administration of empiric broad-spectrum antifungal therapy in a patient with prolonged febrile neutropenia. Voriconazole is an appropriate choice for empiric broad-spectrum therapy in an unstable patient with suspected candidemia, but it has not been shown to be superior to any other agent for prophylaxis against *Candida* in any population. Complicated postoperative surgical patients are at risk of *Candida* infection, and some centers administer prophylaxis to very high-risk patients. However, the widespread use of *Candida* prophylaxis in surgical patients is not recommended because the incidence of disseminated candidiasis is low, the cost-benefit ratio is suboptimal, and there is reasonable rationale to believe that this strategy could increase *Candida* resistance to current medications. *Candida* prophylaxis for HIV-infected patients is recommended to prevent frequent recurrent oropharyngeal or esophageal infection.

IV-201. The answer is C. *(Chap. 203)* Isolation of yeast from the bloodstream can virtually never be considered a contaminant. Presentation may be indolent with malaise only or fulminant with overwhelming sepsis in the neutropenic host. All indwelling catheters need to be removed to ensure clearance of infection, and evaluation for endocarditis and endophthalmitis should be strongly considered, particularly in patients with persistently positive cultures or fever. Both of these complications of fungemia often entail surgical intervention for cure. A positive yeast culture in the urine is often difficult to interpret, particularly in patients taking antibiotics and in the intensive care unit. Most frequently, a positive culture result for yeast represents contamination even if the urinalysis suggests bladder inflammation. An attractive option is to remove the Foley catheter and recheck a culture. Antifungals are indicated if the patient appears ill, in the context of renal transplant in which fungal balls can develop in the graft, and often in neutropenic patients. *Candida* pneumonia is uncommon even in immunocompromised patients. A positive yeast culture of the sputum is usually representative of commensal oral flora and should not be managed as an infection, particularly as in this patient in whom acute bacterial pneumonia is likely.

IV-202. The answer is C. *(Chap. 203)* Candidemia may lead to seeding of other organs. Among nonneutropenic patients, up to 10% develop retinal lesions; therefore, it is very important to perform thorough funduscopy. Focal seeding can occur within 2 weeks of the onset of candidemia and may occur even if the patient is afebrile or the infection clears. The lesions may be unilateral or bilateral and are typically small white retinal exudates. However, retinal infection may progress to retinal detachment, vitreous abscess, or extension into the anterior chamber of the eye. Patients may be asymptomatic initially but may also report blurring, ocular pain, or scotoma. Abdominal abscess are possible but usually occur in patients recovering from profound neutropenia. Fungal endocarditis is also possible but is more common in patients who use intravenous drugs and may have a murmur on cardiac examination. Fungal pneumonia and pulmonary abscesses are very rare and are not likely in this patient.

IV-203. The answer is A. *(Chap. 204)* Aspergillus has a worldwide distribution, typically growing in decomposing plant materials. Immunocompetent individuals generally do not develop disease without intense exposure such as during construction or handling of moldy hay, bark, or compost. Nosocomial outbreaks are usually directly related to contaminated air source in the hospital. HEPA filtration is effective in eliminating infection from operating rooms and units with high-risk patients. Contaminated water sources are the typical reservoir of nosocomial *Legionella* outbreaks. Patient-to-patient spread in waiting rooms has been described for cystic fibrosis patients transmitting *Burkholderia* infection. Provider-to-patient transmission of methicillin-resistant *Staphylococcus aureus* and most other bacteria is reduced with effective use of alcohol-based disinfectant; however, in the case of *Clostridium difficile*, alcohol will not eliminate spores, and effective handwashing with soap and water is necessary.

IV-204. The answer is B. *(Chap. 204)* Diagnosis of invasive *Aspergillus* infection is often difficult because early therapy is essential, and approximately 40% of cases are missed clinically and are diagnosed at autopsy. Sputum culture is positive in only 10% to 30% of patients; the yield is higher when fungal media rather than bacterial agar is used. Thus, specifically requesting fungal culture is necessary. The *Aspergillus* antigen assay relies on galactomannan release during fungal growth. Antigen testing results are positive days before clinical or radiologic abnormalities appear. The test may be falsely positive in patients receiving β-lactam/β-lactamase inhibitor antibiotics. The sensitivity in patients with prolonged neutropenia is likely about 80%. Prior therapeutic or empiric use of antifungal therapy lowers the sensitivity of the serum test. The test can be performed on bronchoalveolar lavage samples. The computed tomography findings in this case are also typical of the "halo sign" often seen in cases of invasive pulmonary aspergillosis. The halo of ground glass infiltrate surrounding an *Aspergillus* nodule represents hemorrhagic infarction. Other fungi may cause the halo sign, but *Aspergillus*, because of the tendency to be angioinvasive, is the most common. The other diagnoses in this case are much less likely given the clinical history and the radiologic signs.

IV-205. The answer is E. *(Chap. 204)* Intravenous voriconazole is currently the preferred therapy for invasive aspergillosis. Caspofungin, posaconazole, and lipid-based formulations of amphotericin are second-line agents. Amphotericin is not active against *Aspergillus terreus* or *Aspergillus nidulans*. Fluconazole is active against *Candida* spp. but not *Aspergillus* spp. Trimethoprim–sulfamethoxazole is used for therapy against *Pneumocystis jiroveci*.

IV-206. The answer is A. *(Chap. 204)* *Aspergillus* infection has many clinical manifestations. Invasive aspergillosis typically occurs in immunocompromised patients and presents as rapidly progressive pulmonary infiltrates. Infection progresses by direct extension across tissue planes. Cavitation may occur. Allergic bronchopulmonary aspergillosis (ABPA) is a different clinical entity. It often occurs in patients with preexisting asthma or cystic fibrosis. It is characterized by an allergic reaction to *Aspergillus* spp. Clinically, it is characterized by intermittent wheezing, bilateral pulmonary infiltrates, brownish sputum, and peripheral eosinophilia. Immunoglobulin E may be elevated, suggesting an allergic process, and a specific reaction to *Aspergillus* spp. that is manifested by serum antibodies or skin testing is common. Although central bronchiectasis and fleeting infiltrates caused by mucus plugging are common radiographic findings in ABPA, the presence of peripheral cavitary lung lesions is not a common feature.

IV-207. The answer is E. *(Chap. 204)* Allergic bronchopulmonary aspergillosis (ABPA) is not a true infection but rather a hypersensitivity immune response to colonizing *Aspergillus* spp. It occurs in about 1% of patients with asthma and in up to 15% of patients with cystic fibrosis. Patients typically have wheezing that is difficult to control with usual agents, infiltrates on chest radiographs caused by mucus plugging of airways, a productive cough often with mucus casts, and bronchiectasis. Eosinophilia is common if glucocorticoids have not been administered. The total immunoglobulin E (IgE) is of value if greater than 1000 IU/mL in that it represents a significant allergic response and is very suggestive of ABPA. In the proper clinical context, a positive skin test result for *Aspergillus* antigen or detection of serum *Aspergillus*-specific IgG or IgE precipitating antibodies are supportive of the diagnosis. Galactomannan enzyme immunoassay is useful for invasive aspergillosis but has not been validated for ABPA. There is no need to try to culture an organism via bronchoalveolar lavage to make the diagnosis of ABPA. Chest computed tomography, which may reveal bronchiectasis, or pulmonary function testing, which will reveal an obstructive defect, will not be diagnostic.

IV-208. The answer is B. *(Chap. 204)* The primary risk factor for developing invasive *Aspergillus* infection is neutropenia and glucocorticoid use (Figure IV-208). Risk is proportional to the degree and length of neutropenia and the dose of glucocorticoid. Stable HIV patients rarely develop invasive aspergillosis. Patients with AIDS are at some risk, typically in the context of prolonged neutropenia or advanced disease. Patients with graft-versus-host disease and uncontrolled leukemia are at particularly elevated risk. The infection is seen in solid organ transplant patients, particularly those requiring high cumulative doses of glucocorticoids for graft rejection. Recent reports describe an increasing incidence of invasive *Aspergillus* infection in medical intensive care units, particularly in patients with preexisiting lung disease such as pneumonia or chronic obstructive pulmonary disease. Glucocorticoid use does not appear to increase the risk of invasive sinus disease, only lung infection. Anti–tumor necrosis factor therapy also increases the risk of invasive *Aspergillus* infection.

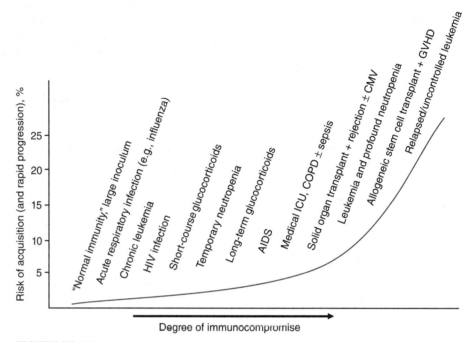

FIGURE IV-208

IV-209. The answer is B. *(Chap. 205)* Mucormycosis refers to life-threatening infection caused by the Mucorales (formerly known as Zygomycetes) family of fungi. The most common fungus accounting for these infections is *Rhizopus oryzae*. The mortality rate of these infections approaches 50%. The Mucorales are environmentally ubiquitous; infection requires a defect in the patient's ability to killing or phagocytic function. The most common predisposing factors are diabetes, glucocorticoid therapy, neutropenia, and iron overload. Free iron supports fungal growth in serum and tissues, enhancing survival and virulence. Deferoxamine therapy predisposes to fatal infection because the chelator acts as a siderophore, directly delivering iron to the fungi. Acidosis also causes dissociation of iron from serum proteins, promoting growth of Mucorales. Patients with diabetic ketoacidosis are at particularly high risk of developing rhinocerebral mucormycosis likely because of the combination of acidosis and phagocytic defects associated with hyperglycemia. Hypoglycemia is not an identified risk factor for mucormycosis.

IV-210. The answer is E. *(Chap. 205)* This patient has evidence of invasive rhinocerebral mucormycosis with risk factors including acute and chronic hyperglycemia and metabolic acidosis caused by chronic renal insufficiency. With a greater than 50% mortality rate, therapy of rhinocerebral mucormycosis requires early diagnosis, reversal of underlying predisposing conditions, surgical debridement, and immediate antifungal therapy. Insulin and hemodialysis should be initiated to correct hyperglycemia and metabolic acidosis. Amphotericin products remain the treatment of choice for mucormycosis. Liposomal amphotericin has improved central nervous system penetration compared with the lipid complex formations. Surgical debridement is also an important component of early therapy. If untreated, the infection quickly spreads from the ethmoid sinus to the orbit and into the cavernous sinus. Development of contralateral signs suggests cavernous sinus thrombosis and portends a very poor prognosis. Differentiation of mucormycosis from *Aspergillus* is important because they tend to infect similar hosts and are rapidly fatal. In contrast to mucormycosis species, the hyphae of *Aspergillus* spp. are septated, are thinner, and branch at acute angles. Voriconazole, the initial therapy for *Aspergillus* infection, is not indicated in mucormycosis and in fact has been shown to exacerbate mucormycosis in animal models. Echinocandin antifungal agents have activity against Mucorales, and animal data suggest that they may have a role in combination with lipid polyene agents.

IV-211. **The answer is E.** (*Chap. 205*) The sites of infection due to Mucorales fungal infection tend to affect patients with specific host defense defects. The most common clinical manifestation of mucormycosis is rhinocerebral. Most cases occur in patients with diabetes or hyperglycemia caused by glucocorticoid therapy (e.g., solid organ transplantation). The initial symptoms usually include facial or orbital pain or numbness, facial suffusion, and soft tissue swelling. The infection usually originates in the ethmoid sinus region and spreads rapidly to the orbit and central nervous system. Painful necrotic lesions may be seen in the mouth. Pulmonary mucormycosis is the second most common manifestation of Mucorales infection. Human stem cell transplantation is a common risk factor for pulmonary mucormycosis. The risk factors and presentation are similar to that of invasive pulmonary *Aspergillus* infection. Differentiation is important because antifungal therapy differs. The two diseases appear similar on chest computed tomography, although the presence of more than 10 nodules, pleural effusion, or concomitant sinusitis makes mucormycosis more likely. Other sites of involvement with mucormycosis are described but less common. Cutaneous disease may result from external implantation (soil-related trauma or plant penetration) or hematogenous dissemination. Implanted cutaneous disease is also highly invasive; the development of fasciitis has a greater than 70% mortality rate. Rapid surgical debridement is essential. Hematogenous dissemination has a very high mortality rate; involvement of the brain has a near 100% mortality rate. Gastrointestinal mucormycosis is most common in neonates with necrotizing enterocolitis.

IV-212. **The answer is E.** (*Chap. 206*) This patient has tinea capitis most likely caused by the dermatophytic mold, *Trichophyton* spp. The other dermatophytes that less frequently cause cutaneous infection include *Microsporum* and *Epidermophyton* spp. They are not part of the normal skin flora but can live in keratinized skin structures. Infections with these organisms are extremely common and are often called ringworm, although the causative organisms are fungi, not worms. They manifest as infection of the head (tinea capitis), feet (tinea pedis), crotch (tinea cruris), and nails (tinea unguium or onychomycosis). Tinea capitis is most common in children ages 3 to 7 years but also occurs in adults. Usually, the typical appearance, as in this case, is diagnostic. Scrapings may be taken from the edge of lesion and stained with KOH to reveal hyphae. Dermatophyte infections often respond to topical therapy. For troublesome infections, itraconazole or terbinafine for 1 to 2 weeks can hasten resolution. Terbinafine is often preferred because of fewer drug interactions.

IV-213. **The answer is D.** (*Chap. 206*) *Sporothrix schenckii* is a thermally dimorphic fungus found in soil, plants, and moss and occurs most commonly in gardeners, farmers, florists, and forestry workers. Sporotrichosis develops after inoculation of the organism into the skin with a contaminated puncture or scratch. The disease typically presents as a fixed cutaneous lesion or with lymphocutaneous spread. The initial lesion typically ulcerates and become verrucous in appearance. The draining lymphatic channels become affected in up to 80% of cases. This presents as painless nodules along the lymphatic channel, which ulcerate. A definitive diagnosis is made by culturing the organism. A biopsy of the lesion may show ovoid or cigar-shaped yeast forms. Treatment for sporotrichosis is systemic therapy. Options include oral itraconazole, saturated solution of potassium iodide, and terbinafine. However, terbinafine has not been approved for this indication in the United States. Topical antifungals are not effective. In cases of serious system disease such as pulmonary sporotrichosis, amphotericin B is the treatment of choice. Caspofungin is not effective against *S. schenckii*.

IV-214. **The answer is C.** (*Chap. 207*) Patients receiving biologic agents, including the tumor necrosis factor antagonists infliximab and etanercept, are at increased risk of multiple infections, including pneumocystis. Pneumocystis is thought to be a worldwide organism with most people exposed before 5 years of age. Airborne transmission has been demonstrated in animal studies, and epidemiologic studies suggest person-person transmission in nosocomial settings. Patients with defects in cell and humoral immunity are at risk for developing pneumonia. Most cases are in HIV-infected patients with CD4 counts less than 200/µL. Others at risk include patients receiving immunosuppressive agents (particularly glucocorticoids) for cancer or organ transplantation, children with immunodeficiency, premature malnourished infants, and patients receiving biologic immunomodulating agents. Pneumocystis pneumonia typically presents in non–HIV-infected patients with several days of dyspnea, fever, and nonproductive cough. Often symptoms develop during or soon after a glucocorticoid taper. Pneumocystis is associated with a reduced diffusing capacity on pulmonary function that typically causes mild hypoxemia and significant oxygen desaturation with exertion. Chest radiography often shows bilateral diffuse infiltrates without pleural effusion. Early in the disease, the radiograph may be unremarkable, but chest computed tomography (CT) will show diffuse ground glass infiltrates as in this case. Patients receiving biologic agents are at risk of pneumonia caused by tuberculosis (the patient was on prophylaxis in this case), *Aspergillus* spp., and *Nocardia* spp. *Aspergillus* spp., *Nocardia* spp., and septic emboli typically appears as nodules on chest CT. Rheumatoid nodules would be unlikely in the context of improving joint disease.

IV-215. **The answer is D.** *(Chap. 207)* Prophylaxis is effective in decreasing the risk of *Pneumocystis* pneumonia. It is clearly indicated in HIV-infected patients with oropharyngeal candidiasis or CD4 count below 200/µL and in HIV-infected or non–HIV-infected patients with a history of prior *Pneumocystis* pneumonia. Prophylaxis may be discontinued in HIV-infected patients who respond to therapy after the CD4 count has risen more than 200/µL for more than 3 months. Indications for primary prophylaxis for at-risk non-HIV infected patients without prior pneumocystis pneumonia (e.g., patients receiving induction chemotherapy or high-dose corticosteroids) are less clear. Trimethoprim–sulfamethoxazole remains the drug of choice for primary and secondary prophylaxis. It also provides protection from opportunistic toxoplasmosis and some bacterial infections.

IV-216. **The answer is E.** *(Chap. 207)* *Pneumocystis jiroveci* lung infection is known to worsen after initiation of treatment, likely caused by lysis of organisms and immune response to their intracellular contents. It is thought that adjunct administration of glucocorticoids may reduce inflammation and subsequent lung injury in patients with moderate to severe pneumonia caused by *P. jiroveci*. Adjunct administration of glucocorticoids in patients with moderate to severe disease as determined by a room air below 70 mmHg or an A –a gradient greater than 35 mmHg has been shown to decrease mortality. Glucocorticoids should be given for a total duration of 3 weeks. Patients often do not improve until many days into therapy and often initially worsen; steroids should be used early in the course of illness rather than waiting for lack of improvement. Pneumothoraces and adult respiratory distress syndrome (ARDS) are common feared complications of *Pneumocystis* infection. If patients present with ARDS caused by *Pneumocystis* pneumonia, they meet the criterion for adjunct glucocorticoids because of the severe nature of disease. The use of glucocorticoids as adjunctive therapy in HIV-infected patients with mild disease or in non–HIV-infected patients remains to be evaluated.

IV-217. **The answer is A.** *(Chap. 208)* Mefloquine remains the preferred drug for malaria prophylaxis in areas where chloroquine resistance is prevalent. High doses may be used for treatment. Drug resistance has been reported in parts of Africa and Southeast Asia. Mefloquine, similar to quinine and chloroquine, is only active against the asexual erythrocytic stages of malarial infection. Mefloquine is poorly water soluble and is not available parenterally. Oral absorption is enhanced when taken with or after food. Mefloquine is excreted mainly in bile and feces. Dosage adjustment is not necessary in patients with renal failure, and the drug is not removed with hemodialysis. Sleep abnormalities, psychosis, and seizures have been reported with mefloquine administration. Mefloquine should not be prescribed to patients with neuropsychiatric conditions, including depression, generalized anxiety disorder, psychosis, or seizure disorders. If acute anxiety, depression, restlessness, or confusion develops during prophylaxis, the drug should be discontinued. Quinine, quinidine, and beta-blockers may interact with mefloquine to cause significant electrocardiographic abnormalities or cardiac arrest. Halofantrine must not be administered with mefloquine within 3 weeks because of the potential for fatal QTc prolongation. Mefloquine may also alter ritonavir pharmacokinetics.

IV-218. The answer is E. *(Chap. 209) Entamoeba histolytica* is a common pathogen in areas of the world with poor sanitation and crowding. Transmission is oral–fecal, and the primary manifestation is colitis, often heme positive. Liver abscess is a common complication, occurring after the organism crosses the colonic border and travels through the portal circulation, subsequently lodging in the liver. At the time of presentation with liver abscess, the primary gastrointestinal infection has usually cleared, and organisms cannot be identified in the stool. Suggestive imaging with a positive serologic test result for *E. histolytica* is diagnostic. When a patient has a diagnostic imaging procedure, a positive amebic serology result is highly sensitive (>94%) and highly specific (>95%) for diagnosis of amebic liver abscess. Treatment for amebic liver abscess is generally with metronidazole. Luminal infection can be treated with paromomycin or iodoquinol. *Campylobacter* is a major cause of foodborne infectious diarrhea. Although usually self-limited, it may cause serious enteritis and inflammatory diarrhea but not liver abscess.

IV-219. The answer is B. *(Chap. 210)* The patient presents with signs of an acute infectious illness in an endemic area for malaria. A thick and thin preparation of her peripheral blood is indicated to evaluate for trophozoites, and indeed they are found in this case. Her neurologic findings suggest cerebral malaria, a defining feature of severe malaria. She is treated with intravenous quinidine. Hypoglycemia is a frequent finding in severe malaria; is associated with a poor prognosis; and may be worsened by quinidine or quinine therapy, which promotes pancreatic insulin secretion. Quinine causes fewer arrhythmias and hypotension with infusion than quinidine, but it is often not available in U.S. hospital pharmacies. Malaria itself causes hypoglycemia through failure of hepatic gluconeogenesis as well as increased glucose consumption by the host and parasite. Seizures may be caused by cerebral malaria but are not a complication of quinidine. Nightmares are frequently found with mefloquine, and retinopathy is a complication of prolonged chloroquine dosing.

IV-220. The answer is C. *(Chap. 210)* Severe malaria is a medical emergency. The patient has infection with *Plasmodium vivax,* which is less likely than *Plasmodium falciparum* to be associated with severe disease. Clinical manifestations of severe disease that cannot be managed as an outpatient include the presence of coma or cerebral malaria, two or more seizures over 24 hours, severe academia or anemia, renal failure, pulmonary edema or adult respiratory distress syndrome, hypoglycemia, hypotension or shock, evidence of disseminated intravascular coagulation, hemoglobinuria, extreme weakness, and jaundice with bilirubin above 3 mg/dL if combined with other organ dysfunction. Finally, if more than 5% of the erythrocytes are affected on the peripheral smear in a non-immune patient, severe malaria is present, and outpatient therapy is not advised.

IV-221. The answer is B. *(Chap. 210)* Artemisinin-containing regimens are now recommended by the World Health Organization as first-line agents for *Plasmodium falciparum* malaria. In severe *P. falciparum* malaria, intravenous (IV) artesunate reduced mortality by 35% compared with IV quinine. Artemether and artemotil are given intramuscularly and are not as effective as artesunate. Although safer and more effective than quinine, artesunate is not available in the United States. In the United States, quinidine or quinine is used as a necessary choice. Intravenous quinine is as effective as and safer than IV quinidine. Quinine causes fewer arrhythmias and hypotension with infusion than quinidine, but it is often not available in U.S. hospital pharmacies. Chloroquine is only effective for *Plasmodium vivax* and in *Plasmodium ovale* and *Plasmodium falciparum* infection in certain pockets of the Middle East and Caribbean where resistance has not yet developed. Mefloquine comes only as an oral formulation. It is most commonly used as a prophylactic agent but is also used for treatment of multidrug-resistant malaria.

IV-222. The answer is E. *(Chap. 210)* Thick and thin smears are a critical part of the evaluation of fever in a person with recent time spent in a *Plasmodium*-endemic region. Thick smears take a longer time to process but increase sensitivity in the setting of low parasitemia. Thin smears are more likely to allow for precise morphologic evaluation to differentiate among the four different types of *Plasmodium* infection and to allow for prognostic calculation of parasitemia. If clinical suspicion is high, repeat smears should be performed if the results are initially negative. If personnel are not available to rapidly interpret a smear, empirical therapy should be strongly considered to ward off the most severe manifestation of *Plasmodium falciparum* infection. Antibody-based diagnostic tests that are sensitive and specific for *P. falciparum* infection have been introduced. The results will remain positive for weeks after infection and do not allow quantification of parasitemia.

IV-223. The answer is C. *(Chap. 211)* The patient is seen in an endemic area for *Babesia microti*, which includes Nantucket, Martha's Vineyard, Block Island, Shelter Island, Long Island, southeastern coastal Massachusetts, Connecticut, and Rhode Island. Her flulike symptoms and tick bite make this disease very likely. Patients generally present with these symptoms or occasionally neck stiffness, sore, throat abdominal pain, and weight loss. Physical examination findings are typically normal with the exception of fever. The presence of erythema chronicum migrans suggests concurrent Lyme disease because a rash is not a feature of babesiosis. Although thick or thin preparation typically demonstrates the ring form of this protozoan, if these are negative, the 18S rRNA may be demonstrated by polymerase chain reaction. The ring forms are distinguished from *Plasmodium falciparum* by the absence of central brownish deposit seen in malarial disease. *Babesia duncani* is typically found on the West Coast of the United States, and *Babesia divergens* have been reported sporadically in Washington state, Missouri, and Kentucky. Therapy for severe *Babesia microti* disease in adults is clindamycin with additional quinine. Red blood cell exchange transfusion may be considered for *B. microti* but is not recommended as it is with *B. divergens*.

IV-224. The answer is C. *(Chap. 212)* Most cases of leishmaniasis occur on the Indian subcontinent and Sudan. The most commonly used technique for diagnosis of visceral leishmaniasis (kala azar) is a rapid immunochromatographic test for recombinant antigen rK39 from *Leishmania infantum*. This is widely available, rapid, and safe, requiring only a fingerprick of blood with results available in approximately 15 minutes. Although splenic aspiration with demonstration of amastigotes in tissue smear is the gold standard for the diagnosis of visceral leishmaniasis and culture may increase the sensitivity, the test is invasive and may be dangerous in inexperienced hands. Polymerase chain reaction for the leishmaniasis nucleic acid is only available at specialized laboratories and is not routinely used clinically. Leishmaniasis is not diagnosed via stool analysis.

IV-225. The answer is C. *(Chap. 213) Trypanosoma cruzi* is the causative agent of Chagas disease or American trypanosomiasis, which only occurs in the Americas. The protozoa is transmitted to mammalian hosts by the reduviid bugs, which become infected by sucking blood from animals or humans with circulating protozoa. The infective form of *T. cruzi* is excreted in the feces and infects humans through contact with breaks in the skin, mucous membranes, or conjunctiva. Infection has also been transmitted from blood transfusion, organ transplant, and ingestion of contaminated food or drink. Acute Chagas disease is typically a mild febrile illness followed by a chronic phase characterized by subpatent parasitemia, antibodies to *T. cruzi*, and no symptoms. About 10% to 30% of patients with chronic Chagas disease develop symptoms, usually related to cardiac or gastrointestinal lesions. Deer flies are the transmission vector of *Loa loa* (filariasis).

IV-226. The answer is D. *(Chap. 213)* This patient most likely has chronic Chagas disease with cardiac involvement and biventricular systolic dysfunction. Chagas disease is a health problem in rural Mexico, Central America, and South America. Most acute cases occur in children, but the epidemiology is uncertain because most cases go undiagnosed. The heart is the organ most often involved in chronic Chagas disease with biventricular systolic dysfunction and conduction abnormalities [right bundle branch block and left anterior hemiblock (LAH)]. Apical aneurysms and mural thrombi may occur. Chronic Chagas disease is diagnosed by demonstration of specific immunoglobulin G antibodies to *Trypanosoma cruzi* antigens. False-positive results may occur in patients with other parasitic infections or autoimmune disease. The World Health Organization recommends a positive test be confirmed with a separate assay. Polymerase chain reaction (PCR) to detect *T. cruzi* DNA in chronically infected patients has not been shown to be superior to serology, and no commercially available PCR tests are available. Given the patient's demographics, lack of coronary artery disease risk factors, and indolent symptoms, acute myocardial infarction, ischemic cardiomyopathy, and hypertensive cardiomyopathy are less likely diagnoses. Right heart catheterization with placement of a Swan-Ganz catheter could quantify left and right heart pressures and cardiac output. Constrictive pericarditis could also be evaluated, but this diagnosis is less likely with the presence of signs of left heart failure.

IV-227. The answer is A. *(Chap. 213)* Current consensus is that all *Trypanosoma cruzi*–infected patients up to 18 years old and all newly infected adults be treated for acute Chagas disease. Unfortunately, the only available drugs, benznidazole and nifurtimox, lack efficacy and have notable side effects. In acute Chagas disease, nifurtimox reduces the duration of symptoms and parasitemia and decreases the acute mortality Rate. However, only approximately 70% of acute infections are cured by a full course of treatment. Benznidazole is at least as effective as nifurtimox and is generally the treatment of choice in Latin America. The role of therapy in patient with indeterminate or chronic asymptomatic Chagas disease is controversial. Some experts recommend that therapy be offered. In contrast, randomized studies have shown benefit of treatment in children. The current antifungal azoles, including voriconazole, do not have adequate efficacy against *T. cruzi,* although newer agents in this class show promise in animal studies. Serologic confirmation with *T. cruzi* immunoglobulin G testing is used to diagnose chronic, not acute, Chagas disease. Malaria is endemic to Honduras below 1000 m elevation, and primaquine is effective therapy in those cases. Thin and thick smears evaluated by experts should not confuse *Plasmodium* spp. with *T. cruzi.*

IV-228. The answer is A. *(Chap. 213)* Human African trypanosomiasis (HAT) or sleeping sickness is caused by the protozoan *Trypanosoma brucei* complex. HAT remains a major public health problem in Africa despite its near-eradication in the 1960s. Although HAT only occurs in sub-Saharan Africa, it is important to distinguish between the West African (*T.b. gambiense*) and East African (*T.b. rhodesiense*) forms. Tsetse flies are the transmission vector for both forms. Humans are the major reservoir of West African trypanosomiasis, and it occurs in rural areas, rarely affecting tourists. Antelope and cattle are the reservoirs for *T.b. rhodesiense,* and infection has been reported in safari tourists. A primary lesion (trypanosomal chancre) typically appears 1 week after the bite of an infected tsetse fly. This is followed by a systemic illness with fever and lymphadenopathy (stage 1 disease). Myocarditis may occur, which can be fatal. Central nervous system (CNS) involvement follows (stage 2 disease) with cerebrospinal fluid (CSF) pleocytosis, elevated protein, and elevated pressure. During this stage, trypanosomes may be found in CSF. *T.b. rhodesiense* tends to be more aggressive with CNS disease developing earlier than *T.b. gambiense.* Symptoms during stage 2 disease include progressive somnolence and indifference sometimes alternating with insomnia and nighttime restlessness. If untreated, symptoms progress to coma and death. Diagnosis requires demonstration of the protozoa from blood, CSF, lymph node material, bone marrow, or chancre fluid. There are serologic tests for *T.b. gambiense,* but they lack the sensitivity or specificity for treatment decisions. There are not yet commercially available polymerase chain reaction tests. All patients with HAT should have a lumbar puncture to evaluate for CNS involvement, which will determine therapy. Suramin is effective for stage 1 East African HAT (*T.b. rhodesiense).* Pentamidine is first-line treatment for stage 1 West African HAT. When the CSF is involved, eflornithine is used for West African HAT and melarsoprol for East African HAT. Melarsoprol is an arsenical that is highly toxic, with a risk of encephalopathy.

IV-229. The answer is C. *(Chap. 214)* The magnetic resonance imaging (MRI) scan shows the classic lesions of encephalitis caused by *Toxoplasma gondii* in a patient with advanced immunosuppression caused by HIV infection. Cats are the definitive host for the sexual phase of *Toxoplasma*, and oocysts are shed in their feces. In the United States, up to 30% of 19-year-old young adults and up to 67% of adults older than 50 years of age have serologic evidence of *Toxoplasma* exposure. Patients with HIV infection are at risk of reactivation of latent toxoplasmosis with resultant encephalitis when the CD4 T-cell count falls below 100/ µL. Patients receiving immunosuppressive medication for lymphoproliferative disease or solid organ transplant are also at risk for reactivation of latent disease. Although the central nervous system (CNS) is the most common site of symptomatic reactivation disease, the lymph nodes, lung, heart, eyes, and gastrointestinal tract may be involved. *Toxoplasma* usually causes encephalitis, not meningitis; therefore, cerebrospinal fluid (CSF) findings may be unremarkable or have modest elevations of cell count and protein (with normal glucose). The treatment of choice for CNS toxoplasmosis is pyrimethamine plus sulfadiazine. Trimethoprim–sulfamethoxazole is an acceptable alternative. The differential diagnosis of encephalitis in patients with AIDS includes lymphoma, metastatic tumor, brain abscess, progressive multifocal leukoencephalopathy, fungal infection, and mycobacterial infection. In this case, given the classic MRI findings, toxoplasmosis is most likely.

IV-230. The answer is C. *(Chap. 215)* Of the listed protozoa, only *Giardia* infection can be diagnosed with stool ova and parasite examination. Stool antigen immunoassay can be used to diagnose *Giardia* and *Cryptosporidium* spp. Fecal acid-fast testing may be used to diagnose *Cryptosporidium*, *Isospora*, and *Cyclospora* spp. Microsporidia require special fecal stains or tissue biopsy for diagnosis.

IV-231. The answer is D. *(Chap. 215)* Trichomoniasis is transmitted via sexual contact with an infected partner. Many men are asymptomatic but may have symptoms of urethritis, epididymitis, or prostatitis. Most women have symptoms of infection that include vaginal itching, dyspareunia, and malodorous discharge. These symptoms do not distinguish *Trichomonas* infection from other forms of vaginitis, such as bacterial vaginosis. Trichomoniasis is not a self-limited infection and should be treated for symptomatic and public health reasons. Wet-mount examination for motile trichomonads has a sensitivity of 50% to 60% in routine examination. Direct immunofluorescent antibody staining of secretions is more sensitive and can also be performed immediately. Culture is not widely available and takes 3 to 7 days. Treatment should consist of metronidazole either as a single 2-g dose or 500-mg doses twice daily for 7 days; all sexual partners should be treated. Trichomoniasis resistant to metronidazole has been reported and is managed with increased doses of metronidazole or with tinidazole.

IV-232. The answer is E. *(Chap. 215)* Giardiasis is diagnosed by detection of parasite antigens in the feces or by visualizing cysts or trophozoites in feces or small intestine. There is no reliable serum test for this disease. Because a wide variety of pathogens are responsible for diarrheal illness, some degree of diagnostic testing beyond the history and physical examination is required for definitive diagnosis. Colonoscopy does not have a role in diagnosing *Giardia* infection. Giardiasis can persist in symptomatic patients and should be treated. Severe symptoms such as malabsorption, weight loss, growth retardation, and dehydration may occur in prolonged cases. Additionally, extraintestinal manifestations such as urticarial, anterior uveitis, and arthritis have been associated with potential giardiasis. A single oral 2-g dose of tinidazole is reportedly more effective than a 5-day course of metronidazole with cure rates above 90% for both. Paromomycin, an oral poorly absorbed aminoglycoside, can be used for symptomatic patients during pregnancy, but its efficacy for eradicating infection is not known. Clindamycin and albendazole do not have a role in treatment of giardiasis. Refractory disease with persistent infection can be treated with a longer duration of metronidazole.

IV-233. The answer is D. *(Chap. 215) Cryptosporidium* typically causes a self-limited diarrheal illness in immunocompetent patients but may cause severe debilitating disease in patients with severe immunodeficiency, such as advanced HIV infection. Outbreaks in immunocompetent hosts are caused by ingestion of oocysts. Infectious oocysts are excreted in human feces, causing human-to-human transmission. Waterborne transmission of oocysts accounts for disease in travelers and common-source outbreaks. Oocysts resist killing by routine chlorination of drinking and recreational water sources. Infection may be asymptomatic in immunocompetent and immunosuppressed hosts. Diarrhea is typically watery and nonbloody and may be associated with abdominal pain, nausea, fever, and anorexia. In immunocompetent hosts, symptoms usually subside in 1 to 2 weeks without therapy. In advanced AIDS with CD4 counts below $100/\mu L$, severe symptoms may develop, leading to significant electrolyte and volume loss. Nitazoxanide is approved for treatment of *Cryptosporidium* but to date has not been shown to be effective in HIV-infected patients. The best available therapy for these patients is antiretroviral therapy to reduce immune suppression. Tinidazole and metronidazole are used to treat giardiasis and trichomoniasis, not cryptosporidiosis.

IV-234. **The answer is D.** *(Chap. 216)* There are roughly 12 cases of trichinellosis reported each year in the United States. Because most infections are asymptomatic, this may be an underestimate. Recent outbreaks in North American have been related to ingestion of wild game, particularly bear. Heavy infections can cause enteritis; periorbital edema; myositis; and, infrequently, death. This infection, caused by ingesting *Trichinella* cysts, occurs when infected meat from pigs or other carnivorous animals is eaten. Laws that prevent feeding pigs uncooked garbage have been an important public health measure in reducing *Trichinella* infection in this country. Person-to-person spread has not been described. The majority of infections are mild and resolve spontaneously.

IV-235. **The answer is E.** *(Chap. 216)* Trichinellosis occurs when infected meat products are eaten, most frequently pork. The organism can also be transmitted through the ingestion of meat from dogs, horses, and bears. Recent outbreaks in the United States and Canada have been related to consumption of wild game, particularly bear meat. During the first week of infection, diarrhea, nausea, and vomiting are prominent features. As the parasites migrate from the gastrointestinal (GI) tract, fever and eosinophilia are often present. Larvae encyst after 2 to 3 weeks in muscle tissue, leading to myositis and weakness. Myocarditis and maculopapular rash are less common features of this illness. In pork, larvae are killed by cooking until the meat is no longer pink or by freezing at $-15°C$ for 3 weeks. However, arctic *Trichinella nativa* larvae in walrus or bear meat are resistant to freezing. *Giardia* and *Campylobacter* are organisms that are frequently acquired by drinking contaminated water; neither produces this pattern of disease. Although both cause GI symptoms (and *Campylobacter* causes fever), neither causes eosinophilia or myositis. *Taenia solium*, or pork tapeworm, shares a similar pathogenesis to *Trichinella* spp. but does not cause myositis. Cytomegalovirus has varied presentations but none that lead to this presentation.

IV-236 and IV-237. **The answers are D and B, respectively.** *(Chap. 216)* Visceral larva migrans, caused in this case by the canine roundworm *Toxocara canis*, most commonly affects young children who are exposed to canine stool. *Toxocara* eggs are ingested and begin their life cycle in the small intestine. They migrate to many tissues in the body. Particularly characteristic of this illness are hepatosplenomegaly and profound eosinophilia, at times close to 90% of the total white blood cell count. Staphylococci will not typically cause eosinophilia. Trichinellosis, caused by ingesting meat from carnivorous animals that has been infected with *Trichinella* cysts, does not cause hepatosplenomegaly and is uncommon without eating a suspicious meal. Giardiasis is characterized by profuse diarrhea and abdominal pain without systemic features or eosinophilia. Cysticercosis typically causes myalgias and can spread to the brain, where it is often asymptomatic but can lead to seizures. The vast majority of *Toxocara* infections are self-limited and resolve without therapy. Rarely, severe symptoms may develop with deaths caused by central nervous system, myocardial, or respiratory disease. Severe myocardial involvement manifests as acute myocarditis. In these patients, glucocorticoids are administered to reduce the inflammatory complications. Antihelminthic drugs such as albendazole, mebendazole, or praziquantel have not been shown conclusively to alter the course of visceral larval migrans. Metronidazole is used for infections caused by *Trichomonas*, not tissue nematodes.

IV-238. The answer is A. (*Chap. 216*) *Angiostrongylus cantonensis*, the rat lungworm, is the most common cause of human eosinophilic meningitis. The infection principally occurs in Southeast Asia and the Pacific Basin, although cases have also been described in Cuba, Australia, Japan, and China. Infective larvae are excreted in rat feces and ingested by land snails and slugs. Humans acquire infection by ingesting the mollusks, vegetables contaminated by mollusk slime, or seafood (crabs, freshwater shrimp) that consumed the mollusks. The larvae migrate to the brain, where they initiate a marked eosinophilic inflammatory response with hemorrhage. Clinical symptoms develop 2 to 35 days after ingestion of larvae, and the initial presentation typically includes headache (indolent or acute), fever, nausea, vomiting, and meningismus. The cerebrospinal fluid (CSF) findings are as in this case with an eosinophil percentage greater than 20%. *A. cantonensis* larvae are only rarely demonstrated in the CSF. The diagnosis usually relies on the presence of eosinophilic meningitis and compatible epidemiology. There is no specific chemotherapy for *A. cantonensis* meningitis. Supportive care includes repeat removal of CSF to control intracranial pressure. Glucocorticoids may reduce inflammation. In most cases, cerebral angiostrongyliasis has a self-limited course with complete recovery. *Gnathostoma spinigerum* is a less common cause of eosinophilic meningoencephalitis. It also causes migratory cutaneous swellings or eye infections. It is also endemic in Southeast Asia and China and is usually transmitted by eating undercooked fish or poultry (som fak in Thailand and sashimi in Japan). *Trichinella murrelli* and *Trichinella nativa* cause trichinosis in North America and the Arctic, respectively. *Trichinella cara* is the cause of larval migrans.

IV-239. The answer is B. (*Chap. 217*) Strongyloides is the only helminth that can replicate in the human host, allowing autoinfection. Humans acquire *Strongyloides* when larvae in fecally contaminated soil penetrate the skin or mucous membranes. The larvae migrate to the lungs via the bloodstream; break through the alveolar spaces; ascend the respiratory airways; and are swallowed to reach the small intestine, where they mature into adult worms. Adult worms may penetrate the mucosa of the small intestine. Strongyloides is endemic in Southeast Asia, sub-Saharan Africa, Brazil, and the Southern United States. Many patients with *Strongyloides* are asymptomatic or have mild gastrointestinal symptoms or the characteristic cutaneous eruption, larval currens, as described in this case. Small bowel obstruction may occur with early heavy infection. Eosinophilia is common with all clinical manifestations. In patients with impaired immunity, particularly glucocorticoid therapy, hyperinfection or dissemination may occur. This may lead to colitis, enteritis, meningitis, peritonitis, and acute renal failure. Bacteremia or gram-negative sepsis may develop because of bacterial translocation through disrupted enteric mucosa. Because of the risk of hyperinfection, all patients with *Strongyloides* infection, even asymptomatic carriers, should be treated with ivermectin, which is more effective than albendazole. Fluconazole is used to treat candidal infections. Mebendazole is used to treat trichuriasis, enterobiasis (pinworm), ascariasis, and hookworm. Mefloquine is used for malaria prophylaxis.

IV-240. The answer is B. (*Chap. 217*) *Ascaris lumbricoides* is the longest nematode (15–40 cm) parasite of humans. It resides in tropical and subtropical regions. In the United States, it is found mostly in the rural Southeast. Transmission is through fecally contaminated soil. Most commonly, the worm burden is low, and it causes no symptoms. Clinical disease is related to larval migration to the lungs or to adult worms in the gastrointestinal tract. The most common complications occur because of a high gastrointestinal adult worm burden, leading to small bowel obstruction (most often in children with a narrow-caliber small bowel lumen) or migration leading to obstructive complications such as cholangitis, pancreatitis, or appendicitis. Rarely, adult worms can migrate to the esophagus and be orally expelled. During the lung phase of larval migration (9–12 days after egg ingestion), patients may develop a nonproductive cough, fever, eosinophilia, and pleuritic chest pain. Eosinophilic pneumonia syndrome (Löffler's syndrome) is characterized by symptoms and lung infiltrates. Meningitis is not a known complication of ascariasis but can occur with disseminated strongyloidiasis in an immunocompromised host.

IV-241. The answer is A. (*Chap. 217*) Ascariasis should always be treated, even in asymptomatic cases, to prevent serious intestinal complications. Albendazole, mebendazole, and ivermectin are effective. These agents should not be administered to pregnant women. Pyrantel is safe in pregnancy. Metronidazole is used for anaerobic bacterial and *Trichomonas* infections. Fluconazole is mostly used to treat *Candida* infections. Diethyl-carbamazine (DEC) is first-line therapy for active lymphatic filariasis. Vancomycin has no effect on nematodes.

IV-242. **The answer is E.** *(Chap. 217)* This patient's most likely diagnosis is anisakiasis. This is a nematode infection in which humans are an accidental host. It occurs hours to days after ingesting eggs that previously settled into the muscles of fish. The main risk factor for infection is eating raw fish. Presentation mimics an acute abdomen. History is critical because upper endoscopy is both diagnostic and curative. The implicated nematodes burrow into the mucosa of·the stomach, causing intense pain, and must be manually removed by endoscope or, on rare occasion, surgery. There is no medical agent known to cure anisakiasis.

IV-243. **The answer is E.** *(Chap. 218)* This patient likely has filariasis with acute lymphadenitis caused by *Wuchereria bancrofti*. It is endemic throughout the tropics and subtropics, including Asia, the Pacific Islands, Africa, parts of South America, and the Caribbean. *W. bancrofti* is the most widely distributed human filarial parasite and is transmitted by infected mosquitoes. Lymphatic infection is common and may be acute or chronic. Chronic lower extremity lymphatic infection causes elephantiasis. Definitive diagnosis requires demonstration of the parasite. Microfilariae may be found in blood, hydrocele, or other body fluid collections by direct microscopic examination. Enzyme-linked immunosorbent assays for circulating antigens are available commercially and have sensitivity of greater than 93% with excellent specificity. Polymerase chain reaction–based assays have been developed that may be as effective. In cases of acute lymphadenitis, ultrasound examination with Doppler may actually reveal motile worms in dilated lymphatics. Live worms have a distinctive movement pattern (filarial dance sign). Worms may be visualized in the spermatic cords of up to 80% of men infected with *W. bancrofti*. Stool ova and parasite examination is not useful for demonstration of *W. bancrofti*.

IV-244. **The answer is B.** *(Chap. 218)* Diethylcarbamazine (DEC), which has macro- and microfilaricidal properties, is the first-line treatment for acute filarial lymphadenitis. Albendazole, doxycycline, and ivermectin are also used to treat microfilarial infections (not macrofilarial). There is growing consensus that virtually all patients with *Wuchereria bancrofti* infection should be treated, even if asymptomatic, to prevent lymphatic damage. Many of these patients have microfilarial infection with subclinical hematuria, proteinuria, and so on. Albendazole and doxycycline have demonstrated macrofilaricidal efficacy. Combinations of DEC with albendazole, ivermectin, and doxycycline have efficacy in eradication programs. The World Health Organization established a global program to eliminate lymphatic filariasis in 1997 using a single annual dose of DEC plus either albendazole (non-African regions) or ivermectin (Africa). Praziquantel is used for treatment of schistosomiasis.

IV-245. **The answer is B.** *(Chap. 218)* This patient has loiasis caused by the African eye worm *Loa loa*. It is endemic to the rain forests of Central and West Africa. Microfilaria circulate periodically in blood with macrofilaria living in subcutaneous tissues including the subconjunctiva. Loiasis is often asymptomatic in indigenous regions with recognition, as in this case, only with visualized macrofilarial migration. Angioedema and swelling may occur in affected areas. Diethylcarbamazine (DEC) is effective treatment for the macrofilarial and microfilarial stages of disease. Multiple courses may be necessary. Albendazole and ivermectin are effective in reducing microfilarial loads but are not approved by the U.S. Food and Drug Administration. There are reports of deaths in patients with heavy loads of microfilaria receiving ivermectin. Terbinafine is the treatment for ringworm. Voriconazole is an antifungal with no activity against worms.

IV-246. **The answer is A.** *(Chap. 219)* Human schistosomiasis is caused by five species of parasitic trematodes. Whereas *Schistosoma mansoni, Schistosoma japonicum, Schistosoma mekongi,* and *Schistosoma intercalatum* are intestinal species, *Schistosoma haematobium* is a urinary species. There are reportedly up to 300 million individuals infected with *Schistosoma*. Figure IV-246 shows the global distribution. *S. haematobium* is not seen in South America. All forms of schistosomiasis are initiated by penetration of infective cercariae released from infected snails into fresh water. After entering the skin, the schistosome migrates via venous or lymphatic vessels to either the intestinal or urinary venous system, depending on the species. Acute skin infection causes dermatitis (swimmer's itch) within 2 to 3 days. Katayama fever, acute schistosomal serum sickness–related to migration, may develop in 4 to 8 weeks. Eosinophilia is common in acute infection. This has become a more common global health problem because travelers are exposed while swimming or boating in infected fresh water bodies. Chronic schistosomiasis depends on the species and the location of infection. The intestinal species are responsible for portal hypertension. *S. haematobium* causes urinary symptoms and a higher risk of urinary tract carcinoma. Immunologic tests are available to diagnose schistosomiasis, and in some cases, stool or urine examination results may be positive.

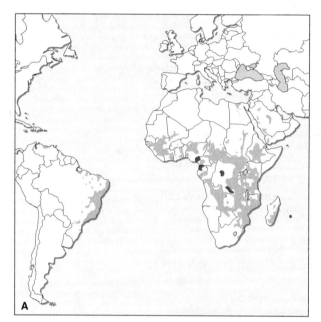 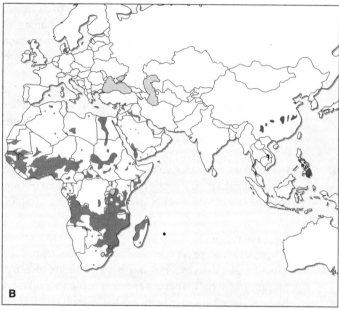

FIGURE IV-246   Global distribution of schistosomiasis. *A. S. mansoni* infection (lightest shade) is endemic in Africa, the Middle East, South America, and a few Caribbean countries. *S. intercalatum* infection (darkest shade) is endemic in sporadic foci in West and Central Africa. *B. S. haematobium* infection (medium shade) is endemic in Africa and the Middle East. The major endemic countries for *S. japonicum* infection (darkest shade) are China, the Philippines, and Indonesia. *S. mekongi* infection (black) is endemic in sporadic foci in Southeast Asia.

IV-247. **The answer is D.** *(Chap. 219)* This patient has Katayama fever caused by infection with *Schistosoma mansoni*. Approximately 4 to 8 weeks after exposure, the parasite migrates through the portal and pulmonary circulations. This phase of the illness may be asymptomatic but in some cases evokes a hypersensitivity response and a serum sickness–type illness. Eosinophilia is usual. Because there is not a large enteric burden of parasites during this phase of the illness, stool study results may not be positive, and serology may be helpful, particularly in patients from nonendemic areas. Praziquantel is the treatment of choice because Katayama fever may progress to include neurologic complications. Praziquantel remains the treatment for most helminthic infections, including schistosomiasis. Chloroquine is used for treatment of malaria; mebendazole for ascariasis, hookworm, trichinosis, and visceral larval migrans; metronidazole for amebiasis, giardiasis, and trichomoniasis; and thiabendazole for *Strongyloides* spp.

IV-248. **The answer is B.** *(Chap. 219)* *Schistosoma mansoni* infection of the liver causes cirrhosis from vascular obstruction resulting from periportal fibrosis but relatively little hepatocellular injury. Hepatosplenomegaly, hypersplenism, and esophageal varices develop quite commonly, and schistosomiasis is usually associated with eosinophilia.

Spider nevi, gynecomastia, jaundice, and ascites are observed less commonly than they are in alcoholic and postnecrotic fibrosis.

IV-249. The answer is B. *(Chap. 220)* This patient has a new onset of seizures caused by neurocysticercosis from infection with *Taenia solium* (pork tapeworm). The computed tomography (CT) scan shows a parenchymal cysticercus with enhancement of the cyst and an internal scolex *(arrow)*. The cyst represents larval oncospheres that have migrated to the central nervous system (CNS). Infections that cause human cystercicosis result from ingestion of *T. solium* eggs, usually from close contact with a tapeworm carrier who developed intestinal infection for ingestion of undercooked pork. Autoinfection may occur if an individual ingests tapeworm eggs excreted in their own feces. Cysticerci may be found anywhere in the body, but clinical manifestations usually arise from lesions in the CNS, cerebrospinal fluid (CSF), skeletal muscle, subcutaneous tissue, or eye. Neurologic manifestations are most common, including generalized or focal seizures from surrounding inflammation, hydrocephalus from CSF outflow occlusion, or arachnoiditis. As shown in Table IV-249, neuroradiologic demonstration of a cystic lesion containing a characteristic scolex is absolute criteria for diagnosis of cysticercosis. Intestinal infection may be detected by fecal examination for eggs. More sensitive enzyme-linked immunosorbent assay, polymerase chain reaction, and serologic testing is not currently commercially available. Treatment of neurocysticercosis after neurologic stabilization is with albendazole or praziquantel. Studies have shown faster resolution of clinical and radiologic findings compared with placebo. Initiation of therapy may be associated with worsening symptoms caused by inflammation that is treated with glucocorticoids. Intestinal *T. solium* infection is treated with a single dose of praziquantel. CNS cystic lesions (but without the visualized scolex) are typical of toxoplasmosis in patients with advanced HIV infection and are treated with pyrimethamine and sulfadiazine. However, in this case, the patient was documented HIV antibody negative, and the CT lesion was typical for cysticercosis. Viral testing for HIV would not be helpful because toxoplasmosis is seen in advanced cases, not acute infection. Echocardiography would be indicated for suspected staphylococcal (or other bacterial) endocarditis with systemic embolization.

TABLE IV-249   **Diagnostic Criteria for Human Cysticercosis**[a]

1. Absolute criteria
   a. Demonstration of cysticerci by histologic or microscopic examination of biopsy material
   b. Visualization of the parasite in the eye by funduscopy
   c. Neuroradiologic demonstration of cystic lesions containing a characteristic scolex
2. Major criteria
   a. Neuroradiologic lesions suggestive of neurocysticercosis
   b. Demonstration of antibodies to cysticerci in serum by enzyme-linked immunoelectrotransfer blot
   c. Resolution of intracranial cystic lesions spontaneously or after therapy with albendazole or praziquantel alone
3. Minor criteria
   a. Lesions compatible with neurocysticercosis detected by neuroimaging studies
   b. Clinical manifestations suggestive of neurocysticercosis
   c. Demonstration of antibodies to cysticerci or cysticercal antigen in cerebrospinal fluid by ELISA
   d. Evidence of cysticercosis outside the central nervous system (e.g., cigar-shaped soft tissue calcifications)
4. Epidemiologic criteria
   a. Residence in a cysticercosis-endemic area
   b. Frequent travel to a cysticercosis-endemic area
   c. Household contact with an individual infected with *Taenia solium*

[a]Diagnosis is confirmed by either one absolute criterion or a combination of two major criteria, one minor criterion, and one epidemiologic criterion. A probable diagnosis is supported by the fulfillment of (1) one major criterion plus two minor criteria, (2) one major criterion plus one minor criterion and one epidemiologic criterion, or (3) three minor criteria plus one epidemiologic criterion.
Abbreviation: ELISA, enzyme-linked immunosorbent assay.
Source: Modified from Del Brutto OH et al: Proposed diagnostic criteria for neurocysticercosis. *Neurology* 57:177, 2001.

IV-250. The answer is B. *(Chap. 220)* Echinococcosis is usually caused by infection of *Echinococcus granulosus* complex or *Echinococcus multilocularis* transmitted to humans via dog feces. *E. granulosus* is found on all continents with high prevalence in China, central Asia, Middle East, Mediterranean region, Eastern Africa, and parts of South America. *E. multilocularis*, which causes multiloculated invasive lung lesions, is found in alpine, sub-Arctic, or Arctic regions, including Canada, the United States, China, Europe, and central Asia. Echinococcal cysts, most commonly in the liver followed by the lung, are typically slowly enlarging and cause symptoms because of space-occupying effects. Cysts are often incidentally discovered on radiologic studies. Compression or leakage into the biliary system may cause symptoms typical for cholelithiasis or cholecystitis. Echinococcal cysts may be characterized by ultrasonography. Demonstration of daughter cysts within a larger cyst is pathognomonic. Serodiagnosis may be helpful in questionable cases for diagnosis of *E. granulosus*. Patients with liver cysts typically have positive serology in more than 90% (but not 100%) of cases. Up to 50% of patients with lung cysts may be seronegative. Biopsy is generally not recommended for cysts close to the liver edge because of the risk of leakage. Small cysts may respond to medical therapy with albendazole or praziquantel. Percutaneous aspiration-injection-resaspiration (PAIR) therapy is recommended for most noncomplex nonsuperficial cysts. Surgical resection is recommended for complex cysts, superficial cysts with risk of leakage, and cysts involving the biliary system. Albendazole therapy is generally administered before and after PAIR or surgical therapy.

SECTION V

Disorders of the Cardiovascular System

DIRECTIONS: Choose the **one best** response to each question.

V-1. A 35-year-old woman is seen in clinic for evaluation of dyspnea. Which of the following physical findings would fit the diagnosis of idiopathic pulmonary arterial hypertension?

A. Elevated neck veins, normal S_1 and S_2, II/VI diastolic blowing murmur heard at the right upper sternal border

B. Elevated neck veins; singular, loud S_2; II/VI systolic murmur left lower sternal border

C. Elevated neck veins; loud, fixed, split S_2; III/VI systolic murmur left lower sternal border

D. Elevated neck veins, expiratory splitting of S_2, II/VI harsh systolic murmur left upper sternal border

E. Elevated neck veins, barrel chest, prolonged expiratory phase

V-2. A 75-year-old woman with widely metastatic non–small cell lung cancer is admitted to the intensive care unit with a systolic blood pressure of 73/25 mmHg. She presented complaining of fatigue and worsening dyspnea over the last 3–5 days. Her physical examination shows elevated neck veins. Chest radiograph shows a massive, water bottle–shaped heart shadow and no new pulmonary infiltrates. Which of the following additional findings is most likely present on physical examination?

A. Fall in systolic blood pressure greater than 10 mmHg with inspiration

B. Lack of fall of the jugular venous pressure with inspiration

C. Late diastolic murmur with opening snap

D. Pulsus parvus et tardus

E. Slow y-descent of jugular venous pressure tracing

V-3. A 78-year-old man is admitted to the intensive care unit with decompensated heart failure. He has long-standing ischemic cardiomyopathy. Electrocardiogram (ECG) shows atrial fibrillation and left bundle branch block. Chest radiograph shows cardiomegaly and bilateral alveolar infiltrates with Kerley's B-lines. Which of the following is least likely to be present on physical examination?

A. Fourth heart sound

B. Irregular heart rate

C. Pulsus alternans

D. Reversed splitting of the second heart sound

E. Third heart sound

V-4. A 45-year-old man is admitted to the intensive care unit with symptoms of congestive heart failure. He is addicted to heroin and cocaine and uses both drugs daily via injection. His blood cultures have yielded methicillin-sensitive *Staphylococcus aureus* in four of four bottles within 12 hours. His vital signs show a blood pressure of 110/40 mmHg and a heart rate of 132 beats/min. There is a IV/VI diastolic murmur heard along the left sternal border. A schematic representation of the carotid pulsation is shown in Figure V-4A. What is the most likely cause of the patient's murmur?

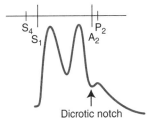

FIGURE V-4A

A. Aortic regurgitation

B. Aortic stenosis

C. Mitral stenosis

D. Mitral regurgitation

E. Tricuspid regurgitation

V-5. A 72-year-old man seeks evaluation for leg pain with ambulation. He describes the pain as an aching to crampy pain in the muscles of his thighs. The pain subsides within minutes of resting. On rare occasions, he has noted numbness of his right foot at rest, and pain in his right leg has woken him at night. He has a history of hypertension and cerebrovascular disease. Four years previously had a transient ischemic attack and underwent right carotid endarterectomy. He currently takes aspirin, irbesartan, hydrochlorothiazide, and atenolol on a daily basis. On examination, he is noted to have diminished dorsalis pedis and posterior tibial pulses bilaterally. The right dorsal pedis pulse is faint. There is loss of hair in the distal extremities. Capillary refill is approximately 5 seconds in the right foot and 3 seconds in the left foot. Which of the following findings would be suggestive of critical ischemia of the right foot?

A. Ankle-brachial index less than 0.3
B. Ankle-brachial index less than 0.9
C. Ankle-brachial index greater than 1.2
D. Lack of palpable dorsalis pedis pulse
E. Presence of pitting edema of the extremities

V-6. A 24-year-old man is referred to cardiology after an episode of syncope while playing basketball. He has no recollection of the event, but he was told that he collapsed while running. He awakened lying on the ground and suffered multiple contusions as a result of the fall. He has always been an active individual but recently has developed some chest pain with exertion that has caused him to restrict his activity. His father died at age 44 while rock climbing. He believes his father's cause of death was sudden cardiac death and recalls being told his father had an enlarged heart. On examination, the patient has a III/VI midsystolic crescendo-decrescendo murmur. His electrocardiogram shows evidence of left ventricular hypertrophy. You suspect hypertrophic cardiomyopathy as the cause of the patient's heart disease. Which of the following maneuvers would be expected to cause an increase in the loudness of the murmur?

A. Handgrip exercise
B. Squatting
C. Standing
D. Valsalva maneuver
E. A and B
F. C and D

V-7. Left bundle branch block is indicative of which of the following sets of conditions?

A. Atrial septal defect, coronary heart disease, aortic valve disease
B. Coronary heart disease, aortic valve disease, hypertensive heart disease
C. Coronary heart disease, aortic valve disease, pulmonary hypertension
D. Pulmonary embolism, cardiomyopathy, hypertensive heart disease
E. Pulmonary hypertension, pulmonary embolism, mitral stenosis

V-8. A 57-year-old man with long-standing ischemic cardiomyopathy is seen in the clinic for a routine visit. He reports good compliance with his diuretic regimen, but has seen his weight fall about 2 kg since his last visit. Routine chemistries are drawn and show a potassium value of 2.0 meq/L. The patient is referred to the emergency department for repletion of potassium. Which of the following is likely to be found on ECG before administration of potassium?

A. Diminution of P wave amplitude
B. Osborne waves
C. Prolongation of QT interval
D. Prominent U waves
E. Scooped ST segments

V-9. A 55-year-old woman from El Salvador is seen in the emergency department because of gradual onset of dyspnea on exertion. She denies chest pain, cough, wheezing, sputum, or fever. Her chest radiograph is notable for large pulmonary arteries and left atrial enlargement, but no parenchymal infiltrate. ECG shows a tall R in lead V_1 and right axis deviation. Which of the following is most likely to be found on her echocardiography?

A. Aortic regurgitation
B. Aortic stenosis
C. Low left ventricular ejection fraction
D. Mitral stenosis
E. Tricuspid stenosis

V-10. A 29-year-old woman is in the intensive care unit with rhabdomyolysis due to compartment syndrome of the lower extremities after a car accident. Her clinical course has been complicated by acute renal failure and severe pain. She has undergone fasciotomies and is admitted to the intensive care unit. An ECG is obtained (shown in Figure V-10). What is the most appropriate course of action at this point?

A. 18-lead ECG
B. Coronary catheterization
C. Hemodialysis
D. Intravenous fluids and a loop diuretic
E. Ventilation/perfusion imaging

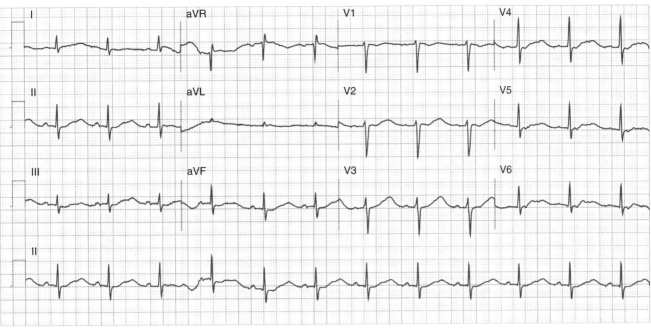

FIGURE V-10

V-11. Acute hyperkalemia is associated with which of the following electrocardiographic changes?

A. Decrease in the PR interval
B. Prolongation of the ST segment
C. Prominent U waves
D. QRS widening
E. T-wave flattening

V-12. The ECG shown below (Figure V-12) was most likely obtained from which of the following patients?

A. A 33-year-old female with acute-onset severe headache, disorientation, and intraventricular blood on head CT scan
B. A 42-year-old male with sudden-onset chest pain while playing tennis
C. A 54-year-old female with a long history of smoking and 2 days of increasing shortness of breath and wheezing
D. A 64-year-old female with end-stage renal insufficiency who missed dialysis for the last 4 days
E. A 78-year-old male with syncope, delayed carotid upstrokes, and a harsh systolic murmur in the right second intercostal space

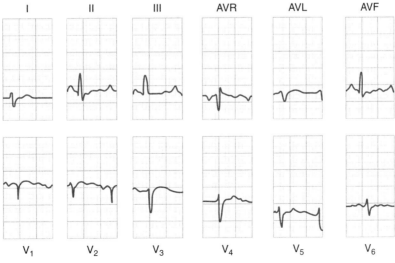

FIGURE V-12

V-13. You are evaluating a new patient in your clinic who has brought in the ECG shown below (Figure V-13) to the visit. The ECG was performed on the patient 2 weeks ago. What complaint do you expect to elicit from the patient?

A. Angina
B. Hemoptysis
C. Paroxysmal nocturnal dyspnea
D. Pleuritic chest pain
E. Tachypalpitations

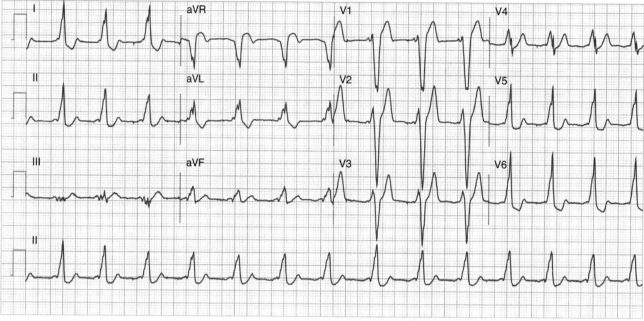

FIGURE V-13

V-14. All the following ECG findings are suggestive of left ventricular hypertrophy EXCEPT:

A. (S in V_1 + R in V_5 or V_6) greater than 35 mm
B. R in aVL greater than 11 mm
C. R in aVF greater than 20 mm
D. (R in I + S in III) greater than 25 mm
E. R in aVR greater than 8 mm

V-15. Based on the electrocardiogram below (Figure V-15), treating which condition might specifically improve this patient's tachycardia?

A. Anemia
B. Chronic obstructive pulmonary disease (COPD)
C. Myocardial ischemia
D. Pain

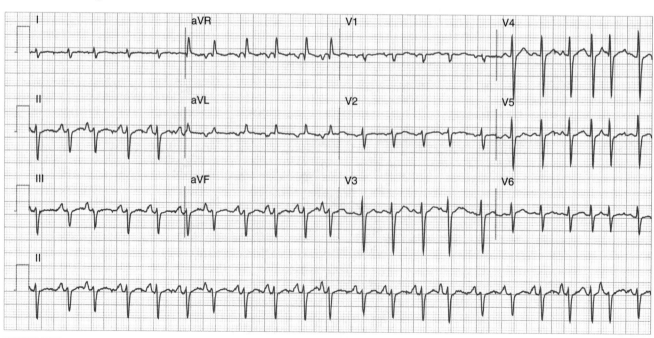

FIGURE V-15

V-16. Doppler echocardiography is most useful for diagnosis of which of the following cardiac lesions?

A. Determination of cardiac mass in a patient with an audible "plop" on examination
B. Determination of left ventricular ejection fraction in a patient with a history of myocardial infarction
C. Diagnosis of myocardial ischemia in a patient with atypical chest pain
D. Diagnosis of pericardial effusion
E. Diastolic filling assessment in a patient with suspected heart failure with preserved ejection fraction

V-17. A 75-year-old man is undergoing routine cardiac catheterization for evaluation of stable angina that has not responded to medical therapy. He is inquiring about the risks associated with the procedure. Which of the following is the most common complication of cardiac catheterization and coronary angiography?

A. Acute renal failure
B. Bradyarrhythmias
C. Myocardial infarction
D. Tachyarrhythmias
E. Vascular access site bleeding

V-18. Which of the following patients is an appropriate candidate for right heart catheterization?

A. A 54-year-old woman with dyspnea of unclear etiology; a loud, fixed split second heart sound; normal chest radiograph; and evidence of bidirectional shunt across her interatrial septum
B. A 54-year-old man with an episode of sustained monomorphic ventricular tachycardia while at the casino terminated with bystander defibrillation. After arrival in the emergency department, the patient is hemodynamically stable.
C. A 63-year-old woman with a history of tobacco abuse, hypercholesterolemia, and Type 2 diabetes mellitus with chest pain at rest, a normal ECG, and mild elevation in serum troponin value
D. A 66-year-old man with a history of diabetes and hypercholesterolemia brought to the emergency department with 1 hour of substernal chest pain and shortness of breath. His blood pressure is 95/60 mmHg with a heart rate of 115 beats/min. An ECG shows a new left bundle branch block since his prior ECG 1 month ago.
E. A 79-year-old man seen in the cardiology clinic for evaluation of severe aortic stenosis found on echocardiography performed for evaluation of dyspnea

V-19. A 55-year-old woman is undergoing evaluation of dyspnea on exertion. She has a history of hypertension since age 32 and is also obese with a body mass index (BMI) of 44 kg/m². Her pulmonary function tests show mild restrictive lung disease. An echocardiogram shows a thickened left-ventricular wall, left-ventricular ejection fraction of 70%, and findings suggestive of pulmonary hypertension with an estimated right-ventricular systolic pressure of

55 mmHg, but the echocardiogram is technically difficult and of poor quality. She undergoes a right heart catheterization that shows the following results:

Mean arterial pressure	110 mmHg
Left-ventricular end-diastolic pressure	25 mmHg
Pulmonary artery (PA) systolic pressure	48 mmHg
PA diastolic pressure	20 mmHg
PA mean pressure	34 mmHg
Cardiac output	5.9 L/min

What is the most likely cause of the patient's dyspnea?

A. Chronic thromboembolic disease
B. Diastolic heart failure
C. Obstructive sleep apnea
D. Pulmonary arterial hypertension
E. Systolic heart failure

V-20. Which of the following is a risk factor for the development of thromboembolism in patients with the tachycardia-bradycardia variant of sick sinus syndrome?

A. Age greater than 50 years
B. Atrial enlargement
C. Diabetes mellitus
D. Prothrombin 20210 mutation
E. None of the above; there is no increased risk of thromboembolism with the tachycardia-bradycardia variant of sick sinus syndrome.

V-21. A 38-year-old man is evaluated for the recent onset of feeling fatigued. He is a busy executive and active triathlete. He competed a challenging course 1 week earlier without difficulty but feels tired at other times. Laboratory examination, including hematocrit and TSH, are unremarkable. Because his wife reports occasional snoring, a sleep study is recommended. There are no notable apneas, but ECG monitoring during the night shows sinus bradycardia. His heart rate varies between 42 and 56 while sleeping. His resting heart rate while awake is 65–72 beats/min. Which of the following is the most appropriate management for his bradycardia?

A. Carotid sinus massage
B. Intermittent nocturnal wakening
C. Measurement of free T_4
D. No specific therapy
E. Referral for pacemaker placement

V-22. All of the following are reversible causes of sinoatrial node dysfunction EXCEPT:

A. Hypothermia
B. Hypothyroidism
C. Increased intracranial pressure
D. Lithium toxicity
E. Radiation therapy

V-23. A 58-year-old man is admitted to the hospital after experiencing 2 days of severe dyspnea. Three weeks ago he had an ST elevation myocardial infarction that was treated with thrombolytics. He reports excellent adherence to his medical regimen that includes atorvastatin, lisinopril, metoprolol, and aspirin. On examination, his heart rate is 44 beats/min, his blood pressure is 100/45 mmHg, his lungs have bilateral crackles, and his cardiac examination is notable for elevated neck veins, bradycardia, and 2+ bilateral leg edema. There are no gallops or new murmurs. ECG shows sinus bradycardia and evidence of the recent infarct, but no acute changes. Which of the following is the most appropriate next management step?

A. Begin dopamine
B. Hold metoprolol
C. Measure TSH
D. Refer for pacemaker placement
E. Refer for urgent coronary angiography

V-24. A 23-year-old college student home for the summer is evaluated in the emergency department for dizziness that began within the last 3 days. He reports a rash on his right leg that looked like a target several days ago, but is otherwise healthy. Physical examination shows bradycardia at 40 beats/min and blood pressure of 88/42 mmHg; oxygen saturation is normal. His examination is otherwise unremarkable except for a bulls-eye rash over the right upper thigh. ECG shows third-degree AV block. Which of the following laboratory studies is most likely to reveal the etiology of his signs and symptoms?

A. ANA
B. HLA B27 testing
C. *Borrelia burgdorferi* ELISA
D. RPR
E. SCL-70

V-25. In the tracing below (Figure V-25), what type of conduction abnormality is present and where in the conduction pathway is the block usually found?

A. First-degree AV block; intranodal
B. Second-degree AV block type 1; intranodal
C. Second-degree AV block type 2; infranodal
D. Second-degree AV block type 2; intranodal

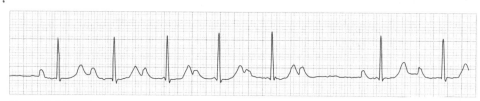

FIGURE V-25

V-26. A 47-year-old woman with a history of tobacco abuse and ulcerative colitis is evaluated for intermittent palpitations. She reports that for the last 6 months every 2–4 days she notes a sensation of her heart "flip-flopping" in her chest for approximately 5 minutes. She has not noted any precipitating factors and has not felt lightheaded or had chest pains with these episodes. Her physical examination is normal. A resting ECG reveals sinus rhythm and no abnormalities. Aside from checking serum electrolytes, which of the following is the most appropriate testing?

A. Abdominal CT with oral and IV contrast
B. Event monitor
C. Holter monitor
D. Reassurance with no further testing needed
E. Referral for EP study

V-27. After further testing, the patient in question V-26 is found to have several episodes of atrial premature contractions. Which of the following statements regarding the dysrhythmia in this patient is true?

A. Atrial premature contractions are less common than ventricular premature contractions on extended ECG monitoring.
B. Echocardiography is indicated to determine if structural heart disease is present.
C. Metoprolol should be initiated for symptom control.
D. The patient should be reassured that this is not a dangerous condition and does not require further evaluation.
E. The patient should undergo a stress test to determine if ischemia is present.

V-28. A 55-year-old man with end-stage COPD is admitted to the intensive care unit with an exacerbation of his obstructive lung disease. Because of hypercarbic respiratory failure, he is intubated and placed on assist-control mechanical ventilation. Despite aggressive sedation, his ventilator alarms several times that peak inspiratory pressures are high. The physician is called to the bedside to evaluate tachycardia. Examination is notable for a blood pressure of 112/68 mmHg and heart rate of 180 beats/min. Cardiac examination shows a regular rhythm, but no other abnormality. Breath sounds are decreased on the right. ECG shows narrow complex tachycardia. With carotid sinus massage, the heart rate transiently drops to 130 beats/min, but then returns to 180 beats/min. Which of the following is the most appropriate next step in management?

A. Adenosine 25-mg IV push
B. Amiodarone 200-mg IV push
C. Chest radiograph
D. Metoprolol 5-mg IV push
E. Sedation followed by cardioversion

V-29. All of the following are risk factors for stroke in a patient with atrial fibrillation EXCEPT:

A. Diabetes mellitus
B. History of congestive heart failure
C. History of stroke
D. Hypertension
E. Left atrial size greater than 4.0 cm

V-30. Which of the following statements regarding restoration of sinus rhythm after atrial fibrillation is true?

A. Dofetilide may be safely started on an outpatient basis.
B. In patients who are treated with pharmacotherapy and are found to be in sinus rhythm, a prolonged Holter monitor should be worn to determine if anticoagulation could be safely stopped.
C. Patients who have pharmacologically maintained sinus rhythm after atrial fibrillation have improved survival compared with patients who are treated with rate control and anticoagulation.
D. Recurrence of atrial fibrillation is uncommon when pharmacotherapy is used to maintain sinus rhythm.

V-31. A 57-year-old woman with a history of a surgically corrected atrial septal defect in childhood presents to the emergency department with palpitations for 3 days. She is found to have a heart rate of 153 beats/min and blood pressure of 128/75 mmHg, and an ECG shows atrial flutter. An echocardiogram demonstrates moderate right and left atrial dilation, postoperative changes from her surgery, and normal left and right ventricular function. Which of the following is true?

A. Anticoagulation with dabigatran should be initiated.
B. If a transesophageal echocardiogram does not demonstrate left atrial thrombus, she may be cardioverted without anticoagulation.
C. Intravenous heparin should be started immediately.
D. She should be immediately cardioverted.
E. Transthoracic echocardiogram is adequate to rule out the presence of left atrial thrombus.

V-32. A patient presents with palpitations and shortness of breath for 6 hours. In the emergency department waiting room an ECG is performed (shown in Figure V-32). Which of the following is most likely to be found on physical examination?

A. Diffuse abdominal tenderness with guarding
B. Diffuse expiratory polyphonic wheezing with poor air movement and hyperinflation
C. Left ventricular heave and third heart sound
D. Supraclavicular lymphadenopathy
E. Vesicular rash over right T5 dermatome

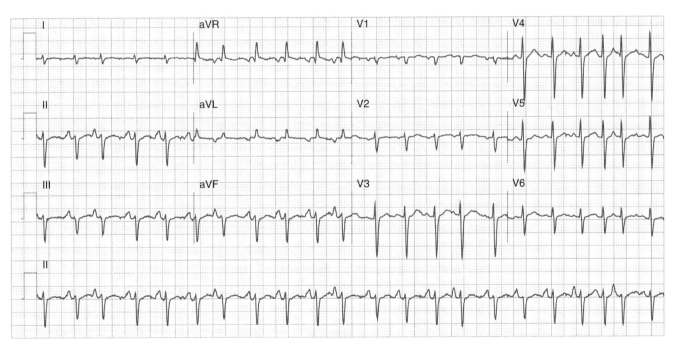

FIGURE V-32

V-33. A 43-year-old woman is seen in the emergency department after sudden onset of palpitations 30 minutes prior to her visit. She was seated at her work computer when the symptoms began. Aside from low back pain, she is otherwise healthy. In triage, her heart rate is 178 beats/min, and blood pressure is 98/56 mmHg with normal oxygen saturation. On physical examination, she has a "frog sign" in her neck and tachycardia, but is otherwise normal. ECG shows a narrow complex tachycardia without identifiable P waves. Which of the following is the most appropriate first step to manage her tachycardia?

A. 5 mg metoprolol IV
B. 6 mg adenosine IV
C. 10 mg verapamil IV
D. Carotid sinus massage
E. DC cardioversion using 100 J

V-34. A 37-year-old man who is healthy aside from a prior knee surgery is evaluated in the emergency department for palpitations that developed suddenly while eating dinner. He is found to have a heart rate of 193 beats/min, blood pressure of 92/52 mmHg, and normal oxygen saturation. His physical examination is normal aside from tachycardia and mild diaphoresis. An ECG obtained before his knee surgery shows delta waves in the early precordial leads. His current ECG shows wide complex tachycardia. Which of the following therapies is contraindicated for treatment of his tachyarrhythmia?

A. Adenosine
B. Carotid sinus massage
C. DC cardioversion
D. Digoxin
E. Metoprolol

V-35. In an ECG with wide complex tachycardia, which of the following clues most strongly supports the diagnosis of ventricular tachycardia?

A. Atrial-ventricular dissociation
B. Classic right bundle branch block pattern
C. Irregularly irregular rhythm with changing QRS complexes
D. QRS duration greater than 120 milliseconds
E. Slowing of rate with carotid sinus massage

V-36. A 40-year-old male with diabetes and schizophrenia is started on antibiotic therapy for chronic osteomyelitis in the hospital. His osteomyelitis has developed just under an ulcer where he has been injecting heroin. He is found suddenly unresponsive by the nursing staff. His electrocardiogram is shown in Figure V-36. The most likely cause of this rhythm is which of the following substances?

A. Furosemide
B. Metronidazole
C. Droperidol
D. Metformin
E. Heroin

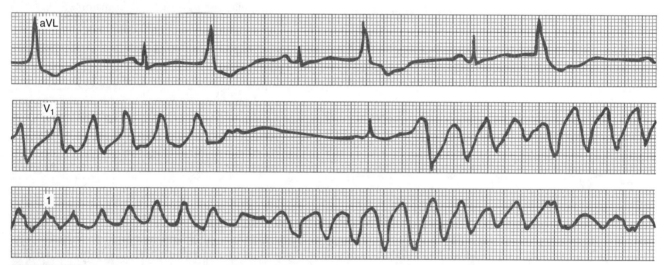

FIGURE V-36

V-37. Normal sinus rhythm is restored with electrical cardioversion in the patient in question V-36. A 12-lead electrocardiogram is notable for a prolonged QT interval. Besides stopping the offending drug, the most appropriate management for this rhythm disturbance should include intravenous administration of which of the following?

A. Amiodarone
B. Lidocaine
C. Magnesium
D. Metoprolol
E. Potassium

V-38. You are caring for a patient with heart rate–related angina. With minor elevations in heart rate, the patient has anginal symptoms that impact his quality of life. On review of a 24-hour Holter monitor, it appears that the patient has sinus tachycardia at the time of his symptoms. What is the mechanism for this patient's arrhythmia?

A. Delayed afterdepolarizations
B. Early afterdepolarizations
C. Increased automaticity
D. Reentry pathway

V-39. Where are the most common drivers of atrial fibrillation anatomically located?

A. Left atrial appendage
B. Mitral annulus
C. Pulmonary vein orifice
D. Sinus venosus
E. Sinus node

V-40. Symptoms of atrial fibrillation vary dramatically from patient to patient. A patient with which of the following clinical conditions will likely be the most symptomatic (e.g., short of breath) if the patient develops atrial fibrillation?

A. Acute alcohol intoxication
B. Hypertrophic cardiomyopathy
C. Hyperthyroidism
D. Hypothermia
E. Postoperative after thoracotomy

V-41. A 47-year-old postmenopausal woman is seen for onset of severe dyspnea over the last few weeks. She reports no preceding chest pain, cough, sputum, or fever, though she does report leg swelling. Physical examination is notable for a blood pressure of 145/78 mmHg and heart rate of 123 beats/min. Exophthalmos is present as well as bilateral inspiratory crackles occupying approximately one-third of the lower chest; neck vein distention; normal cardiac rhythm, though tachycardia is present; and a third heart sound with no murmur. Bilateral lower extremity edema and a fine hand tremor are also present. Which of the following is the most likely pathophysiologic explanation for her heart failure?

A. Anemia with high-output state
B. Chronic systemic hypertension with resultant left ventricular hypertrophy and nonsystolic heart failure
C. Hemochromatosis with subsequent restrictive cardiomyopathy
D. Myocardial infarction with depressed left ventricular systolic function
E. Thyrotoxicosis with high-output state

V-42. Which of the following statements is true regarding measurement of plasma BNP to diagnose heart failure?

A. An elevated plasma BNP in a dyspneic patient confirms the diagnosis of left heart failure.
B. In the presence of renal failure, BNP levels are suppressed even when heart failure is present.
C. Plasma BNP levels may be falsely low in patients with obesity and heart failure.
D. Serial measurement of BNP in the therapy of decompensated heart failure should be used to guide therapy.
E. All of the above are true.

V-43. A 64-year-old man with an ischemic cardiomyopathy, ejection fraction 35%, and stage C heart failure is seen in the cardiology clinic for evaluation of his disease status. The patient reports a regular exercise regimen of walking on the treadmill several times weekly and occasional exacerbations of his leg edema that he manages with an extra dose of furosemide. He has never been hospitalized for heart failure. His current medical regimen includes lisinopril, aspirin, furosemide, atorvastatin, digoxin, spironolactone, and metoprolol. He is interested in stopping medications because of their expense. Which of the following statements is true regarding his medical regimen?

A. ACE inhibition therapy has not been shown to improve heart failure symptoms.
B. Beta blocker therapy in this patient may be exacerbating his occasional need for extra furosemide and therefore should be stopped.
C. He should be switched from spironolactone to eplerenone for improved efficacy, as seen in patients with EF less than 35%.
D. If digoxin is withdrawn, he will likely have worsening symptoms.
E. If he is intolerant to lisinopril because of cough, it would be reasonable to switch him to an angiotensin-receptor blocker.

V-44. A 78-year-old slender woman is seen in the emergency department after several weeks of dyspnea on exertion that progressed to dyspnea at rest following a summer cookout where she consumed multiple pickled vegetables. She also complains of leg swelling, orthopnea, and occasionally awakening at night with dyspnea. Her past medical history is notable for long-standing systemic hypertension, uterine prolapse, and an anxiety disorder. Examination confirms the presence of heart failure with a laterally displaced and sustained point of maximum impulse and a fourth heart sound. She is admitted to the hospital and given diuretics, and an echocardiogram is obtained. Echocardiography reveals severe left ventricular hypertrophy with an ejection fraction of 70%, but there are no focal wall motion abnormalities, and aortic and mitral valvular function is intact. Her right ventricular systolic pressure is estimated to be 45 mmHg. After resolution of her heart failure symptoms with diuresis, the patient is ready for discharge. Which of the following medications have been shown to improve mortality in patients with heart failure with preserved ejection fraction and should be included in this patient's regimen?

A. Digoxin
B. Lisinopril
C. Metoprolol
D. Sildenafil
E. None of the above

V-45. A 68-year-old man with a history of myocardial infarction and congestive heart failure is comfortable at rest. However, when walking to his car he develops dyspnea, fatigue, and sometimes palpitations. He must rest for several minutes before these symptoms resolve. His New York Heart Association classification is which of the following?

A. Class I
B. Class II
C. Class III
D. Class IV

V-46. The husband of a 68-year-old woman with congestive heart failure is concerned because his wife appears to stop breathing for periods of time when she sleeps. He has noticed that she stops breathing for approximately 10 seconds and then follows this with a similar period of hyperventilation. This does not wake her from sleep. She does not snore. She feels well rested in the morning but is very dyspneic with even mild activity. What is your next step in management?

A. Electroencephalography
B. Maximize heart failure management
C. Nasal continuous positive airway pressure (CPAP) during sleep
D. Obtain a sleep study
E. Prescribe bronchodilators

V-47. A 53-year-old man undergoes cardiac transplantation for end-stage ischemic cardiomyopathy due to an underlying familial hypercholesterolemic disorder. His donor was a 23-year-old motor vehicle accident victim. The patient does well for the first 3 years after transplantation with only a single episode of acute rejection. He shows good compliance with his immunosuppression regimen, which includes prednisone and sirolimus. He is evaluated at a routine follow-up visit and reports that he has developed dyspnea on exertion. His pulmonary function tests are unchanged and a chest radiograph is normal. He undergoes right and left heart catheterization with biopsy of the transplanted heart. Severe, diffuse, concentric, and longitudinal coronary artery disease is found on coronary angiography, and histology shows no evidence of acute rejection. Which of the following statements is true regarding the coronary atherosclerosis found in this patient?

A. No immunosuppressive regimen has been shown to have a lower incidence of coronary atherosclerosis after cardiac transplantation.
B. The coronary atherosclerosis is most likely immunologic injury of the vascular endothelium in the transplanted organ.
C. The current coronary atherosclerosis after cardiac transplant is likely due to atherosclerosis present prior to transplantation.
D. The patient's underlying cholesterol disorder did not predispose him to recurrent coronary atherosclerosis after cardiac transplantation.
E. Therapy with statins has not been associated with a reduced incidence of this complication of transplantation.

V-48. Which of the following is a known complication of ventricular assist device placement in patients with end-stage heart failure?

A. Cerebrovascular accident
B. Infection of insertion site
C. Mechanical device failure
D. Thromboembolism
E. All of the above

V-49. All of the following are potential complications of an atrial septal defect in adults EXCEPT:

A. Air embolism from a central venous catheter
B. Arterial oxygen desaturation with exertion
C. Embolic cerebrovascular accident
D. Pulmonary arterial hypertension
E. Unstable angina

V-50. A 32-year-old woman is seen by her primary care physician clinic for routine follow-up of her hypothyroidism. She also has a history of complex congenital heart disease with a partially corrected VSD with predominantly right to left shunt across her patch. She is doing well and is able to work in janitorial services without severe dyspnea. She denies any heart failure or neurologic symptoms, but does have a peripheral oxygen saturation of 78%. A routine CBC is drawn and shows a hematocrit of 65%. Which of the following is the most appropriate management of her elevated hematocrit?

A. Begin oxygen therapy
B. Check co-oximetry on arterial blood gas sample
C. Check serum erythropoietin level
D. Expectant waiting
E. Refer to hematology for phlebotomy

V-51. A 43-year-old man recently was found to have an asymptomatic atrial septal defect that was closed using a percutaneous patch 1 month ago without complication. He is undergoing a root canal at the dentist next week and calls his primary care office to determine if antibiotic prophylaxis is indicated. Which of the following statements is true regarding antibiotic prophylaxis in this patient?

A. Because he had only simple congenital heart disease, no prophylaxis is indicated.
B. Because the lesion is corrected, no prophylaxis is indicated.
C. He should avoid potentially bacteremic dental procedures unless no other alternative is available.
D. Routine antibiotic prophylaxis is indicated for bacteremic dental procedures, particularly if the patch is less than 6 months old.
E. Routine antibiotic prophylaxis is indicated for bacteremic dental procedures whenever foreign material is present.

V-52. A 20-year-old man undergoes a physical examination with chest radiograph for enrollment in the military. He has had a normal childhood without any major illness. There is no history of sinusitis, pneumonia, or chronic respiratory disease. Chest radiograph shows dextrocardia. On closer physical examination, a spleen tip is palpable on the right of the abdomen and the liver can be percussed on the left. Which of the following is true regarding his condition?

A. He is likely to have aortic stenosis.
B. He is likely to have aspermia.
C. He is likely to have an atrial septal defect.
D. He is likely to have a ventriculoseptal defect.
E. He is likely to otherwise be normal.

V-53. A 24-year-old male seeks medical attention for the recent onset of headaches. The headaches are described as "pounding" and occur during the day and night. He has had minimal relief with acetaminophen. Physical examination is notable for a blood pressure of 185/115 mmHg in the right arm, a heart rate of 70 beats/min, arterioventricular (AV) nicking on funduscopic examination, normal jugular veins and carotid arteries, a pressure-loaded PMI with an apical S_4, no abdominal bruits, and reduced pulses in both lower extremities. Review of symptoms is positive only for leg fatigue with exertion. Additional measurement of blood pressure reveals the following:

Right arm	185/115
Left arm	188/113
Right thigh	100/60
Left thigh	102/58

Which of the following diagnostic studies is most likely to demonstrate the cause of the headaches?

A. MRI of the head
B. MRI of the kidney
C. MRI of the thorax
D. 24-hour urinary 5-HIAA
E. 24-hour urinary free cortisol

V-54. The patient described in question V-53 is most likely to have which of the following associated cardiac abnormalities?

A. Bicuspid aortic valve
B. Mitral stenosis
C. Preexcitation syndrome
D. Right bundle branch block
E. Tricuspid atresia

V-55. Mitral stenosis is frequently complicated by pulmonary hypertension. Which of the following is a cause of pulmonary hypertension in mitral stenosis?

A. Interstitial edema in the walls of small pulmonary vessels
B. Passive transmission of elevated left atrial pressure
C. Obliterative changes in the pulmonary vascular bed
D. Pulmonary arteriolar constriction
E. All of the above

V-56. A 58-year-old man with a history of systemic hypertension, hyperlipidemia, and tobacco abuse is admitted to the intensive care unit with crushing chest pain associated with ST-segment elevation and small precordial Q waves. Because his symptoms have been present for 36 hours, he is not a candidate for thrombolytics. On admission to the ICU, his systemic blood pressure is 123/67 mmHg, heart rate is 67 beats/min after beta blockade, and his oxygenation saturation is 93% on 2L nasal cannula. The remainder of the physical examination is normal. He is treated with lisinopril, aspirin, heparin, and metoprolol. Before transfer can be arranged to a tertiary center, the patient reports extreme dyspnea. He is found to be diaphoretic and to have a heart rate of 80 beats/min, blood pressure of 84/56 mmHg, and oxygen saturation of 93% on 100% non-rebreather. His lungs have bilateral crackles throughout, and neck veins are moderately elevated. ECG is unchanged. Chest radiograph shows new alveolar infiltrates in the right lung greater than the left. Which of the following is a likely finding on physical examination?

A. A fourth heart sound, III/VI systolic murmur heard best at the apex with a "cooing" quality that radiates to the axilla
B. A right ventricular heave, loud second heart sound, III/VI murmur increasing with inspiration at the right lower sternal border
C. A third heart sound, III/VI crescendo-decrescendo murmur heard best at the right upper sternal border
D. Diffuse urticarial reaction, wheezing on pulmonary examination
E. Mucosal edema, finger swelling, stridor

V-57. Which of the following is the most appropriate next step in therapy for the patient in question V-56?

A. Aerosolized albuterol
B. Initiation of norepinephrine infusion
C. Intravenous infusion of nitroprusside
D. Intravenous methylprednisolone
E. Placement of intraaortic balloon pump

V-58. A 26-year-old healthy woman is seen for a pap smear at a routine office visit. She feels well and has no complaints and no significant past medical history. Her internist performs a full physical examination and a midsystolic click is heard. No murmur or gallop is present. She is concerned about this finding. Which of the following statements is true regarding her examination finding?

A. In most patients with this disorder, an underlying cause such as a heritable disorder of connective tissue is found.
B. Infective endocarditis prophylaxis is indicated for dental procedures potentially associated with bacteremia.
C. Most patients are asymptomatic from this lesion and will remain so their entire life.
D. She should begin therapy with aspirin 325 mg po daily.
E. This disorder cannot be visualized on echocardiography.

V-59. A 78-year-old man is evaluated for the onset of dyspnea on exertion. He has a long history of tobacco abuse, obesity, and diabetes mellitus. His current medications include metformin, aspirin, and occasional ibuprofen. On physical examination his peripheral pulses show a delayed peak and he has a prominent left ventricular heave. He is in a regular rhythm with a IV/VI midsystolic murmur that is loudest at the base of the heart and radiates to the carotid arteries. A fourth heart sound is present. Echocardiography confirms severe aortic stenosis without other valvular lesions. Which of the following most likely contributed to the development of his cardiac lesion?

A. Congenital bicuspid aortic valve
B. Diabetes mellitus
C. Occult rheumatic heart disease
D. Underlying connective tissue disease
E. None of the above

V-60. A 63-year-old man presents with new-onset exertional syncope and is found to have aortic stenosis. In counseling the patient, you tell him that your therapeutic recommendation is based on the observation that untreated patients with his presentation have a predicted average lifespan of:

A. 5 years
B. 4 years
C. 3 years
D. 2 years
E. 1 year

V-61. Which of the following physical examination findings suggests severe aortic regurgitation?

A. Corrigan's pulse
B. Pulsus alternans
C. Pulsus bigeminus
D. Pulsus paradoxus
E. Pulsus parvus et tardus

V-62. A 41-year-old Somali woman is seen in clinic for onset of hemoptysis in the sixth month of her pregnancy. This is her fourth pregnancy and the others were uncomplicated, though she was 35 years old at the birth of her last child. Prior to this, she had been healthy. She reports mild dyspnea beginning at the fourth month of her pregnancy with onset of mild leg swelling shortly thereafter that she attributed to her pregnancy. The dyspnea has become severe, and she is now limited to walking around her house. She began to cough small amounts of bloody sputum 5 days ago. She had neither fever nor purulent sputum and has not responded to a course of antibiotics prescribed by her obstetrician. Physical examination is notable for a normal temperature, heart rate of 110 beats/min, blood pressure of 108/60 mmHg, and oxygen saturation of 91% on room air. No source of bleeding is seen in her nares or oropharynx. Her lungs have diffuse crackles, and cardiac examination shows moderately elevated neck veins, a regular heart rhythm, a loud second heart sound, and a low-pitched diastolic rumble heard best at the apex. The abdomen has a gravid uterus, and 1+ lower extremity edema is present. Which of the following is most likely to demonstrate the cause of her symptoms?

A. Bronchoscopy
B. Chest CT with contrast
C. Echocardiogram
D. Right heart catheterization
E. Upper airway inspection by an otolaryngologist

V-63. In the patient described in question V-62, which of the following should be prescribed at her visit to alleviate her symptoms?

A. Benazepril
B. Digoxin
C. Furosemide
D. Heparin
E. Levofloxacin

V-64. Which of the following patients with echocardiographic evidence of significant mitral regurgitation has the best indication for surgery with the most favorable likelihood of a positive outcome?

A. A 52-year-old man with an ejection fraction of 25%, NYHA class III symptoms, and a left-ventricular end-systolic dimension of 60 mm
B. A 54-year-old man with an ejection fraction of 30%, NYHA class II symptoms, and pulmonary hypertension
C. A 63-year-old man in sinus rhythm without symptoms, an ejection fraction of 65%, and a normal right heart catheterization
D. A 66-year-old man without symptoms, an ejection fraction of 50%, and left-ventricular end-systolic dimension of 45 mm
E. A 72-year-old asymptomatic woman with newly discovered atrial fibrillation, ejection fraction of 60%, and end-systolic dimension of 35 mm

V-65. All of the following are potential causes of tricuspid regurgitation EXCEPT:

A. Congenital heart disease
B. Infective endocarditis
C. Inferior wall myocardial infarction
D. Pulmonary arterial hypertension
E. Rheumatic heart disease
E. All of the above will cause tricuspid regurgitation.

V-66. All the following are true about cardiac valve replacement EXCEPT:

A. Bioprosthetic valve replacement is preferred to mechanical valve replacement in younger patients because of the superior durability of the valve.
B. Bioprosthetic valves have a low incidence of thromboembolic complications.
C. The risk of thrombosis with mechanical valve replacement is higher in the mitral position than in the aortic position.
D. Mechanical valves are relatively contraindicated in patients who wish to become pregnant.
E. Double-disk tilting mechanical prosthetic valves offer superior hemodynamic characteristics over single-disk tilting valves.

V-67. Which of the following infectious agents have been associated with the development of inflammatory myocarditis?

A.   Coxsackie virus
B.   Diphtheria
C.   Q fever
D.   *Trypanosoma cruzi*
E.   All of the above

V-68. All of the following are risk factors for the development of peripartum cardiomyopathy EXCEPT:

A.   Advanced maternal age
B.   Malnutrition
C.   Primiparity
D.   Twin pregnancy
E.   Use of tocolytics

V-69. A 67-year-old man with a long history of alcohol abuse presents with findings consistent with left ventricular failure including pulmonary edema and congestion. He undergoes right heart catheterization and left heart catheterization. No significant coronary artery disease is found. Which of the following right heart catheterization numbers (see Table V-69) would support a diagnosis of beriberi heart disease?

	Right Atrial Pressure (mmHg)	Mean Pulmonary Arterial Pressure (mmHg)	Pulmonary Capillary Wedge Pressure (mmHg)	Cardiac Output (L/min)	Systemic Vascular Resistance (dyn • s/cm^5)
A.	18	30	24	12	610
B.	4	15	12	6	1050
C.	24	35	28	3	2140
D.	24	48	8	5	2140
E.	2	10	2	4	2140

TABLE V-69

V-70. A 20-year-old basketball player is seen for evaluation prior to beginning another season of competitive sports. A harsh systolic murmur is heard at the left lower sternal border. Which of the following maneuvers will enhance this murmur if hypertrophic cardiomyopathy is the underlying cause?

A.   Hand grip
B.   Leaning forward while sitting
C.   Lying left side down
D.   Squatting
E.   Valsalva maneuver

V-71. A 62-year-old woman presents to your office with dyspnea of 4 months duration. She has a history of monoclonal gammopathy of unclear significance (MGUS) and has been lost to follow-up for the past 5 years. She is able to do only minimal activity before she has to rest but has no symptoms at rest. She has developed orthopnea but denies paroxysmal nocturnal dyspnea. She complains of fatigue, lightheadedness, and lower extremity swelling. On examination, blood pressure is 110/90 mmHg and heart rate is 94 beats/min. Jugular venous pressure is elevated, and the jugular venous wave does not fall with inspiration. An S_3 and S_4 are present, as well as a mitral regurgitation murmur. The point of maximal impulse is not displaced. Abdominal examination is significant for ascites and a large, tender, pulsatile liver. Chest radiograph shows bilateral pulmonary edema. An electrocardiogram

shows an old left bundle branch block. Which clinical features differentiate constrictive pericarditis from restrictive cardiomyopathy?

A.   Elevated jugular venous pressure
B.   Kussmaul's sign
C.   Narrow pulse pressure
D.   Pulsatile liver
E.   None of the above

V-72. You are evaluating a new patient in the clinic. The 25-year-old patient was diagnosed with "heart failure" in another state and has since relocated. He has New York Heart Association class II symptoms and denies angina. He presents for evaluation and management. The patient has been wheelchair bound for many years and has severe scoliosis. He has no family history of hyperlipidemia. His physical examination is notable for bilateral lung crackles, an S_3, and no cyanosis. An electrocardiogram (ECG) is obtained in the clinic and shows tall R waves in V_1 and V_2 with deep Qs in V_5 and V_6. An echocardiogram reports severe global left ventricular dysfunction with reduced ejection fraction. What is the most likely diagnosis?

A.   Amyotrophic lateral sclerosis
B.   Atrial septal defect
C.   Chronic thromboembolic disease
D.   Duchenne's muscular dystrophy
E.   Ischemic cardiomyopathy

V-73. A 35-year-old woman with a history of tobacco abuse presents to the emergency department because of severe chest pain radiating to both arms. The pain began 8 hours ago and is worse with inspiration. She has been unable to lie down as this markedly exacerbates the pain, but she feels better with sitting forward. Examination is notable for a heart rate of 96 beats/min, blood pressure of 145/78 mmHg, and oxygen saturation of 98%. Lungs are clear and a friction rub with three components is audible and is best heard at the left lower sternal border. Which of the following are most likely to be found on her ECG?

A. Diffusely inverted T waves in the precordial leads
B. PR elevation in leads II, III, and aVF
C. Sinus tachycardia
D. ST-segment elevation in I, aVL, and V_2–V_6 with upward concavity and reciprocal depressions in aVR
E. ST-segment elevation V_1–V_6 with convex curvature and reciprocal depressions in aVR

V-74. Which of the following statements is true regarding pulsus paradoxus?

A. It consists of a greater than 15 mmHg increase in systolic arterial pressure with inspiration.
B. It may be found in patients with severe obstructive lung disease.
C. It is the reversal of a normal phenomenon during inspiration.
D. It results from right ventricular distention during expiration resulting in compression of the left ventricular volume and subsequent reduction in systolic pulse pressure.
E. All of the above are true.

V-75. Which of the following are features of Beck's triad in cardiac tamponade?

A. Hypotension, electrical alternans, prominent x-descent in neck veins
B. Hypotension, muffled heart sounds, electrical alternans
C. Hypotension, muffled heart sounds, jugular venous distention
D. Kussmaul's sign, hypotension, muffled heart sounds
E. Muffled heart sounds, hypotension, friction rub

V-76. A 35-year-old woman is admitted to the hospital with malaise, weight gain, increasing abdominal girth, and edema. The symptoms began about 3 months ago and gradually progressed. The patient reports an increase in waist size of approximately 15 cm. The swelling in her legs has gotten increasingly worse such that she now feels her thighs are swollen as well. She has dyspnea on exertion and two-pillow orthopnea. She has a past history of Hodgkin's disease diagnosed at age 18. She was treated at that time with chemotherapy and mediastinal irradiation. On physical examination, she has temporal wasting and appears chronically ill. Her current weight is 96 kg, which reflects an increase of 11 kg over the past 3 months. Her vital signs are normal. Her jugular

venous pressure is approximately 16 cm, and the neck veins do not collapse on inspiration. Heart sounds are distant. There is a third heart sound heard shortly after aortic valve closure. The sound is short and abrupt and is heard best at the apex. The liver is enlarged and pulsatile. Ascites is present. There is pitting edema extending throughout the lower extremities and onto the abdominal wall. Echocardiogram shows pericardial thickening, dilatation of the inferior vena cava and hepatic veins, and abrupt cessation of ventricular filling in early diastole. Ejection fraction is 65%. What is the best approach for treatment of this patient?

A. Aggressive diuresis only
B. Cardiac transplantation
C. Mitral valve replacement
D. Pericardial resection
E. Pericardiocentesis

V-77. A 19-year-old previously healthy hockey player is defending the goal when he is hit in the left chest with a hockey puck. He immediately collapses to the ice. His coach runs to his side and finds him unresponsive and without a pulse. Which of the following is most likely responsible for this syndrome?

A. Aortic rupture
B. Cardiac tamponade
C. Commotio cordis
D. Hypertrophic cardiomyopathy
E. Tension pneumothorax

V-78. A 48-year-old white man is seen in the clinic for a routine physical examination. He reports no complaints. Examination shows a blood pressure of 134/82 mmHg with a normal heart rate. BMI is 31 kg/m². The remainder of his physical examination is normal. Which of the following is true regarding lifestyle modification?

A. Brisk walking for as little as 10 minutes, 4 days per week will lower his blood pressure to within the normal range.
B. Dietary NaCl restriction of less than 6 g per day will reduce his blood pressure.
C. Lifestyle modification will have no effect on his blood pressure.
D. Reduction of alcohol consumption to three or fewer drinks per day will decrease his blood pressure.
E. Weight loss of approximately 9 kg can be expected to bring his blood pressure to within the normal limit.

V-79. A 46-year-old white female presents to your office with concerns about her diagnosis of hypertension 1 month previously. She asks you about her likelihood of developing complications of hypertension, including renal failure and stroke. She denies any past medical history other than hypertension and has no symptoms that suggest secondary causes. She currently is taking hydrochlorothiazide 25 mg/d. She smokes half a pack of cigarettes daily and drinks alcohol no more than once per week. Her family history is significant for hypertension in both parents. Her mother died of a cerebrovascular accident. Her father is alive but has coronary artery disease and is on hemodialysis. Her blood pressure is 138/90 mmHg. Body mass index is 23. She has no retinal exudates or other signs of hypertensive retinopathy. Her point of maximal cardiac impulse is not displaced but is sustained. Her rate and rhythm are regular and without gallops. She has good peripheral pulses. An electrocardiogram reveals an axis of −30 degrees with borderline voltage criteria for left ventricular hypertrophy. Creatinine is 1.0 mg/dL. Which of the following items in her history and physical examination is a risk factor for a poor prognosis in a patient with hypertension?

A. Family history of renal failure and cerebrovascular disease
B. Persistent elevation in blood pressure after the initiation of therapy
C. Ongoing tobacco use
D. Ongoing use of alcohol
E. Presence of left ventricular hypertrophy on ECG

V-80. A 28-year-old female has hypertension that is difficult to control. She was diagnosed at age 26. Since that time she has been on increasing amounts of medication. Her current regimen consists of labetalol 1000 mg bid, lisinopril 40 mg qd, clonidine 0.1 mg bid, and amlodipine 5 mg qd. On physical examination she appears to be without distress. Blood pressure is 168/100 mmHg, and heart rate is 84 beats/min. Cardiac examination is unremarkable, without rubs, gallops, or murmurs. She has good peripheral pulses and has no edema. Her physical appearance does not reveal any hirsutism, fat maldistribution, or abnormalities of genitalia. Laboratory studies reveal a potassium of 2.8 meq/dL and a serum bicarbonate of 32 meq/dL. Fasting blood glucose is 114 mg/dL. What is the likely diagnosis?

A. Congenital adrenal hyperplasia
B. Fibromuscular dysplasia
C. Cushing's syndrome
D. Conn's syndrome
E. Pheochromocytoma

V-81. What is the best way to diagnose this disease in question V-80?

A. Renal vein renin levels
B. 24-hour urine collection for metanephrines
C. Magnetic resonance imaging of the renal arteries
D. 24-hour urine collection for cortisol
E. Plasma aldosterone/renin ratio

V-82. Which of the following patients with aortic dissection or hematoma is best managed *without* surgical therapy?

A. A 74-year-old male with a dissection involving the root of the aorta.
B. A 45-year-old female with a dissection involving the aorta distal to the great vessel origin but cephalad to the renal arteries.
C. A 58-year-old male with aortic dissection involving the distal aorta and the bilateral renal arteries.
D. A 69-year-old male with an intramural hematoma within the aortic root.
E. All of the above patients require surgical management of their aortic disease.

V-83. A 68-year-old male presents to your office for routine follow-up care. He reports that he is feeling well and has no complaints. His past medical history is significant for hypertension and hypercholesterolemia. He continues to smoke a pack of cigarettes daily. He is taking chlorthalidone 25 mg daily, atenolol 25 mg daily, and pravastatin 40 mg nightly. Blood pressure is 133/85 mmHg, and heart rate is 66 beats/min. Cardiac and pulmonary examinations are unremarkable. A pulsatile abdominal mass is felt just to the left of the umbilicus and measures approximately 4 cm. You confirm the diagnosis of abdominal aortic aneurysm by CT imaging. It is located infrarenally and measures 4.5 cm. All the following are true about the patient's diagnosis EXCEPT:

A. The 5-year risk of rupture of an aneurysm of this size is 1–2%.
B. Surgical or endovascular intervention is warranted because of the size of the aneurysm.
C. Infrarenal endovascular stent placement is an option if the aneurysm experiences continued growth in light of the location of the aneurysm infrarenally.
D. Surgical or endovascular intervention is warranted if the patient develops symptoms of recurrent abdominal or back pain.
E. Surgical or endovascular intervention is warranted if the aneurysm expands beyond 5.5 cm.

V-84. A 32-year-old female is seen in the emergency department for acute shortness of breath. A helical CT shows no evidence of pulmonary embolus, but incidental note is made of dilatation of the ascending aorta to 4.3 cm. All the following are associated with this finding EXCEPT:

A. Syphilis
B. Takayasu's arteritis
C. Giant cell arteritis
D. Rheumatoid arthritis
E. Systemic lupus erythematosus

V-85. A 68-year-old man with a history of coronary artery disease is seen in his primary care clinic for complaint of cough with sputum production. His care provider is concerned about pneumonia, so a chest radiograph is ordered. On the chest radiograph, the aorta appears tortuous with a widened mediastinum. A contrast-enhanced CT of the chest confirms the presence of a descending thoracic aortic aneurysm measuring 4 cm with no evidence of dissection. What is the most appropriate management of this patient?

A. Consult interventional radiology for placement of an endovascular stent.
B. Consult thoracic surgery for repair.
C. No further evaluation is needed.
D. Perform yearly contrast-enhanced chest CT and refer for surgical repair when the aneurysm size is greater than 4.5 cm.
E. Treat with beta blockers, perform yearly contrast-enhanced chest CT, and refer for surgical repair if the aneurysm grows more than 1 cm/year.

V-86. A 37-year-old woman with no significant past medical history except for a childhood murmur is evaluated for severe pain of sudden onset in her right lower extremity. Examination is notable for a young, uncomfortable woman with normal vital signs except for a heart rate of 110 beats/min. Right leg has pallor distal to the right knee and is cold to the touch, and the dorsalis pedis pulse is absent. Which of the following studies is likely to diagnose the underlying reason for the patient's presentation?

A. Angiography of right lower extremity
B. Blood cultures
C. Echocardiogram with bubble study
D. Serum c-ANCA
E. Venous ultrasound of right upper extremity

ANSWERS

V-1. **The answer is B.** (*Chaps. 227, 250*) Pulmonary hypertension is associated with a loud second heart sound that is heard to be louder than the first heart sound at the cardiac base. In idiopathic pulmonary arterial hypertension, there is no associated congenital lesion, such as atrial septal defect (ASD). In ASD, the components of the second heart sound, aortic and pulmonic valve closure, do not alter their timing with respect to respiratory cycle and are always widely split, and thus are described as "fixed split." In idiopathic pulmonary arterial hypertension, the components of the second heart sound are nearly superimposed and loud; often there is little respiratory variation. The soft systolic murmur at the left lower sternal border of tricuspid regurgitation is nearly always present in pulmonary hypertension of all etiologies. Idiopathic pulmonary arterial hypertension, by definition, is not associated with a parenchymal lung disease such as emphysema. Patients with idiopathic pulmonary arterial hypertension should not have physical findings associated with chronic airways disease.

V-2. **The answer is A.** (*Chap. 227*) The patient is very likely to have pericardial tamponade from metastatic cancer as suggested by her elevated neck veins, heart shadow shape and size, and predisposing condition. Because of the exaggerated interventricular dependence, the normal (<10 mmHg) fall in systemic blood pressure with inspiration is exaggerated (often >15 mmHg) with cardiac tamponade. This is referred to as pulsus paradoxus, though it is in fact an augmentation of a normal finding. Kussmaul's sign, or a lack of fall of the jugular venous pressure with inspiration, usually denotes a lack of compliance in the right ventricle, as seen most frequently in constrictive pericarditis, though it may be found in restrictive cardiomyopathy or massive pulmonary embolism. A rapid y-descent, which follows the peak of the v wave, of jugular venous pressure tracing is indicative of cardiac tamponade. Pulsus parvus et tardus, or small and slow arterial pulsation, is a late finding in aortic stenosis. Late diastolic murmur and opening snap is found in mitral stenosis.

V-3. **The answer is A.** *(Chap. 227)* A fourth heart sound indicates left ventricular presystolic expansion and is common among patients in whom active atrial contraction is important for ventricular filling. A fourth heart sound is not found in atrial fibrillation. An irregular heart rate is characteristic of atrial fibrillation. The irregular rate is often characterized as "irregularly irregular." A third heart sound occurs during the rapid filling phase of ventricular diastole and indicates heart failure. Reversed splitting of the second heart sound occurs with left bundle branch block, as this patient has. Finally, pulsus alternans is beat-to-beat variability in pulse amplitude. It is present when only every other Korotkoff sound is audible as the cuff pressure is lowered slowly. It is thought to be due to cyclic changes in intracellular calcium and action potential duration and is associated with severe left ventricular failure.

V-4. **The answer is A.** *(Chap. 227)* The presentation of this patient is consistent with the diagnosis of acute valvular dysfunction due to infective endocarditis. The presence of a widened pulse pressure and diastolic murmur heard best along the lower sternal border suggests aortic regurgitation. Panel C of Figure V-4B shows a typical bisferiens pulse that is characteristic of aortic regurgitation. With a bisferiens pulse, there are two distinct pulsations that can be palpated with systole. The initial pulse represents an exaggerated percussion wave reflecting the increased stroke volume that occurs in aortic regurgitation, with the second peak reflecting the tidal, or anacrotic, wave.

Infective endocarditis causes loss of valvular integrity and acutely causes valvular regurgitation. Of the other options, both mitral regurgitation and tricuspid regurgitation (choice E) would cause systolic and not diastolic murmurs. A hyperkinetic pulse may occur in these conditions, particularly if associated with fever or sepsis. With a hyperkinetic pulse the usual dichrotic notch is more pronounced, as seen in panel E of the figure. Mitral stenosis causes a diastolic murmur but is not a common lesion associated with infective endocarditis, unless underlying valvular stenosis was present prior to acquiring the infection. It is not associated with a bisferiens pulse. Aortic stenosis is associated with pulsus parvus et tardus, with a delayed and prolonged carotid upstroke as shown in panel B of the figure. Aortic stenosis has an associated harsh crescendo-decrescendo systolic murmur.

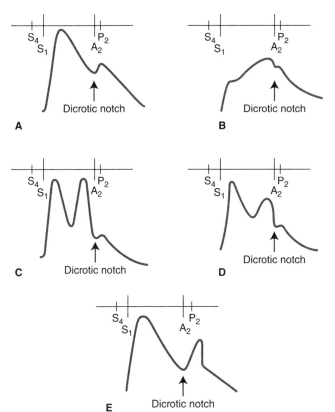

FIGURE V-4B Schematic diagrams of the configurational changes in carotid pulse and their differential diagnoses. Heart sounds are also illustrated. *A.* Normal. S_4, fourth heart sound; S_1, first heart sound; A_2, aortic component of second heart sound; P_2, pulmonic component of second heart sound. *B.* Aortic stenosis. Anacrotic pulse with slow upstroke to a reduced peak. *C.* Bisferiens pulse with two peaks in systole. This pulse is rarely appreciated in patients with severe aortic regurgitation. *D.* Bisferiens pulse in hypertrophic obstructive cardiomyopathy. There is a rapid upstroke to the first peak (percussion wave) and a slower rise to the second peak (tidal wave). *E.* Dicrotic pulse with peaks in systole and diastole. This waveform may be seen in patients with sepsis or during intra-aortic balloon counter-pulsation with inflation just after the dicrotic notch. *[From K Chatterjee, W Parmley (eds): Cardiology: An Illustrated Text/Reference. Philadelphia, JB Lippincott, 1991.]*

V-5.   **The answer is A.** *(Chap. 227)* Peripheral arterial disease (PAD) affects 5–8% of Americans, with increasing incidence with age. Over the age of 65, the incidence of PAD rises to between 12% and 20%. The primary symptom of PAD is claudication. As this patient describes, claudication occurs with ambulation and is often described as a crampy to aching pain that is relieved with rest. On physical examination, those with PAD often have diminished peripheral pulses, delayed capillary refill, and hair loss in the distal extremities. The skin is often cool to the touch with a thin, shiny appearance. In severe PAD, pain in the extremities occurs at rest. Diagnosis of PAD can be suggested by these findings and should be documented by determination of the ankle-brachial index (ABI), as physical examination alone is insufficient to diagnose PAD. Although lack of a palpable pulse suggests critical ischemia, it is not diagnostic. To perform an ABI, blood pressures are determined in the arm and the lower extremities. Either the dorsalis pedis or posterior tibial pulses can be used. The ABI is calculated by dividing the ankle systolic pressure by the brachial systolic pressure. A resting ABI less than 0.9 is abnormal, but critical ischemia with rest pain does not occur until the ABI is less than 0.3. In individuals with heavily calcified blood vessels, the ABI can be abnormally elevated (ABI >1.2) when PAD is present. In this situation, toe pressures to determine ABI or employing imaging techniques such as MRI or arteriography should be considered. Lower extremity edema is suggestive of congestive heart failure, not PAD.

V-6.   **The answer is F.** *(Chap. 227)* When a murmur of uncertain cause is identified on physical examination, a variety of physiologic maneuvers can be used to assist in the elucidation of the cause. Commonly used physiologic maneuvers include change with respiration, Valsalva maneuver, position, and exercise. In hypertrophic cardiomyopathy, there is asymmetric hypertrophy of the interventricular septum, which creates a dynamic outflow obstruction. Maneuvers that decrease left-ventricular filling will cause an increase in the intensity of the murmur, whereas those that increase left-ventricular filling will cause a decrease in the murmur. Of the interventions listed, both standing and a Valsalva maneuver will decrease venous return and subsequently decrease left ventricular filling, resulting in an increase in the loudness of the murmur of hypertrophic cardiomyopathy. Alternatively, squatting will increase venous return and thus decrease the murmur. Maximum handgrip exercise also will result in a decreased loudness of the murmur.

V-7.   **The answer is B.** *(Chap. 228)* Left bundle branch, defined by QRS interval greater than 120 milliseconds with typical pattern in V_1 and V_6, is associated with four conditions: coronary heart disease, hypertensive heart disease, aortic valve disease, and cardiomyopathy. In all cases, the left bundle branch block is associated with increased risk of cardiovascular morbidity and mortality. These conditions share left ventricular pathology. In contrast, right bundle branch block is associated with congenital heart disease, pulmonary vascular disease, and less frequently valvular heart disease.

V-8.   **The answer is D.** *(Chap. 228)* The classic findings of hypokalemia are prominent U waves due to prolonged ventricular repolarization. Scooped ST segments are commonly seen with digoxin toxicity. Low P wave amplitude is found in early hyperkalemia. Prolonged QT intervals are often due to drug toxicity such as tricyclic antidepressant overdose, procainamide, quinidine disopyramide, and phenothiazines. Finally, Osborne waves, or convex elevation of the J point, are found in severe hypothermia and are due to repolarization prolongation.

V-9.   **The answer is D.** *(Chaps. 228, 237, and 250)* The patient presents from a country with likely low rates of treatment for childhood streptococcal infection and was subsequently at high risk for rheumatic heart disease. Her large pulmonary arteries in the absence of parenchymal infiltrates suggests pulmonary hypertension and her ECG shows right ventricular hypertrophy, characterized by a relatively tall R wave in lead V_1, or R greater than or equal to S wave. This is highly likely to be due to mitral stenosis. While aortic stenosis and regurgitation are possible causes, these are less likely. Tricuspid stenosis is not associated with right ventricular hypertrophy. Left ventricular systolic failure may cause pulmonary venous hypertension, but more commonly is associated with evidence of left heart failure on examination.

V-10. **The answer is D.** *(Chaps. 228 and e28)* This ECG shows a short ST segment that is most prominent in V_2, V_3, V_4, and V_5. Hypercalcemia, by shortening the duration of repolarization, abbreviates the total time from depolarization through repolarization. This is manifested on the surface ECG by a short QT interval. In this scenario, the hypercalcemia is due to the rhabdomyolysis and renal failure. Fluids and a loop diuretic are an appropriate therapy for hypercalcemia. Hemodialysis is seldom indicated. Hemodialysis is indicated for significant hyperkalemia, which may also develop after rhabdomyolysis, manifest by "tenting" of the T waves or widening of the QRS. Classic ECG manifestations of a pulmonary embolus (S_1, Q_3, T_3 pattern) are infrequent in patients with pulmonary embolism (PE), though the changes may be seen with massive PE. There are no signs of myocardial ischemia on this ECG, which would make coronary catheterization and 18-lead ECG interpretation of low yield.

V-11. **The answer is D.** *(Chap. 228)* Hyperkalemia leads to partial depolarization of cardiac cells. As a result, there is slowing of the upstroke of the action potential as well as reduced duration of repolarization. The T wave becomes peaked, the RS complex widens and may merge with the T wave (giving a sine-wave appearance), and the P wave becomes shallow or disappears. Prominent U waves are associated with hypokalemia; ST-segment prolongation is associated with hypocalcemia.

V-12. **The answer is C.** *(Chaps. 228 and 238)* The ECG shows slight right axis deviation and low voltage. These changes are typical of emphysema when the thorax is hyperinflated with air and the flattened diaphragm pulls the heart inferiorly and vertically. An acute central nervous system (CNS) event such as a subarachnoid hemorrhage may cause QT prolongation with deep, wide inverted T waves. Hyperkalemia will cause peaked narrowed T waves or a wide QRS complex. Patients with hypertrophic cardiomyopathy will have left ventricular hypertrophy and widespread deep, broad Q waves.

V-13. **The answer is E.** *(Chaps. 228 and e30)* This ECG tracing shows the triad of a short PR interval, wide QRS, and delta waves (seen best in leads I, II, and V_5) consistent with Wolff-Parkinson-White (WPW) syndrome. Patients with WPW syndrome are commonly diagnosed asymptomatically when an ECG is performed showing the classic findings. Symptoms are due to conduction via an accessory pathway and include tachypalpitations, lightheadedness, syncope, cardiopulmonary collapse, and sudden cardiac death. Life-threatening presentations are usually due to the development of atrial fibrillation or atrial flutter with 1:1 conduction, both of which can precipitate ventricular fibrillation. Unstable angina is mainly associated with ST-segment abnormalities, although conduction abnormalities may be seen. Pulmonary embolism, which may cause hemoptysis and pleuritic chest pain, has nonspecific ECG findings including $S_1Q_3T_3$ (acute right ventricular failure) or T-wave abnormalities.

V-14. **The answer is E.** *(Chap. 228)* The limb lead aVR generally has a negative deflection, as the primary vector for ventricular depolarization is directed down and away from this lead. Therefore, in the case of left ventricular hypertrophy the negative deflection, or S wave, would be expected to be larger without an effect on the R wave. There are multiple criteria for diagnosing left ventricular hypertrophy on ECG.

V-15. **The answer is B.** *(Chaps. 228 and e30)* This ECG tracing shows multifocal atrial tachycardia (MAT), right atrial overload, a superior axis, and poor R-wave progression in the precordial leads. There are varying P-wave morphologies (more than three morphologies) and P-P intervals. MAT is most commonly caused by COPD, but other conditions associated with this arrhythmia include coronary artery disease, congestive heart failure, valvular heart disease, diabetes mellitus, hypokalemia, hypomagnesemia, azotemia, postoperative state, and pulmonary embolism. Anemia, pain, and myocardial ischemia are also causes of tachycardia that should be considered when managing a new tachycardia. These states are usually associated with sinus tachycardia.

V-16. **The answer is E.** *(Chap. 229)* Doppler echocardiography uses ultrasound reflecting off moving red blood cells to determine flow velocity within a structure, in this case the heart or great vessels. Thus, it is most useful for determining abnormal flow or flow limitation. Specifically, it is useful in defining valvular regurgitation or stenosis, cardiac output when combined with the cross-sectional area, and diastolic filling of the ventricle. Heart failure with preserved ejection fraction is associated with impaired left ventricle relaxation in early diastole and subsequently there is reduced early transmitral flow compared to normal individuals. Although Doppler might be helpful to determine the physiologic consequence of pericardial effusion, i.e., tamponade, two-dimensional (2D) echocardiography is the preferred mode for effusion diagnosis. Similarly, 2D echocardiography is used to calculate ejection fraction and diagnose cardiac masses. Diagnosis of ischemia can be made with the addition of physiologic or pharmacologic stress to echocardiography, but not with Doppler echocardiography.

V-17. **The answer is E.** *(Chap. 230)* Although myocardial infarction, stroke, and death are complications that have been reported with cardiac catheterization (all with a frequency of <0.1%), the more common complications are tachy- or bradyarrhythmias, acute renal failure, and vascular complications. Vascular access site bleeding is the most common complication of cardiac catheterization, occurring in 1.5–2% of patients. When catheterization is performed in an emergent fashion for acute myocardial infarction or for hemodynamically unstable patients, the complication rate may rise substantially.

V-18. **The answer is A.** *(Chap. 230)* Although right heart catheterization is no longer routinely performed at the time of left heart catheterization, there remain important indications for this procedure. These include evaluation of unexplained dyspnea, especially when there is a suspicion of pulmonary hypertension; diagnosis of valvular heart disease such as mitral regurgitation; pericardial disease; right and/or left ventricular dysfunction, particularly for determination of severity; diagnosis of congenital heart disease; and suspected intracardiac shunts. In this case, the patient likely has an atrial septal defect with physical examination findings of a loud, fixed split second heart sound and perhaps associated dyspnea. During right heart catheterization, the pulmonary arterial pressures will be measured to assess for pulmonary hypertension, and venous saturation will be measured at the inferior vena cava, right atrium, right ventricle, and pulmonary artery to assess for evidence of an increase in saturation suggestive of intracardiac shunt. All the other patients described would be more appropriately served with a left heart catheterization and coronary angiogram.

V-19. **The answer is B.** *(Chaps. 230 and 250)* In the diagnostic algorithm for pulmonary hypertension, the right heart catheterization is important to document the presence and degree of pulmonary hypertension. The right-ventricular systolic pressure (RVSP) on echocardiography provides an estimate of pulmonary arterial pressures, but accurate determination of the RVSP relies on the presence of tricuspid regurgitation and good quality echocardiography. This patient's body habitus is prohibitive in obtaining good windows for echocardiography. Thus, a right heart catheterization is imperative for documenting pulmonary hypertension, as well as for determining the cause. The right heart catheterization demonstrates an elevated mean arterial pressure, elevated left-ventricular end-diastolic pressure (pulmonary capillary wedge pressure), and elevated mean pulmonary artery pressure. In the presence of a normal cardiac output and an elevated left-ventricular ejection fraction, this is consistent with the diagnosis of diastolic heart failure. Systolic heart failure is associated with similar indices on right heart catheterization, but left-ventricular function is depressed in systolic heart failure. The other causes listed as options are known causes of pulmonary hypertension but would not be expected to cause an increase in the left-ventricular end-diastolic pressure. Obstructive sleep apnea is usually associated only with mild elevations in pulmonary artery pressure. This patient's BMI puts her at risk for obstructive sleep apnea but would not be responsible for these right heart catheterization values. Both chronic thromboembolic disease and pulmonary arterial hypertension can cause severe elevations in the pulmonary arterial pressure but have a normal left atrial pressure.

V-20. **The answer is B.** *(Chap. 232)* The tachycardia-bradycardia variant of sick sinus syndrome is associated with an increased risk of thromboembolism, particularly when similar risk factors are present that increase the risk of thromboembolism in patients with atrial fibrillation. Specific risk factors associated with highest risk include age greater than 65 years and prior history of stroke, valvular heart disease, left ventricular dysfunction, or atrial enlargement. Patients with these risk factors should be treated with anticoagulation.

V-21. **The answer is D.** *(Chap. 232)* Bradycardia is frequently present in trained athletes, particularly at night, where heart rates are usually between 40 and 60 beats/min. While sleep apnea can be associated with bradycardia, no apnea was found in this patient on overnight polysomnography. Other possible causes of bradycardia in this patient such as hypothyroidism have been ruled out. Measurement of free T_4 is not indicated with a normal TSH. Pacemaker insertion is not indicated for his normal physiology. Carotid sinus massage is likely to cause further bradycardia. Fatigue is likely due to his stressful job.

V-22. **The answer is E.** *(Chap. 232)* Sinoatrial dysfunction is often divided into intrinsic disease and extrinsic disease of the node. This is a critical distinction, as extrinsic causes are often reversible and pacemaker placement is not required. Drug toxicity is a common cause of extrinsic, reversible sinoatrial dysfunction, with common culprits including beta blockers, calcium channel blockers, lithium toxicity, narcotics, pentamidine, and clonidine. Hypothyroidism, sleep apnea, hypoxia, hypothermia, and increased intracranial pressure are all reversible forms of extrinsic dysfunction. Radiation therapy can result in permanent dysfunction of the node and therefore is an irreversible, or intrinsic, cause of sinoatrial node dysfunction. In symptomatic patients, pacemaker insertion may be indicated.

V-23. **The answer is D.** *(Chap. 232)* When there is evidence of sinoatrial node dysfunction, as manifest in this patient with sinus bradycardia, the first approach is to search for reversible causes. In this case, excessive beta blockade is the most likely explanation for his bradycardia and symptoms. Stopping the metoprolol at least temporarily is in order. There are no urgent indications for temporary or permanent pacemaker placement, as he does not have a high-level AV block, syncope, or shock. His heart failure should reverse when his heart rate increases. Although pharmacologic chronotropic stimulation can increase heart rate temporarily, his moderate symptoms suggest that simply waiting for the beta blocker to be metabolized will be adequate. There is no evidence of new infarction or post-infarct angina; thus the patient does not require urgent revascularization. Once the patient is stabilized, the risks and benefits of restarting the beta blocker at a lower dosage may be considered.

V-24. **The answer is C.** *(Chap. 232)* The patient presents with a classic bulls-eye lesion, or erythema migrans, consistent with Lyme disease. Cardiac conduction abnormalities are common in Lyme disease, often involving the AV node. Temporary pacing may be necessary, but the conduction abnormalities usually resolve. The most common test to diagnose this condition is an ELISA with confirmatory Western blot. Other infectious etiologies can present with heart block such as syphilis and Chagas' disease, but these would not be associated with the characteristic Lyme rash. Autoimmune and infiltrative diseases may also present with conduction system disease such as ankylosing spondylitis, rheumatoid arthritis, scleroderma, and systemic lupus erythematosus.

V-25. **The answer is B.** *(Chap. 232)* Second-degree AV block type 1 (Mobitz type 1) is characterized by a progressive lengthening of the PR interval preceding a pause. The pause in this tracing is between the third and fourth QRS complex. First-degree AV block is a slowing of conduction through the AV junction and is diagnosed when the PR interval is greater than 200 milliseconds. Type 2 second-degree AV block is characterized by intermittent failure of conduction of the P wave without changes in the preceding PR or RR intervals. Second-degree AV block type 2 usually occurs in the distal or infra-His conduction systems.

V-26 and V-27. The answers are B and D, respectively. *(Chap. 233)* The patient has persistent, non–life-threatening palpitations that distress her enough to seek medical attention. A continuous Holter monitor for 24 hours is appropriate for patients in whom the symptoms happen several times a day in which an event monitor is triggered by the patient when symptoms occur and thus can be worn for a longer period of time. There is no indication of gastrointestinal triggers, so abdominal CT would not be helpful. The atrial premature contractions are uncomplicated, do not require additional diagnostic evaluation at this time, and pose no additional health risk. EP referral is indicated for patients with life-threatening or severe symptoms such as syncope.

V-28. **The answer is C.** *(Chap. 233)* The patient has physiologic sinus tachycardia related to a pneumothorax, for which he was at risk from his obstructive lung disease and volume-cycled mechanical ventilation. The increased peak inspiratory pressure on the mechanical ventilator is due to the reduced respiratory system compliance from the pneumothorax. Physiologic sinus tachycardia often comes on slowly and responds poorly to carotid sinus massage with gradual return to original rate. Pharmacologic interventions are usually unsuccessful with correction of the underlying cause required for resolution of the tachycardia. In this case, a tension pneumothorax is confirmed by chest radiograph and, with placement of a chest tube, the tachycardia resolves. Other causes of physiologic sinus tachycardia include pain, hyperthyroidism, anxiety, anemia, hypotension, fever, and exercise.

V-29. **The answer is E.** *(Chap. 233)* Patients at the highest risk for stroke associated with atrial fibrillation include those with a prior history of stroke, TIA, or embolism, and patients with hypertension, diabetes mellitus, congestive heart failure, rheumatic heart disease, LV dysfunction, and marked left atrial dilation of greater than 5.0 cm or age greater than 65 years. Anticoagulation should be strongly considered in these patients. Increased left atrial size is a risk factor for chronic atrial fibrillation.

V-30. **The answer is B.** *(Chap. 233)* The AFFIRM and RACE trials compared outcomes in survival and thromboembolic events in patients with atrial fibrillation using two treatment strategies: rate control and anticoagulation versus pharmacotherapy to maintain sinus rhythm. There was no difference in events in the two groups, which is thought to be due to the inefficiencies of pharmacotherapy, with over half of patients failing drug therapy, and also the high rates of asymptomatic atrial fibrillation in the sinus rhythm group. Thus, when considering discontinuation of anticoagulation in patients who have maintained sinus rhythm, placing a prolonged ECG monitor is recommended to ensure that asymptomatic atrial fibrillation is not present. Because of the risk of QT prolongation and polymorphic ventricular tachycardia, initiation of dofetilide and sotalol in the hospital is recommended.

V-31. **The answer is C.** *(Chap. 233)* The patient has atrial flutter, which has a high risk of thromboembolic events and should be treated the same as atrial fibrillation. If atrial flutter has been present for more than 24–48 hours without anticoagulation, a transesophageal echocardiogram may be performed to rule out left atrial thrombus. If this is not present, cardioversion may be attempted, with anticoagulation continued for 1 month if successful. Transthoracic echocardiography is inadequate to rule out left atrial thrombus. The patient is hemodynamically stable and has no indications for acute cardioversion. Dabigatran is not currently FDA approved for atrial flutter. Intravenous heparin should be started immediately if there are no contraindications, given the greater than 12-hour duration of symptoms.

V-32. **The answer is B.** *(Chap. 233)* The ECG shows at least three different P-wave morphologies with three different PR intervals, which is the hallmark of multifocal atrial tachycardia. This is the signature tachycardia of patients with significant pulmonary disease and is commonly seen in patients with chronic obstructive pulmonary disease, as suggested by diffuse polyphonic expiratory wheezing and hyperinflation.

V-33. **The answer is D.** *(Chap. 233)* The patient has classic symptoms for an AV nodal reentrant tachycardia. The so-called frog sign (prominent venous pulsations in the neck due to cannon A waves seen in AV dissociation) on physical examination is frequently present and suggests simultaneous atrial and ventricular contraction. First-line therapy for these reentrant narrow complex tachyarrhythmias is carotid sinus massage to increase vagal tone. Often this is all that is required to return the patient to sinus rhythm. If that is not successful, IV adenosine 6–12 mg may be attempted. If adenosine fails, intravenous beta blockers or calcium channel blockers may be used (diltiazem or verapamil). Finally, in hemodynamically compromised patients or those who have failed to respond to previous measures, DC cardioversion with 100–200 J is indicated.

V-34. **The answer is D.** *(Chap. 233)* The patient has an accessory conduction pathway, as evidenced by the delta waves on his baseline ECG. He now presents with atrial fibrillation through the accessory pathway. The wide complex is not due to ventricular arrhythmia but rather the aberrant accessory conduction through the accessory pathway. In general, this reentrant tachycardia may be treated as all others, with the exception of avoiding digoxin and verapamil, both of which may cause deterioration to ventricular fibrillation. Digoxin is thought to shorten the refractory period of the accessory pathway and thus can precipitate degeneration to ventricular fibrillation. Verapamil is thought to cause systemic vasodilation, with a resultant increase in sympathetic tone, and thus may precipitate ventricular fibrillation as well.

V-35. **The answer is A.** *(Chap. 233)* Atrial-ventricular dissociation is a classic finding in ventricular tachycardia. Physical examination may show jugular vein cannon A waves when the atria contracts against a closed tricuspid valve and the ECG will manifest this with atrial capture and/or fusion beats. Other findings on ECG of ventricular tachycardia include QRS duration greater than 140 milliseconds for right bundle branch pattern in V_1 or greater than 160 milliseconds for left bundle morphology in lead V_1, frontal plane axis of –90 to 180°, delayed activation during initial phase of the QRS complex, or bizarre QRS pattern that does not mimic typical right or left bundle branch block QRS complex patterns. An irregularly irregular rhythm with changing QRS complexes suggests atrial fibrillation with ventricular preexcitation. Carotid sinus massage, aimed at increasing vagal tone and slowing AV node conduction, is not effective at slowing ventricular tachycardia because the reentrant focus is below the AV node.

V-36 and V-37. **The answers are C and C, respectively.** *(Chap. 233)* The patient's rhythm is torsade de pointes, with polymorphic ventricular tachycardia and QRS complexes with variations in amplitude and cycle length, giving the appearance of oscillation about an axis. Torsades de pointes are associated with a prolonged QT interval; thus, anything that is associated with a prolonged QT can potentially cause torsade. Most commonly, electrolyte disturbances such as hypokalemia and hypomagnesemia, phenothiazines, fluoroquinolones, antiarrhythmic drugs, tricyclic antidepressants, intracranial events, and bradyarrhythmias are associated with this malignant arrhythmia. Management, besides stabilization, which may require electrical cardioversion, consists of removing the offending agent. In addition, success in rhythm termination or prevention has been reported with the administration of magnesium as well as overdrive atrial or ventricular pacing, which will shorten the QT interval. Beta blockers are indicated for patients with congenital long QT syndrome, but are not indicated in this patient.

V-38. **The answer is C.** *(Chap. 233)* There are three main mechanisms by which arrhythmias are initiated and maintained: automaticity, afterdepolarizations, and reentry. Automaticity, such as that seen with sinus tachycardia, atrial premature complexes, and some atrial tachycardias, is due to an increase in the slope of phase 4 of the action potential. The depolarization threshold is reached more quickly and repeatedly. Afterdepolarizations are associated with an increase in cellular calcium accumulation, leading to repeated myocardial depolarization during phase 3 (early) and phase 4 (delayed) of the action potential. Early afterdepolarizations may be related to the initiation of torsades de pointes. Delayed afterdepolarizations are responsible for arrhythmias related to digoxin toxicity and for catecholamine-induced ventricular tachycardia. Reentry is due to inhomogeneities in myocardial conduction and refractory periods. With reentry, conduction is blocked in one pathway, allowing slow conduction in the other. This allows for sufficient delay so that the blocked site has time for reentry and propagation of the tachycardia within the two pathways. Reentry appears to be the mechanism for most supraventricular and ventricular tachycardias.

V-39. **The answer is C.** *(Chap. 233)* The mechanisms for atrial fibrillation initiation and maintenance are still debated; however, there are anatomic structures that play a role in both of these processes. Muscularized tissue at the orifices of the pulmonary vein inlets are the predominant anatomic drivers of atrial fibrillation, although metabolic disturbances (e.g., hyperthyroidism, inflammation, infection) are also very common. Radiofrequency ablation of the tissue in the area of the pulmonary vein inlets can terminate atrial fibrillation; however, recurrences are not uncommon and other anatomic drivers may be present. The left atrial appendage is an important site of thrombus formation in patients with atrial fibrillation. Any focus within the left or right atrium can be a focus of reentry of focal atrial tachycardia, including the mitral annulus or sinus venosus. Increased automaticity of the sinus node is the mechanism for sinus tachycardia.

V-40. **The answer is B.** *(Chap. 233)* Symptoms of atrial fibrillation vary dramatically. The most common symptom is tachypalpitations; however, the hemodynamic effects account for symptoms of impaired left ventricular filling. In atrial fibrillation, there is not an effective atrial contraction to augment late-diastolic left ventricular filling. In patients with impaired ventricular diastolic function, this loss of effective atrial contraction causes impaired left ventricular filling, increased left atrial filling pressures, and pulmonary congestion. These hemodynamic effects are more common in the elderly and in patients with long-standing hypertension, hypertrophic cardiomyopathy, and obstructive aortic valve disease. The tachycardia of atrial fibrillation further compromises left ventricular filling and increases atrial filling pressures. Atrial fibrillation may occur with acute alcohol intoxication, with warming of hypothermic patients, and postoperatively after thoracic surgery. The magnitude of the hemodynamic effect and symptoms will be related to ventricular rate (a slower rate allows more time for left ventricular filling) and underlying cardiac function.

V-41. **The answer is E.** *(Chap. 234)* The patient presents with evidence of heart failure by history, and physical examination confirms this diagnosis. Physical examination also shows exophthalmos and a fine tremor, which are suggestive of hyperthyroidism. Thyrotoxicosis, along with anemia, nutritional disorders, and systemic arteriovenous shunting, can all cause high-output heart failure. Although systolic and diastolic dysfunction are more common causes of heart failure, disorders associated with a high-output state are often reversible, and therefore a diagnosis should be pursued when clinical clues suggest this may be present.

V-42. **The answer is C.** *(Chap. 234)* Circulating levels of natriuretic peptides may be a useful adjunctive tool in the diagnosis of heart failure, but they cannot replace clinical judgment. BNP or N-terminal BNP are most commonly used and are released from the failing heart, though their release is not specific to left or right heart failure; thus, elevations are commonly seen in cor pulmonale associated with pulmonary vascular disease as well as in patients with left heart failure. Additionally, there are a number of factors that may affect the level of BNP that is normally released from the failing heart. Age and renal dysfunction increase plasma BNP levels. Obesity is associated with falsely low BNP levels. Although BNP levels may normalize after therapy, serial monitoring of this peptide is not presently recommended as a guide for heart failure therapy.

V-43. **The answer is E.** *(Chap. 234)* Several drugs have been shown to prevent disease progression in heart failure including ACE inhibitors, angiotensin receptor blockers, beta blockers, and aldosterone antagonists. ACE inhibition has been shown to improve symptoms and survival, reduce cardiac hypertrophy, and reduce hospitalizations. Its use is often complicated by cough related to kinin potentiation, which is an acceptable reason to switch to an angiotensin receptor blocker. Digoxin therapy has not been shown to improve survival, may be associated with dose toxicity, and in patients with stable disease who are not frequently hospitalized, can usually be withdrawn. Beta blocker therapy may occasionally be associated with worsening heart failure symptoms at the time of initiation, but this can usually be managed with increased diuretics. The benefits of beta blockers would far outweigh the nuisance of occasional extra diuretics in this patient. Aldosterone antagonists such as spironolactone and eplerenone are recommended for patients with EF less than 35% who are receiving standard therapy as above. There is no known benefit to one member of this class of drugs over another.

V-44. **The answer is E.** *(Chap. 234)* Although there is a wealth of information on which drugs will improve symptoms and survival in heart failure with reduced ejection fraction, little is known about heart failure with preserved ejection fraction. In fact, there are no proven or approved pharmacologic therapies for patients with heart failure and preserved ejection fraction. Therapy should be aimed at treating the predisposing factors for development of this condition, i.e., treat systemic hypertension if present, reverse ischemia if appropriate, etc. Precipitating factors, such as dietary indiscretion in this patient, atrial fibrillation, or infection, may be addressed to improve symptoms. Sildenafil is currently only approved for therapy of pulmonary arterial hypertension and is not proven to be useful for pulmonary hypertension associated with heart failure with preserved ejection fraction.

V-45. **The answer is C.** *(Chap. 234)* The New York Heart Association (NYHA) classification is a tool to define criteria that describe the functional ability and clinical manifestations of patients in heart failure. It is also used in patients with pulmonary hypertension. These criteria have been shown to have prognostic value with worsening survival as class increases. They are also useful to clinicians when reading studies to understand the entry and exclusion criteria of large clinical trials. Class I is used for patients with no limiting symptoms; class II for patients with slight or mild limitation; class III implies no symptoms at rest but dyspnea or angina or palpitations with little exertion—patients are moderately limited; class IV is used for severely limited patients in whom even minimal activity causes symptoms. Treatment guidelines also frequently base recommendations on these clinical stages. This patient has symptoms with mild exertion but is comfortable at rest; therefore, he is NYHA class III.

V-46. **The answer is B.** *(Chap. 234)* Patients with severe congestive heart failure often exhibit Cheyne-Stokes breathing, defined as intercurrent short periods of hypoventilation and hyperventilation. The mechanism is thought to relate to the prolonged circulation time between the lungs and the respiratory control centers in the brain, leading to poor respiratory control of $PaCO_2$. The degree of Cheyne-Stokes breathing is related to the severity of heart failure. This pattern of breathing is different from obstructive sleep apnea, which is notable for loud snoring, periods of apnea, and sudden waking. Patients are also often hypersomnolent during the day. While sleep apnea is managed with weight loss and overnight CPAP, Cheyne-Stokes breathing is difficult to address as it is often a sign of advanced systolic dysfunction and implies a poor prognosis. All efforts to further maximize heart failure management are indicated. A sleep study would demonstrate this pattern of breathing, but this history and clinical presentation is typical. There is no role for bronchodilators or an electroencephalogram.

V-47. **The answer is B.** *(Chap. 235)* Coronary artery disease is a common late complication after cardiac transplantation and is thought to be due to a primary immunologic injury of the vascular endothelium, though it is influenced by nonimmunologic factors such as dyslipidemia, diabetes mellitus, and cytomegalovirus infection. Use of mycophenolate mofetil and the mammalian target of rapamycin sirolimus have been associated with a lower short-term incidence of coronary intimal thickening. Similarly, statin use has been shown to reduce the incidence of this complication. Because donors are generally young, the coronary artery disease after transplantation is not thought to be due to coronary lesions present pretransplantation.

V-48. **The answer is E.** *(Chap. 234)* Ventricular assist device therapy can be used either as a "bridge" to transplantation in eligible candidates or as a final destination in patients with end-stage heart failure who are not transplant candidates. There are four FDA-approved devices, all of which share common complications including thromboembolism, cerebrovascular accident, device failure, and infection.

V-49. **The answer is E.** *(Chap. 236)* Atrial septal defect (ASD) is a not uncommon simple congenital heart disease lesion that is often diagnosed in adults. Because of chronic left-to-right shunting of intracardiac blood, pulmonary arterial hypertension is a well-recognized common complication. With the development of pulmonary arterial hypertension, the potential for paradoxical embolization of either air or thrombotic material from the right atrium to the systemic circulation is increased. Similarly, with exertion in the context of pulmonary arterial hypertension and ASD, blood may shunt right to left, leading to systemic arterial oxygen desaturation. Atrial fibrillation or other supraventricular arrhythmias may occur, also as a result of atrial stretching with the lesion. While atherosclerosis and unstable angina may certainly occur in adults, is not a reported complication of ASD.

V-50. **The answer is D.** *(Chap. 236)* The patient has secondary erythrocytosis due to Eisenmenger's syndrome and chronic arterial hypoxemia. Her partially corrected left-to-right shunt resulted in chronic pulmonary circulation overflow and the subsequent development of pulmonary arterial hypertension. With a rise in pulmonary vascular pressure, the shunt reverses to become predominantly right to left, which causes systemic oxygen desaturation. Because hypoxemia is caused by shunt and not ventilation/perfusion mismatch (as in typical COPD), it is not responsive to oxygen therapy. Peripheral desaturation results in decreased oxygen delivery to the kidneys, increased erythropoietin secretion, and resultant erythrocytosis. Erythropoietin levels would be expected to be elevated in this case (in contrast to polycythemia vera rubra). Phlebotomy is only used for patients with symptomatic erythrocytosis; hyperviscosity symptoms, including neurologic symptoms such as transient ischemic attack; epistaxis or bleeding symptoms; or visual changes. Because iron depletion may worsen viscosity even at a lower hematocrit, it is considered as only a temporary therapy for management of erythrocytosis in Eisenmenger's syndrome. This patient had no symptoms referable to erythrocytosis; therefore, expectant management is most appropriate.

V-51. **The answer is D.** *(Chap. 236)* Routine antibiotic prophylaxis is indicated for bacteremic dental procedures or instrumentation through an infected site in most patients with operated congenital heart disease, particularly whenever foreign material is present. The one exception is patches that don't have a post-placement high-grade leak, where prophylaxis is only required for 6 months until endothelialization.

V-52. **The answer is E.** *(Chap. 236)* The patient presents with dextrocardia on his chest radiograph and situs inversus, or complete mirror image situs inversus on examination. When dextrocardia occurs in isolation without situs inversus, multiple cardiac abnormalities are frequently present. Alternatively, when dextrocardia occurs with situs inversus, other cardiac defects are unlikely. Kartagener's syndrome with mucociliary dysfunction may underlie situs inversus, but it is associated with sinusitis and chronic bronchitis, which this patient did not have.

V-53 and V-54. **The answers are C and A, respectively.** *(Chap. 236)* This patient has a coarctation of the aorta presenting with marked hypertension proximal to the lesion. The narrowing most commonly occurs distal to the origin of the left subclavian artery, explaining the equal pressure in the arms and reduced pressure in the legs. Coarctations account for approximately 7% of congenital cardiac abnormalities, occur more frequently (2×) in men than in women, and are associated with gonadal dysgenesis and bicuspid aortic valves. Adults will present with hypertension, manifestations of hypertension in the upper body (headache, epistaxis), or leg claudication. Physical examination reveals diminished and/or delayed lower extremity pulses, enlarged collateral vessels in the upper body, or reduced development of the lower extremities. Cardiac examination may reveal findings consistent with left ventricular (LV) hypertrophy. There may be no murmur, a midsystolic murmur over the anterior chest and back, or an aortic murmur with a bicuspid valve. Transthoracic (suprasternal/parasternal) or transesophageal echocardiography, contrast CT or MRI of the thorax, or cardiac catheterization can be diagnostic. MRI of the head would not be useful diagnostically. The clinical picture is not consistent with renal artery stenosis, pheochromocytoma, carcinoid, or Cushing's syndrome.

V-55. **The answer is E.** *(Chap. 237)* Mitral stenosis is one of the leading causes of pulmonary hypertension worldwide, particularly in developing countries where the treatment of streptococcal disease is less available. The primary determinants of pulmonary artery pressure are left atrial pressure, pulmonary vascular resistance, and flow. Mitral stenosis may restrict flow from the left atrium to the left ventricle, and thus is associated with left atrial hypertension and passive pulmonary hypertension (due to back pressure). Additionally, the pulmonary vascular bed may actively vasoconstrict in response to left atrial hypertension. Additional contributors to pulmonary hypertension in mitral stenosis include interstitial edema in the walls of small pulmonary vessels and, in end-stage disease, obliterative changes in the pulmonary vascular bed as may be seen in some forms of pulmonary arterial hypertension. Pulmonary hypertension related to mitral stenosis is generally reversible with correction of the valvular lesion.

V-56 and V-57. **The answers are A and E, respectively.** *(Chap. 237)* The patient presents with a relatively stable ST elevation myocardial infarction. He likely has extensive necrosis given the duration of symptoms and ECG findings, and thus is at risk for complication of myocardial infarction. In this case, his acute dyspnea, worsening oxygenation, and asymmetric edema on chest radiograph all point to acute mitral regurgitation from papillary muscle rupture. An allergic reaction to a medication should not cause severe hypoxemia. It may cause rather mild reversible hypoxemia, and should not cause an abnormal chest radiograph. The classic finding of acute mitral regurgitation is a relatively loud systolic murmur heard best at the apex and radiating to the axilla. The murmur is described as having a "cooing" or "seagull-like" quality. A fourth heart sound is also common. Management of acute mitral regurgitation includes afterload and preload reduction, if possible, often with intravenous nitroprusside. If patients are unable to tolerate medical interventions to achieve this because of systemic hypotension, as in this patient, an intraaortic balloon pump is indicated. Albuterol and methylprednisolone are indicated for acute bronchospasm due to primary airways disease, but would not be helpful for the management of cardiogenic shock.

V-58. **The answer is C.** *(Chap. 237)* The patient has classic physical examination findings for mitral valve prolapse with a midsystolic click that may or may not be associated with a systolic murmur. Mitral valve prolapse is generally thought to be a benign lesion, with most patients never developing symptoms during their lifetimes. While many patients with heritable connective tissue disorders such as Marfan's syndrome have mitral valve prolapse, in the majority of cases, a cause is not identified. Mitral valve prolapse may be seen on echocardiography by systolic displacement of the mitral valve leaflets by at least 2 mm into the left atrium. Doppler imaging may also be helpful to define the condition. Because the lesion is generally benign, endocarditis prophylaxis is generally not indicated unless the patient has a prior history of endocarditis. Although some patients develop atrial arrhythmias in conjunction with mitral valve prolapse, prophylactic antiplatelet agents or warfarin are not recommended, as most patients do not have complications.

V-59. **The answer is B.** *(Chap. 237)* The patient has aortic stenosis that presented late in life. While bicuspid aortic valve underlies nearly half of all aortic stenosis cases, this lesion typically presents earlier in life, and only 40% of patients greater than 70 years old with aortic stenosis who undergo surgery have a bicuspid valve. Rheumatic heart disease may cause aortic stenosis, but almost invariably mitral stenosis is also present. Underlying connective tissue disease is not known to be associated. Modern research on the development of aortic stenosis has shown that several traditional atherosclerotic risk factors are present such as diabetes mellitus, smoking, chronic kidney disease, and the metabolic syndrome.

Polymorphisms of the vitamin D receptor have also been demonstrated in patients with symptomatic aortic stenosis.

V-60. **The answer is C.** *(Chap. 237)* Exertional syncope is a late finding in aortic stenosis (AS) and portends a poor prognosis. Patients with this symptom or with angina pectoris have an average time to death of 3 years. Patients with dyspnea have 2 years, and patients with heart failure have an average time to death of 1.5–2 years. Because of these data, patients with severe AS and symptoms should be strongly considered for surgical therapy.

V-61. **The answer is A.** *(Chap. 237)* Patients with severe aortic regurgitation will have a "water-hammer" pulse that collapses suddenly as arterial pressure rapidly falls during late systole and diastole, a so-called Corrigan's pulse. Capillary pulsations seen in the nail bed in severe aortic regurgitation are named Quincke's pulse. Traube's sign, or a pistol shot sound, may be heard over the femoral arteries and Duroziez's sign, with a to-and-fro murmur over the femoral artery, have also been described. Pulsus parvus et tardus is found in severe aortic stenosis. Pulsus bigeminus occurs when there is a shorter interval after a normal beat with a following low volume pulse, often with a premature ventricular beat. Pulsus paradoxus has been described with pericardial tamponade or severe obstructive lung disease. Pulsus alternans is alternating large and small volume pulses seen in severe heart failure.

V-62 and V-63. **The answers are C and C, respectively.** *(Chap. 237)* The patient presents with heart failure during her second trimester from a region with high rates of rheumatic fever. She is therefore at risk for rheumatic mitral stenosis, which often presents during the second trimester of pregnancy as the cardiac output must rise to accommodate the fetus and intravascular volume expands substantially. The stenotic valve cannot accommodate the increased flow demands of pregnancy, and congestive heart failure ensues with secondary pulmonary venous hypertension. The patient has evidence of heart failure on examination with pulmonary hypertension. Her diastolic rumble is characteristic of mitral stenosis. Finally, hemoptysis is a not infrequent finding in severe mitral stenosis and may be due to the rupture of pulmonary-bronchial venous connections secondary to pulmonary venous hypertension. Occasionally, pink frothy sputum can be found in patients with frank alveolar hemorrhage related to elevated pulmonary capillary pressure. Mitral stenosis is readily demonstrated by echocardiography. While right heart catheterization may demonstrate pulmonary hypertension and an elevated pulmonary capillary wedge pressure, the etiology of these findings will remain unknown without imaging of the left heart. Short-term management of mitral stenosis with heart failure should include diuretics. As the patient does not have left ventricular failure, ACE inhibition and digoxin are not likely to alleviate her symptoms. Occasionally, beta blockade may improve symptoms, particularly in patients with symptomatic atrial arrhythmias. Anticoagulation is not indicated in mitral stenosis alone unless atrial arrhythmias or pulmonary embolism is present. As infection does not underlie the patient's hemoptysis, further antibiotics will not be helpful.

V-64. **The answer is D.** *(Chap. 237)* Indications for surgical repair of mitral regurgitation are dependent on left-ventricular function, ventricular size, and the presence of sequelae of chronic mitral regurgitation. The experience of the surgeon and the likelihood of successful mitral valve repair are also important considerations. The management strategy for chronic severe mitral regurgitation depends on the presence of symptoms, left-ventricular function, left-ventricular dimensions, and the presence of complicating factors such as pulmonary hypertension and atrial fibrillation. With very depressed left-ventricular function (<30% or end-systolic dimension >55 mm), the risk of surgery increases, left-ventricular recovery is often incomplete, and long-term survival is reduced. However, since medical therapy offers little for these patients, surgical repair should be considered if there is a high likelihood of success (>90%). When ejection fraction is between 30% and 60%, and end-systolic dimension rises above 40 mm, surgical repair is indicated even in the absence of symptoms, owing to the excellent long-term results achieved in this group. Waiting for worsening left-ventricular function leads to irreversible left-ventricular remodeling. Pulmonary hypertension and atrial fibrillation are important to consider as markers for worsening regurgitation. For asymptomatic patients with normal left-ventricular function and dimensions, the presence of new pulmonary hypertension or atrial fibrillation in patients with normal ejection fraction and end-systolic dimensions are class IIa indications for mitral valve repair.

V-65.   **The answer is F.** *(Chap. 237)* Tricuspid regurgitation is most commonly caused by dilation of the tricuspid annulus due to right-ventricular enlargement of any cause. Any cause of left-ventricular failure that results in right-ventricular failure may lead to tricuspid regurgitation. Congenital heart diseases or pulmonary arterial hypertension leading to right-ventricular failure will dilate the tricuspid annulus. Inferior wall infarction may involve the right ventricle. Rheumatic heart disease may involve the tricuspid valve, although less commonly than the mitral valve. Infective endocarditis, particularly in IV drug users, will infect the tricuspid valve, causing vegetations and regurgitation. Other causes of tricuspid regurgitation include carcinoid heart disease, endomyocardial fibrosis, congenital defects of the atrioventricular canal, and right-ventricular pacemakers.

V-66.   **The answer is A.** *(Chap. 237)* Bioprosthetic valves are made from human, porcine, or bovine tissue. The major advantage of a bioprosthetic valve is the low incidence of thromboembolic phenomena, particularly 3 months after implantation. Although in the immediate postoperative period some anticoagulation may occur, after 3 months there is no further need for anticoagulation or monitoring. The downside is the natural history and longevity of the bioprosthetic valve. Bioprosthetic valves tend to degenerate mechanically. Approximately 50% will need replacement at 15 years. Therefore, these valves are useful in patients with contraindications to anticoagulation, such as elderly patients with comorbidities and younger patients who desire to become pregnant. Elderly people may also be spared the need for repeat surgery, as their life span may be shorter than the natural history of the bioprosthesis. Mechanical valves offer superior durability. Hemodynamic parameters are improved with double-disk valves compared with single-disk or ball-and-chain valves. However, thrombogenicity is high and chronic anticoagulation is mandatory. Younger patients with no contraindications to anticoagulation may be better served by mechanical valve replacement.

V-67.   **The answer is E.** *(Chap. 238)* Many infectious etiologies have been associated with the development of inflammatory myocarditis including viral agents (coxsackie, adenovirus, HIV, hepatitis C) and parasitic agents, with Chagas disease or *T. cruzi* being most prominent, but also toxoplasmosis. Additionally, bacterial etiologies like diphtheria, spirochetal disease like *Borrelia burgdorferi*, rickettsial disease, and fungal infections have been associated.

V-68.   **The answer is C.** *(Chap. 238)* Peripartum cardiomyopathy is a rare complication of pregnancy and can occur during the last trimester or within the first 6 months postpartum. Risk factors include advanced age, increased parity, twin pregnancy, malnutrition, use of tocolytic therapy for premature labor, and preeclampsia.

V-69.   **The answer is A.** *(Chap. 238)* Beriberi heart disease is a dilated cardiomyopathy due to thiamine deficiency. While uncommon in developed countries, this condition still occurs in patients who derive most of their calories from alcohol and has been reported in teenagers who eat only highly processed foods. This condition involves systemic vasodilation with a very high cardiac output in its early stages. In advanced disease, a low-output state can occur. Thiamine repletion can lead to a complete recovery. Patient A has evidence of heart failure with systemic vasodilation and elevated cardiac output, as would be found in beriberi. Alternatively, patient B has normal hemodynamics. Patient C has evidence of low-output heart failure with systemic vasoconstriction. Patient D has elevated pulmonary arterial pressures with right heart failure in conjunction with normal pulmonary capillary wedge pressure, consistent with primary pulmonary vascular disease, e.g., pulmonary arterial hypertension. Patient E has low right heart filling pressures, with somewhat low cardiac output and elevated systemic vascular resistance, as might be found in hypovolemic shock.

V-70. **The answer is E.** *(Chap. 238)* Hypertrophic cardiomyopathy usually presents between age 20 and 40 years, with the most common symptom being dyspnea. Many patients are, however, asymptomatic and the only clue to the presence of this potentially deadly disease is physical examination. Physical examination will show a harsh systolic murmur heard best at the left lower sternal border arising from both the outflow tract turbulence during ventricular ejection and the often concomitant mitral regurgitation. Maneuvers that decrease ventricular volume such as Valsalva or moving from squatting to standing will enhance the murmur. Conversely, maneuvers that increase left ventricular volume will decrease the murmur's intensity. These include hand grip and squatting. Having the patient lie with the left side down and leaning forward may make the friction rub of pericarditis more audible.

V-71. **The answer is E.** *(Chap. 238)* A common diagnostic dilemma is differentiating constrictive pericarditis from a restrictive cardiomyopathy. Elevated jugular venous pressure is almost universally present in both. Kussmaul's sign (increase or no change in jugular venous pressure with inspiration) can be seen in both conditions. Other signs of heart failure do not reliably distinguish the two conditions. In restrictive cardiomyopathy, the apical impulse is usually easier to palpate than in constrictive pericarditis, and mitral regurgitation is more common. These clinical signs, however, are not reliable to differentiate the two entities. In conjunction with clinical information and additional imaging studies of the left ventricle and pericardium, certain pathognomic findings increase diagnostic certainty. A thickened or calcified pericardium increases the likelihood of constrictive pericarditis. Conduction abnormalities are more common in infiltrating diseases of the myocardium. In constrictive pericarditis, measurements of diastolic pressures will show equilibrium between the ventricles, while unequal pressures and/or isolated elevated left ventricular pressures are more consistent with restrictive cardiomyopathy. The classic "square root sign" during right heart catheterization (deep, sharp drop in right ventricular pressure in early diastole, followed by a plateau during which there is no further increase in right ventricular pressure) can be seen in both restrictive cardiomyopathy and constrictive pericarditis. The presence of a paraprotein abnormality (MGUS, myeloma, amyloid) makes restrictive cardiomyopathy more common.

V-72. **The answer is D.** *(Chap. 238)* Cardiac involvement is common in many of the neuromuscular diseases. The ECG pattern of Duchenne's muscular dystrophy is unique and consists of tall R waves in the right precordial leads with an R/S ratio greater than 1.0, often with deep Q waves in the limb and precordial leads. These patients often have a variety of supraventricular and ventricular arrhythmias, and are at risk for sudden death due to the intrinsic cardiomyopathy as well as the low ejection fraction. Implantable cardioverter defibrillators should be considered in the appropriate patient. Global left ventricular dysfunction is a common finding in dilated cardiomyopathies, whereas focal wall motion abnormalities and angina are more common if there is ischemic myocardium. This patient is at risk for venous thromboembolism; however, chronic thromboembolism would not account for the severity of the left heart failure and would present with findings consistent with pulmonary hypertension. Amyotrophic lateral sclerosis is a disease of motor neurons and does not involve the heart. This patient would be young for that diagnosis. An advanced atrial septal defect would present with cyanosis and heart failure (Eisenmenger's physiology).

V-73. **The answer is D.** *(Chap. 239)* The patient has a classic presentation for acute pericarditis with constant or pleuritic chest pain, exacerbated by lying flat and alleviated by sitting forward. Serum biomarkers may show mild evidence of myocardial injury from myocardial inflammation, but are generally not substantially elevated. Friction rub is frequently present, has three components, and is best heard while the patient is upright and leaning forward. In the acute stages, ECG classically shows ST-segment elevation with upward concavity in two or three standard limb leads and V_2 through V_6 with reciprocal changes in aVR. Convex curvature is more commonly found in acute myocardial infarction. PR depression may be found. After several days, the ST changes resolve and T waves become inverted. After weeks to months, the ECG returns to normal.

V-74. **The answer is B.** (*Chap. 239*) Pulsus paradoxus is an exaggeration of the normal phenomenon in which systolic blood pressure declines 10 mmHg or less with inspiration. Pulsus paradoxus is typically seen in patients with pericardial tamponade and in patients with severe obstructive lung disease (COPD, asthma). In pulsus paradoxus due to pericardial tamponade, the inspiratory systolic blood pressure decline is greater due to the tight incompressible pericardial sac. The right ventricle distends with inspiration, compressing the left ventricle and resulting in decreased systolic pulse pressure in the systemic circulation. In severe obstructive lung disease, the inspiratory decline of systolic blood pressure may be due to the markedly negative pleural pressure either causing left ventricular compression (due to increased RV venous return) or increased LV impedance to ejection (increased afterload).

V-75. **The answer is C.** (*Chap. 239*) Beck's triad can be used to alert clinicians to the potential presence of cardiac tamponade. The principal features are hypotension, muffled or absent heart sounds, and elevated neck veins, often with prominent x-descent and absent y-descent. These are due to the failure of ventricular filling and limited cardiac output. Kussmaul's sign is seen in restrictive cardiomyopathy and pericardial constriction, not tamponade. Friction rub may be seen in any condition associated with pericardial inflammation.

V-76. **The answer is D.** (*Chap. 239*) This patient's presentation and physical examination are most consistent with the diagnosis of constrictive pericarditis. The most common cause of constrictive pericarditis worldwide is tuberculosis, but given the low incidence of tuberculosis in the United States, constrictive pericarditis is a rare condition in this country. With the increasing ability to cure Hodgkin's disease with mediastinal irradiation, many cases of constrictive pericarditis in the United States involve patients who received curative radiation therapy 10–20 years prior. These patients are also at risk for premature coronary artery disease. Risks for these complications include dose of radiation and radiation windows that include the heart. Other rare causes of constrictive pericarditis are recurrent acute pericarditis, hemorrhagic pericarditis, prior cardiac surgery, mediastinal irradiation, chronic infection, and neoplastic disease. Physiologically, constrictive pericarditis is characterized by the inability of the ventricles to fill because of the noncompliant pericardium. In early diastole, the ventricles fill rapidly, but filling stops abruptly when the elastic limit of the pericardium is reached. Clinically, patients present with generalized malaise, cachexia, and anasarca. Exertional dyspnea is common, and orthopnea is generally mild. Ascites and hepatomegaly occur because of increased venous pressure. In rare cases, cirrhosis may develop from chronic congestive hepatopathy. The jugular venous pressure is elevated, and the neck veins fail to collapse on inspiration (Kussmaul's sign). Heart sounds may be muffled. A pericardial knock is frequently heard. This is a third heart sound that occurs 0.09–0.12 seconds after aortic valve closure at the cardiac apex. Right heart catheterization would show the "square root sign" characterized by an abrupt y-descent followed by a gradual rise in ventricular pressure. This finding, however, is not pathognomonic of constrictive pericarditis and can be seen in restrictive cardiomyopathy of any cause. Echocardiogram shows a thickened pericardium, dilatation of the inferior vena cava and hepatic veins, and an abrupt cessation of ventricular filling in early diastole. Pericardial resection is the only definitive treatment of constrictive pericarditis. Diuresis and sodium restriction are useful in managing volume status preoperatively, and paracentesis may be necessary. Operative mortality ranges from 5–10%. Underlying cardiac function is normal; thus, cardiac transplantation is not indicated. Pericardiocentesis is indicated for the diagnostic removal of pericardial fluid and cardiac tamponade, which is not present on the patient's echocardiogram. Mitral valve stenosis may present similarly with anasarca, congestive hepatic failure, and ascites. However, pulmonary edema and pleural effusions are also common. Examination would be expected to demonstrate a diastolic murmur, and echocardiogram should show a normal pericardium and a thickened immobile mitral valve. Mitral valve replacement would be indicated if mitral stenosis were the cause of the patient's symptoms.

V-77. **The answer is C.** (*Chap. 240*) Blunt, nonpenetrating trauma such as that described here can result in commotio cordis, which occurs when the trauma impacts the heart during the susceptible phase of repolarization just before the peak of the T wave and results in ventricular fibrillation. This syndrome is most common in young athletes who are playing hockey, football, baseball, or lacrosse, for example. Treatment is prompt defibrillation. While aortic rupture, myocardial rupture with cardiac tamponade, and tension pneumothorax may occur with chest wall trauma, their presentation should be less immediate after the trauma. Hypertrophic cardiomyopathy may present with sudden cardiac death, as in this case, but the preceding chest trauma makes commotio cordis more likely.

V-78. **The answer is E.** *(Chap. 247)* The patient presents with prehypertension, as evidenced by systolic blood pressure of 120–139 mmHg or diastolic blood pressure of 80–89 mmHg. Although at this blood pressure medication therapy is not indicated, the MRFIT trial clearly showed a graded influence of both systolic and diastolic blood pressure on cardiovascular mortality including down to within normal range at 120 mmHg systolic. Thus, lifestyle modification is in order for the patient described here. Alcohol consumption is recommended to be two or fewer drinks per day for men and one drink or less per day for women. NaCl consumption of less than 6 g per day has been shown to reduce blood pressure in patients with established hypertension and in certain ethnic groups. To reduce blood pressure, regular moderate to intense aerobic activity for 30 minutes 6–7 days per week is recommended. Finally, a weight loss of 9.2 kg has been shown to drop blood pressure on average 6/3 mmHg.

V-79. **The answer is C.** *(Chap. 247)* Several factors have been shown to confer an increased risk of complications from hypertension. In the patient described here there is only one: ongoing tobacco use. Epidemiologic factors that have poorer prognosis include African-American race, male sex, and onset of hypertension in youth. In addition, comorbid factors that independently increase the risk of atherosclerosis worsen the prognosis in patients with hypertension. These factors include hypercholesterolemia, obesity, diabetes mellitus, and tobacco use. Physical and laboratory examination showing evidence of end organ damage also may portend a poorer prognosis. This includes evidence of retinal damage or hypertensive heart disease with cardiac enlargement or congestive heart failure. Furthermore, electrocardiographic evidence of ischemia or left ventricular strain but not left ventricular hypertrophy alone may predict worse outcomes. A family history of hypertensive complications does not worsen the prognosis if diastolic blood pressure is maintained at less than 110 mmHg.

V-80 and V-81. **The answers are D and E, respectively.** *(Chap. 247)* This patient presents at a young age with hypertension that is difficult to control, raising the question of secondary causes of hypertension. The most likely diagnosis in this patient is primary hyperaldosteronism, also known as Conn's syndrome. The patient has no physical features that suggest congenital adrenal hyperplasia or Cushing's syndrome. In addition, there is no glucose intolerance, as is commonly seen in Cushing's syndrome. The lack of episodic symptoms and the labile hypertension make pheochromocytoma unlikely. The findings of hypokalemia and metabolic alkalosis in the presence of difficult to control hypertension yield the likely diagnosis of Conn's syndrome. Diagnosis of the disease can be difficult, but the preferred test is the plasma aldosterone/renin ratio. This test should be performed at 8 a.m., and a ratio above 30 to 50 is diagnostic of primary hyperaldosteronism. Caution should be taken in interpreting this test while the patient is on ACE inhibitor therapy, as ACE inhibitors can falsely elevate plasma renin activity. However, a plasma renin level that is undetectable or an elevated aldosterone/renin ratio in the presence of ACE inhibitor therapy is highly suggestive of primary hyperaldosteronism. Selective adrenal vein renin sampling may be performed after the diagnosis to help determine if the process is unilateral or bilateral. Although fibromuscular dysplasia is a common secondary cause of hypertension in young females, the presence of hypokalemia and metabolic alkalosis should suggest Conn's syndrome. Thus, magnetic resonance imaging of the renal arteries is unnecessary in this case. Measurement of 24-hour urine collection for potassium wasting and aldosterone secretion can be useful in the diagnosis of Conn's syndrome. The measurement of metanephrines or cortisol is not indicated.

V-82. **The answer is B.** *(Chap. 248)* For all patients with aortic dissection or hematoma, appropriate management includes reduction of shear stress with beta blockade and management of systemic hypertension to reduce tension on the dissection. However, emergent or urgent surgical therapy is indicated to patients with ascending aortic dissection and intramural hematomas (type A), and for complicated type B dissections (distal aorta). Complications that would warrant surgical intervention include propagation despite medical therapy, compromise of major branches, impending rupture, or continued pain. Thus, patient B has a distal dissection without evidence of complications and is the best candidate for medical therapy.

V-83. **The answer is B.** *(Chap. 248)* Abdominal aortic aneurysms (AAAs) affect 1–2% of men older than age 50. Most AAAs are asymptomatic and are found incidentally on physical examination. The predisposing factors for AAA are the same as those for other cardiovascular disease, with over 90% being associated with atherosclerotic disease. Most AAAs are located infrarenally, and recent data suggest that an uncomplicated infrarenal AAA may be treated with endovascular stenting instead of the usual surgical grafting. Indications for proceeding to surgery include any patient with symptoms or an aneurysm that is growing rapidly. Serial ultrasonography or CT imaging is imperative, and all aneurysms larger than 5.5 cm warrant intervention because of the high mortality associated with repair of ruptured aortic aneurysms. The rupture rate of an AAA is directly related to size, with the 5-year risk of rupture being 1–2% with aneurysms less than 5 cm and 20–40% with aneurysms greater than 5 cm. The mortality of patients undergoing elective repair is 1–2% and is greater than 50% for the emergent treatment of a ruptured AAA. Preoperative cardiac evaluation before elective repair is imperative, as coexisting coronary artery disease is common.

V-84. **The answer is E.** *(Chap. 248)* Aortitis and ascending aortic aneurysms are commonly caused by cystic medial necrosis and mesoaortitis that result in damage to the elastic fibers of the aortic wall with thinning and weakening. Many infectious, inflammatory, and inherited conditions have been associated with this finding, including syphilis, tuberculosis, mycotic aneurysm, Takayasu's arteritis, giant cell arteritis, rheumatoid arthritis, and the spondyloarthropathies (ankylosing spondylitis, psoriatic arthritis, Reiter's syndrome, Behçet's disease). In addition, it can be seen with the genetic disorders Marfan's syndrome and Ehlers-Danlos syndrome.

V-85. **The answer is E.** *(Chap. 248)* Descending aortic aneurysms are most commonly associated with atherosclerosis. The average growth rate is approximately 0.1–0.2 cm yearly. The risk of rupture and subsequent management are related to the size of the aneurysm as well as symptoms related to the aneurysm. However, most thoracic aortic aneurysms are asymptomatic. When symptoms do occur, they are frequently related to mechanical complications of the aneurysm causing compression of adjacent structures. This includes the trachea and esophagus, and symptoms can include cough, chest pain, hoarseness, and dysphagia. The risk of rupture is approximately 2–3% yearly for aneurysms less than 4 cm and increases to 7% per year once the size is greater than 6 cm. Management of descending aortic aneurysms includes blood pressure control. Beta blockers are recommended because they decrease the contractility of the heart and thus decrease aortic wall stress, potentially slowing aneurysmal growth. Individuals with thoracic aortic aneurysms should be monitored with chest imaging at least yearly, or more frequently if new symptoms develop. This can include CT angiography, MRI, or transesophageal echocardiography. Operative repair is indicated if the aneurysm expands by more than 1 cm in a year or reaches a diameter of more than 5.5–6.0 cm. Endovascular stenting for the treatment of thoracic aortic aneurysms is a relatively new procedure with limited long-term results available. The largest study to date included more than 400 patients with a variety of indications for thoracic endovascular stents. In 249 patients, the indication for stent was thoracic aortic aneurysm. This study showed an initial success rate of 87.1%, with a 30-day mortality rate of 10%. However, if the procedure was done emergently, the mortality rate at 30 days was 28%. At 1 year, data were available on only 96 of the original 249 patients with degenerative thoracic aneurysms. In these individuals, 80% continued to have satisfactory outcomes with stenting and 14% showed growth of the aneurysm (LJ Leurs, *J Vasc Surg* 40:670, 2004). Ongoing studies with long-term follow-up are needed before endovascular stenting can be recommended for the treatment of thoracic aortic aneurysms, although in individuals who are not candidates for surgery, stenting should be considered.

V-86. **The answer is C.** *(Chap. 249)* The patient presents with classic signs of arterial occlusion with limb pain, physical examination showing pallor, and a pulseless, cold leg. She has no risk factors for central or peripheral atherosclerotic disease; thus angiogram would simply confirm the diagnosis of arterial occlusion, not demonstrate her predisposing condition. In the absence of fever or systemic symptoms, vasculitis and endocarditis are unlikely sources of arterial embolization. She likely had a paradoxical embolism in the context of an atrial septal defect, which was the source of her childhood murmur. Because many of these patients develop pulmonary hypertension with time, she is now at risk for a paradoxical embolism. Although in this context, arterial emboli frequently originate from venous thrombus, the thrombi cannot produce a paradoxical embolism in the absence of right-to-left shunt, such as in a large patent foramen ovale or an atrial septal defect.

SECTION VI

Disorders of the Respiratory System

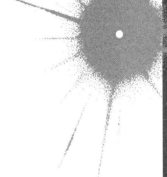

QUESTIONS

DIRECTIONS: Choose the **one best** response to each question.

VI-1. Which of the following statements regarding auscultation of the chest is TRUE?

A. Absence of breath sounds in a hemithorax is almost always associated with a pneumothorax.

B. An astute clinician should be able to differentiate "wet" from "dry" crackles.

C. "Cardiac asthma" refers to wheezing associated with alveolar edema in congestive heart failure.

D. Rhonchi are a manifestation of obstruction of medium-sized airways.

E. The presence of egophony can be used to distinguish pulmonary fibrosis from alveolar filling.

VI-2. A 72-year-old male with a long history of tobacco use is seen in the clinic for 3 weeks of progressive dyspnea on exertion. He has had a mild nonproductive cough and anorexia but denies fevers, chills, or sweats. On physical examination, he has normal vital signs and normal oxygen saturation on room air. Jugular venous pressure is normal, and cardiac examination shows decreased heart sounds but no other abnormality. The trachea is midline, and there is no associated lymphadenopathy. On pulmonary examination, the patient has dullness over the left lower lung field, decreased tactile fremitus, decreased breath sounds, and no voice transmission. The right lung examination is normal. After obtaining chest plain film, appropriate initial management at this point would include which of the following?

A. Intravenous antibiotics

B. Thoracentesis

C. Bronchoscopy

D. Deep suctioning

E. Bronchodilator therapy

VI-3. At what lung volume does the outward recoil of the chest wall equal the inward elastic recoil of the lung?

A. Expiratory reserve volume

B. Functional residual capacity

C. Residual volume

D. Tidal volume

E. Total lung capacity

VI-4. A 65-year-old man is evaluated for progressive dyspnea on exertion that has occurred over the course of the past 3 months. His medical history is significant for an episode of necrotizing pancreatitis that resulted in multiorgan failure and acute respiratory distress syndrome. He required mechanical ventilation for 6 weeks prior to his recovery. He also has a history of 30 pack-years of tobacco, quitting 15 years previously. He is not known to have chronic obstructive pulmonary disease. On physical examination, a low-pitched inspiratory and expiratory wheeze is heard that is loudest over the mid-chest area. On pulmonary function testing, the forced expiratory volume in 1 second is 2.5 L (78% predicted), forced vital capacity is 4.00 L (94% predicted), and the FEV_1/FVC ratio is 62.5%. The flow volume curve is shown in Figure VI-4. What is the most likely cause of the patient's symptoms?

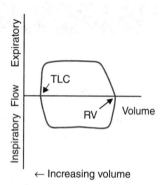

FIGURE VI-4

A. Aspirated foreign body
B. Chronic obstructive pulmonary disease
C. Idiopathic pulmonary fibrosis
D. Subglottic stenosis
E. Unilateral vocal cord paralysis

VI-5. A 32-year-old woman presents to the emergency department in her 36th week of pregnancy complaining of acute dyspnea. She has had an uncomplicated pregnancy and has no other medical problems. She is taking no medications other than prenatal vitamins. On examination, she appears dyspneic. Her vital signs are as follows: blood pressure 128/78, heart rate 126 beats/min, respiratory rate 28 breaths/min, and oxygen saturation is 96% on room air. She is afebrile. Her lung and cardiac examinations are normal. There is trace bilateral pitting pedal edema. A chest x-ray performed with abdominal shielding is normal, and the ECG demonstrates sinus tachycardia. An arterial blood gas is performed. The pH is 7.52, $PaCO_2$ is 26 mmHg, and PaO_2 is 85 mmHg. What is the next best step in the diagnosis and management of this patient?

A. Initiate therapy with amoxicillin for acute bronchitis.
B. Perform a CT pulmonary angiogram.
C. Perform an echocardiogram.
D. Reassure the patient that dyspnea is normal during this stage of pregnancy and no abnormalities are seen on testing.
E. Treat with clonazepam for a panic attack.

VI-6. Match each of the following pulmonary function test results with the respiratory disorder for which they are the most likely findings.

A. Increased total lung capacity (TLC), decreased vital capacity (VC), decreased FEV_1/FVC ratio
B. Decreased TLC, decreased VC, decreased residual volume (RV), increased FEV_1/FVC ratio, normal maximum inspiratory pressure (MIP)
C. Decreased TLC, increased RV, normal FEV_1/FVC ratio, decreased MIP
D. Normal TLC, normal RV, normal FEV_1/FVC ratio, normal MIP

1. Myasthenia gravis
2. Idiopathic pulmonary fibrosis
3. Familial pulmonary hypertension
4. Chronic obstructive pulmonary disease

VI-7. A 78-year-old woman is admitted to the medical intensive care unit with multilobar pneumonia. On initial presentation to the emergency room, her initial oxygen saturation was 60% on room air and only increased to 82% on a nonrebreather face mask. She was in marked respiratory distress and intubated in the emergency room. Upon admission to the intensive care unit, she was sedated and paralyzed. The ventilator is set in the assist-control mode with a respiratory rate of 24, tidal volume of 6 mL/kg, FiO_2 of 1.0, and positive end-expiratory pressure of 12 cmH_2O. An arterial blood gas measurement is performed on these settings; the results are pH 7.20, PCO_2 of 32 mmHg, and PO_2 of 54 mmHg. What is the cause of the hypoxemia?

A. Hypoventilation alone
B. Hypoventilation and ventilation-perfusion mismatch
C. Shunt
D. Ventilation-perfusion mismatch

VI-8. A 65-year-old man is evaluated for progressive dyspnea on exertion and dry cough that have worsened over the course of 6 months. He has not had dyspnea at rest and denies wheezing. He has not experienced chest pain. He has a history of coronary artery disease and atrial fibrillation, and underwent coronary artery bypass surgery 12 years ago. His medications include metoprolol, aspirin, warfarin, and enalapril. He previously smoked one pack of cigarettes daily for 40 years, quitting 5 years previously. His vital signs are blood pressure 122/68, heart rate 68 beats/min, respiratory rate 18 breaths/min, and oxygen saturation 92% on room air. His chest examination demonstrates bibasilar crackles present about one-third of the way up bilaterally. No wheezing is heard. He has an irregularly irregular rhythm with a II/VI holosystolic murmur at the apex. The jugular venous pressure is not elevated. No edema is present, but clubbing is noted. Pulmonary function testing reveals a forced expiratory volume in 1 second 65% predicted, forced vital capacity of 67% predicted, FEV_1/FVC ratio of 74%, total lung capacity 68% predicted, and diffusion capacity for carbon monoxide of 62% predicted. Which test is most likely to determine the etiology of the patient's dyspnea?

A. Bronchoscopy with transbronchial lung biopsy
B. CT pulmonary angiography
C. Echocardiography
D. High-resolution CT scan of the chest
E. Nuclear medicine stress test

VI-9. A 24-year-old woman is seen for a complaint of shortness of breath and wheezing. She reports the symptoms to be worse when she has exercised outdoors and is around cats. She has had allergic rhinitis in the spring and summer for many years and suffered from eczema as a child. On physical examination, she is noted to have expiratory wheezing. Her pulmonary function tests demonstrate a forced expiratory volume in 1 second (FEV_1) of 2.67 (79% predicted), forced vital capacity of 3.81 L (97% predicted), and an FEV_1/FVC ratio of 70% (predicted value 86%). Following administration of albuterol, the FEV_1 increases to 3.0 L (12.4%). Which of the following statements regarding the patient's disease process is TRUE?

A. Confirmation of the diagnosis will require methacholine challenge testing.
B. Mortality due to the disease has been increasing over the past decade.
C. The most common risk factor in individuals with the disorder is genetic predisposition.
D. The prevalence of the disorder has not changed in the last several decades.
E. The severity of the disease does not vary significantly within a given patient with the disease.

VI-10. A 38-year-old woman is brought to the emergency room for status asthmaticus. She rapidly deteriorates and dies of her disease. All of the following pathologic findings would likely be seen in this individual EXCEPT:

A. Infiltration of the airway mucosa with eosinophils and activated T-lymphocytes
B. Infiltration of the alveolar spaces with eosinophils and neutrophils
C. Occlusion of the airway lumen by mucous plugs
D. Thickening and edema of the airway wall
E. Thickening of the basement membrane of the airways with subepithelial collagen deposition

VI-11. A 25-year-old woman is seen for follow-up of persistent asthma symptoms despite treatment with inhaled fluticasone 88 μg twice daily for the past 3 months. According to the National Asthma Education and Prevention Program guidelines endorsed by the National Institutes of Health, which of the following changes in therapy can be considered?

A. Addition of a leukotriene antagonist.
B. Addition of a long-acting beta-agonist.
C. Addition of low-dose theophylline.
D. Increase the dosage of inhaled corticosteroid.
E. Any of the above can be considered.

VI-12. Which of the following patients is appropriately diagnosed with asthma?

A. A 24-year-old woman treated with inhaled corticosteroids for cough and wheezing that has persisted for 6 weeks following a viral upper respiratory infection.
B. A 26-year-old man who coughs and occasionally wheezes following exercise in cold weather.
C. A 34-year-old woman evaluated for chronic cough with an FEV_1/FVC ratio of 68% with an FEV_1 that increases from 1.68 L (52% predicted) to 1.98 L (61% predicted) after albuterol (18% change in FEV_1).
D. A 44-year-old man who works as a technician caring for the mice in a medical research laboratory complains of wheezing, shortness of breath, and cough that are most severe at the end of the week.
E. A 60-year-old man who has smoked two packs of cigarettes per day for 40 years who has dyspnea and cough, and airway hyperreactivity in response to methacholine.

VI-13. A 40-year-old woman with moderate persistent asthma has been under good control for 3 months and is currently using her albuterol MDI for symptomatic control once weekly. She awakens at night twice monthly with asthma symptoms, but continues to exercise regularly without difficulties. Her other medications include fluticasone inhaled 88 μg/puff twice daily and salmeterol 50 μg twice daily. Her FEV_1 is currently at 83% of her personal best. Which action is most appropriate at the present time?

A. Add montelukast 10 mg once daily, as the current albuterol usage suggests poor asthma control.
B. Decrease the fluticasone to 44 μg/puff twice daily.
C. Discontinue the fluticasone.
D. Discontinue the salmeterol.
E. Do nothing, as the current albuterol usage suggests poor asthma control.

VI-14. You are considering omalizumab therapy for a patient with severe persistent asthma who is requiring oral prednisone at 5–10 mg daily in addition to high-dose inhaled corticosteroids, long-acting bronchodilators, and montelukast to control her symptoms. Which of the following is necessary prior to initiating omalizumab?

A. Discontinuation of oral prednisone
B. Demonstrated elevation in immunoglobulin E levels to greater than 1000 IU/L
C. Normalization of FEV_1 or peak expiratory flow rates
D. Presence of sensitivity to a perennial aeroallergen
E. Switch oral prednisone to intravenous prednisolone

VI-15. A 76-year-old woman is evaluated for acute onset of shortness of breath and dry cough for the past 2 days. She also has had a fever to as high as 102.5°F (39.2°C). Her past medical history includes hypothyroidism and diabetes mellitus. She currently is taking metformin 1000 mg twice daily. Her levothyroxine dose was increased to 100 μg daily 1 month ago, and she was prescribed nitrofurantoin 100 mg twice daily 3 days ago for a urinary tract infection. Her vital signs show a blood pressure of 115/82, heart rate of 96 beats per minute, respiratory rate of 24 breaths per minute, temperature of 101.3°F (38.5°C), and oxygen saturation of 94% on room air. There is dullness to percussion and decreased breath sounds at the right lung base. Crackles are heard bilaterally as well. A chest radiograph shows a moderate right-sided pleural effusion, and patchy bilateral lung infiltrates are seen. The patient is admitted to the hospital. A thoracentesis is performed demonstrating an exudative effusion. The fluid has a white cell count of 3500/mm³ with a differential of 60% polymorphonuclear cells, 30% eosinophils, and 10% lymphocytes. A bronchoscopy is performed that shows a differential of 50% polymorphonuclear cells, 15% eosinophils, and 35% alveolar macrophages. Which of the following would be the most important next step in the treatment of this patient?

A. Await pleural fluid cultures before making a treatment recommendation.
B. Decrease levothyroxine dose.
C. Discontinue nitrofurantoin.
D. Increase levothyroxine dose.
E. Initiate treatment with high-dose steroid therapy (methylprednisolone 1 g daily).

VI-16. A 34-year-old female seeks evaluation for a complaint of cough and dyspnea on exertion that has gradually worsened over 3 months. The patient has no past history of pulmonary complaints and has never had asthma. She started working in a pet store approximately 6 months ago. Her duties there include cleaning the reptile and bird cages. She reports occasional low-grade fevers but has had no wheezing. The cough is dry and nonproductive. Before 3 months ago the patient had no limitation of exercise tolerance, but now she reports that she gets dyspneic climbing two flights of stairs. On physical examination the patient appears well. She has an oxygen saturation of 95% on room air at rest but desaturates to 89% with ambulation. Temperature is 37.7°C (99.8°F). The pulmonary examination is unremarkable. No clubbing or cyanosis is present. The patient has a normal chest radiogram. A high-resolution chest CT shows diffuse ground-glass infiltrates in the lower lobes with the presence of centrilobular nodules. A transbronchial biopsy shows an interstitial alveolar infiltrate of plasma cells, lymphocytes, and occasional eosinophils. There are also several loose noncaseating granulomas. All cultures are negative for bacterial, viral, and fungal pathogens. What is the diagnosis?

A. Aspergillosis
B. Hypersensitivity pneumonitis
C. Nonspecific interstitial pneumonitis related to collagen vascular disease
D. Psittacosis
E. Sarcoidosis

VI-17. What treatment do you recommend for the patient in question VI-16?

A. Amphotericin
B. Doxycycline
C. Glucocorticoids
D. Glucocorticoids plus azathioprine
E. Glucocorticoids plus removal of antigen

VI-18. A 75-year-old man is evaluated for a new left-sided pleural effusion and shortness of breath. He worked as an insulation worker at a shipyard for more than 30 years and did not wear protective respiratory equipment. He has a 50 pack-year history of tobacco with known moderate COPD (FEV₁ 55% predicted) and prior history of myocardial infarction 10 years previously. His current medications include aspirin, atenolol, benazepril, tiotropium, and albuterol. His physical examination is consistent with a left-sided effusion with dullness to percussion and decreased breath sounds occurring over one-half of the hemithorax. On chest x-ray, there is a moderate left-sided pleural effusion with bilateral pleural calcifications and left apical pleural thickening. No lung mass is seen. A chest CT confirms the findings on chest x-ray and also fails to show a mass. There is compressive atelectasis of the left lower lobe. A thoracentesis is performed that demonstrates an exudative effusion with 65% lymphocytes, 25% mesothelial cells, and 10% neutrophils. Cytology does not demonstrate any malignancy. Which of the following statements regarding the most likely cause of the patient's effusion is TRUE?

A. Cigarette smoking increases the likelihood of developing the condition.
B. Death in this disease is usually related to diffuse metastatic disease.
C. Exposure to the causative agent can be as little as 1–2 years, and latency to expression of disease may be as great as 40 years.
D. Repeated pleural fluid cytology will most likely lead to a definitive diagnosis.
E. Therapy with a combination of surgical resection and adjuvant chemotherapy significantly improves long-term survival.

VI-19. Chronic silicosis is related to an increased risk of which of the following conditions?

A. Infection with invasive *Aspergillus*
B. Infection with *Mycobacterium tuberculosis*
C. Lung cancer
D. Rheumatoid arthritis
E. All of the above

VI-20. All of the following occupational lung diseases are correctly matched with their exposure EXCEPT:

A. Berylliosis—High-technology electronics
B. Byssinosis—Cotton milling
C. Farmer's lung—Moldy hay
D. Progressive massive fibrosis—Shipyard workers
E. Metal fume fever—Welding

VI-21. A 45-year-old male is evaluated in the clinic for asthma. His symptoms began 2 years ago and are characterized by an episodic cough and wheezing that responded initially to inhaled bronchodilators and inhaled corticosteroids but now require nearly constant prednisone tapers. He notes that the symptoms are worst on weekdays but cannot pinpoint specific triggers. His medications are an albuterol MDI, a fluticasone MDI, and prednisone 10 mg po daily. The patient has no habits and works as a textile worker. Physical examination is notable for mild diffuse polyphonic expiratory wheezing but no other abnormality. Which of the following is the most appropriate next step?

A. Exercise physiology testing
B. Measurement of FEV_1 before and after work
C. Methacholine challenge testing
D. Skin testing for allergies
E. Sputum culture for *Aspergillus fumigatus*

VI-22. A 53-year-old male is seen in the emergency department with sudden-onset fever, chills, malaise, and shortness of breath, but no wheezing. He has no significant past medical history and is a farmer. Of note, he worked earlier in the day stacking hay. PA and lateral chest radiography show bilateral upper lobe infiltrates. Which organism is most likely to be responsible for this presentation?

A. *Nocardia asteroides*
B. *Histoplasma capsulatum*
C. *Cryptococcus neoformans*
D. *Actinomyces*
E. *Aspergillus fumigatus*

VI-23. All of the following conditions are associated with an increased risk of methicillin-resistant *Staphylococcus aureus* as a cause of health care–associated pneumonia EXCEPT:

A. Antibiotic therapy in the preceding 3 months
B. Chronic dialysis
C. Home wound care
D. Hospitalization for more than 2 days in the preceding 3 months
E. Nursing home residence

VI-24. Which of the following statements regarding the diagnosis of community-acquired pneumonia is TRUE?

A. Directed therapy specific to the causative organism is more effective than empirical therapy in hospitalized patients who are not in intensive care.
B. Five percent to 15% of patients hospitalized with community-acquired pneumonia will have positive blood cultures.
C. In patients who have bacteremia caused by *Streptococcus pneumoniae*, sputum cultures are positive in more than 80% of cases.
D. Polymerase chain reaction tests for identification of *Legionella pneumophila* and *Mycoplasma pneumoniae* are widely available and should be utilized for diagnosis in patients hospitalized with community-acquired pneumonia.
E. The etiology of community-acquired pneumonia is typically identified in about 70% of cases.

VI-25. A 55-year-old man presents to his primary care physician with a 2-day history of cough and fever. His cough is productive of thick, dark green sputum. His past medical history is significant for hypercholesterolemia treated with rosuvastatin. He does not smoke cigarettes and is generally quite healthy, exercising several times weekly. He has no ill contacts and cannot recall the last time he was treated with any antibiotics. On presentation, his vital signs are as follows: temperature 102.1°F (38.9°C), blood pressure 132/78, heart rate 87 beats/min, respiratory rate 20 breaths/min, and oxygen saturation 95% on room air. Crackles are present in the right lung base with egophony. A chest radiograph demonstrates segmental consolidation of the right lower lobe with air bronchograms. What is the most appropriate approach to the ongoing care of this patient?

A. Obtain a sputum culture and await results prior to initiating treatment.
B. Perform a chest CT to rule out postobstructive pneumonia.
C. Refer to the emergency department for admission and treatment with intravenous antibiotics.
D. Treat with doxycycline 100 mg twice daily.
E. Treat with moxifloxacin 400 mg daily.

VI-26. A 65-year-old woman is admitted to the intensive care unit for management of septic shock associated with an infected hemodialysis catheter. She was initially intubated on hospital day 1 for acute respiratory distress syndrome. She has slowly been improving such that her FIO_2 was weaned to 0.40, and she was no longer febrile or requiring vasopressors. On hospital day 7, she develops a new fever to 39.4°C (102.9°F) with increased thick, yellow-green sputum from her endotracheal tube. You suspect the patient has ventilator-associated pneumonia. What is the best way to make a definitive diagnosis in this patient?

A. Endotracheal aspirate yielding a new organism typical of a ventilator-associated pneumonia.
B. Presence of a new infiltrate on chest radiograph.
C. Quantitative cultures from an endotracheal aspirate yielding more than 10^6 organisms typical of ventilator-associated pneumonia.
D. Quantitative culture from a protected brush specimen yielding more than 10^3 organisms typical of ventilator-associated pneumonia.
E. There is no single set of criteria that is reliably diagnostic of pneumonia in a ventilated patient.

VI-27. Which of the following associations correctly pairs clinical scenarios and community-acquired pneumonia (CAP) pathogens?

A. Aspiration pneumonia: *Streptococcus pyogenes*
B. Heavy alcohol use: Atypical pathogens and *Staphylococcus aureus*
C. Poor dental hygiene: *Chlamydia pneumoniae, Klebsiella pneumoniae*
D. Structural lung disease: *Pseudomonas aeruginosa, S. aureus*
E. Travel to southwestern United States: *Aspergillus* spp.

VI-28. Which of the following is the most common cause of diffuse bronchiectasis worldwide?

A. Cystic fibrosis
B. Immunoglobulin deficiency
C. *Mycobacterium avium-intracellulare* infection
D. *Mycobacterium tuberculosis* infection
E. Rheumatoid arthritis

VI-29. A 54-year-old woman presents complaining of chronic cough that has worsened over a period of 6–12 months. She reports the cough to be present day and night, and productive of a thick green sputum. Over the course of the day, she estimates that she produces as much as 100 mL of sputum daily. Bilateral coarse crackles are heard in the lower lung zones. Pulmonary function tests demonstrate an FEV_1 of 1.68 L (53.3% predicted), FVC of 3.00 L (75% predicted), and FEV_1/FVC ratio of 56%. A chest radiograph is unremarkable. What would you recommend as the next step in the evaluation of this patient?

A. Bronchoscopy with bronchoalveolar lavage
B. Chest CT with intravenous contrast
C. High-resolution chest CT
D. Serum immunoglobulin levels
E. Treatment with a long-acting bronchodilator and inhaled corticosteroid

VI-30. A 48-year-old man is admitted to the hospital with fever and cough. He suffers from alcoholism and is homeless. He does not routinely obtain any health care. He reports that he has felt poorly for about 8 weeks. He has fatigue and generalized malaise. He states that he lost weight over this period as his clothing is very loose, but he cannot quantify the weight loss. He has felt feverish at times. During this period, he has been having increasing cough with malodorous sputum production. He coughs at least 3 tablespoons of dark sputum daily that has been blood streaked at times. He takes no medications, but drinks about 1 L of vodka daily. He also smokes one pack of cigarettes daily. On physical examination, the patient is disheveled and appears chronically ill. His vital signs are heart rate 98 beats/min, blood pressure 110/73, respiratory rate 20 breaths/min, temperature 38.2°C (100.8°F), and oxygen saturation of 94% on room air. He has evidence of temporal wasting with very poor dentition. A foul odor is present on his breath. Amphoric breath sounds are heard posteriorly in the right lower lung field. A chest x-ray shows a 4-cm cavitary lung lesion in the right lower lobe. The patient is admitted and placed on respiratory isolation. Sputum cultures for bacteria, mycobacteria, and fungus are ordered. What is the best initial choice for therapy in this patient?

A. Ampicillin-sulbactam 3 g intravenously every 6 hours
B. Isoniazid, rifampin, pyrazinamide, and ethambutol orally
C. Metronidazole 500 mg orally four times daily
D. Percutaneous drainage of the cavity
E. Piperacillin-tazobactam 2.25 g intravenously every 4 hours in combination with tobramycin 5 mg/kg intravenously daily

VI-31. A 35-year-old male is seen in the clinic for evaluation of infertility. He has never fathered any children, and after 2 years of unprotected intercourse his wife has not achieved pregnancy. Sperm analysis shows a normal number of sperm, but they are immotile. Past medical history is notable for recurrent sinopulmonary infections, and the patient recently was told that he has bronchiectasis. Chest radiography is likely to show which of the following?

A. Bihilar lymphadenopathy
B. Bilateral upper lobe infiltrates
C. Normal findings
D. Situs inversus
E. Water balloon–shaped heart

VI-32. A 28-year-old woman is evaluated for recurrent lung and sinus infections. She recalls having at least yearly episodes of bronchitis beginning in her early teens. She states that for the past 5 years she has been on antibiotics at least three times yearly for respiratory or sinus infections. She also reports that she has had difficulty gaining weight and has always felt short compared to her peers. On physical examination, the patient has a body mass index of 18.5 kg/m^2. Her oxygen saturation is 94% on room air at rest. Nasal polyps are present. Coarse rhonchi and crackles are heard in the bilateral upper lung zones. Mild clubbing is seen. A chest radiograph shows bilateral upper lobe bronchiectasis with areas of mucous plugging. You are concerned about the possibility of undiagnosed cystic fibrosis (CF). Which of the following tests would provide the strongest support for the diagnosis of CF in this individual?

A. DNA analysis demonstrating one copy of the delta F508 allele
B. Decreased baseline nasal potential difference
C. Presence of *Pseudomonas aeruginosa* on repeated sputum cultures
D. Sweat chloride values greater than 35 meq/L
E. Sweat chloride values greater than 70 meq/L

VI-33. A 22-year-old man with cystic fibrosis is seen for a routine follow-up exam. He is currently treated with recombinant human DNAse and albuterol by nebulization twice daily. His primary sputum clearance technique is aerobic exercise five times weekly and autogenic drainage. He is feeling well overall, and his examination is normal. Pulmonary function testing demonstrates an FEV$_1$ of 4.48 L (97% predicted), an FVC of 5.70 L (103% predicted), and an FEV$_1$/FVC ratio of 79%. A routine sputum culture grows *Pseudomonas aeruginosa*. The only organism isolated on prior cultures has been *Staphylococcus aureus*. What do you recommend for this patient?

A. High-frequency chest wall oscillation
B. Hypertonic saline (7%) nebulized twice daily
C. Inhaled tobramycin 300 mg twice daily every other month
D. Intravenous cefepime and tobramycin for 14 days
E. Return visit in 3 months with repeat sputum cultures and treatment only if there is persistent *P. aeruginosa*

VI-34. Which of the following organisms is unlikely to be found in the sputum of a patient with cystic fibrosis?

A. *Haemophilus influenzae*
B. *Acinetobacter baumannii*
C. *Burkholderia cepacia*
D. *Aspergillus fumigatus*
E. *Staphylococcus aureus*

VI-35. All of the following are risk factors for chronic obstructive pulmonary disease EXCEPT:

A. Airway hyperresponsiveness
B. Coal dust exposure
C. Passive cigarette smoke exposure
D. Recurrent respiratory infections
E. Use of biomass fuels in poorly ventilated areas

VI-36. A 65-year-old woman is evaluated for dyspnea on exertion and chronic cough. She has a long history of tobacco use, smoking 1.5 packs of cigarettes daily since the age of 20. She is a thin woman in no obvious distress. Her oxygen saturation on room air is 93% with a respiratory rate of 22/min. The lungs are hyperexpanded on percussion with decreased breath sounds in the upper lung fields. You suspect chronic obstructive pulmonary disease. What are the expected findings on pulmonary function testing (see Table VI-36)?

	FEV$_1$	FVC	FEV$_1$/FVC Ratio	TLC	DLCO
A.	Decreased	Normal or decreased	Decreased	Decreased	Decreased
B.	Decreased	Normal or decreased	Decreased	Increased	Decreased
C.	Decreased	Decreased	Normal	Decreased	Decreased
D.	Decreased	Normal or decreased	Decreased	Increased	Normal or increased

TABLE VI-36

VI-37. A 70-year-old man with known chronic obstructive pulmonary disease is seen for follow-up. He has been clinically stable without an exacerbation for the past 6 months. However, he generally feels in poor health and is limited in what he can do. He reports dyspnea with usual activities. He is currently being managed with an albuterol metered-dose inhaler twice daily and as needed. He has a 50 pack-year history of smoking and quit 5 years previously. His other medical problems include peripheral vascular disease, hypertension, and benign prostatic hyperplasia. He is managed with aspirin, lisinopril, hydrochlorothiazide, and tamsulosin. On examination, the patient has a resting oxygen saturation of 93% on room air. He is hyperinflated to percussion with decreased breath sounds at the apices and faint expiratory wheezing. His pulmonary function tests demonstrate an FEV_1 of 55% predicted, an FVC of 80% predicted, and an $FEV_1/$FVC ratio of 50%. What is the next best step in the management of this patient?

A. Initiate a trial of oral glucocorticoids for a period of 4 weeks and initiate inhaled fluticasone if there is a significant improvement in pulmonary function.
B. Initiate treatment with inhaled fluticasone 110 μg/puff twice daily.
C. Initiate treatment with inhaled fluticasone 250 μg/puff in combination with inhaled salmeterol 50 mg/puff twice daily.
D. Initiate treatment with inhaled tiotropium 18 μg/daily.
E. Perform exercise and nocturnal oximetry, and initiate oxygen therapy if these demonstrate significant hypoxemia.

VI-38. A 56-year-old woman is admitted to the intensive care unit with a 4-day history of increasing shortness of breath and cough with copious sputum production. She has known severe COPD with an FEV_1 of 42% predicted. On presentation, she has a room air blood gas with a pH 7.26, $PaCO_2$ 78 mmHg, and PaO_2 50 mmHg. She is in obvious respiratory distress with the use of accessory muscles and retractions. Breath sounds are quiet with diffuse expiratory wheezing and rhonchi. No infiltrates are present on chest radiograph. Which of the following therapies has been demonstrated to have the greatest reduction in mortality for patients with these findings?

A. Administration of inhaled bronchodilators
B. Administration of intravenous glucocorticoids
C. Early administration of broad-spectrum antibiotics with coverage of *Pseudomonas aeruginosa*
D. Early intubation with mechanical ventilation
E. Use of noninvasive positive pressure ventilation

VI-39. A 63-year-old male with a long history of cigarette smoking comes to see you for a 4-month history of progressive shortness of breath and dyspnea on exertion. The symptoms have been indolent, with no recent worsening. He denies fever, chest pain, or hemoptysis. He has a daily cough of 3–6 tablespoons of yellow phlegm. The patient says he has not seen a physician for over 10 years. Physical examination is notable for normal vital signs, a prolonged expiratory

phase, scattered rhonchi, elevated jugular venous pulsation, and moderate pedal edema. Hematocrit is 49%. Which of the following therapies is most likely to prolong his survival?

A. Atenolol
B. Enalapril
C. Oxygen
D. Prednisone
E. Theophylline

VI-40. A 62-year-old man is evaluated for dyspnea on exertion that has progressively worsened over a period of 10 months. He has a 50 pack-year history of tobacco, quitting 10 years ago. His physiologic and radiologic evaluation demonstrates a restrictive ventilatory defect with diffuse fibrosis that is worse in the subpleural region and at the bases. A surgical lung biopsy is performed, which is consistent with usual interstitial pneumonia. No autoimmune or drug-related cause is found. What is the recommended treatment for this patient?

A. Azathioprine 125 mg daily plus prednisone 60 mg daily
B. Cyclophosphamide 100 mg daily
C. N-acetylcysteine 600 mg twice daily plus prednisone 60 mg daily
D. Prednisone 60 mg daily
E. Referral for lung transplantation

VI-41. What would be the expected finding on bronchoalveolar lavage in a patient with diffuse alveolar hemorrhage?

A. Atypical hyperplastic type II pneumocytes
B. Ferruginous bodies
C. Hemosiderin laden macrophages
D. Lymphocytosis with an elevated CD4:CD8 ratio
E. Milky appearance with foamy macrophages

VI-42. A 42-year-old male presents with progressive dyspnea on exertion, low-grade fevers, and weight loss over 6 months. He also is complaining of a primarily dry cough, although occasionally he coughs up thick mucoid sputum. There is no past medical history. He does not smoke cigarettes. On physical examination, the patient appears dyspneic with minimal exertion. The patient's temperature is 37.9°C (100.3°F). Oxygen saturation is 91% on room air at rest. Faint basilar crackles are heard. On laboratory studies, the patient has polyclonal hypergammaglobulinemia and a hematocrit of 52%. A CT scan reveals bilateral alveolar infiltrates that are primarily perihilar in nature with a mosaic pattern. The patient undergoes bronchoscopy with bronchoalveolar lavage. The effluent appears milky. The cytopathology shows amorphous debris with periodic acid–Schiff (PAS)-positive macrophages. What is the diagnosis?

A. Bronchiolitis obliterans organizing pneumonia
B. Desquamative interstitial pneumonitis
C. Nocardiosis
D. *Pneumocystis carinii* pneumonia
E. Pulmonary alveolar proteinosis

VI-43. What treatment is most appropriate at this time for the patient in question VI-42?

A. Doxycycline
B. Prednisone
C. Prednisone and cyclophosphamide
D. Trimethoprim-sulfamethoxazole
E. Whole-lung saline lavage

VI-44. A 68-year-old man presents for evaluation of dyspnea on exertion. He states that he first noticed the symptoms about 2 years ago. At that time, he had to stop walking the golf course and began to use a cart, but he was still able to complete a full 18 holes. Over the past year, he has stopped golfing altogether because of breathlessness and states that he has difficulty walking to and from his mailbox, which is about 50 yards from his house. He also has a dry cough that occurs on most days. It is not worse at night, and he can identify no triggers. He denies wheezing. He has had no fevers, chills, or weight loss. He denies any joint symptoms. He is a former smoker of about 50 pack-years, but quit 8 years previously after being diagnosed with coronary artery disease. On physical examination, he appears breathless after walking down the hallway to the examination room, but quickly recovers upon resting. Vital signs are as follows: blood pressure 118/67 mmHg, heart rate 88 beats/min, respiratory rate 20 breaths/min. His SaO$_2$ is 94% at rest and decreases to 86% after ambulating 300 ft. His lung examination shows normal percussion and expansion. There are Velcro-like crackles at both bases, and they are distributed halfway through both lung fields. No wheezing is noted. Cardiovascular examination is normal. Digital clubbing is present. A chest CT is performed and is shown in Figure VI-44. He is referred for surgical lung biopsy. Which pathologic description is most likely to be seen in this patient's disease?

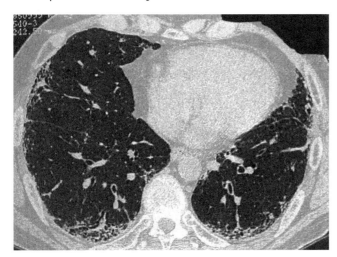

FIGURE VI-44

A. Dense amorphous fluid within the alveoli diffusely that stains positive with periodic acid–Schiff stain
B. Destruction of alveoli with resultant emphysematous areas, predominantly in the upper lobes
C. Diffuse alveolar damage
D. Formation of noncaseating granulomas
E. Heterogeneous collagen deposition with fibroblast foci and honeycombing

VI-45. All the following are pulmonary manifestations of systemic lupus erythematosus EXCEPT:

A. Cavitary lung nodules
B. Diaphragmatic dysfunction with loss of lung volumes
C. Pleuritis
D. Pulmonary hemorrhage
E. Pulmonary vascular disease

VI-46. A 56-year-old woman presents for evaluation of dyspnea and cough for 2 months. During this time, she has also had intermittent fevers, malaise, and a 5.5-kg (12-lb) weight loss. She denies having any ill contacts and has not recently traveled. She works as a nurse, and a yearly PPD test performed 3 months ago was negative. She denies any exposure to organic dusts and does not have any birds as pets. She has a history of rheumatoid arthritis and is currently taking hydroxychloroquine, 200 mg twice daily. There has been no worsening in her joint symptoms. On physical examination, diffuse inspiratory crackles and squeaks are heard. A CT scan of the chest reveals patchy alveolar infiltrates and bronchial wall thickening. Pulmonary function testing reveals mild restriction. She undergoes a surgical lung biopsy. The pathology shows granulation tissue filling the small airways, alveolar ducts, and alveoli. The alveolar interstitium has chronic inflammation and organizing pneumonia. What is the most appropriate therapy for this patient?

A. Azathioprine 100 mg daily
B. Discontinuation of hydroxychloroquine and observation
C. Infliximab IV once monthly
D. Methotrexate 15 mg weekly
E. Prednisone 1 mg/kg daily

VI-47. In which of the following patients presenting with acute dyspnea would a positive D-dimer prompt additional testing for a pulmonary embolus?

A. A 24-year-old woman who is 32 weeks pregnant.
B. A 48-year-old man with no medical history who presents with calf pain following prolonged air travel. The alveolar-arterial oxygen gradient is normal.
C. A 56-year-old woman undergoing chemotherapy for breast cancer.
D. A 62-year-old man who underwent hip replacement surgery 4 weeks previously.
E. A 72-year-old man who had an acute myocardial infarction 2 weeks ago.

VI-48. A 62-year-old woman is hospitalized following an acute pulmonary embolism. All of the following would typically indicate a massive pulmonary embolism EXCEPT:

A. Elevated serum troponin levels
B. Initial presentation with hemoptysis
C. Initial presentation with syncope
D. Presence of right ventricular enlargement on CT scan of the chest
E. Presence of right ventricular hypokinesis on echocardiogram

VI-49. Which of the following statements regarding diagnostic imaging in pulmonary embolism is TRUE?

A. A high probability ventilation-perfusion scan is one that has at least one segmental perfusion defect in the setting of normal ventilation.

B. If a patient has a high probability ventilation-perfusion scan, there is a 90% likelihood that the patient does indeed have a pulmonary embolism.

C. Magnetic resonance angiography provides excellent resolution for both large proximal and smaller segmental pulmonary emboli.

D. Multidetector-row spiral CT imaging is suboptimal for detecting small peripheral emboli, necessitating the use of invasive pulmonary angiography.

E. None of the routinely used imaging techniques provide adequate evaluation of the right ventricle to assist in risk stratification of the patient.

VI-50. A 53-year-old woman presents to the hospital following an episode of syncope, with ongoing lightheadedness and shortness of breath. She had a history of antiphospholipid syndrome with prior pulmonary embolism and has been nonadherent to her anticoagulation medication recently. She has been prescribed warfarin, 7.5 mg daily, but reports taking it only intermittently. She does not know her most recent INR. On presentation to the emergency room, she appears diaphoretic and tachypneic. Her vital signs are as follows: blood pressure 86/44 mmHg, heart rate 130 beats/min, respiratory rate 30 breaths/min, and oxygen saturation of 85% on room air. Cardiovascular examination shows a regular tachycardia without murmurs, rubs, or gallops. The lungs are clear to auscultation. On extremity examination, there is swelling of her left thigh with a positive Homan's sign. Chest CT angiography confirms a saddle pulmonary embolus with ongoing clot seen in the pelvic veins on the left. Anticoagulation with unfractionated heparin is administered. After a fluid bolus of 1 L, the patient's blood pressure remains low at 88/50 mmHg. Echocardiogram demonstrates hypokinesis of the right ventricle. On 100% non-rebreather mask, the oxygen saturation is 92%. What is the next best step in the management of this patient?

A. Continue current management.

B. Continue IV fluids at 500 mL/h for a total of 4 L of fluid resuscitation.

C. Refer for inferior vena cava filter placement and continue current management.

D. Refer for surgical embolectomy.

E. Treat with dopamine and recombinant tissue plasminogen activator, 100 mg IV.

VI-51. A 42-year-old woman presents to the emergency room with acute onset of shortness of breath. She recently had been to visit her parents out of state and rode in a car for about 9 hours each way. Two days ago, she developed mild calf pain and swelling, but she thought that this was not unusual after having been sitting with her legs dependent for the recent trip. On arrival to the emergency room, she is noted to be tachypneic. The vital signs are as follows:

blood pressure 98/60 mmHg, heart rate 114 beats/min, respiratory rate 28 breaths/min, oxygen saturation of 92% on room air, weight 89 kg. The lungs are clear bilaterally. There is pain in the right calf with dorsiflexion of the foot, and the right leg is more swollen when compared to the left. An arterial blood gas measurement shows a pH of 7.52, PCO_2 25 mmHg, and PO_2 68 mmHg. Kidney and liver function are normal. A helical CT scan confirms a pulmonary embolus. All of the following agents can be used alone as initial therapy in this patient EXCEPT:

A. Enoxaparin 1 mg/kg SC twice daily

B. Fondaparinux 7.5 mg SC once daily

C. Tinzaparin 175 U/kg SC once daily

D. Unfractionated heparin IV adjusted to maintain activated partial thromboplastin time (aPTT) two to three times the upper limit of normal

E. Warfarin 7.5 mg po once daily to maintain INR at 2–3

VI-52. A 62-year-old woman is admitted to the hospital with a community-acquired pneumonia with a 4-day history of fever, cough, and right-sided pleuritic chest pain. The admission chest x-ray identifies a right lower and middle lobe infiltrate with an associated effusion. All of the following characteristics of the pleural effusion indicate a complicated effusion that may require tube thoracostomy EXCEPT:

A. Loculated fluid

B. Pleural fluid pH less than 7.20

C. Pleural fluid glucose less than 60 mg/dL

D. Positive Gram stain or culture of the pleural fluid

E. Recurrence of fluid following the initial thoracentesis

VI-53. A 58-year-old man is evaluated for dyspnea and is found to have a moderate right-sided pleural effusion. He undergoes thoracentesis with the following characteristics:

Appearance	Serosanguinous
pH	7.48
Protein	5.8 g/dL (serum protein 7.2 g/dL)
LDH	285 IU/L (serum LDH 320 IU/L)
Glucose	66 mg/dL
WBC	3800/mm^3
RBC	24,000/mm^3
PMNs	10%
Lymphocytes	80%
Mesothelial cells	10%
Cytology	Lymphocytosis with chronic inflammation and no malignant cells or organisms identified

Which of the following is an unlikely cause of the pleural effusion in this patient?

A. Cirrhosis

B. Lung cancer

C. Mesothelioma

D. Pulmonary embolism

E. Tuberculosis

VI-54. A 66-year-old woman is evaluated for dyspnea. One month previously, she had undergone an esophagectomy for adenocarcinoma of the esophagus. On physical examination, the patient appears tachypneic with difficulty speaking in full sentences. She has a respiratory rate of 28/min and an oxygen saturation of 88% on room air. There is dullness to percussion with absent breath sounds in the left hemithorax. A chest radiograph confirms a large left-sided pleural effusion with mediastinal shift to the right. A thoracentesis removes 1.5 L of a milky-appearing fluid. The protein of the fluid is 6.2 mg/dL, LDH is 368 IU/L, and the WBC count is 1500/μL (20% PMNs, 80% lymphocytes). The triglyceride level is 168 mg/dL. Cultures and cytology are negative. Which of the following is the best management for this patient?

A. Placement of a chest tube plus octreotide
B. Placement of a chest tube to wall suction until drainage decreases to less than 100 mL daily
C. Reexploration of the chest with surgical correction of the likely defect
D. Referral for palliative care
E. Repeat thoracentesis for cytologic examination

VI-55. A 28-year-old man presents to the emergency room with acute-onset shortness of breath and pleuritic chest pain on the right that began 2 hours previously. He is generally healthy and has no medical history. He has smoked one pack of cigarettes daily since the age of 18. On physical examination, he is tall and thin with a body mass index of 19.2 kg/m^2. He has a respiratory rate of 24/min with an oxygen saturation of 95% on room air. He has slightly decreased breath sounds at the right lung apex. A chest x-ray demonstrates a 20% pneumothorax on the right side. Which of the following is TRUE regarding pneumothorax in this patient?

A. A CT scan is likely to show emphysematous changes.
B. If the patient were to develop recurrent pneumothoraces, thorascopy with pleural abrasion has a success rate of nearly 100% for prevention of recurrence.
C. Most patients with this presentation require tube thoracostomy to resolve the pneumothorax.
D. The likelihood of recurrent pneumothorax is about 25%.
E. The primary risk factor for the development of spontaneous pneumothorax is a tall and thin body habitus.

VI-56. The most common cause of a pleural effusion is:

A. Cirrhosis
B. Left ventricular failure
C. Malignancy
D. Pneumonia
E. Pulmonary embolism

VI-57. A patient with mild amyotrophic lateral sclerosis is followed by a pulmonologist for respiratory dysfunction associated with his neuromuscular disease. Which of the following symptoms in addition to PaCO$_2$ of 45 mmHg or greater would necessitate therapy with noninvasive positive pressure ventilation for hypoventilation?

A. Orthopnea
B. Poor quality sleep
C. Impaired cough
D. Dyspnea in activities of daily living
E. All of the above

VI-58. A 27-year-old man with muscular dystrophy is evaluated by his primary care physician for hypoxemia. He reports feeling at his baseline and is not short of breath. On physical examination, finger pulse oximetry is 86% on room air, his lungs are clear, and aside from stigmata of muscular dystrophy, is normal. Chest radiograph shows low lung volumes. Which of the following is most likely the source of his low oxygen saturation?

A. Atelectasis
B. Mucous plug
C. Elevated PaCO$_2$
D. Pneumonia
E. Methemoglobinemia

VI-59. Patients with chronic hypoventilation disorders often complain of a headache upon wakening. What is the cause of this symptom?

A. Arousals from sleep
B. Cerebral vasodilation
C. Cerebral vasoconstriction
D. Polycythemia
E. Nocturnal microaspiration and cough

VI-60. A 47-year-old woman with idiopathic pulmonary arterial hypertension has failed medical therapy including intravenous epoprostenol. She has advanced right heart failure with severe right ventricular dysfunction on echocardiography and a cardiac index of 1.7 L/min per m^2. She is referred for lung transplantation. Which of the following statements is true?

A. She will require heart-lung transplantation for her advanced right heart failure.
B. Idiopathic pulmonary arterial hypertension patients have worse 5-year survival than other transplant recipients.
C. Single-lung transplantation is the preferred surgical procedure for idiopathic pulmonary arterial hypertension.
D. Her own right ventricular function will recover after lung transplantation.
E. She is at risk for recurrent pulmonary arterial hypertension after lung transplantation.

VI-61. A 25-year-old woman with cystic fibrosis is referred for lung transplantation. She is concerned about her long-term outcomes. Which of the following is the main impediment to long-term survival after lung transplantation?

A. Bronchiolitis obliterans syndrome
B. Cytomegalovirus infection
C. Chronic kidney disease
D. Primary graft dysfunction
E. Post-transplant lymphoproliferative disorder

VI-62. A 30-year-old man with end-stage cystic fibrosis undergoes lung transplantation. Three years later, he has a 6-month progressive decline in his renal function. Which of the following medications is the most likely etiology of this?

A. Prednisone
B. Tacrolimus
C. Albuterol
D. Mycophenolate mofetil
E. None of the above

VI-63. A 22-year-old man has cystic fibrosis. He currently is hospitalized about three times yearly for infectious exacerbations. He is colonized with *Pseudomonas aeruginosa*

and *Staphylococcus aureus*, but has never had *Burkholderia cepacia* complex. He remains active and is in college studying architecture. He requires 2 L of oxygen with exertion. The most recent pulmonary function tests demonstrate an FEV_1 that is 28% of the predicted value and an FEV_1/FVC ratio of 44%. Measurement of his arterial blood gas or room air is pH 7.38, PCO_2 36 mmHg, and PO_2 62 mmHg. Which of these characteristics is an indication for referral for lung transplantation?

A. Colonization with *Pseudomonas aeruginosa*
B. FEV_1 less than 30% predicted
C. FEV_1/FVC ratio less than 50%
D. PCO_2 less than 40 mmHg
E. Use of oxygen with exertion

ANSWERS

VI-1. **The answer is E.** *(Chap. 251)* An experienced clinician should be able to gain significant insight into the cause of dyspnea or cough in a patient by a thorough pulmonary examination. Wheezes are most commonly high-pitched sounds heard predominantly on expiration and are indicative of obstruction of small airways. The most frequent cause of wheezing is asthma, which results in polyphonic wheezing due to the dynamic variability in airway obstruction throughout the lung fields. However, many other diseases cause wheezing, including congestive heart failure. This so-called "cardiac asthma" is due to peribronchiolar edema that results in narrowing of the adjacent airways. In contrast, rhonchi are caused by obstruction of medium-sized airways and are associated with a lower pitch and more coarse sound. The most common cause of rhonchi is secretions in the airways. Stridor is another breath sound that is commonly labeled as wheezing, but is indicative of upper airway obstruction. When compared to wheezing associated with small airway disease, stridor is loudest during inspiration, although it can be heard during expiration as well.

Crackles (or rales) are predominantly heard during inspiration and are considered a sign of alveolar or interstitial lung disease. A variety of diseases cause crackles including pneumonia, pulmonary edema, and any cause of interstitial lung fibrosis. Some clinicians attempt to distinguish between the "wet" crackles of pulmonary edema or pneumonia compared to the "dry" crackles of interstitial lung disease. However, this is not a reliable finding. A better way to differentiate between the alveolar and interstitial causes of crackles is to test for the presence of egophony. When alveolar filling is present, the "EEE" sound will be heard as a "AH" sound; however, in interstitial lung disease the "EEE" sound will be preserved. Whispered pectoriloquy will also be intensified in alveolar filling processes, but not interstitial lung disease.

The lack of breath sounds is important to note, but can be caused by many factors including severe bullous lung disease, emphysema, pneumothorax, or pleural effusion.

VI-2. **The answer is B.** *(Chap. 251)* This patient presents with subacute-onset dyspnea and an examination consistent with pleural effusion. Dullness to percussion can be seen with consolidation, atelectasis, and pleural effusion. With consolidation, voice transmission is increased during expiration so that one may hear whispered pectoriloquy or egophony. However, in both pleural effusion and atelectasis, breath sounds are diminished and there is no augmentation of voice transmission. Although this patient could have either atelectasis or pleural effusion, the lack of tracheal deviation points to pleural effusion. Atelectasis would have to be of many segments to account for these findings, and such significant airway collapse would generally cause ipsilateral tracheal deviation. The clinician would expect to find pleural effusion on chest film, and the most appropriate next management step would be thoracentesis to aid in the diagnosis of the etiology and for symptomatic relief. With a lack of symptoms to suggest infection, antibiotics are not indicated. Similarly, in the absence of wheezing or significant sputum production, bronchodilators and deep suctioning are unlikely to be helpful. Bronchoscopy may be indicated ultimately in the management of this patient, particularly if malignancy is suspected; however, the most appropriate first attempt at diagnosis is by means of thoracentesis.

VI-3.   **The answer is B.** *(Chap. 252)* The functional residual capacity of the lung refers to the volume of air that remains in the lung following a normal tidal respiration. This volume of air represents the point at which the outward recoil of the chest wall is in equilibrium with the inward elastic recoil of the lungs. The lungs would remain at this volume if not for the actions of the respiratory muscles. The functional residual capacity is comprised of two lung volumes: the expiratory reserve volume and the residual volume. The expiratory reserve volume represents the additional volume of air that can be exhaled from the lungs when acted upon by the respiratory muscles of exhalation. The residual volume is the volume of air that remains in the lung following a complete exhalation and is determined by the closing pressure of the small airways.

VI-4.   **The answer is D.** *(Chap. 252)* This patient presents with subacute dyspnea, stridor, and airflow obstruction, which are consistent with a diagnosis of subglottic stenosis related to his prior prolonged mechanical ventilation. This is confirmed by the finding of fixed airflow obstruction on the flow-volume loop. Flow-volume loops are derived from spirometry. Following a maximum inspiratory effort from residual volume, an individual forces the maximum volume of air from the lungs, and the resultant flows are plotted against the volume. By convention, inspiration is shown on the lower portion of the curve and expiration is on the top. There are characteristic patterns of airflow obstruction that can be evaluated by examining this curve. A fixed central airflow obstruction results in flattening of the flow-volume loop in both inspiration and expiration, yielding the characteristic boxlike effect in this patient. Examples of fixed airflow obstruction include tracheal stenosis and an obstructing central airway tumor. Other patterns of large airway obstruction are a variable intrathoracic obstruction and variable extrathoracic obstruction. In these situations, flattening of the flow-volume curve occurs on only one limb of the flow-volume loop, and the pattern of flattening can be explained by the dynamic changes in pressure that affect the trachea. A variable intrathoracic obstruction causes flattening of the flow-volume curve only on expiration. During inspiration the pleural pressure is more negative than the tracheal pressure, and the trachea remains unimpeded to flow. However, when pleural pressure rises on expiration relative to tracheal pressure, there is collapse of the trachea and flattening of the flow-volume curve. An example of a variable intrathoracic obstruction is tracheomalacia. In contrast, the variable extrathoracic defect leads to flattening of the flow-volume loop on inspiration but not expiration. The relevant pressure acting on airflow in the trachea in an extrathoracic obstruction is atmospheric pressure. During inspiration, the tracheal pressure drops below atmospheric pressure, leading to compromised airflow and the characteristic flattening of the flow-volume loop. However, tracheal pressure rises above atmospheric pressure during expiration, leading to a normal expiratory curve.

VI-5.   **The answer is B.** *(Chap. 252)* Pregnancy is a known risk factor for the development of venous thromboembolic disease and should be suspected in any pregnant patient presenting with acute dyspnea. Determining the need for further testing in a pregnant patient should take into account the potential risks of radiation exposure on the fetus. Unfortunately, the signs and symptoms of pulmonary embolism are often nonspecific. Most chest x-rays are normal, and sinus tachycardia may be the only finding on electrocardiogram. In addition, in the pregnant patient dyspnea is common due to a variety of factors including increased size of the uterus and the effects of progesterone as a central respiratory stimulant. The normal arterial blood gas in pregnancy shows a chronic respiratory alkalosis with a pH ranging as high as 7.47 and $PaCO_2$ between 30 and 32 mmHg. Calculation of the alveolar-arterial gradient (A-a gradient) can be helpful in this situation. It is easy to be fooled by the presence of a normal oxygen saturation and partial pressure of oxygen on arterial blood gas, but the A-a gradient may still be elevated in the presence of respiratory alkalosis. To calculate the A-a gradient, one first must calculate the alveolar oxygen tension with the alveolar gas equation shown below:

$PaO_2 = PiO_2 - (PaCO_2/R)$ where,

PiO_2 = inspired partial pressure of oxygen = $FiO_2 \times (P_{bar} - P_{H2O})$, and

R = respiratory quotient = carbon dioxide production/oxygen consumption = ~0.8

In this patient, calculation of the $PaO_2 = [0.21 \times (760 - 47)] - (26/0.8) = 117.23$ mmHg. At the same time the measured arterial partial pressure of oxygen was 85. Thus, the A-a gradient is elevated at 32 mmHg and should prompt the physician to perform further workup for pulmonary embolism. The choice of test for diagnosis of pulmonary embolism in pregnant patients is most commonly CT pulmonary angiography, although ventilation-perfusion scanning may also be used.

VI-6.   **The answers are 1. C; 2. B; 3. D; 4. A.** *(Chap. 252)* Ventilatory function can be easily measured with lung volume measurement and the FEV_1/FVC ratio. A decreased FEV_1/FVC ratio diagnoses obstructive lung disease. Alternatively, low lung volumes, specifically decreased TLC, and occasionally decreased RV diagnose restrictive lung disease. With extensive air trapping in obstructive lung disease, TLC is often increased and RV may also be increased. VC is proportionally decreased. MIP measures respiratory muscle strength and is decreased in patients with neuromuscular disease. Thus, myasthenia gravis will produce low lung volumes and decreased MIP, whereas patients with idiopathic pulmonary fibrosis will have normal muscle strength and subsequently a normal MIP, but decreased TLC and RV. In some cases of pulmonary parenchymal restrictive lung disease, the increase in elastic recoil results in an increased FEV_1/FVC ratio.

VI-7.   **The answer is C.** *(Chap. 252)* In this patient presenting with multilobar pneumonia, hypoxemia is present that does not correct with increasing the concentration of inspired oxygen. The inability to overcome hypoxemia or the lace of a notable increase in PaO_2 with increasing fraction of inspired oxygen to 1.0 physiologically defines a shunt. A shunt occurs when deoxygenated blood is transported to the left heart and systemic circulation without having the capability of becoming oxygenated. Causes of shunt include alveolar collapse (atelectasis), intra-alveolar filling processes, intrapulmonary vascular malformations, or structural cardiac disease leading to right-to-left shunt. In this case, the patient has multilobar pneumonia leading to alveoli that are being perfused but are unable to participate in gas exchange because they are filled with pus and inflammatory exudates. Acute respiratory distress syndrome is another common cause of shunt physiology. Ventilation-perfusion mismatch is the most common cause of hypoxemia and results when there are some alveolar units with low ratios (low ventilation to perfusion) that fail to fully oxygenate perfused blood. When blood is returned to the left heart, the poorly oxygenated blood admixes with blood from normal alveolar units. The resultant hypoxemia is less severe than with shunt and can be corrected with increasing the inspired oxygen concentration. Hypoventilation with or without other causes of hypoxemia is not present in this case as the $PaCO_2$ is less than 40 mmHg, indicating hyperventilation. The acidosis present in this case is of a metabolic rather than a pulmonary source. Because the patient is paralyzed, she is unable to increase her respiratory rate above the set rate to compensate for the metabolic acidosis.

VI-8.   **The answer is D.** *(Chap. 253)* This patient presents with a slowly progressive illness manifested by dyspnea on exertion, dry cough, clubbing, and the presence of crackles on examination. In addition, the pulmonary function tests demonstrate restrictive lung disease. This scenario is characteristic of an individual with interstitial lung disease, most commonly idiopathic pulmonary fibrosis in individuals at this age. A more thorough history should be obtained to determine if there are any other exposures or symptoms that could identify other causes of interstitial lung disease. The next step in the evaluation of this patient is to perform a high-resolution computed tomography scan (HRCT) of the chest. The high-resolution technique for CT imaging employs thinner cross-sectional images at approximately 1–2 mm rather than the usual 7–10 mm. This creates more visible details and is particularly useful for recognizing subtle changes of the interstitium and small airways including interstitial lung disease, bronchiolitis, and bronchiectasis. Bronchoscopy with transbronchial biopsy typically does not provide the detail required to adequately diagnose interstitial lung disease. It may be considered if there are specific features on HRCT that would suggest an alternative diagnosis. However, in most instances, the pathologic diagnosis of interstitial lung disease requires a surgical lung biopsy to provide a definitive diagnosis. This patient's symptoms do not suggest coronary artery disease or congestive heart failure. Thus, echocardiography and nuclear stress testing are not indicated.

CT scanning has evolved over the years to offer several different techniques that are useful in a variety of circumstances. Standard CT imaging is most useful for the evaluation and staging of lung masses. Helical CT scanning requires only a single breath hold and provides continuous collection of data with improved contrast enhancement and thinner collimation. Once the data are obtained, the images can be reconstructed into other views including sagittal and coronal planes as well as 3D volumetric representations. A recent use of this technology is employed in the setting of "virtual bronchoscopy" to aid in the planning and performance of bronchoscopy. Multidetector CT scans can obtain multiple slices in a single rotation that are thinner than the usual cuts. Multidetector CT scanners are used in the performance of the CT pulmonary angiogram.

VI-9.   **The answer is E.** (*Chap. 254*) The patient in this clinical scenario presents with symptoms typical of asthma, including shortness of breath and wheezing. She also manifests evidence of atopy, the most common risk factor for developing asthma, with sensitivity to outdoor allergens and cats. In addition, the patient has a history of allergic rhinitis and eczema, both of which are commonly seen in individuals with asthma. Indeed, over 80% of asthma patients have a concomitant diagnosis of allergic rhinitis. Atopy is present in 40–50% of the population of affluent countries, but only a small proportion of these individuals develop asthma. Many studies have shown a genetic predisposition via family history and recent genome-wide screens, but no single genetic profile has show high positive predictive value. Overall, the prevalence of asthma in developed countries has increased over the past 30 years, but recently has leveled off with a prevalence of about 15% in children and 10–12% in adults. Asthma deaths remain rare and have decreased in recent decades. In the 1960s, asthma deaths did increase with an overuse of short-acting beta-agonist medications. However, since the introduction of inhaled corticosteroids as maintenance therapy, deaths have declined. Risk factors for fatal asthma include frequent use of rescue inhalers, lack of therapy with inhaled corticosteroids, and prior hospitalizations for asthma. Interestingly, the overall disease severity does not vary significantly within a given patient over the course of the disease. Individuals who have mild asthma typically continue to have mild asthma, whereas as those with severe disease present with severe disease. Diagnosis of asthma can be made by demonstrating airflow obstruction with significant reversibility on bronchodilator administration. In this case, the FEV_1/FVC ratio is decreased to 70%, which is low. In addition, the FEV_1 increases by 12.4% and 230 mL. This meets the criteria for bronchodilator reversibility of an increase of at least 200 mL and 12%. Bronchoprovocation testing with methacholine may be considered in individuals who have suspected asthma but have normal pulmonary function tests.

VI-10.   **The answer is B.** (*Chap. 254*) The pathology of asthma has largely been determined by examining bronchial biopsies of patients with asthma as well as the lungs of individuals who die from asthma. These pathologic changes are centered around the airways with sparing of the alveolar spaces. The airways are infiltrated by eosinophils, activated T lymphocytes, and activated mucosal mast cells. However, the degree of inflammation does not correlate with the severity of asthma. Another common finding in all asthmatics and individuals with eosinophilic bronchitis is thickening of the basement membrane due to collagen deposition in the subepithelium. The airway smooth muscle is hypertrophied as well. Overall, this leads to thickening of the airway wall, which may also exhibit edematous fluid, particularly in those with fatal asthma. In cases of fatal asthma, it is also common to find multiple airways that are occluded by mucous plugs. However, the disease is limited to the airways, and infiltration of the alveolar spaces by inflammatory cells is not seen.

VI-11. **The answer is E.** *(Chap. 254)* A step up in asthma therapy should be considered when a patient continues to have symptoms after 3 months on appropriate therapy. Symptoms to consider when determining whether asthma therapy should be increased include presence of daily symptoms, nocturnal awakening more than once weekly, and limitations in daily activity. Physicians should also review the use of rescue inhalers and lung function when making decisions to step up therapy. In addition, the use of standard asthma severity questionnaires such as the Asthma Control Score may be helpful. When stepping up therapy in mild persistent asthma, the preferred next step in therapy is increasing to medium-dose inhaled corticosteroids or adding a long-acting beta-agonist. However, an alternate therapy that can be considered is adding a leukotriene antagonist, low-dose theophylline, or the leukotriene synthesis inhibitor zileuton to low-dose inhaled corticosteroids.

VI-12. **The answer is C.** *(Chap. 254)* The preferred method for diagnosing asthma is demonstration of airflow obstruction on spirometry that is at least partially reversible. This is demonstrated in option C with a decreased FEV_1/FVC ratio, decreased FEV_1, and a significant increase in FEV_1 following administration of albuterol. For an individual to be considered responsive to a bronchodilator, the individual should experience an increase in either FEV_1 or FVC of at least 200 mL and 12%. Option A describes someone with postviral cough syndrome, which can persist for several weeks following a viral upper respiratory infection. Option B describes someone with exercise-induced bronchoconstriction (EIB), which, in the absence of other symptoms to suggest asthma, should not be diagnosed as asthma. Isolated EIB lacks the characteristic airway inflammation of asthma and does not progress to asthma. While it is estimated that 80–90% of individuals with asthma experience EIB, many individuals who have EIB do not also have asthma. EIB is caused by hyperventilation with inhalation of cool, dry air that leads to bronchospasm. Option D describes someone with occupational asthma that has occurred after working with animals in the medical laboratory for many years. Symptoms that are characteristic of occupational asthma are symptoms only while at work that improve on the weekends and during holidays. Option E describes a patient with chronic obstructive pulmonary disease (COPD). In COPD, 25–48% of individuals can demonstrate bronchial hyperresponsiveness in response to methacholine.

VI-13. **The answer is D.** *(Chap. 254)* A step-down in asthma therapy can be considered when an individual has been clinically stable for 3–6 months. Factors demonstrating appropriate asthma control include daytime symptoms 2 or fewer times weekly, nighttime symptoms 2 or fewer times monthly, use of rescue inhaler 2 or fewer times weekly, FEV_1 or peak expiratory flow rate at least 80% of personal best, or appropriate control by validated asthma control questionnaires such as the Asthma Control Test or Asthma Therapy Assessment Questionnaire. When stepping down therapy, it is important to review the medications and their dosages. This patient is currently being managed with low-dose inhaled corticosteroids plus a long-acting beta-agonist. At this point, the best course of therapy is to stop the long-acting beta-agonist salmeterol. Since the dose of fluticasone the patient is receiving is already at a low dose, it would not be recommended to decrease it further, and it is never appropriate to treat with a long-acting beta-agonist alone without inhaled corticosteroids. In a large clinical trial, asthma mortality increased in individuals treated with long-acting beta-agonists in the absence of therapy with inhaled corticosteroids. Adding another medication is not indicated as the patient is demonstrating good asthma control.

VI-14. **The answer is D.** *(Chap. 254)* Omalizumab is a blocking antibody that binds to and neutralizes circulating immunoglobulin E (IgE) to inhibit IgE-mediated reactions. Omalizumab therapy can be considered for the outpatient treatment of severe, persistent asthma requiring high-dose inhaled corticosteroids in the presence of sensitivity to an aeroallergen. In clinical trials, treatment with omalizumab has been demonstrated to decrease the number of exacerbations in individual experiences and most individuals are also able to decrease the amount of oral or inhaled corticosteroids they are using. Elevations in serum IgE are frequently seen in asthmatic patients, and omalizumab can be considered in individuals whose IgE ranges from 30 to 700 IU/L. However, the manufacturer recommends not giving omalizumab therapy with marked elevations in IgE (>700 IU/L). Omalizumab is given as an injection every 2–4 weeks and must be given in an office setting because rare anaphylactic reactions can occur. If an individual is experiencing an acute exacerbation of asthma, omalizumab is typically held. However, it is not necessary to normalize lung function or discontinue oral steroids prior to initiating therapy with omalizumab.

VI-15. **The answer is C.** *(Chap. 255)* This patient has an acute presentation with pulmonary infiltrates and a pleural effusion, both of which have an increased percentage of eosinophils. In the United States, drug reactions are the most common cause of pulmonary infiltrates with eosinophilia (PIE syndrome), and among the drugs that can cause eosinophilia, nitrofurantoin is the most common. Nitrofurantoin is known to cause two types of pulmonary drug reaction. The acute drug reaction occurs within hours to days of starting nitrofurantoin. Patients present with dry cough, dyspnea, and fever. Chest radiograph demonstrates bilateral infiltrates. In a minority of cases, a pleural effusion is seen. Differential cell count demonstrates eosinophilia in both the pleural and bronchoalveolar lavage fluids. Treatment of nitrofurantoin-associated pulmonary eosinophilia consists primarily of stopping the medication. In severe cases, oral corticosteroids can be used as well, but this does not supersede the need to discontinue the nitrofurantoin. High doses of steroids are typically not required for drug-related pulmonary eosinophilia. While pulmonary infections can cause pulmonary eosinophilia, this patient has a typical time course and presentation for nitrofurantoin-associated lung disease. Therefore, one would not wait for cultures before recommending stopping the nitrofurantoin. Multiple drugs have been associated with eosinophilic pulmonary reactions. In addition to nitrofurantoin, they include sulfonamides, NSAIDs, penicillins, thiazides, tricyclic antidepressants, hydralazine, and chlorpropamide, among others. Levothyroxine, however, is not known to cause any lung disease. Both hypo- and hyperthyroidism can be associated with pleural effusions from the primary disease or associated heart failure. However, they are not associated with eosinophilic lung disease, and adjusting the levothyroxine dose is not indicated.

VI-16 and VI-17. **The answers are B and E, respectively.** *(Chap. 249)* The patient has a subacute presentation of hypersensitivity pneumonitis related to exposure to bird droppings and feathers at work. Hypersensitivity pneumonitis is a delayed-type hypersensitivity reaction that has a variety of presentations. Some people develop acute onset of shortness of breath, fevers, chills, and dyspnea within 6–8 hours of antigen exposure. Others may present subacutely with worsening dyspnea on exertion and dry cough over weeks to months. Chronic hypersensitivity pneumonitis presents with more severe and persistent symptoms with clubbing. Progressive worsening is common with the development of chronic hypoxemia, pulmonary hypertension, interstitial pulmonary fibrosis, and respiratory failure. The diagnosis relies on a variety of tests. Peripheral eosinophilia is not a feature of this disease as the disease is mediated through T-cell inflammation. Other nonspecific markers of inflammation may be elevated, including the erythrocyte sedimentation rate, C-reactive protein, rheumatoid factor, and serum immunoglobulins. Neutrophilia and lymphopenia may be seen. If a specific antigen is suspected, serum precipitins directed toward that antigen may be demonstrated. However, these tests are neither sensitive nor specific for the presence of disease. Chest radiography may be normal or show a diffuse reticulonodular infiltrate. High-resolution chest CT is the imaging modality of choice and shows ground-glass infiltrates in the lower lobes. Centrilobular infiltrates are often seen as well. In the chronic stages, patchy emphysema is the most common finding. Histopathologically, interstitial alveolar infiltrates predominate, with a variety of lymphocytes, plasma cells, and occasional eosinophils and neutrophils being seen. Loose, noncaseating granulomas are typical.

Treatment requires removing the individual from exposure to the antigen. If this is not possible, the patient should wear a mask that prevents small-particle inhalation during exposure. In patients with mild disease, removal from antigen exposure alone may be sufficient to treat the disease. More severe symptoms require therapy with glucocorticoids at an equivalent prednisone dose of 1 mg/kg daily for 7–14 days. The steroids are then gradually tapered over 2–6 weeks.

VI-18. **The answer is C.** *(Chap. 256)* Mesothelioma is a rare malignancy of the pleura and peritoneum with almost all cases associated with asbestos exposure. It is notable that the exposure to asbestos could seem almost minimal, but still confer significant risk. Exposures of less than 1–2 years or those that have occurred more than 40 years in the past have been demonstrated to confer an increased risk of mesothelioma. While tobacco smoking in association with asbestos exposure increases the risk of lung cancer several fold, there is no additive or exponential risk of mesothelioma in those who smoke. Mesothelioma most often presents with a persistent unilateral pleural effusion that may mask the underlying pleural tumor. However, the pleura may be diffusely thickened. Even with large effusions, no mediastinal shift is seen on chest radiograph because the pleural thickening associated with the disease leads to a fixed chest cavity size and thoracic restriction. The most difficult diagnostic dilemma in these patients is to differentiate mesothelioma from metastatic lung carcinoma (usually adenocarcinoma), as many patients are at risk for both tumors, and lung cancer is far and away the most common malignancy seen in those individuals with asbestos exposure and cigarette smoking. Pleural fluid cytology is not adequate for the diagnosis of most individuals with mesothelioma, with samples being positive for the disease in less than 50% of individuals. Most often video-assisted thoracoscopy is required to directly visualize the pleural surfaces and direct biopsy sampling. Unfortunately, there is no proven effective therapy for mesothelioma, and most patients die from local extension of the disease.

VI-19. **The answer is E.** *(Chap. 256)* Silicosis results from the inhalation of free silica (or crystalline quartz) and is associated with mining, stonecutting, foundry work, and quarrying. The chronic form of silicosis has been associated with an increased risk of a variety of diseases. Silica is known to be cytotoxic to alveolar macrophages and thus places patients at increased risk of pulmonary infections that rely on cellular immunity, including *Mycobacterium tuberculosis*, atypical mycobacteria, and fungus. In addition, silicosis is associated with the development of connective tissue disorders including rheumatoid arthritis with rheumatoid nodules (Caplan syndrome) and scleroderma. Finally, silica is listed as a probable lung carcinogen.

VI-20. **The answer is D.** *(Chap. 256)* Occupational lung diseases have been associated with a wide variety of organic and inorganic exposures in the workplace and clinically can range from primarily an airways disease to progressive pulmonary fibrosis. When evaluating a patient for a new pulmonary diagnosis, it is important to perform a detailed occupational history to determine if there is a possibility that the patient's profession may be causing or perpetuating the disease process. Specific clinical syndromes are associated with well-defined clinical exposures. The inorganic dusts include asbestos, silica, coal dust, beryllium, and a variety of other metals. Asbestos and silica are among the most common exposures. Asbestos exposure is associated with mining, construction, and ship repair. In areas near where asbestos mining has occurred, the general population also has shown an increased risk of asbestos-related lung disease. Clinically, asbestos exposure is associated with a range of clinical syndromes including asbestosis, benign pleural plaques and pleural effusions, lung cancer, and mesothelioma. Silica exposure is common among miners, stone masons, and individuals involved in sand blasting or quarrying. A variety of clinical syndromes can occur with silica exposure, the most severe being progressive massive fibrosis with masslike upper-lobe consolidating nodules (>1 cm). Coal mining is also associated with a clinical picture similar to silicosis and progressive massive fibrosis. Beryllium is a lightweight metal that is highly conductive and is used in high-tech industries. The classic disease associated with beryllium exposure is a chronic granulomatous disease similar in clinical appearance to sarcoidosis. Other metals can produce any number of clinical syndromes. Welders of galvanized metal who utilize zinc oxide are susceptible to metal fume fever and present with an acute self-limited influenza-like illness.

Organic dusts that can lead to occupational lung disease include cotton dust, grain dust, toxic chemicals, and other agricultural dusts, among many others. Cotton milling and processing can present with a clinical syndrome known as byssinosis, which has asthma-like features. Many of the organic dust exposures also lead to hypersensitivity pneumonitis. Examples of hypersensitivity pneumonitis syndromes related to occupational exposures include farmer's lung, pigeon breeder's lung, and malt worker's lung. Typically, a specific antigen can be identified as the culprit for the development of hypersensitivity pneumonitis. In farmer's lung, the most common cause is thermophilic *Actinomyces* species found in moldy hay.

VI-21. **The answer is B.** *(Chaps. 254 and 256)* The patient presents with typical asthma symptoms; however, the symptoms are escalating and now require nearly constant use of oral steroids. It is of note that the symptoms are worse during weekdays and better on weekends. This finding suggests that there is an exposure during the week that may be triggering the patient's asthma. Often textile workers have asthma resulting from the inhalation of particles. The first step in diagnosing a work-related asthma trigger is to check FEV_1 before and after the first shift of the workweek. A decrease in FEV_1 would suggest an occupational exposure. Skin testing for allergies would not be likely to pinpoint the work-related exposure. Although *A. fumigatus* can be associated with worsening asthma from allergic bronchopulmonary aspergillosis, this would not result in a fluctuation in symptoms throughout the week. The patient does not require further testing to diagnose that he has asthma; therefore, a methacholine challenge is not indicated. Finally, the exercise physiology test is generally used to differentiate between cardiac and pulmonary causes or deconditioning as etiologies for shortness of breath.

VI-22. **The answer is D.** *(Chap. 256)* The patient presents with acute-onset pulmonary symptoms, including wheezing, with no other medical problems. He is a farmer and was recently handling hay. The clinical presentation and radiogram are consistent with farmer's lung, a hypersensitivity pneumonitis caused by *Actinomyces*. In this disorder, spores of actinomycetes in moldy hay are inhaled and produce a hypersensitivity pneumonitis. The disorder is seen most commonly in rainy periods, when the spores multiply. Patients present generally 4–8 hours after exposure with fever, cough, and shortness of breath without wheezing. Chest radiograms often show patchy, bilateral, often upper-lobe infiltrates. The exposure history will differentiate this disorder from other types of pneumonia.

VI-23. **The answer is A.** *(Chap. 257)* Health care–associated pneumonia (HCAP) has emerged as a new category of pneumonia distinct from community-acquired pneumonia (CAP), as individuals at risk of HCAP frequently have multidrug-resistant organisms more typical of hospital-acquired pneumonia (HAP). Several risk factors have been identified for HCAP, and specific organisms are more commonly seen in specific situations. For example, methicillin-resistant *Staphylococcus aureus* (MRSA) has not only been associated with hospitalization for more than 48 hours, but also any hospitalization for 2 or more days in the preceding 3 months, as well as with individuals residing in nursing homes or extended care facilities, chronic dialysis, home infusion therapy, home wound care, or a family member with a multidrug-resistant infection. Antibiotic therapy in the preceding 3 months is not associated with the development of MRSA as a cause of HCAP, but is associated with *Pseudomonas aeruginosa* and multidrug-resistant (MDR) *Enterobacteriaceae* as causes of HCAP.

VI-24. **The answer is B.** *(Chap. 257)* The diagnosis and treatment of community-acquired pneumonia (CAP) often incorporate a combination of clinical, radiographic, and laboratory features to determine the most likely etiology and treatment. In most instances of CAP, outpatient treatment is sufficient, and definitive etiologic diagnosis of the causative organism is not required, nor is it cost-effective. However, the outpatient diagnosis of CAP most often does require confirmation by chest radiograph, as the sensitivity and specificity of the findings on physical examination are about 58% and 67%, respectively. In addition, chest radiograph may identify risk factors for more severe clinical courses such as multifocal infiltrates. Moreover, outside of the 2% of individuals admitted to intensive care for treatment of CAP, there are no data that treatment directed against the specific causative organism is superior to empiric therapy. In some instances, one may decide to attempt to determine a causative organism for CAP, particularly in individuals who have risk factors for resistant organisms or if the patient fails to respond appropriately to initial antibiotic therapy. The most common way CAP is diagnosed is via sputum culture with Gram stain. The primary purpose of the Gram stain is to ensure that the sputum is an adequate lower respiratory sample for culture with fewer than 10 squamous epithelial cells and more than 25 neutrophils per high-powered field. However, at times it can suggest a specific diagnosis based on the appearance. Generally, the yield from sputum culture is 50% or less, even in cases of bacteremic pneumococcal pneumonia. The yield from blood cultures is also low, even when collected prior to initiation of antibiotics, at 5–14%. More recently, antigen tests or polymerase chain reaction (PCR) testing directed against specific organisms has gained favor. The most common antigen test that is performed is for *Legionella pneumophila*, as this organism does not grow in culture unless performed on specific media. Antigen and PCR tests are also available for *Streptococcus pneumoniae* and *Mycoplasma pneumoniae*, but given the costs they are not frequently performed

VI-25. **The answer is D.** *(Chap. 257)* Determining the appropriate empiric coverage for community-acquired pneumonia (CAP) initially requires determining if the severity of illness warrants admission to the hospital. Clinical rules for determining the potential severity of pneumonia have been developed including the Pneumonia Severity Index (PSI) and the CURB-65 criteria. While the PSI has the largest body of research to support its use, the model includes 20 variables, which may be impractical in a busy clinical practice. The CURB-65 criteria include only five variables: (1) **C**onfusion; (2) **U**rea greater than 7 mmol/L; (3) **R**espiratory rate greater than or equal to 30/min; (4) **B**lood pressure less than or equal to 90/60; and (5) age of **65** or older. This patient meets none of the criteria for hospitalization and is not hypoxemic or in a high-risk group for complications from CAP. Therefore, he can safely be treated as an outpatient without further diagnostic workup, as his history, physical examination, and chest radiograph are all consistent with the diagnosis of CAP. The empiric antibiotic regimen recommended by the Infectious Diseases Society of America and the American Thoracic Society for individuals who are previously healthy and have not received antibiotics in the prior 3 months is either doxycycline or a macrolide such as azithromycin or clarithromycin. In outpatients with significant medical comorbidities or antibiotics within the prior 3 months, the suggested antibiotic therapy is either a respiratory fluoroquinolone or a beta-lactam plus a macrolide.

VI-26. **The answer is E.** *(Chap. 257)* Ventilator-associated pneumonia (VAP) is a common complication of endotracheal intubation and mechanical ventilation. Prevalence estimates indicate that 70% of patients requiring mechanical ventilation for 30 days or longer will have at least one instance of VAP. However, the epidemiology of VAP has been difficult to accurately study as no single set of criteria is reliably diagnostic of VAP. Generally, it is thought that VAP has a tendency to be overdiagnosed for a variety of reasons, including the high rates of tracheal colonization with pathogenic organisms and the multiple alternative causes of fevers and/or pulmonary infiltrates in critically ill patients. Quantitative cultures have gained favor, as the quantitative nature is thought to discriminate better between colonization and active infection. A variety of approaches have been advocated including endotracheal aspirates yielding more than 10^6 organisms or protected brush specimens from distal airways yielding more than 10^3 organisms. However, the quantitative yield of these tests can be highly influenced by even a single dose of antibiotics, and antibiotic changes are common in critically ill patients, particularly when a new fever has emerged. Thus, the lack of growth on quantitative culture may be difficult to interpret in this setting. More recently, there has been growing use of the Clinical Pulmonary Infection Score (CPIS), which incorporates a variety of clinical, radiographic, and laboratory factors to determine the likelihood of VAP, although its true utility in clinical practice remains to be fully determined.

VI-27. **The answer is D.** *(Chap. 257)* Aspiration can lead to anaerobic infection and chemical pneumonitis. The etiologic differential diagnosis of community-acquired pneumonia (CAP) in a patient with a history of recent travel to the southwestern United States should include *Coccidioides*. *Aspergillus* has a worldwide distribution and is not a cause of CAP syndrome. Alcohol use predisposes patients to anaerobic infection, likely due to aspiration, as well as *S. pneumoniae*. *Klebsiella* is classically associated with CAP in alcoholic patients, but in reality this is rarely seen. Patients with structural lung disease, such as cystic fibrosis or bronchiectasis, are at risk for a unique group of organisms including *P. aeruginosa* and *S. aureus*. Poor dental hygiene is associated with anaerobic infections.

VI-28. **The answer is D.** *(Chap. 258)* Bronchiectasis occurs when there is irreversible dilation of the distal airways and can occur in a focal or diffuse fashion. The most common cause of diffuse bronchiectasis worldwide is prior granulomatous infection due to *Mycobacterium tuberculosis*. In the developed world, tuberculosis is a less common cause of bronchiectasis, with nontuberculous mycobacteria such as *Mycobacterium avium-intracellulare* complex being a more common cause, particularly in the midlung fields. Other potential etiologies of diffuse bronchiectasis include cystic fibrosis, postradiation pneumonitis, immunoglobulin deficiency, end-stage fibrotic lung disease, and recurrent aspiration. However, despite extensive workup, as many as 25–50% of cases remain idiopathic.

VI-29. **The answer is C.** *(Chap. 258)* Bronchiectasis is a disorder with a variable presentation depending on cause. In inherited disorders such as cystic fibrosis, the symptoms of bronchiectasis most often begin in early childhood. However, in general, the incidence of bronchiectasis increases with age, typically affecting women more than men. The primary clinical symptom of bronchiectasis is a daily productive cough. Classically, the sputum is described as large volume with a thick tenacious character. Hemoptysis may also occur in association with bronchiectasis. The physical examination may demonstrate crackles or wheezing with mild to moderate airflow obstruction on pulmonary function testing. In more advanced cases, digital clubbing may be seen. The diagnosis of bronchiectasis is often suspected based on clinical symptoms, but confirmation of diagnosis on high-resolution CT imaging of the chest is recommended. The chest radiograph may show tram tracking, but is frequently normal and is of insufficient sensitivity to definitively make the diagnosis. On high-resolution chest CT imaging, bronchiectatic airways appear dilated more than 1.5 times the size of the adjacent pulmonary artery. In addition, the airways fail to taper in the periphery, and airways may be identifiable within 1 cm of the pleural surface, which is clearly abnormal. Bronchial wall thickening and inspissated secretions may also be seen. Contrast administration is not necessary to visualize bronchiectasis. Once bronchiectasis is confirmed as the etiology of the patient's chronic cough, workup for the underlying etiology of the bronchiectasis should be performed and would likely include sputum cultures for mycobacteria and bacteria, serum immunoglobulin, and α_1 antitrypsin levels, among others.

VI-30. **The answer is A.** *(Chap. 258)* This patient presents with a clinical history that is consistent with a polymicrobial lung abscess with infection by anaerobic bacteria. Often individuals present with an indolent course and nonspecific symptoms including fever, fatigue, and weight loss. Cough with a foul-smelling sputum production may also be seen. Individuals presenting with lung abscess often have risk factors for aspiration and evidence of periodontal infection. In more advanced cases, the lung abscess can erode into the pleura, creating an empyema with associated pleuritic chest pain. Although chest radiograph often demonstrates a cavitary lesion, a CT may be performed to determine the extent of the disease and whether there are associated lesions. Bacterial, mycobacterial, and fungal cultures should be performed, but this should not delay treatment of the most likely cause of the lung abscess. A sputum culture on an expectorated sample will only detect aerobic organisms, and the detection of anaerobes would be confounded by the presence of multiple oral anaerobes that could contaminate an expectorated specimen. Initial treatment should be directed primarily at anaerobic organisms. Recommended antibiotics are clindamycin IV 600 mg four times daily or a β-lactam/β-lactamase inhibitor combination (ampicillin-sulbactam, amoxicillin-clavulanic acid). Metronidazole is not recommended because it has poor activity against the microaerophilic streptococci that commonly infect lung abscesses. The duration of treatment is not well defined. Some experts recommend continuing therapy until the abscess has entirely healed. Persistence of fever beyond 5–7 days should prompt the clinician to investigate further. Potential complications include development of empyema or a bronchopleural fistula. In addition, one should consider performing bronchoscopy to rule out an obstructing lesion. Percutaneous or surgical intervention is generally not required unless the patient fails to respond to antibiotic therapy or has a lung abscess greater than 6 cm.

VI-31. **The answer is D.** *(Chap. 258)* The combination of infertility and recurrent sinopulmonary infections should prompt consideration of an underlying disorder of ciliary dysfunction that is termed primary ciliary dyskinesia. These disorders account for approximately 5–10% of cases of bronchiectasis. A number of deficiencies have been described, including malfunction of dynein arms, radial spokes, and microtubules. All organ systems that require ciliary function are affected. The lungs rely on cilia to beat respiratory secretions proximally and subsequently to remove inspired particles, especially bacteria. In the absence of this normal host defense, recurrent bacterial respiratory infections occur and can lead to bronchiectasis. Otitis media and sinusitis are common for the same reason. In the genitourinary tract, sperm require cilia to provide motility. Kartagener's syndrome is a combination of sinusitis, bronchiectasis, and situs inversus. It accounts for approximately 50% of patients with primary ciliary dyskinesia. Cystic fibrosis is associated with infertility and bilateral upper-lobe infiltrates. It causes a decreased number of sperm or absent sperm on analysis because of the congenital absence of the vas deferens. Sarcoidosis, which is often associated with bihilar adenopathy, is not generally a cause of infertility. A water balloon–shaped heart is found in those with pericardial effusions, which one would not expect in this patient.

VI-32. **The answer is E.** *(Chap. 259)* Cystic fibrosis (CF) is a common autosomal-recessive disorder that affects 1 out of every 3000 live births in the Caucasian population of North America and Europe. There have been more than 1500 mutations identified in the gene for the cystic fibrosis transmembrane conductance regulator (CFTR)—the abnormal protein identified in CF. This protein is a large transmembrane protein involved in the transport of chloride and other ions, and abnormalities of the CFTR lead to abnormalities of salt and water transport. The primary clinical manifestations of CF are due to the effects of the mutated CFTR in the lungs, gastrointestinal tract, and pancreas. In the lungs, abnormal CFTR leads to thick, sticky mucus with abnormal mucociliary clearance. A patient will have recurrent respiratory infections with development of cystic bronchiectasis over time. The presenting manifestation in infancy is often meconium ileus and can lead to constipation and distal intestinal obstruction in adults. Failure of the CFTR in the pancreas prevents appropriate release of pancreatic enzymes to allow for proper digestion of food, especially fatty foods, with resultant malnutrition and steatorrhea. While most patients with CF present in infancy or childhood, about 5% of all individuals with CF will not be diagnosed until adulthood. Presenting symptoms in adulthood can be myriad and often result from minor mutations of the CFTR gene. These symptoms can include recurrent lung and sinus infections, malnutrition, sinus disease, and infertility, especially absence of the vas deferens in men. The standard test for the diagnosis of CF is the sweat chloride test. Elevated values are pathognomonic for CF, with a cutoff of greater than 70 meq/L in adults being diagnostic. Values greater than approximately 35 meq/L fall within the indeterminate range. DNA analysis for common CF mutations is often performed, and one would want to demonstrate two alleles known to cause CF before making the diagnosis, as the disease is autosomal recessive. Identification of only one allele only identifies the carrier state. In some individuals, the diagnosis can remain elusive. In such cases, referral to a tertiary center for nasal potential difference (PD) testing can be helpful, as CF patients demonstrate an elevated baseline nasal PD with failure to respond to stimulation with beta-agonists. Presence of *Pseudomonas aeruginosa* is common in adults with CF, but is not specific for the diagnosis of the disease as bronchiectasis from any cause can lead to *P. aeruginosa* colonization.

VI-33. **The answer is C.** *(Chap. 259)* Individuals with cystic fibrosis (CF) experience recurrent pulmonary and sinus infections. In childhood, the most commonly isolated organisms are *Haemophilus influenzae* and *Staphylococcus aureus*. However, over time, most adults demonstrate *Pseudomonas aeruginosa*. It is now recognized that chronic colonization with *Pseudomonas*, especially multidrug-resistant organisms, is associated with a more rapid decline in lung function. The Cystic Fibrosis Foundation recommends quarterly office visits with a physician, with assessment of respiratory cultures at each visit. When *Pseudomonas* is initially detected, attempts to eradicate the organism should be undertaken. Clinical trials have not definitively determined the best regimen for eradicating *Pseudomonas*, but the most common utilized treatment is the aminoglycoside antibiotic tobramycin given as a nebulized solution twice daily every other month with follow-up cultures at the next office visit to determine if the therapy should be continued. For all patients chronically colonized with *Pseudomonas*, inhaled tobramycin every other month should be continued on an indefinite basis. In addition, azithromycin 500 mg three times weekly or 250 mg daily is also utilized. Whether azithromycin primarily exerts its beneficial effect through anti-inflammatory or antimicrobial actions is not definitively known at the present time. As the patient is clinically well without any symptoms of acute exacerbation, the use of intravenous antibiotics is not required. Chest wall oscillation and hypertonic saline are both mechanisms to improve airway clearance. By history and lung function, the patient is achieving adequate airway clearance at the present time, so escalation of care in this area is not required.

VI-34. **The answer is B.** *(Chap. 259)* Patients with cystic fibrosis are at risk for colonization and/or infection with a number of pathogens, and in general these infections have a temporal relationship. In childhood, the most frequently isolated organisms are *Haemophilus influenzae* and *Staphylococcus aureus*. As patients age, *Pseudomonas aeruginosa* becomes the predominant pathogen. Interestingly, *Aspergillus fumigatus* is found in the airways of up to 50% of cystic fibrosis patients. All these organisms merely colonize the airways but occasionally can also cause disease. *Burkholderia* (previously called *Pseudomonas*) *cepacia* can occasionally be found in the sputum of cystic fibrosis patients, where it is always pathogenic and is associated with a rapid decline in both clinical parameters and pulmonary function testing. Atypical mycobacteria can occasionally be found in the sputum but are often merely colonizers. *Acinetobacter baumannii* is not associated with cystic fibrosis; rather, it is generally found in nosocomial infections.

VI-35. **The answer is D.** *(Chap. 260)* Chronic obstructive pulmonary disease (COPD) affects more than 10 million Americans and is currently the fourth leading cause of death in the United States. Worldwide, COPD is also increasing as cigarette smoking, the primary risk factor for the development of COPD, is increasing in prevalence throughout the world. While cigarette smoking is clearly identified as a risk factor for COPD, other factors have also been identified to contribute to the risk of COPD. In many developing countries, the prevalence of smoking among women remains low. However, the incidence of COPD is increasing in women as well as men. In many developing countries, this increased incidence of COPD in women is attributable to the use of biomass fuels in poorly ventilated areas for heat and cooking. In addition, passive cigarette smoke exposure may also contribute. Occupational exposures also lead to an increased risk of COPD. While some exposures such as cotton textile dust and gold mining have not been definitively associated with COPD, coal dust exposure is a risk factor for emphysema in both smokers and nonsmokers. Inherent properties of the airways also affect the risk of COPD. Airway hyperresponsiveness increases the risk of lung function decline and is a risk factor for COPD. While there is much interest in the role of chronic or recurrent infections as a risk factor for COPD, there has been no proven link.

VI-36. **The answer is B.** *(Chap. 260)* Chronic obstructive pulmonary disease (COPD) is a disease process encompassing the clinical entities of emphysema and chronic bronchitis. COPD is defined pathophysiologically by the presence of irreversible airflow obstruction with hyperinflation and impaired gas exchange. The airflow obstruction occurs for several reasons including decreased elastic recoil of the lungs, increased airway inflammation, and increased closure of small airways due to loss of tethering in emphysematous lungs. This leads to early closure of airways in expiration with air trapping and hyperinflation. Finally, the loss of alveoli in emphysematous lungs leads to a progressive decline in gas exchange with alterations of ventilation-perfusion relationships. On pulmonary function testing, these pathophysiologic changes result in a typical pattern, with the primary characteristic of COPD being a decrease in the FEV_1/FVC ratio and FEV_1. The severity of airflow obstruction is graded by the degree of decline in the percentage predicted FEV_1. The FVC may or may not be decreased. With hyperinflation, the total lung capacity increases with a concomitant increase in residual volume. Finally, the diffusion capacity for carbon monoxide is also characteristically decreased in most cases of COPD. Some patients with pure chronic bronchitis without any emphysematous component may have a preserved carbon monoxide diffusing capacity (DLCO). This same pattern of pulmonary function testing can be seen in asthma with the exception of the DLCO, which is normal or increased in asthma.

VI-37. **The answer is D.** *(Chap. 260)* This patient has a known diagnosis of chronic obstructive pulmonary disease (COPD) with worsening symptoms and pulmonary function testing consistent with a moderate degree of disease. By the Global Initiative for Lung Disease (GOLD) criteria, the patient would have stage II disease. He is currently undermanaged with a short-acting beta-agonist only in the setting of limiting symptoms. Unfortunately, there is no medical therapy that alters mortality or definitively decreases the rate of decline in lung function in COPD, with the exception of smoking cessation, oxygen for chronic hypoxemia, and lung volume reduction surgery in a small subset of highly selected patients. Therefore, the goal of therapy in COPD is to improve symptoms and quality of life. The best initial medication for this patient would be to add a long-acting bronchodilator in the form of the antimuscarinic agent tiotropium. In large randomized controlled trials, tiotropium has been demonstrated to improve symptoms and decrease exacerbations in COPD. Ipratropium, a short-acting anticholinergic medication, also improves symptoms, but has not been similarly shown to decrease exacerbation rate. Combinations of long-acting beta-agonists and inhaled glucocorticoids have also been shown to decrease exacerbations and improve quality of life in those with COPD. The largest trial of these medications to date has demonstrated a trend toward improved mortality. Currently the recommendation for initiation of long-acting beta-agonist and inhaled glucocorticoid combinations is to consider starting the medication if the patient has two or more exacerbations yearly or demonstrates significant acute bronchodilator reactivity on pulmonary function testing. At one time, physicians considered prescribing long-term oral glucocorticoids if a patient demonstrated significant improvement in lung function in response to a trial of oral steroids. However, long-term treatment with steroids has an unfavorable risk-benefit ratio including weight gain, osteoporosis, and increased risk of infection, especially pneumonia. Oxygen therapy improves outcomes in individuals who are hypoxemic at rest or have borderline hypoxemia with evidence of end-organ damage (pulmonary hypertension, polycythemia, etc.). While oxygen may be prescribed for individuals with isolated exercise or nocturnal hypoxemia, research to date has not demonstrated any change in outcomes with oxygen in these settings.

VI-38. **The answer is E.** *(Chap. 260)* Acute exacerbations of chronic obstructive pulmonary disease (COPD) are marked by an increase in dyspnea, an increase in sputum, and a change in sputum color. Acute exacerbations of COPD account for more than $10 billion in health care expenditures annually in the United States, with a significant morbidity and mortality associated with these exacerbations. Prompt treatment can improve symptoms and decrease hospitalizations and mortality in this setting. In patients presenting with hypercarbic respiratory failure in the setting of an acute exacerbation, the treatment that has demonstrated the strongest reduction in mortality is noninvasive positive pressure ventilation (NIPPV) when compared to traditional mechanical ventilation. NIPPV also decreases the need for endotracheal intubation, complications, and length of stay in the hospital. Antibiotics, bronchodilators, and glucocorticoids are all cornerstones of therapy in the treatment of acute exacerbations in COPD, but have not been demonstrated in clinical trials to have similar mortality benefits in the situation of acute hypercarbic respiratory failure. Specifically, no benefit is demonstrated for intravenous versus oral corticosteroids. Likewise, the choice of antibiotic should be made based on local susceptibility patterns, and the need for broad-spectrum antibiotics that cover *Pseudomonas* is not typically indicated.

VI-39. **The answer is C.** *(Chap. 260)* The only therapies that have been proven to improve survival in patients with COPD are smoking cessation, oxygen in patients with resting hypoxemia, and lung volume reduction surgery in a very small subset of highly selected patients. This patient probably has resting hypoxemia resulting from the presence of an elevated jugular venous pulse, pedal edema, and an elevated hematocrit. Theophylline has been shown to increase exercise tolerance in patients with COPD through a mechanism other than bronchodilation. Oral glucocorticoids are not indicated in the absence of an acute exacerbation and may lead to complications if they are used indiscriminately. Atenolol and enalapril have no specific role in therapy for COPD but are often used when there is concomitant hypertension or cardiovascular disease.

VI-40. **The answer is E.** *(Chap. 261)* Usual interstitial pneumonia is the pathologic hallmark of idiopathic pulmonary fibrosis (IPF), but can occur in rheumatologic disorders or secondary to exposures. If no other cause is identified on history or serologic workup, then the patient is given the diagnosis of IPF. IPF is a disease that typically presents with progressive dyspnea on exertion and dry cough in an older individual. It is rare in individuals younger than 50. On physical examination, inspiratory crackles and clubbing are common. Pulmonary function tests demonstrate restrictive ventilatory defect with a low DLCO. High-resolution chest CT shows interstitial fibrosis that is worse in the bases and begins in the subpleural areas. Bronchoscopy is insufficient for histologic confirmation, and a surgical lung biopsy is required for definitive diagnosis. The natural history of IPF is one of continued progression of disease and a high mortality rate. Acute exacerbations also occur with a rapid progression of symptoms associated with a pattern of diffuse ground-glass opacities on CT. These are associated with a high mortality. Unfortunately, no therapy has been found to be effective for the treatment of IPF. Referral for lung transplantation or participation in clinical trials should be considered in all patients with a diagnosis of IPF.

VI-41. **The answer is C.** *(Chap. 261)* In many cases of interstitial lung disease, bronchoscopy can offer some clues to the cause of the disease. Diffuse alveolar hemorrhage (DAH) is a pathologic process that can occur in many diseases including vasculitis, Goodpasture's syndrome, systemic lupus erythematosus, crack cocaine use, mitral stenosis, and idiopathic pulmonary hemosiderosis, among many others. On bronchoscopy, one would expect to see a progressively increasing bloody return on sequential aliquots of lavage fluid. Microscopic examination would show hemosiderin-laden macrophages and red blood cells. Atypical hyperplastic type II pneumocytes are seen in diffuse alveolar damage or cases of drug toxicity. Ferruginous bodies and dust particles are found in asbestos-related pulmonary disease. Lymphocytosis is common to hypersensitivity pneumonitis and sarcoidosis. Hypersensitivity pneumonitis has a low CD4:CD8 ratio, whereas sarcoidosis has an elevated CD4:CD8 ratio. The bronchoalveolar lavage fluid in pulmonary alveolar proteinosis has a milky appearance with foamy macrophages.

VI-42 and VI-43. **The answers are E and E, respectively.** *(Chap. 261)* Pulmonary alveolar proteinosis (PAP) is a rare disorder with an incidence of approximately one per million. The disease usually presents in those between the ages of 30 and 50 and is slightly more common in men. Three distinct subtypes have been described: congenital, acquired, and secondary (most frequently caused by acute silicosis or hematologic malignancies). Interestingly, the pathogenesis of the disease has been associated with antibodies to granulocyte-macrophage colony-stimulating factor (GM-CSF) in most cases of acquired disease in adults. The pathobiology of the disease is failure of clearance of pulmonary surfactant. These patients typically present with subacute dyspnea on exertion with fatigue and low-grade fevers. Associated laboratory abnormalities include polycythemia, hypergammaglobulinemia, and increased LDH levels. Classically, the CT appearance is described as "crazy pavement" with ground-glass alveolar infiltrates in a perihilar distribution and intervening areas of normal lung. Bronchoalveolar lavage is diagnostic, with large amounts of amorphous proteinaceous material seen. Macrophages filled with periodic acid–Schiff (PAS)-positive material are also frequently seen. The treatment of choice is whole-lung lavage through a double-lumen endotracheal tube. Survival at 5 years is higher than 95%, although some patients will need a repeat whole-lung lavage. Secondary infection, especially with *Nocardia*, is common, and these patients should be followed closely.

VI-44. **The answer is E.** *(Chap. 261)* This patient's clinical presentation and CT imaging are consistent with the diagnosis of idiopathic pulmonary fibrosis (IPF), which is manifested histologically as usual interstitial pneumonitis (UIP). On microscopic examination, UIP is characterized by a heterogeneous appearance on low magnification with normal-appearing alveoli adjacent to severely fibrotic alveoli. There is lymphocytic infiltrate and scattered foci of fibroblasts within the alveolar septae. End-stage fibrosis results in honeycombing with loss of all alveolar structure. The typical clinical presentation of IPF/UIP is slowly progressive exertional dyspnea with a nonproductive cough. Clinical examination reveals dry crackles and digital clubbing. Patients with IPF are usually older than 50 years, and more than two-thirds have a history of current or former tobacco use. In the typical clinical situation of an older individual, a high-resolution CT scan of the chest can be diagnostic and shows subpleural pulmonary fibrosis that is greatest at the lung bases. As disease progresses, traction bronchiectasis and honeycombing are characteristic on CT scan. The cause of UIP is unknown, and no therapies have been shown to improve survival in this disease, with the exception of lung transplantation.

The presence of a dense, amorphous material in alveolar spaces that is periodic acid–Schiff positive is characteristic of pulmonary alveolar proteinosis. Pulmonary alveolar proteinosis is an interstitial lung disease that presents with progressive dyspnea, and CT imaging shows characteristic "crazy paving" with ground-glass infiltrates and thickened alveolar septae. Fibrosis is not present. Alveolar destruction with emphysematous changes would be seen in chronic obstructive pulmonary disease (COPD). The presence of crackles without wheezing or hyperinflation on examination does not suggest COPD. Furthermore, clubbing is not typically seen in COPD. Diffuse alveolar damage is seen in acute interstitial pneumonitis and acute respiratory distress syndrome (ARDS). These disorders present with a rapid, acute course that is not present in this case. The formation of non-caseating granulomas is typical of sarcoidosis, a systemic disease that usually presents in younger individuals. It is more common in those of African-American race. A typical CT in sarcoidosis would show interstitial infiltrates and hilar lymphadenopathy. End-stage disease may result in pulmonary fibrosis, but it is greatest in the upper lobes. Poorly formed granulomas may be seen in hypersensitivity pneumonitis.

VI-45. **The answer is A.** *(Chap. 261)* Pulmonary complications are common in patients with systemic lupus erythematosus (SLE). The most common manifestation is pleuritis with or without effusion. Other possible manifestations include pulmonary hemorrhage, diaphragmatic dysfunction with loss of lung volumes (the so-called shrinking lung syndrome), pulmonary vascular disease, acute interstitial pneumonitis, and bronchiolitis obliterans organizing pneumonia. Other systemic complications of SLE also cause pulmonary complications, including uremic pulmonary edema and infectious complications. Chronic progressive pulmonary fibrosis is not a complication of SLE. Cavitary lung nodules are typical of Wegener's granulomatosis but may also be seen in a variety of necrotizing lung infections.

VI-46. **The answer is E.** *(Chap. 261)* This patient with rheumatoid arthritis (RA) is presenting with pulmonary symptoms, and the biopsy shows a pattern of cryptogenic organizing pneumonia (COP), a known pulmonary manifestation of rheumatoid arthritis. COP (formerly bronchiolitis obliterans organizing pneumonia, BOOP) usually presents in the fifth or sixth decade with a flulike illness. Symptoms include fever, malaise, weight loss, cough, and dyspnea. Inspiratory crackles are common, and late inspiratory squeaks may also be heard. Pulmonary function testing reveals restrictive lung disease. The typical pattern on high-resolution chest CT is patchy areas of airspace consolidation, nodular opacities, and ground-glass opacities that occur more frequently in the lower lung zones. Pathology shows the presence of granulation tissue plugging airways, alveolar ducts, and alveoli. There is frequently chronic inflammation in the alveolar interstitium. Treatment with high-dose steroids is effective in two-thirds of individuals, with most individuals being able to be tapered to lower doses over the first year. Azathioprine is an immunosuppressive therapy that is commonly used in interstitial lung disease due to usual interstitial pneumonitis. While it may be considered in COP that is unresponsive to glucocorticoids, it would not be a first-line agent used without concomitant steroid therapy. RA has multiple pulmonary complications. However, therapy with infliximab or methotrexate, which is useful for severe RA, is not used in the treatment of COP. Methotrexate also has pulmonary side effects and may cause pulmonary fibrosis. Hydroxychloroquine is frequently useful for joint symptoms in autoimmune disorders. Its major side effect is retinal toxicity, and it is not known to cause COP.

VI-47. **The answer is B.** (*Chap. 262*) The D-dimer measured by enzyme-linked immunosorbent assay (ELISA) is elevated in the setting of breakdown of fibrin by plasmin, and the presence of a positive D-dimer can prompt the need for additional imaging for deep venous thrombosis and/or pulmonary embolus in specific clinical situations where the patient would be considered to have an elevation in D-dimer. However, one must be cautious about placing value on an elevated D-dimer in other situations where there can be an alternative explanation for the elevated level. Of the scenarios listed in the question, the only patient who would be expected to have a negative D-dimer would be the patient with calf pain and recent air travel. The presence of a normal alveolar-arterial oxygen gradient cannot reliably differentiate between those with and without pulmonary embolism. In all the other scenarios, elevations in D-dimer could be related to other medical conditions and provide no diagnostic information to inform the clinician regarding the need for further evaluation. Some common clinical situations in which the D-dimer is elevated include sepsis, myocardial infarction, cancer, pneumonia, the postoperative state, and the second and third trimesters of pregnancy.

VI-48. **The answer is B.** (*Chap. 262*) Clinically, individuals with massive pulmonary embolus present with hypotension, syncope, or cyanosis. The hypotension and syncope occur due to acute right ventricular overload, and elevated troponin or NT-pro-brain natriuretic peptide can result from this right ventricular strain. Both elevated troponin and NT-pro-brain natriuretic peptide predict worse outcomes in pulmonary embolism. Further prognostic signs of massive pulmonary embolism include the presence of right ventricular enlargement on CT of the chest or right ventricular hypokinesis on echocardiogram. The presence of hemoptysis, pleuritic chest pain, or cough in association with pulmonary embolism most commonly indicates a small peripheral lesion.

VI-49. **The answer is B.** (*Chap. 262*) For many years, ventilation-perfusion imaging (V-Q) was the standard for the diagnosis of pulmonary embolism (PE). Determination of abnormal V-Q imaging can be difficult. To call a V-Q scan a high-probability scan, one needs to see two or more segmental perfusion defects in the setting of normal ventilation. In patients with underlying lung disease, however, ventilation is frequently abnormal, and most patients with PE do not actually have high-probability V-Q scans. When there is a high-probability V-Q scan, the likelihood of PE is 90% or greater. Alternatively, patients with normal perfusion imaging have a very low likelihood of PE. Most patients fall into either the low or intermediate probability of having a PE by V-Q imaging. In this setting, 40% of patients with a high clinical suspicion of PE are determined by pulmonary angiography to indeed have a PE despite having a low-probability V-Q scan. At the present time, V-Q scanning is largely supplanted by multidetector-row spiral CT angiography of the chest. When compared to conventional CT scanning with intravenous contrast, the multidetector spiral CT can provide evaluation of the pulmonary arteries to the sixth-order branches, a level of resolution that is as good as or exceeds that of conventional invasive pulmonary angiography. In addition, the CT allows evaluation of the right and left ventricles as well as the lung parenchyma to provide additional information regarding prognosis in acute PE or alternative diagnosis in the patient with dyspnea. Magnetic resonance angiography is a rarely used alternative to the above modalities in patients with contrast dye allergy. This technique provides the ability to detect large proximal PEs, but lacks reliability for segmental and subsegmental PE.

VI-50. **The answer is E.** *(Chap. 262)* This patient is presenting with massive pulmonary embolus with ongoing hypotension, right ventricular dysfunction, and profound hypoxemia requiring 100% oxygen. In this setting, continuing with anticoagulation alone is inadequate, and the patient should receive circulatory support with fibrinolysis if there are no contraindications to therapy. The major contraindications to fibrinolysis include hypertension greater than 180/110 mmHg, known intracranial disease or prior hemorrhagic stroke, recent surgery, or trauma. The recommended fibrinolytic regimen is recombinant tissue plasminogen activator (rTPA), 100 mg IV over 2 hours. Heparin should be continued with the fibrinolytic to prevent a rebound hypercoagulable state with dissolution of the clot. There is a 10% risk of major bleeding with fibrinolytic therapy, with a 1–3% risk of intracranial hemorrhage. The only indication approved by the U.S. Food and Drug Administration for fibrinolysis in pulmonary embolus (PE) is for massive PE presenting with life-threatening hypotension, right ventricular dysfunction, and refractory hypoxemia. In submassive PE presenting with preserved blood pressure and evidence of right ventricular dysfunction on echocardiogram, the decision to pursue fibrinolysis is made on a case-by-case basis. In addition to fibrinolysis, the patient should also receive circulatory support with vasopressors. Dopamine and dobutamine are the vasopressors of choice for the treatment of shock in PE. Caution should be taken with ongoing high-volume fluid administration, as a poorly functioning right ventricle may be poorly tolerant of additional fluids. Ongoing fluids may worsen right ventricular ischemia and further dilate the right ventricle, displacing the interventricular septum to the left to worsen cardiac output and hypotension. If the patient had contraindications to fibrinolysis and was unable to be stabilized with vasopressor support, referral for surgical embolectomy should be considered. Referral for inferior vena cava filter placement is not indicated at this time. The patient should be stabilized hemodynamically as a first priority. The indications for inferior vena cava filter placement are active bleeding, precluding anticoagulation, and recurrent deep venous thrombosis on adequate anticoagulation.

VI-51. **The answer is E.** *(Chap. 262)* Warfarin should not be used alone as initial therapy for the treatment of venous thromboembolic disease (VTE) for two reasons. First, warfarin does not achieve full anticoagulation for at least 5 days, as its mechanism of action is to decrease the production of vitamin K–dependent coagulation factors in the liver. Second, a paradoxical reaction that promotes coagulation may also occur upon initiation of warfarin as it also decreases the production of the vitamin K–dependent anticoagulants protein C and protein S, which have shorter half-lives than the procoagulant factors. For many years, unfractionated heparin delivered IV was the treatment of choice for VTE. However, it requires frequent monitoring of activated partial thromboplastin time (aPTT) levels and hospitalization until therapeutic international normalized ratio (INR) is achieved with warfarin. There are now several safe and effective alternatives to unfractionated heparin that can be delivered SC. Low-molecular-weight heparins (enoxaparin, tinzaparin) are fragments of unfractionated heparin with a lower molecular weight. These compounds have a greater bioavailability, longer half-life, and more predictable onset of action. Their use in renal insufficiency should be considered with caution because low-molecular-weight heparins are renally cleared. Fondaparinux is a direct factor Xa inhibitor that, like low-molecular-weight heparins, requires no monitoring of anticoagulant effects and has been demonstrated to be safe and effective in treating both deep venous thrombosis and pulmonary embolism.

VI-52. **The answer is E.** *(Chap. 263)* Parapneumonic effusions are one of the most common causes of the exudative pleural effusion. When an effusion is identified in association with pneumonia, it is prudent to perform a thoracentesis if the fluid can be safely accessed. One way to know if there is enough fluid for thoracentesis is to perform a lateral decubitus film and observe if there is 10 mm of free flowing fluid along the chest wall-pleural interface. However, if the fluid does not layer, this may indicate that it is a complex loculated fluid. A loculated effusion often indicates an infected effusion and may require chest tube drainage or surgical intervention. Other factors that are associated with the need for more invasive procedures include pleural fluid pH less than 7.20, pleural fluid glucose less than 60 mg/dL (<3.3 mmol/L), positive Gram stain or culture of the pleural fluid, and presence of gross pus in the pleural space (empyema). Fluid recurrence following initial thoracentesis does indicate a complicated pleural effusion, but a repeat thoracentesis should be performed to ensure that no concerning features have developed.

VI-53. **The answer is A.** *(Chap. 263)* The characteristics of the pleural fluid in this patient are consistent with an exudate by Light's criteria. These criteria are as follows: pleural fluid protein/serum protein greater than 0.5, pleural fluid LDH/serum LDH greater than 0.6, and pleural fluid LDH more than two-thirds of the upper limit of normal serum values. If one of the criteria is met, then the effusion would be classified as an exudate. This patient clearly meets the criteria for an exudate. Exudative pleural effusions occur when there are alterations in the local environment that change the formation and absorption of pleural fluid. The most common causes of exudative pleural effusion are infection and malignancy. Other less common causes include pulmonary embolism, chylothorax, autoimmune diseases, asbestos exposure, drug reactions, hemothorax, and postoperative cardiac surgery or other cardiac injury, among others. Unfortunately, 25% of transudative effusions can be incorrectly identified as exudates by these criteria. Most often this occurs when the effusion has an increased number of cells to cause an elevation in the LDH or has been treated with diuretics to cause an increase in pleural fluid protein. Transudative effusions are most often caused by heart failure, but can also be seen in cirrhosis, nephrotic syndrome, and myxedema.

VI-54. **The answer is A.** *(Chap. 263)* The pleural fluid characteristics are typical of a chylothorax, which occurs when there has been an injury to the thoracic duct leading to accumulation of chyle in the pleural space. The most common cause of chylothorax is traumatic disruption of the thoracic duct, especially following surgeries. The surgeries that have been associated most often with chylothorax are esophagectomy and correction of congenital heart disease. The patient often presents with rapidly progressive shortness of breath within a few weeks of the surgery and has large pleural effusions. The appearance of a milky fluid on thoracentesis should alert one to the possibility of chylothorax and prompt measurement of triglyceride levels of the pleural fluid. A triglyceride level of more than 110 mg/dL (1.2 mmol/L) is characteristic of chylothorax. The treatment of chylothorax is placement of a chest tube with administration of octreotide, a somatostatin analogue. While it is not entirely clear why this is effective, the hypothesis is that octreotide decreases splanchnic blood flow and thereby decreases triglyceride production and thoracic duct flow. Patients are often also asked to stop all oral intake to further decrease chyle production. If conservative measures fail, the thoracic duct ligation can be performed. Prolonged chest tube drainage is contraindicated, however, as the high protein content in the drained fluid can lead to malnutrition and increased infection risk.

VI-55. **The answer is B.** *(Chap. 263)* A primary spontaneous pneumothorax occurs in the absence of trauma to the thorax. Most individuals who present with a primary spontaneous pneumothorax are young, and primary spontaneous pneumothorax occurs almost exclusively in cigarette smokers, with cigarette smoking being the primary risk factor. Primary spontaneous pneumothorax is also more common in men and has been associated with a tall, thin body habitus. The primary cause is the rupture of small apical pleural blebs or cysts, and the CT scan of the chest is often normal. About half of individuals will experience more than one primary spontaneous pneumothorax. The initial treatment is simple needle aspiration, which is most commonly done with ultrasound or CT guidance. Oxygen is given simultaneously to speed resorption of the residual air in the pleural space. If conservative treatment fails, tube thoracostomy can be performed. Pneumothoraces that fail to resolve or are recurrent often require thoracoscopy with stapling of blebs and pleural abrasion, a treatment that is effective in almost 100% of cases.

VI-56. **The answer is B.** *(Chap. 263)* The most common cause of pleural effusion is left ventricular failure. Pleural effusions occur in heart failure when there are increased hydrostatic forces increasing the pulmonary interstitial fluid and the lymphatic drainage is inadequate to remove the fluid. Right-sided effusions are more common than left-sided effusions in heart failure. Thoracentesis would show a transudative fluid. Pneumonia can be associated with a parapneumonic effusion or empyema. Parapneumonic effusions are the most common cause of exudative pleural effusions and are second only to heart failure as a cause of pleural effusions. Empyema refers to a grossly purulent pleural effusion. Malignancy is the second most common cause of exudative pleural effusion. Breast and lung cancers and lymphoma cause 75% of all malignant pleural effusions. On thoracentesis, the effusion is exudative. Cirrhosis and pulmonary embolus are far less common causes of pleural effusions.

VI-57. **The answer is E** *(Chap. 264)* Patients with amyotrophic lateral sclerosis (ALS) often develop hypoventilation due to involvement of their respiratory pump muscles, e.g., diaphragm, intercostal muscles, and sternocleidomastoids. Noninvasive positive pressure ventilation (NIPPV) has been used successfully in the therapy of patients with hypoventilation such as ALS. Nocturnal NIPPV can improve daytime hypercapnea, prolong survival, and improve health-related quality of life. Current ALS guidelines are to institute NIPPV if symptoms of hypoventilation exist and $PaCO_2$ is 45 mmHg or greater, nocturnal desaturation to less than 89% is documented for 5 consecutive minutes, maximal inspiratory pressure is less than 60 cmH$_2$O, or FVC is less than 50% predicted. Symptoms of hypoventilation are not particular to ALS and may include the following: dyspnea during activities of daily living, orthopnea in diseases that affect diaphragm function, poor quality sleep, daytime hypersomnolence, early morning headaches, anxiety, and impaired cough in neuromuscular disease.

VI-58. **The answer is C.** *(Chap. 264)* The patient has muscular dystrophy and is at risk for the development of hypoventilation. Many patients with hypoventilation are relatively asymptomatic or only endorse symptoms after pointed questions about sleep quality, morning headache, or orthopnea due to diaphragmatic weakness if present. The patient described here has asymptomatic hypoxemia and a normal chest radiograph aside from low lung volumes. Ventilation-perfusion mismatch and shunt are unlikely to be present without infiltrates, thus atelectasis, mucous plug, and pneumonia are not the correct answers. The patient has no risk factors described for methemoglobinemia. The most likely explanation is the presence of hypoventilation with alveolar hypoxia due to elevated $PaCO_2$ through the alveolar gas equation. An arterial blood gas measurement would confirm this with elevation in $PaCO_2$, depressed PaO_2, and a normal A-a gradient.

VI-59. **The answer is B.** *(Chap. 264)* The physiologic effects of hypoventilation are typically magnified during sleep because of a further reduction in central respiratory drive. Hypercapnia causes cerebral vasodilation, which manifests as headache upon wakening. The headache typically resolves soon after awakening as cerebral vascular tone returns to normal with increased ventilation. Patients with frequent nocturnal arousals from sleep and patients with nocturnal hypoventilation commonly complain of daytime somnolence and may also exhibit confusion and fatigue. Hypoventilation causes an increase in PCO_2 and an obligatory fall in PO_2. The hypoxemia can stimulate erythropoiesis and result in polycythemia. With central hypoventilation disorders, patients may also have impaired cranial nerve reflexes or muscular function, causing aspiration.

VI-60. **The answer is D.** *(Chap. 266)* Common indications for lung transplantation include chronic obstructive pulmonary disease, idiopathic pulmonary fibrosis, suppurative lung disease such as cystic fibrosis, and pulmonary arterial hypertension. Five-year survival is similar for all indications for lung transplantation at approximately 50%. For most indications, double-lung transplantation is the preferred procedure, and it is mandatory for patients with suppurative lung disease like cystic fibrosis. In general, in patients with idiopathic pulmonary arterial hypertension, double-lung transplantation is preferred because of concern of overcirculation in the low-resistance vascular bed of the transplanted lung when a native lung is present with markedly elevated pulmonary vascular resistance. It is very rare for the primary disease to recur after transplantation, and this has not been described in idiopathic pulmonary arterial hypertension. The right ventricle is highly plastic and will generally recover function after elevated pulmonary vascular resistance is removed by lung transplantation. Subsequently, it is rare to perform heart-lung transplantation in pulmonary arterial hypertension patients unless there is concomitant complex congenital heart disease that cannot be repaired at the time of lung transplantation.

VI-61. **The answer is A.** *(Chap. 266)* The long-term complications of lung transplantation are multisystem and range from the diseases that affect the lung and are complications of a foreign body in the chest to distant organ disease, either due to infections or complications of immunosuppressive therapy. Although osteoporosis, post-transplant lymphoproliferative disorders, and chronic kidney disease are important complications of steroids, calcineurin inhibitors, and other agents used for immunosuppression, the major complications post-transplant are in the lung. Primary graft dysfunction is a form of acute lung injury immediately after lung transplantation and is relatively rare, with severe disease occurring in only 10–20% of cases. Airway complications such as anastomotic dehiscence or stenosis have similar occurrence rates, but can usually be managed bronchoscopically with good survival. Rejection of transplanted organ is very common and is the main limitation to better medium- and long-term outcomes. Rejection occurs as acute cellular rejection often presenting with cough, low-grade fever, dyspnea, infiltrates on radiographs, and declining lung function. In contrast, chronic rejection typically presents with advancing obstruction on pulmonary function testing, no infiltrates, and worsening dyspnea on exertion. This constellation in post-transplant patients is termed bronchiolitis obliterans syndrome. Fifty percent of lung transplant patients have some degree of bronchiolitis obliterans syndrome, and it is the main impediment to better long-term survival. Therapy is often with augmented immunosuppression, although there is no consensus of how to do this or the duration of this augmentation.

VI-62. **The answer is B** *(Chap. 266)* Chronic kidney disease is a common finding in patients after lung transplantation and is associated with poorer outcomes. While rarely patients may have hemolytic-uremic syndrome underlying the kidney disease, it is usually acute, and the most common etiology of gradually progressive decline in renal function is calcineurin inhibitor neuropathy. Cyclosporine and tacrolimus are calcineurin inhibitors commonly used in immunosuppressive regimens after lung transplantation. The exact mechanism of this toxicity is unclear but may include a direct toxicity of inhibition of the calcineurin-NFAT system within the kidney, alteration in glomerular blood flow, and host/environment interactions within the kidney with calcineurin inhibitors. Prednisone, albuterol, and mycophenolate mofetil are not known to be nephrotoxic.

VI-63. **The answer is B.** *(Chap. 266)* The optimal timing for lung transplantation is critical to improve survival and add quality-adjusted life years. Individuals with cystic fibrosis should be considered for lung transplantation when the FEV_1 is less than 30% predicted or is rapidly falling. Other indications for lung transplantation in cystic fibrosis include oxygen-dependent respiratory failure, hypercapnia, and pulmonary hypertension.

SECTION VII
Disorders of the Kidney and Urinary Tract

QUESTIONS

DIRECTIONS: Choose the **one best** response to each question.

VII-1. Which of the following is a potential etiology for ischemic acute renal failure?

A. Apoptosis and necrosis of tubular cells
B. Decreased glomerular vasodilation in response to nitric oxide
C. Increased glomerular vasoconstriction in response to elevated endothelin levels
D. Increased leukocyte adhesion within the glomerulus
E. All of the above

VII-2. A 47-year-old man with a history of diabetes mellitus, hyperlipidemia, tobacco abuse, and coronary artery disease undergoes emergency appendectomy. Which of the following conditions predisposes this patient to postoperative acute kidney injury?

A. Abdominal procedure, emergency surgery, and hyperlipidemia
B. Age greater than 40, abdominal procedure, and emergency surgery
C. Age greater than 40, emergency surgery, and diabetes mellitus
D. Coronary artery disease, tobacco abuse, and abdominal procedure
E. Diabetes mellitus and emergency procedure

VII-3. A 57-year-old man with a history of diabetes mellitus and chronic kidney disease with a baseline creatinine of 1.8 mg/dL undergoes cardiac catheterization for acute myocardial infarction. He is subsequently diagnosed with acute kidney injury related to iodinated contrast. All of the following statements are true regarding his kidney injury EXCEPT:

A. Fractional excretion of sodium will be low.
B. His creatinine is likely to peak within 3–5 days.
C. His diabetes mellitus predisposed him to develop contrast nephropathy.
D. Transient tubule obstruction with precipitated iodinated contrast contributed to the development of his acute kidney injury.
E. White blood cell casts are likely on microscopic examination of urinary sediment.

VII-4. Which of the following acute kidney injury patients is most likely to have evidence of hydronephrosis on ultrasound evaluation of the kidneys?

A. A 19-year-old man with purpura fulminans associated with gonococcal sepsis
B. A 37-year-old woman undergoing chemotherapy and radiation for advanced cervical cancer
C. A 53-year-old man with *E. coli* 0157:H7 associated thrombotic thrombocytopenic purpura
D. An 85-year-old nursing home resident with pyelonephritis and sepsis
E. None of the above

VII-5. In evaluation for acute kidney injury in a patient who has recently undergone cardiopulmonary bypass during mitral valve replacement, which of the following findings on urine microscopy is most suggestive of cholesterol emboli as the source of renal failure?

A. Calcium oxalate crystals
B. Eosinophiluria
C. Granular casts
D. Normal sediment
E. White blood cell casts

VII-6. A 54-year-old man is admitted to the medical intensive care unit with sepsis associated with pneumococcal pneumonia. He requires mechanical ventilation as well as norepinephrine to maintain a mean arterial pressure greater than 60 mmHg. Invasive hemodynamics show adequate left-heart filling pressures and he is not known to have left ventricular dysfunction. On the third hospital day, his urine output drops and his creatinine increases to 3.4 mg/dL. Acute tubular injury is diagnosed. Which of the following agents has been shown to improve outcomes associated with his acute tubular injury?

A. Furosemide
B. Bosentan
C. Low-dose dopamine
D. Insulin-like growth factor
E. None of the above

VII-7. It is hospital day 5 for a 65-year-old patient with prerenal azotemia secondary to dehydration. His creatinine was initially 3.6 mg/dL on admission, but it has improved today to 2.1 mg/dL. He complains of mild lower back pain, and you prescribe naproxen to be taken intermittently. By what mechanism might this drug further impair his renal function?

A. Afferent arteriolar vasoconstriction
B. Afferent arteriolar vasodilatation
C. Efferent arteriolar vasoconstriction
D. Proximal tubular toxicity
E. Ureteral obstruction

VII-8. Preoperative assessment of a 55-year-old male patient for coronary angiography shows an estimated glomerular filtration rate of 33 mL/min per 1.73 m^2 and poorly controlled diabetes. He is currently on no nephrotoxic medications, and the nephrologist assures you that he does not currently have acute renal failure. The surgery is due to begin in 4 hours, and you would like to prevent contrast nephropathy. Which agent will definitely reduce the risk of contrast nephropathy?

A. Dopamine
B. Fenoldopam
C. Indomethacin
D. *N*-acetylcysteine
E. Sodium bicarbonate

VII-9. In stage 5 chronic kidney disease the glomerular filtration rate is below:

A. 50 mL/min per 1.73 m^2
B. 25 mL/min per 1.73 m^2
C. 15 mL/min per 1.73 m^2
D. 5 mL/min per 1.73 m^2
E. 0 mL/min per 1.73 m^2 (anuria)

VII-10. What is the leading cause of death in patients with chronic kidney disease?

A. Cardiovascular disease
B. Hyperkalemia
C. Infection
D. Malignancy
E. Uremia

VII-11. All of the following statements regarding the use of exogenous erythropoietin in patients with chronic kidney disease are true EXCEPT:

A. Exogenous erythropoietin should be administered with a target hemoglobin concentration of 100–115 g/L.
B. The use of exogenous erythropoietin is associated with improved cardiovascular outcomes.
C. The use of exogenous erythropoietin is associated with increased risk of stroke in patients with concomitant Type 2 diabetes mellitus.
D. The use of exogenous erythropoietin may be associated with faster progression to the need for dialysis.
E. The use of exogenous erythropoietin is associated with an increased incidence of thromboembolic events.

VII-12. A patient is followed closely by her nephrologist for stage IV chronic kidney disease associated with focal segmental glomerulosclerosis. Which of the following is an indication for initiation of maintenance hemodialysis?

A. Acidosis controlled with daily bicarbonate administration
B. Bleeding diathesis
C. BUN greater than 110 mg/dL without symptoms
D. Creatinine greater than 5 mg/dL without symptoms
E. Hyperkalemia controlled with sodium polystyrene

VII-13. A 27-year-old woman with chronic kidney disease is undergoing hemodialysis and is found to be hypotensive during her treatment. Which of the following are potential mechanisms for hypotension during hemodialysis?

A. Antihypertensive agents
B. Excessive ultrafiltration
C. Impaired autonomic responses
D. Osmolar shifts
E. All of the above

VII-14. A 35-year-old woman with hypertensive kidney disease progresses to end-stage renal disease. She was initiated on peritoneal dialysis 1 year ago and has done well with relief of her uremic symptoms. She is brought to the emergency department with fever, altered mental status, diffuse abdominal pain, and cloudy dialysate. Her peritoneal fluid is withdrawn through her catheter and sent to the laboratory for analysis. The fluid white blood cell count is 125/mm^3 with 85% polymorphonuclear neutrophils. Which organism is most likely to be found on culture of the peritoneal fluid?

A. *C. albicans*
B. *E. coli*
C. *M. tuberculosis*
D. *P. aeruginosa*
E. *S. aureus*

VII-15. A 45-year-old woman begins hemodialysis for end-stage renal disease associated with diabetes mellitus. Which of the following is the most likely eventual cause of her death?

A. Dementia
B. Major bleeding episode
C. Myocardial infarction
D. Progressive uremia
E. Sepsis

VII-16. The "dose" of dialysis is currently defined as:

A. The counter-current flow rate of the dialysate
B. The fractional urea clearance
C. The hours per week of dialysis
D. The number of sessions actually completed in a month

VII-17. Your patient with end-stage renal disease on hemodialysis has persistent hyperkalemia. He has a history of total bilateral renal artery stenosis, which is why he is on hemodialysis. He has electrocardiogram changes only when his potassium rises above 6.0 meq/L, which occurs a few times per week. You admit him to the hospital for further evaluation. Your laboratory evaluation, nutrition counseling, and medication adjustments have not impacted his serum potassium. What is the next reasonable step to undertake for this patient?

A. Adjust the dialysate.
B. Administer a daily dose of furosemide.
C. Perform "sodium modeling."
D. Implant an automatic defibrillator.
E. Perform bilateral nephrectomy.

VII-18. Which of the following statements is true regarding kidney transplantation?

A. Five-year survival rates are similar for recipients of living donor kidneys and deceased donor kidneys.
B. Deceased donor age does not influence graft survival.
C. Renal transplantation offers no cost benefit compared to hemodialysis.
D. When first-degree relatives are donors, the graft survival rate at 1 year is 5–7% greater than that for deceased donors.
E. When followed for more than 20 years, renal complications in single kidney donors are common.

VII-19. All of the following are likely causes of glomerular damage leading to renal failure EXCEPT:

A. Diabetes mellitus
B. Fanconi's syndrome
C. Lupus nephritis
D. Malignant hypertension
E. Mutation of TRPC6 cation channel

VII-20. A 21-year-old man is diagnosed with post-streptococcal glomerulonephritis. Which of the following is likely to be found in his urine?

A. Greater than 3 g/24-hour proteinuria without hematuria
B. Macroscopic hematuria and 24-hour urinary albumin of 227 mg
C. Microscopic hematuria with leukocytes and 24-hour urinary albumin of 227 mg
D. Positive urine culture for *Streptococcus*
E. Sterile pyuria without proteinuria

VII-21. The condition of a 50-year-old obese female with a 5-year history of mild hypertension controlled by a thiazide diuretic is being evaluated because proteinuria was noted during her routine yearly medical visit. Physical examination disclosed a height of 167.6 cm (66 in.), weight of 91 kg (202 lb), blood pressure of 130/80 mmHg, and trace pedal edema. Laboratory values are as follows:

Serum creatinine: 106 μmol/L (1.2 mg/dL)
BUN: 6.4 mmol/L (18 mg/dL)
Creatinine clearance: 87 mL/min
Urinalysis: pH 5.0; specific gravity 1.018; protein 3+; no glucose; occasional coarse granular cast
Urine protein excretion: 5.9 g/d

A renal biopsy demonstrates that 60% of the glomeruli have segmental scarring by light microscopy, with the remainder of the glomeruli appearing unremarkable (see Figure VII-21).

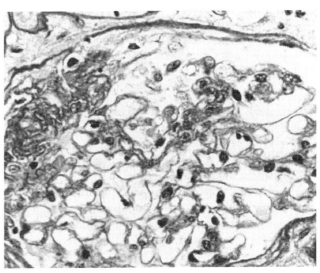

FIGURE VII-21

The most likely diagnosis is:

A. Hypertensive nephrosclerosis
B. Focal and segmental sclerosis
C. Minimal-change (nil) disease
D. Membranous glomerulopathy
E. Crescentic glomerulonephritis

VII-22. Which of the following is an extrarenal manifestation of autosomal dominant polycystic kidney disease?

A. Aortic regurgitation
B. Aortic root dilation
C. Colonic diverticulae
D. Intracranial aneurysm
E. All of the above

VII-23. A 21-year-old male college student is evaluated for profound fatigue that has been present for several years but has recently become debilitating. He also reports several foot spasms and cramps, and occasional sustained muscle contractions that are uncontrollable. He is otherwise healthy, takes no medications, and denies tobacco or alcohol use. On examination he is well developed with normal vital signs including blood pressure. The remainder of the examination is normal. Laboratory evaluation shows a sodium of 138 meq/L, potassium of 2.8 meq/L, chloride of 90 meq/L, and bicarbonate of 30 mmol/L. Magnesium level is normal. Urine screen for diuretics is negative and urine chloride is elevated. Which of the following is the most likely diagnosis?

A. Bulimia nervosa
B. Diuretic abuse
C. Gitelman's syndrome
D. Liddle's syndrome
E. Type 1 pseudohypoaldosteronism

VII-24. A 28-year-old woman was recently diagnosed with autosomal dominant polycystic kidney disease after an episode of hematuria. She is concerned about her intracranial aneurysm risk. Which of the following statements is true regarding this risk?

A. Family history of ruptured intracranial aneurysms does not increase risk of rupture.
B. Prior intracranial hemorrhage does not increase risk of subsequent hemorrhage.
C. The size of the aneurysm does not correlate with its risk of spontaneous rupture.
D. There is no increased risk of intracranial aneurysm in this condition.
E. Uncontrolled hypertension augments the risk of spontaneous rupture.

VII-25. A patient with a history of Sjögren's syndrome has the following laboratory findings: plasma sodium 139 meq/L, chloride 112 meq/L, bicarbonate 15 meq/L, and potassium 3.0 meq/L; urine studies show a pH of 6.0, sodium of 15 meq/L, potassium of 10 meq/L, and chloride of 12 meq/L. The most likely diagnosis is:

A. Type I renal tubular acidosis (RTA)
B. Type II RTA
C. Type III RTA
D. Type IV RTA
E. Chronic diarrhea

VII-26. A 16-year-old female star gymnast presents to your office complaining of fatigue, diffuse weakness, and muscle cramps. She has no previous medical history and denies tobacco, alcohol, or illicit drug use. There is no significant family history. Examination shows a thin female with normal blood pressure. Body mass index (BMI) is 18 kg/m². Oral examination shows poor dentition. Muscle tone is normal, and neurologic examination is normal.

Laboratory studies show hematocrit of 38.5%, creatinine of 0.6 mg/dL, serum bicarbonate of 30 meq/L, and potassium of 2.7 meq/L. Further evaluation should include which of the following?

A. Urinalysis and urine culture
B. Plasma renin and aldosterone levels
C. Urine toxicology screen for opiates
D. Urine toxicology screen for diuretics
E. Serum magnesium level

VII-27. In which of the following cases would treatment for biopsy-proven interstitial nephritis with corticosteroids be most likely to impact long-term renal recovery?

A. A 37-year-old woman with sarcoidosis
B. A 48-year-old man with slowly progressing interstitial nephritis over 2 months with fibrosis found on biopsy
C. A 54-year-old man with diabetes mellitus and recent salmonella infection
D. A 63-year-old man with allergic interstitial nephritis after cephalosporin antibiotic use
E. None of the above

VII-28. A 58-year-old woman undergoes a hysterectomy and postoperatively develops acute respiratory distress syndrome. She is treated with mechanical ventilation and broad-spectrum antibiotics. Aside from hypothyroidism, she has no underlying medical conditions. On day 5 of her hospitalization her urine output is noted to fall and her serum creatinine rises from 1.2 mg/dL to 2.5 mg/dL. Allergic interstitial nephritis from cephalosporin antibiotics is suspected. Which of the following findings will confirm this diagnosis?

A. Hematuria
B. Peripheral blood eosinophilia
C. Urinary eosinophils on urine microscopy
D. White blood cell casts on urine microscopy
E. None of the above

VII-29. A 44-year-old obese woman undergoes elective cholecystectomy for cholelithiasis. Postoperatively she does well and is discharged after 3 days. Two days after discharge she develops altered mental status and fever, and is brought to the emergency department by her family. She takes an antidepressant, but is otherwise healthy. Her temperature is 103°F, pulse is 127 beats/min, blood pressure is 110/78 mmHg, and respiratory rate and oxygen saturation are normal. Examination is notable for confusion and a well-healed surgical incision. Routine chemistries are drawn and show normal electrolytes, BUN of 80 mg/dL, creatinine of 2.5 mg/dL, white blood cell count of 17.3 thousand/μL, hematocrit of 30%, and platelet count of 25 thousand/μL. A peripheral blood smear shows schistocytes and confirms low platelets without clumping. Which of the following statements regarding her condition is true?

A. Low activity of the metalloprotease ADAMTS13 is likely present in her peripheral blood.

B. Plasma exchange is unlikely to be helpful.

C. This was likely caused by an occult *E. coli* 0157:H7 infection.

D. This condition is more common in men than women.

E. Untreated mortality from this condition is low.

VII-30. A 35-year-old female presents with complaints of bilateral lower extremity edema, polyuria, and moderate left-sided flank pain that began approximately 2 weeks ago. There is no past medical history. She is taking no medications and denies tobacco, alcohol, or illicit drug use. Examination shows normal vital signs, including normal blood pressure. There is 2+ edema in the bilateral lower extremities. The 24-hour urine collection is significant for 3.5 g of protein. Urinalysis is bland except for the proteinuria. Serum creatinine is 0.7 mg/dL, and ultrasound examination shows the left kidney measuring 13 cm and the right kidney measuring 11.5 cm. You are concerned about renal vein thrombosis. What test do you choose for the evaluation?

A. Computed tomography of the renal veins

B. Contrast venography

C. Magnetic resonance venography

D. ^{99}Tc-labeled pentetic acid (DPTA) imaging

E. Ultrasound with Doppler evaluation of the renal veins

VII-31. A 48-year-old man with diabetes mellitus and hyperlipidemia presents to the emergency department for evaluation of right flank pain and groin pain that has been severe and present for approximately 3 hours. He is diagnosed with a kidney stone. Which of the following is most likely to be found as the constituent of his stone?

A. Calcium

B. Cysteine

C. Oxalic acid

D. Struvite

E. Uric acid

VII-32. A 54-year-old woman with a history of colon cancer treated with resection 2 years prior and chemotherapy is admitted to the hospital after routine lab work at her primary care physician's office showed a BUN of 65 mg/dL and a creatinine of 4.5 mg/dL. She reports mild fatigue and recent lower back pain, but otherwise feels well. She does admit to recent NSAID use, but has not taken more than the recommended quantity. Aside from stopping NSAIDs and avoiding nephrotoxins, which of the following studies should be ordered first?

A. CT of the abdomen/pelvis with oral contrast

B. Post-void residual volume of bladder

C. Retrograde urography

D. Ultrasound of the abdomen/kidney

E. Urinary fractional excretion of sodium

VII-33. A 67-year-old man presents to the emergency department with severe abdominal distention and pain. He is found to have a palpable bladder, and after Foley catheter placement 1.5 L of urine passes. His prostate-specific antigen (PSA) is not elevated, but he does report that he has had difficulty passing his urine for several weeks, culminating in no urination for 2 days. His BUN is 89 mg/dL and creatinine is 6.4 mg/dL. Over the next 4 days of hospitalization, his BUN and Cr fall, but his urine output is found to be rising. He is not receiving intravenous fluids. He passes 6 L of urine on the third and fourth hospital days. Which is the most likely explanation for the increased urine output?

A. Cerebral salt wasting

B. Decreased medullary osmolarity

C. Increased activation of the renin-angiotensin-aldosterone system

D. Increased tubule pressure

E. Postobstructive diuresis

VII-34. The patient in question VII-33 is at risk for which of the following complications?

A. Erythrocytosis

B. Hyperchloremic metabolic acidosis

C. Hyperkalemia

D. Prerenal azotemia

E. Systemic hypertension

VII-35. The pain associated with acute urinary tract obstruction is a result of which of the following?

A. Compensatory natriuresis

B. Decreased medullary blood flow

C. Increased renal blood flow

D. Vasodilatory prostaglandins

VII-36. You are evaluating a 28-year-old man from Peru with abdominal pain. As part of the diagnostic workup, an abdominal ultrasound shows bilateral hydronephrosis and hydroureters. Which of the following conditions is least likely in this patient?

A. Lymphoma

B. Meatal stenosis

C. Phimosis

D. Retroperitoneal fibrosis

ANSWERS

VII-1. **The answer is E.** *(Chap. 279)* Ischemic acute renal failure has many potential etiologies. Microvascular disorders include increased vasoconstriction from endothelin and other mediators, decreased nitric oxide, prostaglandin- or bradykinin-mediated vasodilation, increased endothelial and vascular smooth muscle cell damage, and increased leukocyte adhesion. Tubular factors include cytoskeletal breakdown, loss of polarity, apoptosis and necrosis, desquamation of viable and necrotic cells, tubular obstruction, and backleak. Inflammatory and vasoactive mediators may affect both tubular and microvascular pathophysiologic mechanisms.

VII-2. **The answer is E.** *(Chap. 279)* The risk for acute kidney injury is less well studied for abdominal procedures compared to cardiac surgery, but appears to be relatively comparable. Abdominal procedures, however, are not thought to be of particular risk compared with other major chest or orthopedic procedures. Common risk factors for postoperative acute kidney injury include underlying chronic kidney disease, older age, diabetes mellitus, congestive heart failure, and emergency procedures. Most commonly, postoperative acute kidney injury is multifactorial.

VII-3. **The answer is E.** *(Chap. 279)* Iodinated contrast agents that are commonly used in cardiovascular and CT imaging are a major cause of acute kidney injury. Underlying mechanisms leading to kidney injury include transient tubular obstruction by contrast material, hypoxia in the other renal medulla due to alterations in renal microcirculation and occlusion of small vessels, and cytotoxic damage to the tubules directly or through the generation of free radicals by contrast material. Risk factors for contrast-associated nephropathy include diabetes mellitus, congestive heart failure, preexisting chronic kidney disease, and multiple myeloma–associated renal failure. Serum creatinine begins to rise at 24–48 hours and will peak at 3–5 days, usually with resolution within a week. Urinary sediment is bland, without casts. The fractional excretion of sodium is low in many cases, particularly early before tubular injury is extensive because of the microvascular source of injury.

VII-4. **The answer is B.** *(Chap. 279)* Postrenal obstruction is an important and potentially reversible cause of acute kidney injury. Ultrasound evaluation of the kidneys classically demonstrates bilateral hydronephrosis, as unilateral obstruction is unlikely to cause kidney injury unless a single functioning kidney is present, chronic kidney disease preexists, or rarely, there is reflex vasospasm of the unobstructed kidney. Advanced cervical cancer with invasion into the urinary system or retroperitoneum is a common cause of obstructive uropathy. Thrombotic thrombocytopenic purpura (TTP), disseminated gonococcus with sepsis, and pyelonephritis are intrinsic causes of acute kidney failure and will not cause bilateral hydronephrosis.

VII-5. **The answer is B.** *(Chap. 279)* Cholesterol emboli are an important cause of acute kidney injury in patients who have undergone cardiac procedures that may disrupt aortic atherosclerotic disease and shower cholesterol emboli. Livedo reticularis is a common finding on physical examination and peripheral blood eosinophilia may be present. When found, eosinophiluria is highly suggestive. The other major cause of eosinophiluria is acute interstitial nephritis. White blood cell casts suggest interstitial nephritis, pyelonephritis, glomerulonephritis, or malignant infiltration of the kidney; calcium oxalate crystals are found in ethylene glycol intoxication; and granular casts are suggestive of acute ischemic kidney injury (acute tubular necrosis), glomerulonephritis, vasculitis, or tubulointerstitial nephritis.

VII-6. **The answer is E.** *(Chap. 279)* Multiple studies have demonstrated that acute kidney injury is an independent poor prognostic indicator in critically ill patents with multiple medical conditions. Unfortunately, care of critically ill patients with acute kidney injury is supportive, as no specific therapy has been shown to improve outcomes. Agents that have specifically been shown to have no benefit in the treatment of acute tubular injury include atrial natriuretic peptide, low-dose dopamine, endothelin antagonists, loop diuretics, calcium channel blockers, α-adrenergic receptor blockers, prostaglandin analogs, antioxidants, insulin-like growth factor, and antibodies against leukocyte adhesion molecules. Volume repletion is critical to ensure adequate perfusion, and diuretics are only indicated in patients with replete fluid status and low urinary flow rates.

VII-7.   **The answer is A.** (*Chap. 279*) Nonsteroidal anti-inflammatory drugs (NSAIDs) do not alter glomerular filtration rate in normal individuals. However, in states of mild to moderate hypoperfusion (as in prerenal azotemia) or in the presence of chronic kidney disease, glomerular perfusion and filtration fraction are preserved through several compensatory mechanisms. In response to a reduction in perfusion pressures, stretch receptors in afferent arterioles trigger a cascade of events that lead to afferent arteriolar dilatation and efferent arteriolar vasoconstriction, thereby preserving glomerular filtration fraction. These mechanisms are partly mediated by the vasodilators prostaglandin E_2 and prostacyclin. NSAIDs can impair the kidney's ability to compensate for a low perfusion pressure by interfering with local prostaglandin synthesis and inhibiting these protective responses. Ureteral obstruction is not the mechanism by which NSAIDs impair renal function in this scenario. NSAIDs are not known to be proximal tubule toxins.

VII-8.   **The answer is E.** (*Chap. 279*) Radiocontrast agents cause renal injury through intrarenal vasoconstriction and the generation of oxygen radicals, causing acute tubular necrosis. These medications cause an acute decrease in renal blood flow and glomerular filtration rate. Patients with chronic kidney disease, diabetes mellitus, heart failure, multiple myeloma, and volume depletion are at the highest risk of contrast nephropathy. It is clear that hydration with normal saline is an effective measure to prevent contrast nephropathy. Of the other measures mentioned here, only sodium bicarbonate or *N*-acetylcysteine could be recommended for clinical use to reduce the risk of contrast nephropathy. Dopamine has been proven an ineffective agent to prevent contrast nephropathy. Fenoldopam, a D_1-receptor agonist, has been tested in several clinical trials and does not appear to reduce the incidence of contrast nephropathy. Although several small clinical studies have suggested a clinical benefit to the use of *N*-acetylcysteine, a meta-analysis has been inconclusive, and the medication should be administered well in advance of the procedure. Sodium bicarbonate begun within 1 hour of the procedure has shown a significant benefit in a single-center, randomized controlled trial. Due to the time limitations, and based on the evidence, only sodium bicarbonate would be helpful in this patient.

VII-9.   **The answer is C.** (*Chap. 280*) Chronic kidney disease is classified by glomerular filtration rate. In stage 0 patients, GFR is greater than 90 mL/min per 1.73 m^2, stage 2 GFR is 60–89 mL/min per 1.73 m^2, stage 3 GFR is 30–59 mL/min per 1.73 m^2, and stage 4 GFR is 15–29 mL/min per 1.73 m^2. Stage 5 GFR is less than 15 mL/min per 1.73 m^2.

VII-10.   **The answer is A.** (*Chap. 280*) The leading cause of morbidity and mortality in patients with chronic kidney disease regardless of stage is cardiovascular disease. The presence of chronic kidney disease is a major risk factor for ischemic heart disease; in addition to traditional cardiovascular risk factors, patients with chronic kidney disease have additional risk factors including anemia, hyperphosphatemia, hyperparathyroidism, sleep apnea, and systemic inflammation. Left ventricular hypertrophy and dilated cardiomyopathy are also frequently present in those with chronic kidney disease and are strongly associated with cardiovascular morbidity and mortality.

VII-11.   **The answer is B.** (*Chap. 280*) Anemia is a common consequence of chronic kidney disease and may be multifactorial, with etiologies including relative erythropoietin deficiency, iron deficiency, chronic inflammation, diminished red cell survival, and bleeding diathesis. Several trials of erythropoietin supplementation in patients with chronic kidney disease have failed to show improved cardiovascular outcomes with this therapy. Indeed, these trials have shown a higher incidence of thromboembolic events, stroke in Type 2 diabetics, and potentially faster progression to need for dialysis. Because of these concerning findings, erythropoietin use has been altered from prior recommendations, and current practice is to target a hemoglobin concentration of 100–115 g/L.

VII-12. The answer is B. *(Chap. 281)* The commonly accepted criteria for initiating patients on maintenance dialysis include the presence of uremic symptoms, the presence of hyperkalemia unresponsive to conservative management, persistent extracellular volume expansion despite diuretics, acidosis refractory to medical therapy, bleeding diathesis, or a creatinine clearance or estimated GFR below 10 mL/min per 1.73m². BUN or creatinine values alone are inadequate to initiate dialysis.

VII-13. The answer is E. *(Chap. 281)* Hypotension is the most common complication of hemodialysis. There are many potential etiologies of hypotension including antihypertensive use, excessive ultrafiltration, impaired vasoactive or autonomic responses, impaired cardiac reserve, and osmolar shifts. Less common causes include dialyzer reactions and high-output heart failure related to large arteriovenous (AV) fistulae. Manipulation of buffer for dialysate, alterations of timing of ultrafiltration, and midodrine may be used to improve hemodynamic tolerance to hemodialysis. Patients with unexpected or new hypotension during stable dialysis should also be evaluated for graft infection and bacteremia.

VII-14. The answer is E. *(Chap. 281)* The major complication of peritoneal dialysis therapy is peritonitis, though other complications include catheter-associated non-peritonitis infections, weight gain, metabolic derangements, and residual uremia. Peritonitis is usually a result from a failure of sterile technique during the exchange procedure. Transvisceral infection from the bowel is much less common. Because of the high dextrose used in dialysate, the environment is conducive for the development of bacterial infection. This can be diagnosed by the presence of more than 100/mm³ leukocytes with more than 50% polymorphonuclear cells on microscopy. Cloudy dialysate and abdominal pain are the most common symptoms. The most commonly isolated bacteria are skin flora such as *Staphylococcus*. Gram-negative organisms, fungi, and mycobacteria have also been described. A recent Cochrane review (Wiggins KJ et al: Treatment for peritoneal dialysis-associated peritonitis. *Cochrane Database of Systematic Reviews* 2008, Issue 1. Art. No.: CD005284. DOI: 10.1002/14651858.CD005284.pub2) concluded that intraperitoneal administration of antibiotics was more effective than intravenous administration, and that adjunctive treatment with urokinase or peritoneal lavage offers no advantage. Intraperitoneal vancomycin is common initial empiric therapy.

VII-15. The answer is C. *(Chap. 281)* The most common cause of mortality in patients with end-stage renal disease is cardiovascular disease (stroke and myocardial infarction). Although the underlying mechanisms driving this association are under active investigation, the shared risk factors of diabetes, hypertension, and dyslipidemia in addition to specific risks such as increased inflammation, hyperhomocysteinemia, anemia, and altered vascular function are thought to play an important role. Inefficient or inadequate dialysis is a risk for patients with difficult vascular access or poor adherence to therapy. Patients receiving hemodialysis are at risk and often develop neurologic, hematologic, and infectious complications. Nevertheless, the biggest risk to survival in these patients is also the most common cause of death in the general population.

VII-16. The answer is B. *(Chap. 281)* Although the dose is currently defined as a derivation of the fractional urea clearance, factors that are also important include patient size, residual kidney function, dietary protein intake, comorbid conditions, and the degree of anabolism/catabolism. The efficiency of dialysis depends on the counter-current flow rate of the dialysate. The number of hours/sessions prescribed for a patient is derived from the dialysis dose and is individualized.

VII-17. The answer is A. *(Chap. 281)* The potassium concentration of dialysate is usually 2.5 meq/L but may be varied depending on the predialysis serum potassium. This patient may need a lower dialysate potassium concentration. Sodium modeling is an adjustment of the dialysate sodium that may lessen the incidence of hypotension at the end of a dialysis session. Aldosterone defects, if present, are not likely to play a role in this patient since his kidneys are not being perfused. Therefore, nephrectomy is not likely to control his potassium. Similarly, since the patient is likely anuric, there is no efficacy in utilizing loop diuretics to effect kaluresis. This patient has no approved indications for implantation of a defibrillator.

VII-18. **The answer is D.** *(Chap. 282)* Both deceased and living donor kidney transplantations are highly successful. When compared to hemodialysis there are substantial cost-benefit advantages to individuals and society related to decreased morbidity, subsequent hospitalizations, and mortality. When first-degree relatives are donors, the graft survival rates are higher than those of deceased donors by 5–7% at 1 year. This difference persists for up to 10 years. There are few reported complications for donors, particularly in the absence of hypertension or diabetes mellitus. For deceased donors, older age, the presence of preexisting renal damage, or prolonged ischemia decreases the longevity of the graft.

VII-19. **The answer is B.** *(Chap. 283)* There are a wide variety of diseases that can cause glomerular injury to the kidney, ranging from genetic conditions such as TRPC6 mutation causing cation channel dysfunction and associated focal segmental glomerulosclerosis to glomerular stress from systemic hypertension and/or diabetes mellitus. Inflammatory disease such as lupus nephritis, Wegener's granulomatosis, and poststreptococcal glomerulonephritis may also cause glomerular disease. Fanconi's syndrome is a classic disease of tubular dysfunction with associated aminoaciduria, type 2 renal tubular acidosis, and rickets, not glomerular disease.

VII-20. **The answer is C.** *(Chap. 283)* The hallmark of glomerular renal disease is microscopic hematuria and proteinuria. IgA nephropathy and sickle cell disease are the exception to this when gross hematuria may be present. Proteinuria may be heavy (>3 g/24 hours) or lower quantity with microalbuminuria (30–300 mg/24 hours) depending on the underlying disease or site of the immune lesion. Patients with post-streptococcal glomerulonephritis often have pyuria, but cultures are not expected to be positive as the infection is usually skin or mucosal, and it is the immune reaction that drives the renal lesion.

VII-21. **The answer is B.** *(Chap. 283)* The characteristic pattern of focal (not all glomeruli) and segmental (not the entire glomerulus) glomerular scarring is shown. The history and laboratory features are also consistent with this lesion: some associated hypertension, diminution in creatinine clearance, and a relatively inactive urine sediment. The "nephropathy of obesity" may be associated with this lesion secondary to hyperfiltration; this condition may be more likely to occur in obese patients with hypoxemia, obstructive sleep apnea, and right-sided heart failure. Hypertensive nephrosclerosis exhibits more prominent vascular changes and patchy, ischemic, totally sclerosed glomeruli. In addition, nephrosclerosis seldom is associated with nephrotic-range proteinuria. Minimal-change disease usually is associated with symptomatic edema and normal-appearing glomeruli, as demonstrated on light microscopy. This patient's presentation is consistent with that of membranous nephropathy, but the biopsy is not. With membranous glomerular nephritis all glomeruli are uniformly involved with subepithelial dense deposits. There are no features of crescentic glomerulonephritis present.

VII-22. **The answer is E.** *(Chap. 284)* Autosomal polycystic kidney disease is a common genetic disorder accounting for up to 4% of end-stage renal disease cases in the United States. Although the most common manifestations of this condition are renal cysts, hematuria, urinary tract infection, and occasionally nephrolithiasis, there are several common extrarenal manifestations including intracranial aneurysm, aortic root and annulus dilatation, valvular heart disease including aortic regurgitation and mitral valve prolapse, hepatic cysts, hernias, and colonic diverticulae with a high propensity to perforate.

VII-23. **The answer is C.** *(Chap. 284)* The patient presents with hypokalemia and hypochloremic metabolic alkalosis in the absence of hypertension. This is most commonly due to surreptitious vomiting or diuretic abuse, but in this case the urine diuretic screen was negative. In patients with surreptitious vomiting, urine chloride levels are low to preserve intravascular volume and this was not present in this patient. Those with Bartter's syndrome and Gitelman's syndrome have hypokalemia and hypochloremic metabolic alkalosis with inappropriately elevated urine chloride levels. Gitelman's syndrome is less severe and presents later in life than Bartter's, which is commonly found in childhood due to failure to thrive. Additionally, those with Gitelman's syndrome have more prominent fatigue and muscle cramping. Most forms of Bartter's syndrome also include associated hypomagnesemia and hypocalciuria. Those with type 1 pseudohypoaldosteronism have severe renal salt wasting and hyperkalemia. Liddle's syndrome presents with apparent aldosterone excess with severe hypertension, hypokalemia, and metabolic alkalosis.

VII-24. **The answer is E.** *(Chap. 284)* Patients with autosomal dominant polycystic kidney disease have a two- to fourfold increased risk of subarachnoid or cerebral hemorrhage compared to the general population. Hemorrhage tends to occur before age 50 in patients with a family history of intracranial hemorrhage, patients with a personal history of intracranial hemorrhage, aneurysms larger than 10 mm, or patients with uncontrolled hypertension.

VII-25. **The answer is A.** *(Chap. 284)* This patient has a normal anion gap metabolic acidosis (anion gap = 12). The calculated urine anion gap ($Na^+ + K^+ - Cl^-$) is +3; thus the acidosis is unlikely to be due to gastrointestinal bicarbonate loss. In this patient the diagnosis is type I renal tubular acidosis, or distal RTA. This is a disorder in which the distal nephron does not lower pH normally. It is associated with a urine pH greater than 5.5, hypokalemia, and lack of bicarbonaturia. This condition may be associated with calcium phosphate stones and nephrocalcinosis. Type II RTA, or proximal RTA, includes a pH less than 5.5, hypokalemia, a positive urine anion gap, bicarbonaturia, hypophosphatemia, and hypercalciuria. This condition results from the defective resorption of bicarbonate. Type III RTA is rare and most commonly is seen in children. Type IV RTA is also referred to as hyperkalemic distal RTA. Hyporeninemic hypoaldosteronism is the most common cause of type IV RTA and is usually associated with diabetic nephropathy.

VII-26. **The answer is D.** *(Chap. 284)* In any patient with hypokalemia the use of diuretics must be excluded. This patient has multiple warning signs for the use of agents to alter her weight, including her age, gender, and participation in competitive sports. Her BMI is low, and the oral examination may suggest chronic vomiting. Chronic vomiting may be associated with a low urine chloride level. Once diuretic use and vomiting are excluded, the differential diagnosis of hypokalemia and metabolic alkalosis includes magnesium deficiency, Liddle's syndrome, Bartter's syndrome, and Gitelman's syndrome. Liddle's syndrome is associated with hypertension and undetectable aldosterone and renin levels. It is a rare autosomal-dominant disorder. Classic Bartter's syndrome has a presentation similar to that of this patient. It may also include polyuria and nocturia because of hypokalemia-induced diabetes insipidus. Gitelman's syndrome can be distinguished from Bartter's syndrome by hypomagnesemia and hypocalciuria.

VII-27. **The answer is A.** *(Chap. 285)* Acute interstitial nephritis is a common cause of both acute and chronic kidney dysfunction. Many causes of interstitial nephritis are successfully treated with glucocorticoids with improved rates of long-term renal recovery including Sjögren's syndrome, sarcoidosis, systemic lupus erythematosus, adults with tubulointerstitial nephritis with uveitis, and idiopathic or other granulomatous interstitial nephritis. In patients with gradually progressive disease or fibrosis on biopsy, the benefit is less clear. Additionally, allergic interstitial nephritis recovery may be accelerated with glucocorticoid therapy, but long-term renal recovery has not been proven to improve. Postinfectious interstitial nephritis has been associated with many bacterial and viral pathogens, but generally resolves with treatment of the underlying condition.

VII-28. **The answer is E.** *(Chap. 285)* Allergic interstitial nephritis is a common cause of unexplained acute renal failure. This is generally a clinical diagnosis with acute renal failure in the context of exposure to a potential offending agent (often NSAIDs, antibiotics, anticonvulsants, or proton pump inhibitors) and improvement in renal function with withdrawal of the agent. Peripheral blood eosinophilia supports the diagnosis, but is rarely found. Urine microscopy often shows white blood cell casts and hematuria, but these are not specific findings. Urine eosinophils are neither sensitive nor specific for allergic interstitial nephritis. A renal biopsy is generally not required but may show extensive tubulointerstitial infiltration of white cells including eosinophils.

VII-29. **The answer is A.** *(Chap. 286)* The patient presents with the classic pentad for thrombotic thrombocytopenic purpura (TTP), including fever, neurologic findings, renal failure, hemolytic anemia, and thrombocytopenia. This condition is more common in women than men, and in black than white patients, and may be triggered by a number of factors including pregnancy, infection, surgery, and pancreatitis. Several drugs have been implicated in the pathogenesis of TTP such as immunosuppressive agents, chemotherapeutic agents, and antiplatelet drugs. TTP may be differentiated from hemolytic uremic syndrome (HUS) by the demographics, with HUS typically affecting young children and TTP being more common in middle-aged persons. Additionally, HUS is generally triggered by a diarrheal illness, which is much less common in TTP. On a molecular level, the metalloprotease ADAMTS13 specific for von Willebrand factor (vWF) is generally low if not absent in activity in TTP. The development of HUS is likely driven by bacterial toxins such as shiga toxin or shiga-like toxin, often from *E. coli* 0157:H7. Because TTP is associated with low protein levels that may be driven by autoantibodies, plasma exchange serves the dual purpose of removing the aberrant antibody and repleting protein levels. With appropriate therapy, 1-month mortality is approximately 20%. Untreated mortality nears 90%, primarily from microvascular thrombosis and multiorgan failure.

VII-30. **The answer is C.** *(Chap. 286)* Renal vein thrombosis occurs in 10–15% of patients with nephrotic syndrome accompanying membranous glomerulopathy and oncologic disease. The clinical manifestations can be variable but may be characterized by fever, lumbar tenderness, leukocytosis, and hematuria. Magnetic resonance venography is the most sensitive and specific noninvasive form of imaging to make the diagnosis of renal vein thrombosis. Ultrasound with Doppler is operator dependent and therefore may be less sensitive. Contrast venography is the gold standard for diagnosis, but it exposes the patient to a more invasive procedure and contrast load. Nuclear medicine screening is not performed to make this diagnosis.

VII-31. **The answer is A.** *(Chap. 287)* Calcium stones account for 75–85% of all kidney stones. Although they are most commonly caused by idiopathic hypercalciuria, hypocitraturia, hyperuricosuria, and primary hyperparathyroidism are also causes. Uric acid stones are the next most common stone, followed by cysteine and struvite. Oxalic acid does not form stones without complexing with a positive cation, such as calcium. Struvite stones are precipitated by bacterial infections, such as *Proteus*, that promote conversion of urea to ammonium and raise urinary pH. General management for calcium stones includes increasing consumption of water, low protein, and low calcium. If this is ineffective, thiazide diuretics may be used.

VII-32. **The answer is D.** *(Chap. 289)* Urinary tract obstruction is an important and potentially reversible cause of kidney failure. This patient is at risk for urinary obstruction based on her history of colon cancer. Although recent NSAID use may be contributing to the rapidity of her kidney damage, routine dosing is less likely to cause acute kidney injury in the absence of preexisting renal dysfunction. Ultrasound of the kidneys is the best screening test for obstruction. Hydroureter and/or hydronephrosis may be found and suggest the presence of obstruction. Although obstruction may be unilateral, it rarely causes clinically significant renal failure in the absence of underlying renal disease. CT of the abdomen is useful after ultrasound to evaluate the site and etiology of obstruction. Post-void residual is useful if functional causes of obstruction are suspected, such as urinary retention. After the obstruction site is located, retrograde urography with stent placement may be indicated, but only after defining the presence or absence of obstruction.

VII-33 and VII-34. The answers are E and D, respectively. *(Chap. 289)* The patient has relief of recent urinary obstruction and is now making an inappropriately large amount of urine. This is likely due to postobstructive diuresis, which results from release of obstruction, increase in GFR over the course of days, decreased tubule pressure, and increased solute load per nephron, resulting in increased urine output. Decreased medullary osmolarity is a feature of chronic obstruction and persistent obstruction. The patient has not had recent head trauma or neurosurgical procedure and is unlikely to have cerebral salt wasting. Increased activation of the renin-angiotensin-aldosterone system is associated with chronic, unrelieved obstruction. Patients with postobstructive diuresis are at risk for volume depletion with possible development of prerenal azotemia and resultant acute kidney injury, as well as electrolyte imbalance, particularly due to losses of Na, K, PO_4, Mg, and free water. Erythrocytosis may be seen in patients with obstruction, but is a rare feature and is not associated with postobstructive diuresis. Systemic hypotension is more common than hypertension due to volume depletion.

VII-35. The answer is C. *(Chap. 289)* In acute urinary tract obstruction, pain is due to distention of the collecting system or renal capsule. Acutely, there is a compensatory increase in renal blood flow when kidney function is impaired by obstruction, which further exacerbates capsular stretch. Eventually, vasodilatory prostaglandins act to preserve renal function when glomerular filtration rate has decreased. Medullary blood flow decreases as the pressure of the obstruction further inhibits the renal parenchyma from perfusing; however, the ensuing chronic renal destruction may occur without substantial pain. When an obstruction has been relieved, there is a postobstructive diuresis that is mediated by relief of tubular pressure, increased solute load (per nephron), and natriuretic factors. There can be an extreme amount of diuresis, but this is not painful.

VII-36. The answer is D. *(Chap. 289)* The level of obstruction is important when considering urinary tract obstruction. Bilateral hydronephrosis and hydroureter suggest either a systemic process or mechanical obstruction at or below the level of the uretero-vesical junctions. While retroperitoneal fibrosis can cause such a picture, it is most common among middle-aged men. In patients of reproductive age, genital tract infections can cause meatal stenosis if left untreated or if infections are recurrent. Retroperitoneal lymphomas can cause bilateral hydroureter, as can more distal obstructions like phimosis. In the developing world, one may also consider schistosomiasis and genitourinary tuberculosis.

SECTION VIII
Disorders of the Gastrointestinal System

DIRECTIONS: Choose the **one best** response to each question.

VIII-1. The advantages of endoscopy over barium radiography in the evaluation of dysphagia include all of the following EXCEPT:

A. Ability to intervene as well as diagnose

B. Ability to obtain biopsy specimens

C. Increased sensitivity for the detection of abnormalities identified by color, e.g., Barrett's metaplasia

D. Increased sensitivity for the detection of mucosal lesions

E. No meaningful risk to procedure

VIII-2. A 47-year-old man is evaluated in the emergency department for chest pain that developed at a restaurant after swallowing a piece of steak. He reports intermittent episodes of meat getting stuck in his lower chest over the past 3 years, but none as severe as this event. He denies food regurgitation outside of these episodes or heartburn symptoms. He is able to swallow liquids without difficulty and has not had any weight loss. Which of the following is the most likely diagnosis?

A. Achalasia

B. Adenocarcinoma of the esophagus

C. Esophageal diverticula

D. Plummer-Vinson syndrome

E. Schatzki's ring

VIII-3. Which of the following has a well-established association with gastroesophageal reflux?

A. Chronic sinusitis

B. Dental erosion

C. Pulmonary fibrosis

D. Recurrent aspiration pneumonia

E. Sleep apnea

VIII-4. A 36-year-old female with AIDS and a CD4 count of 35/mm^3 presents with odynophagia and progressive dysphagia. The patient reports daily fevers and a 20-lb weight loss. She has been treated with clotrimazole troches without relief. On physical examination the patient is cachectic with a body mass index (BMI) of 16 and a weight of 86 lb. She has a temperature of 38.2°C (100.8°F) and is noted to be orthostatic by blood pressure and pulse. Examination of the oropharynx reveals no evidence of thrush. The patient undergoes esophagogastroduodenoscopy (EGD), which reveals serpiginous ulcers in the distal esophagus without vesicles. No yellow plaques are noted. Multiple biopsies are taken that show intranuclear and intracytoplasmic inclusions in large endothelial cells and fibroblasts. What is the best treatment for this patient's esophagitis?

A. Ganciclovir

B. Glucocorticoids

C. Fluconazole

D. Foscarnet

E. Thalidomide

VIII-5. A 57-year-old man is evaluated with an esophagogastroduodenoscopy after an episode of hematemesis. The patient reports a history of tobacco use and hypercholesterolemia, but is otherwise healthy. He has had lower back pain for the past month and has been intermittently using acetaminophen 1000 mg for relief. His endoscopy shows a 3-cm duodenal ulcer. Which of the following statements is correct regarding this finding?

A. The lesion should be biopsied as duodenal ulcers have an elevated risk of being due to carcinoma.

B. First-line therapy should be discontinuation of acetaminophen use.

C. The patient is not at risk for any associated cancers.

D. Poor socioeconomic status is a risk factor for development of this condition.

E. Antral gastritis is rarely found with this condition.

VIII-6. A 58-year-old man is evaluated for abdominal pain by his primary care physician. He reports severe stress at his job for the last 3 months and has since noted that he has epigastric pain that is relieved by eating and drinking milk. He has not had food regurgitation, dysphagia, or bloody emesis or bowel movements. He denies any symptoms in his chest. Peptic ulcer disease is suspected. Which of the following statements regarding noninvasive testing for *Helicobacter pylori* is true?

A. There is no reliable noninvasive method to detect *H. pylori*.
B. Stool antigen testing is appropriate for both diagnosis of and proof of cure after therapy for *H. pylori*.
C. Plasma antibodies to *H. pylori* offer the greatest sensitivity for diagnosis of infection.
D. Exposure to low-dose radiation is a limitation to the urea breath test.
E. False-negative testing using the urea breath test may occur with recent use of NSAIDs.

VIII-7. A 44-year-old woman complains of 6 months of epigastric pain that is worst between meals. She also reports symptoms of heartburn. The pain is typically relieved by over-the-counter antacid medications. She comes to the clinic after noting her stools darkening. She has no significant past medical history and takes no medications. Her physical examination is normal except for diffuse midepigastric pain. Her stools are heme positive. She undergoes EGD, which demonstrates a well-circumscribed 2-cm duodenal ulcer that is positive for *H. pylori*. Which of the following is recommended initial therapy given these findings?

A. Lansoprazole plus clarithromycin plus amoxicillin for 14 days
B. Pantoprazole plus amoxicillin for 21 days
C. Pantoprazole plus clarithromycin for 14 days
D. Omeprazole plus bismuth plus tetracycline plus metronidazole for 14 days
E. Omeprazole plus metronidazole plus clarithromycin for 7 days

VIII-8. A 57-year-old man with peptic ulcer disease experiences transient improvement with *Helicobacter pylori* eradication. However, 3 months later symptoms recur despite acid-suppressing therapy. He does not take nonsteroidal anti-inflammatory agents. Stool analysis for *H. pylori* antigen is negative. Upper GI endoscopy reveals prominent gastric folds together with the persistent ulceration in the duodenal bulb previously detected and the beginning of a new ulceration 4 cm proximal to the initial ulcer. Fasting gastrin levels are elevated and basal acid secretion is 15 meq/h. What is the best test to perform to make the diagnosis?

A. No additional testing is necessary.
B. Blood sampling for gastrin levels following a meal.
C. Blood sampling for gastrin levels following secretin administration.
D. Endoscopic ultrasonography of the pancreas.
E. Genetic testing for mutations in the MEN1 gene.

VIII-9. A 23-year-old woman is evaluated by her primary care physician for diffuse, crampy abdominal pain. She reports that she has had abdominal pain for the last several years, but it is getting worse and is now associated with intermittent diarrhea without flatulence. This does not waken her at night. Stools do not float and are not hard to flush. She has not noted any worsening with specific foods, but she does have occasional rashes on her lower legs. She has lost about 5 kg over the last year. She is otherwise healthy and takes no medications. Which of the following is the most appropriate recommendation at this point?

A. Increased dietary fiber intake
B. Measurement of antiendomysial antibody
C. Measurement of 24-hour fecal fat
D. Referral to gastroenterologist for endoscopy
E. Trial of lactose-free diet

VIII-10. All of the following are direct complications of short bowel syndrome EXCEPT:

A. Cholesterol gallstones
B. Coronary artery disease
C. Gastric acid hypersecretion
D. Renal calcium oxalate calculi
E. Steatorrhea

VIII-11. A 54-year-old man is evaluated by a gastroenterologist for diarrhea that has been present for approximately 1 month. He reports stools that float and are difficult to flush down the toilet; these can occur at any time of day or night, but seem worsened by fatty meals. In addition, he reports pain in many joints that lasts days to weeks and is not relieved by ibuprofen. His wife notes that the patient has had difficulty with memory for the last few months. He has lost 30 pounds and reports intermittent low-grade fevers. He takes no medications and is otherwise healthy. Endoscopy is recommended. Which of the following is the most likely finding on small-bowel biopsy?

A. Dilated lymphatics
B. Flat villi with crypt hyperplasia
C. Mononuclear cell infiltrate in the lamina propria
D. Normal small-bowel biopsy
E. PAS-positive macrophages containing small bacilli

VIII-12. A 54-year-old male presents with 1 month of diarrhea. He states that he has 8–10 loose bowel movements a day. He has lost 4 kg during this time. Vital signs and physical examination are normal. Serum laboratory studies are normal. A 24-hour stool collection reveals 500 g of stool with a measured stool osmolality of 200 mosmol/L and a calculated stool osmolality of 210 mosmol/L. Based on these findings, what is the most likely cause of this patient's diarrhea?

A. Celiac sprue
B. Chronic pancreatitis
C. Lactase deficiency
D. Vasoactive intestinal peptide tumor
E. Whipple's disease

VIII-13. Cobalamin absorption may occur in all of the following diseases EXCEPT:

A. Bacterial overgrowth syndrome
B. Chronic pancreatitis
C. Crohn's disease
D. Pernicious anemia
E. Ulcerative colitis

VIII-14. Which of the following statements regarding the epidemiology of inflammatory bowel disease is correct?

A. Monozygotic twins are highly concordant for ulcerative colitis.
B. Oral contraceptive use decreases the incidence of Crohn's disease.
C. Persons of Asian descent have the highest rates of ulcerative colitis and Crohn's disease.
D. Smoking may decrease the incidence of ulcerative colitis.
E. Typical age of onset for Crohn's disease is 40–50 years old.

VIII-15. A 24-year-old woman is admitted to the hospital with a 1-year history of severe abdominal pain and chronic diarrhea, which has been bloody for the past 2 months. She reports a 20-lb weight loss, frequent fevers, and night sweats. She denies vomiting. Her abdominal pain is crampy and primarily involves her right lower quadrant. She is otherwise healthy. Examination is concerning for an acute abdomen with rebound and guarding present. CT shows free air in the peritoneum. She is urgently taken to the operating room for surgical exploration, where she is found to have multiple strictures and a perforation of her bowel in the terminal ileum. The rectum was spared and a fissure from the duodenum to the jejunum is found. The perforated area is resected and adhesions lysed. Which of the following findings on pathology of her resected area confirms her diagnosis?

A. Crypt abscesses
B. Flat villi
C. Noncaseating granuloma throughout the bowel wall
D. Special stain for *Clostridium difficile* toxin
E. Transmural acute and chronic inflammation

VIII-16. A 45-year-old man with ulcerative colitis has been treated for the past 5 years with infliximab with excellent resolution of his bowel symptoms and endoscopic evidence of normal colonic mucosa. He is otherwise healthy. He is evaluated by a dermatologist for a lesion that initially was a pustule over his right lower extremity but has since progressed in size with ulceration. The ulcer is moderately painful. He does not recall any trauma to the area. On examination the ulcer measures 15 cm by 7 cm and central necrosis is present. The edges of the ulcer are violaceous. No other lesions are identified. Which of the following is the most likely diagnosis?

A. Erythema nodosum
B. Metastatic Crohn's disease
C. Psoriasis
D. Pyoderma gangrenosum
E. Pyoderma vegetans

VIII-17. Inflammatory bowel disease (IBD) may be caused by exogenous factors. Gastrointestinal flora may promote an inflammatory response or may inhibit inflammation. Probiotics have been used to treat IBD. Which of the following organisms has been used in the treatment of IBD?

A. *Campylobacter* spp.
B. *Clostridium difficile*
C. *Escherichia* spp.
D. *Lactobacillus* spp.
E. *Shigella* spp.

VIII-18. Your 33-year-old patient with Crohn's disease (CD) has had a disappointing disease response to glucocorticoids and 5-ASA agents. He is interested in steroid-sparing agents. He has no liver or renal disease. You prescribe once-weekly methotrexate injections. In addition to monitoring hepatic function and complete blood count, what other complication of methotrexate therapy do you advise the patient of?

A. Disseminated histoplasmosis
B. Lymphoma
C. Pancreatitis
D. Pneumonitis
E. Primary sclerosing cholangitis

VIII-19. Which of the following patients requires no further testing before making the diagnosis of irritable bowel syndrome and initiating treatment?

A. A 76-year-old woman with 6 months of intermittent crampy abdominal pain that is worse with stress and associated with bloating and diarrhea.
B. A 25-year-old woman with 6 months of abdominal pain, bloating, and diarrhea that has worsened steadily and now awakes her from sleep at night to move her bowels.
C. A 30-year-old man with 6 months of lower abdominal crampy pain relieved with bowel movements, usually loose. Symptoms are worse during the daytime at work and better on the weekend. Weight loss is not present.
D. A 19-year-old female college student with 2 months of diarrhea and worsening abdominal pain with occasional blood in her stool.
E. A 27-year-old woman with 6 months of intermittent abdominal pain, bloating, and diarrhea without associated weight loss. Crampy pain and diarrhea persist after a 48-hour fast.

VIII-20. A 29-year-old woman comes to see you in the clinic because of abdominal discomfort. She feels abdominal discomfort on most days of the week, and the pain varies in location and intensity. She notes constipation as well as diarrhea, but diarrhea predominates. In comparison to 6 months ago, she has more bloating and flatulence than she has had before. She identifies eating and stress as aggravating factors, and her pain is relieved by defecation. You suspect irritable bowel syndrome (IBS). Laboratory data include white blood cell (WBC) count 8000/μL, hematocrit 32%, platelets 210,000/μL, and erythrocyte sedimentation rate (ESR) of 44 mm/h. Stool studies show the presence of lactoferrin but no blood. Which intervention is appropriate at this time?

A. Antidepressants
B. Ciprofloxacin
C. Colonoscopy
D. Reassurance and patient counseling
E. Stool bulking agents

VIII-21. After a careful history and physical, and a cost-effective workup, you have diagnosed a 24-year-old female patient with irritable bowel syndrome. What other condition would you reasonably expect to find in this patient?

A. Abnormal brain anatomy
B. Autoimmune disease
C. History of sexually transmitted diseases
D. Psychiatric diagnosis
E. Sensory hypersensitivity to peripheral stimuli

VIII-22. A 78-year-old woman is admitted to the hospital with fever, loss of appetite, and left lower quadrant pain. She is not constipated, but has not moved her bowels recently. Laboratory examination is notable for an elevated WBC count. These symptoms began approximately 3 days ago and have steadily worsened. Which of the following statements regarding the use of radiologic imaging to evaluate her condition is true?

A. Air-fluid levels are commonly seen on plain abdominal films.
B. Barium enema should not be performed because of the risk of perforation.
C. Lower gastrointestinal bleeding will likely be visualized on CT angiography.
D. A thickened colonic wall is not required on CT for the diagnosis of her likely condition.
E. Ultrasound of the pelvis is the best modality to visualize the likely pathologic process.

VIII-23. Which of the following patients is *MOST* appropriate for surgical management of their acute diverticulitis?

A. A 45-year-old woman with rheumatoid arthritis treated with infliximab and prednisone.
B. A 63-year-old woman with diverticulitis in the descending colon and a distal stricture.
C. A 70-year-old woman with end-stage renal disease with colonic wall thickening of 8 mm on CT scan.
D. A 77-year-old man with two episodes of diverticulitis in the past 2 years.
E. None of the above patients requires surgical management.

VIII-24. A 67-year-old man is evaluated in the emergency department for blood in the toilet bowl after moving his bowels. Blood was also present on the toilet paper after wiping. He reports straining and recent constipation. He has a history of systemic hypertension and hyperlipidemia. Vital signs are normal and he is not orthostatic. Anoscopy shows external hemorrhoids. Hematocrit is normal and bleeding does not recur during his 6-hour emergency department stay. Which of the following is the most appropriate management?

A. Ciprofloxacin and metronidazole
B. Cortisone suppositories, fiber supplementation
C. Hemorrhoidal banding
D. Operative hemorrhoidectomy
E. Upper endoscopy

VIII-25. Which of the following statements regarding anorectal abscess is true?

A. Anorectal abscess is more common in diabetic patients.
B. Anorectal abscess is more common in women.
C. Difficulty voiding is uncommon and should prompt further evaluation of anorectal abscess.
D. Examination in the operating room under anesthesia is required for adequate exploration in most cases.
E. The peak incidence is the seventh decade of life.

VIII-26. An 88-year-old woman is brought to your clinic by her family because she has become increasingly socially withdrawn. The patient lives alone and has been reluctant to visit or be visited by her family. Family members, including seven children, also note a foul odor in her apartment and on her person. She has not had any weight loss. Alone in the examining room, she only complains of hemorrhoids. On mental status examination, she has signs of depression. Which of the following interventions is most appropriate at this time?

A. Head CT scan
B. Initiate treatment with an antidepressant medication
C. Physical examination including genitourinary and rectal examination
D. Screening for occult malignancy
E. Serum thyroid-stimulating hormone

VIII-27. A 37-year-old woman presents with abdominal pain, anorexia, and fever of 4 days' duration. The abdominal pain is mostly in the left lower quadrant. Her past medical history is significant for irritable bowel syndrome, diverticulitis treated 6 months ago, and status post-appendectomy. Since her last bout of diverticulitis she has increased her fiber intake and avoids nuts and popcorn. Review of systems is positive for weight loss, daily chills and sweats, and "bubbles" in her urinary stream. Her temperature is 39.6°C. A limited CT scan shows thickened colonic wall (5 mm) and inflammation with pericolic fat stranding. She is admitted with a presumptive diagnosis of diverticulitis. What is the most appropriate management for this patient?

A. A trial of rifaximin and a high-fiber diet
B. Bowel rest, ciprofloxacin, metronidazole, and ampicillin
C. Examination of the urine sediment
D. Measurement of 24-hour urine protein
E. Surgical removal of the affected colon and exploration

VIII-28. An 85-year-old woman is brought to a local emergency department by her family. She has been complaining of abdominal pain off and on for several days, but this morning states that this is the worst pain of her life. She is able to describe a sharp, stabbing pain in her abdomen. Her family reports that she has not been eating and seems to have no appetite. She has a past medical history of atrial fibrillation and hypercholesterolemia. She has had two episodes of vomiting and in the ER experiences diarrhea that is hemoccult positive. On examination she is afebrile, with a heart rate of 105 beats/min and blood pressure of 111/69 mmHg. Her abdomen is mildly distended and she has hypoactive bowel sounds. She does not exhibit rebound tenderness or guarding. She is admitted for further management. Several hours after admission she becomes unresponsive. Blood pressure is difficult to obtain and at best approximation is 60/40 mmHg. She has a rigid abdomen. Surgery is called and the patient is taken for emergent laparotomy. She is found to have acute mesenteric ischemia. Which of the following is true regarding this diagnosis?

A. Mortality for this condition is greater than 50%.
B. Risk factors include low-fiber diet and obesity.
C. The "gold standard" for diagnosis is CT scan of the abdomen.
D. The lack of acute abdominal signs in this case is unusual for mesenteric ischemia.
E. The splanchnic circulation is poorly collateralized.

VIII-29. All of the following are potential causes of appendix obstruction and appendicitis EXCEPT:

A. Ascaris infection
B. Carcinoid tumor
C. Cholelithiasis
D. Fecalith
E. Measles infection

VIII-30. Which of the following organisms is most likely to be causative in acute appendicitis?

A. *Clostridium* species
B. *Escherichia coli*
C. *Mycobacterium tuberculosis*
D. *Staphylococcus aureus*
E. *Yersinia enterocolitica*

VIII-31. A 32-year-old woman is evaluated in the emergency department for abdominal pain. She reports a vague loss of appetite for the past day and has had progressively severe abdominal pain, initially at her umbilicus, but now localized to her right lower quadrant. The pain is crampy. She has not moved her bowels or vomited. She reports that she is otherwise healthy and has had no sick contact. Exam is notable for a temperature of 100.7°F, heart rate of 105 beats/min, and otherwise normal vital signs. Her abdomen is tender in the right lower quadrant and pelvic examination is normal. Urine pregnancy test is negative. Which of the following imaging modalities is most likely to confirm her diagnosis?

A. CT of the abdomen without contrast
B. Colonoscopy
C. Pelvic ultrasound
D. Plain film of the abdomen
E. Ultrasound of the abdomen

VIII-32. A 38-year-old male is seen in the urgent care center with several hours of severe abdominal pain. His symptoms began suddenly, but he reports several months of pain in the epigastrium after eating, with a resultant 10-lb weight loss. He takes no medications besides over-the-counter antacids and has no other medical problems or habits. On physical examination temperature is 38.0°C (100.4°F), pulse 130 beats/min, respiratory rate 24 breaths/min, and blood pressure 110/50 mmHg. His abdomen has absent bowel sounds and is rigid with involuntary guarding diffusely. A plain film of the abdomen is obtained and shows free air under the diaphragm. Which of the following is most likely to be found in the operating room?

A. Necrotic bowel
B. Necrotic pancreas
C. Perforated duodenal ulcer
D. Perforated gallbladder
E. Perforated gastric ulcer

VIII-33. Which of the following is the source of the peritonitis of the patient in question VIII-32?

A. Bile
B. Blood
C. Foreign body
D. Gastric contents
E. Pancreatic enzymes

VIII-34. Which of the following is the most common symptom or sign of liver disease?

A. Fatigue
B. Itching
C. Jaundice
D. Nausea
E. Right upper quadrant pain

VIII-35. In women, what is the average amount of reported daily alcohol intake that is associated with the development of chronic liver disease?

A.   1 drink
B.   2 drinks
C.   3 drinks
D.   6 drinks
E.   12 drinks

VIII-36. Elevations in all of the following laboratory studies would be indicative of liver disease EXCEPT:

A.   5′-nucleotidase
B.   Aspartate aminotransferase
C.   Conjugated bilirubin
D.   Unconjugated bilirubin
E.   Urine bilirubin

VIII-37. A 61-year-old male is admitted to your service for swelling of the abdomen. You detect ascites on clinical examination and perform a paracentesis. The results show a white blood cell count of 300 leukocytes/µL with 35% polymorphonuclear cells. The peritoneal albumin level is 1.2 g/dL, protein is 2.0 g/dL, and triglycerides are 320 mg/dL. Peritoneal cultures are pending. Serum albumin is 2.6 g/dL. Which of the following is the most likely diagnosis?

A.   Congestive heart failure
B.   Peritoneal tuberculosis
C.   Peritoneal carcinomatosis
D.   Chylous ascites
E.   Bacterial peritonitis

VIII-38. A 26-year-old male resident is noticed by his attending physician to have yellow eyes after his 24-hour call period. When asked, the resident states he has no medical history, but on occasion he has thought he might have mild jaundice when he is stressed or has more than 4–5 alcoholic drinks. He never sought medical treatment because he was uncertain, and his eyes would return fully to normal within 2 days. He denies nausea, abdominal pain, dark urine, light-colored stools, pruritus, or weight loss. On examination he has a body mass index of 20.1 kg/m², and his vital signs are normal. Scleral icterus is present. There are no stigmata of chronic liver disease. The patient's abdomen is soft and nontender. The liver span is 8 cm to percussion. The liver edge is smooth and palpable only with deep inspiration. The spleen is not palpable. Laboratory examinations are normal except for a total bilirubin of 3.0 mg/dL. Direct bilirubin is 0.2 mg/dL. Aspartate aminotransferase (AST), alanine aminotransferase (ALT), and alkaline phosphatase are normal. Hematocrit, lactate dehydrogenase (LDH), and haptoglobin are normal. Which of the following is the most likely diagnosis?

A.   Autoimmune hemolytic anemia
B.   Crigler-Najjar syndrome type 1
C.   Choledocholithiasis
D.   Dubin-Johnson syndrome
E.   Gilbert's syndrome

VIII-39. What is the next step in the evaluation and management of the patient in question VIII-38?

A.   Genotype studies
B.   Peripheral blood smear
C.   Prednisone
D.   Reassurance
E.   Right upper quadrant ultrasound

VIII-40. A 34-year-old man presents to the physician complaining of yellow eyes. For the past week, he has felt ill with decreased oral intake, low-grade fevers (~100°F), fatigue, nausea, and occasional vomiting. With the onset of jaundice, he has noticed pain in his right upper quadrant. He currently uses marijuana and ecstasy, and has a prior history of injection drug use with cocaine. He has no other past medical history, but he was unable to donate blood 4 years previously for reasons that he cannot recall. His social history is remarkable for working as a veterinary assistant. On sexual history, he reports five male sexual partners over the past 6 months. He does not consistently use condoms. On physical examination, he appears ill and has obvious jaundice with scleral icterus. His liver is 15 cm to percussion and is palpable 6 cm below the right costal margin. The edge is smooth and tender to palpation. The spleen is not enlarged. There are no stigmata of chronic liver disease. His AST is 1232 U/L, ALT is 1560 U/L, alkaline phosphatase is 394 U/L, total bilirubin is 13.4 mg/dL, and direct bilirubin is 12.2 mg/dL. His INR is 2.3, and aPTT is 52 seconds. Hepatitis serologies are sent and reveal the following:

Hepatitis A IgM negative
Hepatitis A IgG negative
Hepatitis B core IgM positive
Hepatitis B core IgG negative
Hepatitis B surface antigen positive
Hepatitis B surface antibody negative
Hepatitis B e antigen positive
Hepatitis B e antibody negative
Hepatitis C antibody positive

What is the cause of the patient's current clinical presentation?

A.   Acute hepatitis A infection
B.   Acute hepatitis B infection
C.   Acute hepatitis C infection
D.   Chronic hepatitis B infection
E.   Drug-induced hepatitis

VIII-41. In the scenario described in question VIII-40, what would be the best approach to prevent development of chronic hepatitis?

A.   Administration of anti-hepatitis A virus IgG.
B.   Administration of lamivudine.
C.   Administration of pegylated interferon α plus ribavirin.
D.   Administration of prednisone beginning at a dose of 1 mg/kg daily.
E.   Do nothing and observe, as 99% of individuals with this disease recover.

VIII-42. Which of the following viral causes of acute hepatitis is most likely to cause fulminant hepatitis in a pregnant woman?

A. Hepatitis A
B. Hepatitis B
C. Hepatitis C
D. Hepatitis D
E. Hepatitis E

VIII-43. A 16-year-old woman had visited your clinic 1 month ago with jaundice, vomiting, malaise, and anorexia. Two other family members were ill with similar symptoms. Based on viral serologies, including a positive anti-hepatitis A virus (HAV) IgM, a diagnosis of hepatitis A was made. The patient was treated conservatively, and 1 week after first presenting, she appeared to have made a full recovery. She returns to your clinic today complaining of the same symptoms she had 1 month ago. She is jaundiced, and an initial panel of laboratory tests returns elevated transaminases. Which of the following offers the best explanation of what has occurred in this patient?

A. Coinfection with hepatitis C
B. Inappropriate treatment of initial infection
C. Incorrect initial diagnosis; this patient likely has hepatitis B
D. Reinfection with hepatitis A
E. Relapse of hepatitis A

VIII-44. A 26-year-old woman presents to your clinic and is interested in getting pregnant. She seeks your advice regarding vaccines she should obtain, and in particular asks about the hepatitis B vaccine. She works as a receptionist for a local business, denies alcohol or illicit drug use, and is in a monogamous relationship. Which of the following is true regarding hepatitis B vaccination?

A. Hepatitis B vaccine consists of two IM doses 1 month apart.
B. Only patients with defined risk factors need to be vaccinated.
C. Pregnancy is not a contraindication to the hepatitis B vaccine.
D. This patient's hepatitis serologies should be checked before vaccination.
E. Vaccination should not be administered to children under 2 years old.

VIII-45. An 18-year-old man presents to a rural clinic with nausea, vomiting, anorexia, abdominal discomfort, myalgias, and jaundice. He describes occasional alcohol use and is sexually active. He describes using heroin and cocaine "a few times in the past." He works as a short-order cook in a local restaurant. He has lost 15.5 kg since his last visit to the clinic and appears emaciated and ill. On examination he is noted to have icteric sclerae and a palpable, tender liver below the right costal margin. In regard to acute hepatitis, which of the following is true?

A. A distinction between viral etiologies cannot be made using clinical criteria alone.
B. Based on age and risk factors, he is likely to have hepatitis B infection.
C. He does not have hepatitis E virus, as this infects only pregnant women.
D. This patient cannot have hepatitis C because his presentation is too acute.
E. This patient does not have hepatitis A because his presentation is too fulminant.

VIII-46. A 36-year-old male presents with fatigue and tea-colored urine for 5 days. Physical examination reveals jaundice and tender hepatomegaly, but is otherwise unremarkable. Laboratories are remarkable for an aspartate aminotransferase (AST) of 2400 U/L and an alanine aminotransferase (ALT) of 2640 U/L. Alkaline phosphatase is 210 U/L. Total bilirubin is 8.6 mg/dL. Which of the following diagnoses is least likely to cause this clinical picture and these laboratory abnormalities?

A. Acute hepatitis A infection
B. Acute hepatitis B infection
C. Acute hepatitis C infection
D. Acetaminophen ingestion
E. Budd-Chiari syndrome

VIII-47. Which of the following drugs has a direct toxic effect on hepatocytes?

A. Acetaminophen
B. Chlorpromazine
C. Halothane
D. Isoniazid
E. Rosuvastatin

VIII-48. A 32-year-old woman is admitted to the intensive care unit following an overdose of acetaminophen with coingestion of alcohol. She was known to be alert and interactive about 4 hours before her presentation when she had a fight with her boyfriend who then left the home. When he returned 6 hours later, he found an empty bottle of acetaminophen 500 mg capsules as well as an empty vodka bottle. The exact number of pills in the bottle is unknown but the full bottle held as much as 50 capsules. The patient was unresponsive and had vomited, so her boyfriend called 911. Upon arrival to the emergency department, the patient is stuporous. Her vital signs are as follows: pulse 109 beats/min, respiratory rate 20 breaths/min, blood pressure 96/52 mmHg, and oxygen saturation 95% on room air. Her examination shows mild nonspecific abdominal pain with palpation. The liver is not enlarged. Her initial laboratory values show a normal CBC, and normal electrolytes and kidney function. The AST is 68 U/L, ALT is 46 U/L, alkaline phosphatase is 110 U/L, and total bilirubin is 1.2 mg/dL. Glucose and coagulation studies are normal. The serum alcohol level is 210 g/dL. The acetaminophen level is 350 μg/mL. What is the most appropriate next step in the treatment of this patient?

A. Administration of activated charcoal or cholestyramine.
B. Administration of *N*-acetylcysteine 140 mg/kg followed by 70 mg/kg every 4 hours for a total of 15–20 doses.
C. Continued monitoring of liver function, glucose, and coagulation studies every 4 hours with administration of *N*-acetylcysteine if these begin to change.
D. Do nothing as normal liver function tests and coagulation studies are indicative of only a minor ingestion.
E. Initiate hemodialysis for toxin clearance.

VIII-49. A 38-year-old woman is evaluated for elevated transaminase levels that were identified during routine laboratory testing for life insurance. She is originally from Thailand and immigrated to the United States 10 years previously. She has been married to an American for the past 12 years, having met him while he was living abroad for business. She previously worked in Thailand as a deputy tourism minister for the government, but is not currently employed. She has no significant past medical history. She had one uncomplicated pregnancy at the age of 22. When queried about risk factors for liver disease, she denies alcohol intake or drug abuse. She has never had a blood transfusion. She recalls an episode of jaundice that she did not seek evaluation for about 15 years ago. It resolved spontaneously. She currently feels well, and her husband wished to have her added to his life insurance policy. There are no stigmata of chronic liver disease. Her laboratory studies reveal an AST of 346 U/L, ALT of 412 U/L, alkaline phosphatase of 98 U/L, and total bilirubin of 1.5 mg/dL. Further workup includes the following viral studies: hepatitis A IgG +, hepatitis B surface antigen +, hepatitis B e antigen +, anti-HBV core IgG +, and hepatitis C IgG negative. The HBV DNA level

is 4.8×10^4 IU/mL. What treatment do you recommend for this patient?

A. Entecavir.
B. Pegylated interferon.
C. Pegylated interferon plus entecavir.
D. No treatment is necessary.
E. Either A or C.

VIII-50. A 46-year-old man is known to have chronic hepatitis C virus (HCV) infection. He is a former IV drug user for more than 20 years who has been abstinent from drug use for 1 year. He is asking whether he should receive treatment for his HCV infection. He has a prior history of hepatitis B virus (HBV) and has positive antibody to HBV surface antigen. He was treated for tricuspid valve endocarditis 3 years previously. He has no other medical history. He does not know when he acquired HCV. His laboratory studies show a positive HCV IgG antibody with a viral load of greater than 1 million copies. The virus is genotype 1. His AST is 62 U/L, and his ALT is 54 U/L. He undergoes liver biopsy, which demonstrates a moderate degree of bridging fibrosis. What do you tell him regarding his likelihood of progression and possibilities regarding treatment?

A. As he is infected with genotype 1, the likelihood of response to pegylated interferon and ribavirin is less than 40%.
B. Following 12 weeks of treatment, the expected viral load should be undetectable.
C. Given his normal liver enzymes on laboratory testing, he is unlikely to develop progressive liver injury.
D. If the patient elects to undergo treatment, the best regimen for individuals with genotype 1 disease is pegylated interferon and ribavirin for 24 weeks.
E. The presence of bridging fibrosis on liver biopsy is the most predictive factor of the development of cirrhosis over the next 10–20 years.

VIII-51. A 34-year-old woman is evaluated for fatigue, malaise, arthralgias, and a 10-lb weight loss over the past 6–8 weeks. She has no past medical history. Since feeling poorly, she has taken approximately one or two tablets of acetaminophen 500 mg daily. On physical examination, her temperature is 100.2°F, respiratory rate is 18 breaths/min, blood pressure is 100/48 mmHg, heart rate is 92 beats/min, and oxygen saturation is 96% on room air. She has scleral icterus. Her liver edge is palpable 3 cm below the right costal margin. It is smooth and tender. The spleen is not enlarged. She has mild synovitis in the small joints of her hands. Her AST is 542 U/L, ALT is 657 U/L, alkaline phosphatase is 102 U/L, total bilirubin is 5.3 mg/dL, and direct bilirubin is 4.8 mg/dL. Which of the following tests would be LEAST likely to be positive in this diagnosis?

A. Antinuclear antibodies in a homogeneous pattern
B. Anti-liver/kidney microsomal antibodies
C. Antimitochondrial antibodies
D. Hypergammaglobulinemia
E. Rheumatoid factor

VIII-52. In chronic hepatitis B virus (HBV) infection, the presence of hepatitis B e antigen (HBeAg) signifies which of the following?

A. Development of liver fibrosis leading to cirrhosis.
B. Dominant viral population is less virulent and less transmissible.
C. Increased likelihood of an acute flare in the next 1–2 weeks.
D. Ongoing viral replication.
E. Resolving infection.

VIII-53. A 32-year-old woman is admitted to the hospital with fever, abdominal pain, and jaundice. She drinks approximately 6 beers daily and has recently increased her alcohol intake to more than 12 beers daily. She has no other substance abuse history and has no history of alcoholic liver disease or pancreatitis. She is not taking any medications. On physical examination, she appears ill and disheveled with a fruity odor to her breath. Her vital signs are as follows: heart rate 122 beats/min, blood pressure 95/56 mmHg, respiratory rate 22 breaths/min, temperature 101.2°F, and oxygen saturation 98% on room air. She has scleral icterus, and spider angiomata are present on the trunk. The liver edge is palpable 10 cm below the right costal margin. It is smooth and tender to palpation. The spleen is not palpable. No ascites or lower extremity edema is present. Laboratory studies demonstrate an AST of 431 U/L, ALT of 198 U/L, bilirubin of 8.6 mg/dL, alkaline phosphatase of 201 U/L, amylase of 88 U/L, and lipase of 50 U/L. Total protein is 6.2 g/dL, and albumin is 2.8 g/dL. The prothrombin time is 28.9 seconds. What is the best approach to treatment of this patient?

A. Administer IV fluids, thiamine, and folate, and observe for improvement in laboratory tests and clinical condition.
B. Administer IV fluids, thiamine, folate, and imipenem while awaiting blood culture results.
C. Administer prednisone 40 mg daily for 4 weeks before beginning a taper.
D. Consult surgery for management of acute cholecystitis.
E. Perform an abdominal CT with IV contrast to assess for necrotizing pancreatitis.

VIII-54. A 48-year-old woman presents complaining of fatigue and itching. She has been tired for the past 6 months and has recently developed diffuse itching. It is worse in the evening hours, but it is intermittent. She does not note it to be worse following hot baths or showers. Her past medical history is significant only for hypothyroidism for which she takes levothyroxine 125 μg daily. On physical examination, she has mild jaundice and scleral icterus. The liver is enlarged to 15 cm on palpation and is palpable 5 cm below the right costal margin. Xanthomas are seen on both elbows. Hyperpigmentation is noticeable on the trunk and arms where the patient has excoriations. Laboratory

studies demonstrate the following: WBC 8900/μL, hemoglobin 13.3 g/dL, hematocrit 41.6%, and platelets 160,000/μL. The creatinine is 1.2 mg/dL. The AST is 52 U/L, ALT is 62 U/L, alkaline phosphatase is 216 U/L, total bilirubin is 3.2 mg/dL, and direct bilirubin is 2.9 mg/dL. The total protein is 8.2 g/dL, and albumin is 3.9 U/L. The thyroid-stimulating hormone is 4.5 U/mL. Antimitochondrial antibodies are positive. P-ANCA and C-ANCA are negative. What is the most likely cause of the patient's symptoms?

A. Lymphoma
B. Polycythemia vera
C. Primary biliary cirrhosis
D. Primary sclerosis cholangitis
E. Uncontrolled hypothyroidism

VIII-55. A 63-year-old man presents to the emergency department complaining of hematemesis. The vomiting began abruptly and was not preceded by any abdominal pain or other symptoms. He describes the vomiting as about 500 mL of bright red blood. He has not had melena or bright red blood per rectum. He has known alcoholic cirrhosis and continues to drink at least 12 beers daily. He does not seek regular medical care, and he has not previously had an endoscopy to screen for varices. When he is initially evaluated in the emergency department, he is noted to be tachycardic with a heart rate of 125 beats/min and a blood pressure of 76/40. After 1 L of IV saline, his blood pressure increases to 92/56. He has an additional 300 mL of hematemesis upon arriving in the emergency department. The initial hematocrit is 32%. All of the following should be a part of the initial management of this patient EXCEPT:

A. Administration of octreotide 100 μg/h by continuous IV infusion
B. Administration of propranolol 10 mg four times daily
C. Emergent GI consult for upper endoscopy
D. Ongoing volume resuscitation with saline and packed red blood cells as needed to maintain adequate blood pressure
E. Placement of large-bore IV access in the antecubital fossae or large central vein

VIII-56. A 42-year-old man with cirrhosis related to hepatitis C and alcohol abuse has ascites requiring frequent large-volume paracentesis. All of the following therapies would be indicated for this patient EXCEPT:

A. Fluid restriction to less than 2 L daily
B. Furosemide 40 mg daily
C. Sodium restriction to less than 2 g daily
D. Spironolactone 100 mg daily
E. Transjugular intrahepatic portosystemic shunt if medical therapy fails

VIII-57. Which of the following statements about cardiac cirrhosis is TRUE?

A. AST and ALT levels may mimic the very high levels seen in acute viral hepatitis.

B. Budd-Chiari syndrome cannot be distinguished clinically from cardiac cirrhosis.

C. Echocardiography is the gold standard for diagnosing constrictive pericarditis as a cause of cirrhosis.

D. Prolonged passive congestion from right-sided heart failure results first in congestion and necrosis of portal triads, resulting in subsequent fibrosis.

E. Venoocclusive disease can be confused with cardiac cirrhosis and is a major cause of morbidity and mortality in patients undergoing liver transplantation.

VIII-58. You are asked to consult on a 62-year-old white female with pruritus for 4 months. She has noted progressive fatigue and a 5-lb weight loss. She has intermittent nausea but no vomiting and denies changes in her bowel habits. There is no history of prior alcohol use, blood transfusions, or illicit drug use. The patient is widowed and had two heterosexual partners in her lifetime. Her past medical history is significant only for hypothyroidism, for which she takes levothyroxine. Her family history is unremarkable. On examination she is mildly icteric. She has spider angiomata on her torso. You palpate a nodular liver edge 2 cm below the right costal margin. The remainder of the examination is unremarkable. A right upper quadrant ultrasound confirms your suspicion of cirrhosis. You order a complete blood count and a comprehensive metabolic panel. What is the most appropriate next test?

A. 24-hour urine copper

B. Antimitochondrial antibodies (AMA)

C. Endoscopic retrograde cholangiopancreatography (ERCP)

D. Hepatitis B serologies

E. Serum ferritin

VIII-59. A 58-year-old man is evaluated for a new diagnosis of cirrhosis. The patient has a medical history of diabetes mellitus, hypertriglyceridemia, and hypertension. He takes pioglitazone, rosuvastatin, lisinopril, and atenolol. He is a lifetime nonsmoker and has never used IV drugs. He drinks about one glass of wine weekly. For about 4–8 years in his 20s, he admits to binge drinking as much as 12–18 beers on the weekends, but has not drunk more than two glasses of wine weekly for many years. He has never had a blood transfusion and has been in a monogamous sexual relationship for 30 years. He has no family history of liver disease. He works as a machinist in a factory making airplane engines. He denies chemical exposures. His physical examination is notable for a body mass index of 45.9 kg/m². He has stigmata of chronic liver disease including spider angiomata and caput medusa. Moderate ascites is present. Workup has shown no evidence of viral hepatitis, hemochromatosis, Wilson's disease, autoimmune hepatitis, or α₁ antitrypsin deficiency. He undergoes liver biopsy, which shows fibrosis in a perivenular and perisinusoidal distribution. Which of the following statements is TRUE regarding the cause of the patient's cirrhosis?

A. As opposed to individuals with metabolic syndrome alone, these individuals do not show significant insulin resistance.

B. The aspartate aminotransferase is commonly elevated to more than twice the alanine aminotransferase level.

C. The lack of steatohepatitis on liver biopsy rules out nonalcoholic fatty liver disease as a cause of the patient's cirrhosis.

D. The prevalence of the milder form of this disorder is between 10 and 20% in the United States and Europe, with as much as 10–15% of affected individuals developing cirrhosis in some series.

E. Treatment with ursodeoxycholic acid and HMG-CoA reductase inhibitors has been demonstrated to improve outcomes in this disorder.

VIII-60. Which of the following statements regarding liver transplantation is TRUE?

A. Individuals with cholangiocarcinoma should be referred early for consideration of liver transplantation.

B. Living donor transplantation is only performed in children.

C. Reinfection with hepatitis B typically occurs in 35% or more of patients with liver transplantation.

D. The 5-year survival rate for orthotopic liver transplantation is about 50%.

E. The most common indication for liver transplantation is chronic hepatitis B infection.

VIII-61. A 55-year-old male with cirrhosis is seen in the clinic for follow-up of a recent hospitalization for spontaneous bacterial peritonitis. He is doing well and finishing his course of antibiotics. He is taking propranolol and lactulose. Besides complications of end-stage liver disease, he has well-controlled diabetes mellitus and had a basal cell carcinoma resected 5 years ago. The cirrhosis is thought to be due to alcohol abuse, and his last drink of alcohol was 2 weeks ago. He and his wife ask if he is a liver transplant candidate. He can be counseled in which of the following ways?

A. Because he had a skin cancer he is not a transplant candidate.

B. Because he has diabetes mellitus he is not a transplant candidate.

C. He is appropriate for liver transplantation and should be referred immediately.

D. He is not a transplant candidate as he has a history of alcohol dependence.

E. He is not a transplant candidate now, but may be after a sustained period of proven abstinence from alcohol.

VIII-62. A 44-year-old woman is evaluated for complaints of abdominal pain. She describes the pain as a postprandial burning pain. It is worse with spicy or fatty foods and is relieved with antacids. She is diagnosed with a gastric ulcer and is treated appropriately for *Helicobacter pylori.* During the course of her evaluation for her abdominal pain, the patient had a right upper quadrant ultrasound that demonstrated the presence of gallstones. Following treatment of *H. pylori,* her symptoms have resolved. She is requesting your opinion regarding whether treatment is required for the finding of gallstone disease. Upon review of the ultrasound report, there were numerous stones in the gallbladder, including in the neck of the gallbladder. The largest stone measures 2.8 cm. What is your advice to the patient regarding the risk of complications and the need for definitive treatment?

A. Given the size and number of stones, prophylactic cholecystectomy is recommended.

B. No treatment is necessary unless the patient develops symptoms of biliary colic frequently and severely enough to interfere with the patient's life.

C. The only reason to proceed with cholecystectomy is the development of gallstone pancreatitis or cholangitis.

D. The risk of developing acute cholecystitis is about 5–10% per year.

E. Ursodeoxycholic acid should be given at a dose of 10–15 mg/kg daily for a minimum of 6 months to dissolve the stones.

VIII-63. A 62-year-old man has been hospitalized in intensive care for the past 3 weeks following an automobile accident resulting in multiple long-bone fractures and acute respiratory distress syndrome. He has been slowly improving, but remains on mechanical ventilation. He is now febrile and hypotensive, requiring vasopressors. He is being treated empirically with cefepime and vancomycin. Multiple blood cultures are negative. He has no new infiltrates or increasing secretions on chest radiograph. His laboratory studies demonstrated a rise in his liver function tests, bilirubin, and alkaline phosphatase. Amylase and lipase are normal. A right upper quadrant ultrasound shows sludge in the gallbladder, but no stones. The bile duct is not dilated. What is the next best step in the evaluation and treatment of this patient?

A. Discontinue cefepime.

B. Initiate treatment with clindamycin.

C. Initiate treatment with metronidazole.

D. Perform hepatobiliary scintigraphy.

E. Refer for exploratory laparotomy.

VIII-64. All of the following are associated with an increased risk for cholelithiasis EXCEPT:

A. Chronic hemolytic anemia

B. Female sex

C. High-protein diet

D. Obesity

E. Pregnancy

VIII-65. A 41-year-old female presents to your clinic with a week of jaundice. She notes pruritus, icterus, and dark urine. She denies fever, abdominal pain, or weight loss. The examination is unremarkable except for yellow discoloration of the skin. Total bilirubin is 6.0 mg/dL, and direct bilirubin is 5.1 mg/dL. AST is 84 U/L, and ALT is 92 U/L. Alkaline phosphatase is 662 U/L. CT scan of the abdomen is unremarkable. Right upper quadrant ultrasound shows a normal gallbladder but does not visualize the common bile duct. What is the most appropriate next management step?

A. Antibiotics and observation

B. Endoscopic retrograde cholangiopancreatography (ERCP)

C. Hepatitis serologies

D. HIDA scan

E. Serologies for antimitochondrial antibodies

VIII-66. A 27-year-old woman is admitted to the hospital with acute-onset severe right upper quadrant pain that radiates to the back. The pain is constant and not relieved with eating or bowel movements. Her labs show a marked elevation in amylase and lipase, and acute pancreatitis is diagnosed. Which of the following is the best first test to demonstrate the etiology of her pancreatitis?

A. Right upper quadrant ultrasound

B. Serum alcohol level

C. Serum triglyceride level

D. Technetium HIDA scan

E. Urine drug screen

VIII-67. A 58-year-old man with severe alcoholism is admitted to the hospital with acute pancreatitis. His symptoms have been present for 3 days and he has continued to drink heavily. He now has persistent vomiting and feels dizzy upon standing. On examination he has severe epigastric and right upper quadrant tenderness and decreased bowel sounds, and appears uncomfortable. A faint blue discoloration is present around the umbilicus. What is the significance of this finding?

A. A CT of the abdomen is likely to show severe necrotizing pancreatitis.

B. Abdominal plain film is likely to show pancreatic calcification.

C. Concomitant appendicitis should be ruled out.

D. He likely has a pancreatico-aortic fistula.

E. Pancreatic pseudocyst is likely present.

VIII-68. A 36-year-old man is admitted to the hospital with acute pancreatitis. In order to determine the severity of disease and risk of mortality, the BISAP (Bedside Index of Severity in Acute Pancreatitis) is calculated. All of the following variables are used to calculate this score EXCEPT:

A. Age greater than 60 years

B. BUN greater than 35

C. Impaired mental status

D. Pleural effusion

E. White blood cell count greater than 15,000 leukocytes/μL

VIII-69. A 54-year-old man is admitted to the intensive care unit with severe pancreatitis. His BMI is 30 or above and he has a prior history of diabetes mellitus. A CT of the abdomen is obtained and shows severe necrotizing pancreatitis. He is presently afebrile. Which of the following medications has been shown to be effective in the treatment of acute necrotizing pancreatitis?

A. Calcitonin
B. Cimetidine
C. Glucagon
D. Imipenem
E. None of the above

VIII-70. Which of the following statements is true regarding enteral feeding in acute pancreatitis?

A. A patient with persistent evidence of pancreatic necrosis on CT 2 weeks after acute presentation should be maintained on bowel rest.

B. All patients with elevations of amylase and lipase and CT evidence of pancreatitis should be fasted until amylase and lipase normalize.

C. Enteral feeding with a nasojejunal tube has been demonstrated to have fewer infectious complications than total parenteral nutrition in the management of patients with acute pancreatitis.

D. Patients requiring surgical removal of infected pancreatic pseudocysts should be treated with total parental nutrition.

E. Total parenteral nutrition has been shown to maintain integrity of the intestinal tract in acute pancreatitis.

VIII-71. A 47-year-old woman presents to the emergency department with severe mid-abdominal pain radiating to her back. The pain began acutely and is sharp. She denies cramping or flatulence. She has had two episodes of emesis of bilious material since the pain began, but this has not lessened the pain. She currently rates the pain as a 10 out of 10 and feels the pain is worse in the supine position. For the past few months, she has had intermittent episodes of right upper and mid-epigastric pain that occurs after eating but subsides over a few hours. This is associated with a feeling of excess gas. She denies any history of alcohol abuse. She has no medical history of hypertension or hyperlipidemia. On physical examination, she is writhing in distress and slightly diaphoretic. Vital signs are as follows: heart rate 127 beats/min, blood pressure 92/50 mmHg, respiratory rate 20 breaths/min, temperature 37.9°C, and 88% oxygen saturation on room air. Her body mass index is 29 kg/m². The cardiovascular examination reveals a regular tachycardia. The chest examination shows dullness to percussion at bilateral bases with a few scattered crackles. On abdominal examination, bowel sounds are hypoactive. There is no rash or bruising evident on inspection of the abdomen. There is voluntary guarding on palpation. The pain with palpation is greatest in the periumbilical and epigastric areas without rebound tenderness. There is no evidence of jaundice, and the liver span is

about 10 cm to percussion. Amylase level is 750 IU/L, and lipase level is 1129 IU/L. Other laboratory values include aspartate aminotransferase (AST) 168 U/L, alanine aminotransferase (ALT) 196 U/L, total bilirubin 2.3 mg/dL, alkaline phosphatase level 268 U/L, lactate dehydrogenase (LDH) 300 U/L, and creatinine 1.9 mg/dL. The hematocrit is 43%, and white blood cell (WBC) count is 11,500/μL with 89% neutrophils. An arterial blood gas shows a pH of 7.32, PCO_2 of 32 mmHg, and a PO_2 of 56 mmHg. An ultrasound confirms a dilated common bile duct with evidence of pancreatitis manifested as an edematous and enlarged pancreas. A CT scan shows no evidence of necrosis. After 3 L of normal saline, her blood pressure comes up to 110/60 mmHg with a heart rate of 105 beats/min. Which of the following statements best describes the pathophysiology of this disease?

A. Intrapancreatic activation of digestive enzymes with autodigestion and acinar cell injury

B. Chemoattraction of neutrophils with subsequent infiltration and inflammation

C. Distant organ involvement and systemic inflammatory response syndrome related to release of activated pancreatic enzymes and cytokines

D. All of the above

VIII-72. A 25-year-old female with cystic fibrosis is diagnosed with chronic pancreatitis. She is at risk for all of the following complications EXCEPT:

A. Vitamin B_{12} deficiency
B. Vitamin A deficiency
C. Pancreatic carcinoma
D. Niacin deficiency
E. Steatorrhea

VIII-73. A 64-year-old man seeks evaluation from his primary care physician because of chronic diarrhea. He reports that he has two or three large loose bowel movements daily. He describes them as markedly foul smelling, and they often leave an oily ring in the toilet. He also notes that the bowel movements often follow heavy meals, but if he fasts or eats low-fat foods, the stools are more formed. Over the past 6 months, he has lost about 18 kg. In this setting, he reports intermittent episodes of abdominal pain that can be quite severe. He describes the pain as sharp and in a mid-epigastric location. He has not sought evaluation of the pain previously, but when it occurs he will limit his oral intake and treat the pain with nonsteroidal anti-inflammatory drugs. He notes the pain has not lasted for more than 48 hours and is not associated with meals. His past medical history is remarkable for peripheral vascular disease and tobacco use. He currently smokes one pack of cigarettes daily. In addition, he drinks 2–6 beers daily. He has stopped all alcohol intake for up to a week at a time in the past without withdrawal symptoms. His current medications are aspirin 81 mg daily and albuterol metered dose inhaler (MDI) on an as-needed basis. On physical examination, the patient is thin but appears well. His body mass index is 18.2 kg/m^2. Vital signs are normal. Cardiac and pulmonary examinations are normal. The abdominal examination shows mild epigastric tenderness without rebound or guarding. The liver span is 12 cm to percussion and palpable 2 cm below the right costal margin. There is no splenomegaly or ascites present. There are decreased pulses in the lower extremities bilaterally. An abdominal radiograph demonstrates calcifications in the epigastric area, and CT scan confirms that these calcifications are located within the body of the pancreas. No pancreatic ductal dilatation is noted. Amylase level is 32 U/L, and lipase level is 22 U/L. What is the next most appropriate step in diagnosing and managing this patient's primary complaint?

A.   Advise the patient to stop all alcohol use and prescribe pancreatic enzymes.
B.   Advise the patient to stop all alcohol use and prescribe narcotic analgesia and pancreatic enzymes.
C.   Perform angiography to assess for ischemic bowel disease.
D.   Prescribe prokinetic agents to improve gastric emptying.
E.   Refer the patient for endoscopic retrograde cholangiopancreatography (ERCP) for sphincterotomy.

ANSWERS

VIII-1. The answer is E. *(Chap. 292)* Endoscopy, also known as esophagogastroduodenoscopy (EGD), is the best test for the evaluation of the proximal gastrointestinal tract. Because of high-quality images, disorders of color such as Barrett's metaplasia, and mucosal irregularities are easily demonstrated. The sensitivity of endoscopy is superior to that of barium radiography for mucosal lesions. Because the endoscope has an instrumentation channel, biopsy specimens are easily obtained and dilation of strictures can also be performed. The only advantage that barium radiography confers is the absence of the requirement for sedation, which, in some populations at risk for conscious sedation, is an important consideration.

VIII-2. The answer is E. *(Chap. 292)* Intermittent solid food dysphagia is a classic symptom in Schatzki's ring in which a distal esophageal ring occurs at the squamocolumnar mucosal junction. The origin of these rings is unknown, and smaller rings with a lumen of greater than 13 mm are common in the general population (up to 15%). When the lumen is less than 13 mm, dysphagia may occur. Schatzki's rings typically occur in persons older than 40 years and often cause "steakhouse syndrome" from meat getting stuck at the ring. The rings are easily treated with dilation. Plummer-Vinson syndrome also includes esophageal rings, but typically the rings occur in the proximal esophagus, are associated with iron-deficiency anemia, and occur in middle-aged women. Achalasia involves both solid and liquid dysphagia often with regurgitation. Adenocarcinoma often includes solid and liquid dysphagia at later stages. Most esophageal diverticulae are asymptomatic.

VIII-3. The answer is B. *(Chap. 292)* Aside from the discomfort and local complications of gastroesophageal reflux disease (GERD), a number of other non-GI–related sites may have a complication related to it. Syndromes with a well-established association with GERD include chronic cough, laryngitis, asthma, and dental erosions. Other diseases have implicated GERD as potentially contributory, but the role of GERD is less well established. These include pharyngitis, pulmonary fibrosis, chronic sinusitis, cardiac arrhythmias, sleep apnea, and recurrent aspiration pneumonia.

VIII-4. The answer is A. *(Chap. 292)* This patient has symptoms of esophagitis. In patients with HIV, various infections can cause this disease, including herpes simplex virus (HSV), cytomegalovirus (CMV), varicella-zoster virus (VZV), *Candida*, and HIV itself. The lack of thrush does not rule out *Candida* as a cause of esophagitis, and EGD is necessary for diagnosis. CMV classically causes serpiginous ulcers in the distal esophagus that may coalesce to form giant ulcers. Brushings alone are insufficient for diagnosis, and biopsies must be performed. Biopsies reveal intranuclear and intracytoplasmic inclusions with enlarged nuclei in large fibroblasts and endothelial cells. Given her notable swallowing symptoms, IV ganciclovir is the treatment of choice. Valganciclovir is an effective oral preparation. Foscarnet is useful in treating ganciclovir-resistant CMV. Herpes simplex virus manifests as vesicles and punched-out lesions in the esophagus, with the characteristic finding on biopsy of ballooning degeneration with ground-glass changes in the nuclei. It can be treated with acyclovir or foscarnet in resistant cases. Candida esophagitis has the appearance of yellow nodular plaques with surrounding erythema. Treatment usually requires fluconazole therapy. Finally, HIV alone can cause esophagitis that can be quite resistant to therapy. On EGD these ulcers appear deep and linear. Treatment with thalidomide or oral glucocorticoids is employed, and highly active antiretroviral therapy should be considered.

VIII-5. The answer is D. *(Chap. 293)* The patient has a duodenal ulcer, which is almost universally due to *H. pylori* infection, although in a minority of cases NSAID use may either facilitate development or be the only identified cause. The patient was taking acetaminophen and not a traditional NSAID, making *H. pylori*–associated peptic ulcer disease the most likely cause of the findings. *H. pylori* infection is closely correlated with advancing age, low socioeconomic status, and low education levels. After initial infection, antral gastritis is very common, and in a portion of cases, duodenal or gastric ulcers form. Associated with these conditions is the development of gastric cancer or MALT lymphoma. Duodenal ulcers are rarely cancerous, although this is a not an uncommon finding in gastric cancers. After discovery of the ulcer, first-line therapy is eradication of *H. pylori* in addition to acid suppression.

VIII-6. The answer is D. *(Chap. 293)* Noninvasive testing for *H. pylori* infection is recommended in patients with suggestive symptoms and no other indication for endoscopy, e.g., GI bleeding, atypical symptoms. Several tests have good sensitivity and specificity, including plasma serology for *H. pylori*, ^{14}C or ^{13}C-urea breath test, and the fecal *H. pylori* antigen test. Sensitivity and specificity are greater than 80% and greater than 90%, respectively, for serology, while the urea breath test and fecal antigen testing are greater than 90% for both. Serology is not useful for early follow-up after therapy completion, as antibody titers will take several weeks to months to fall. The urea breath test, which relies on the presence of urease secreted by *H. pylori* to digest the swallowed radioactive urea and liberate ^{14}C or ^{13}C as part of ammonia, is simple and rapid. It is useful for early follow-up, as it requires living bacteria to secrete urease and produce a positive test. The limitations to the test include the requirement for ingestion of radioactive materials, albeit low dose, and false-negative results with recent use of PPI, antibiotics, or bismuth compounds. Stool antigen testing is cheap and convenient, but is not established for proof of eradication.

VIII-7. The answer is A. *(Chap. 293)* *H. pylori* should be eradicated in patients with documented peptic ulcer disease no matter the number of episodes, severity, presence of confounding factors (e.g., NSAID ingestion), or symptomatic status. Documented eradication of *H. pylori* is associated with substantially lower recurrence rates and symptom improvement. Treating patients with GERD who require long-term acid reduction therapy and the role of *H. pylori* eradication to prevent gastric cancer are controversial. Fourteen-day regimens are most effective. Shorter duration of therapy with current agents available has high recurrence rates. Dual-therapy regimens are not recommended because of eradication rates of less than 80%. A number of combinations are available (Table VIII-7). Triple-therapy regimens (one antacid plus two antibiotics) for 14 days have an eradication rate of 85–90%. Antibiotic resistance is the most common cause of failure to eradicate in compliant patients. Unfortunately, there is no currently available test for *H. pylori* sensitivity to direct therapy. Quadruple therapy should be reserved for patients with failure to eradicate after an effective initial course.

TABLE VIII-7   Regimens Recommended for Eradication of *H. Pylori* Infection

Drug	Dose
Triple Therapy	
1. Bismuth subsalicylate *plus*	2 tablets qid
Metronidazole *plus*	250 mg qid
Tetracycline[a]	500 mg qid
2. Ranitidine bismuth citrate *plus*	400 mg bid
Tetracycline *plus*	500 mg bid
Clarithromycin or metronidazole	500 mg bid
3. Omeprazole (lansoprazole) *plus*	20 mg bid (30 mg bid)
Clarithromycin *plus*	250 or 500 mg bid
Metronidazole[b] *or*	500 mg bid
Amoxicillin[c]	1 g bid
Quadruple Therapy	
Omeprazole (lansoprazole)	20 mg (30 mg) daily
Bismuth subsalicylate	2 tablets qid
Metronidazole	250 mg qid
Tetracycline	500 mg qid

[a]Alternative: use prepacked Helidac.
[b]Alternative: use prepacked Prevpac.
[c]Use either metronidazole or amoxicillin, not both.

VIII-8. The answer is C. (*Chap. 293*) Fasting gastrin levels can be elevated in a variety of conditions including atrophic gastritis with or without pernicious anemia, G-cell hyperplasia, and acid suppressive therapy (gastrin levels increase as a consequence of loss of negative feedback). The diagnostic concern in a patient with persistent ulcers following optimal therapy is Zollinger-Ellison syndrome (ZES). The result is not sufficient to make a diagnosis because gastrin levels may be elevated in a variety of conditions. Elevated basal acid secretion also is consistent with ZES, but up to 12% of patients with peptic ulcer disease may have basal acid secretion as high as 15 meq/h. Thus, additional testing is necessary. Gastrin levels may go up with a meal (>200%), but this test does not distinguish G-cell hyperfunction from ZES. The best test in this setting is the secretin stimulation test. An increase in gastrin levels greater than 200 pg within 15 minutes of administering 2 μg/kg of secretin by IV bolus has a sensitivity and specificity of greater than 90% for ZES. Endoscopic ultrasonography is useful in locating the gastrin-secreting tumor once the positive secretin test is obtained. Genetic testing for mutations in the gene that encodes the menin protein can detect the fraction of patients with gastrinomas that are a manifestation of multiple endocrine neoplasia type I (Wermer's syndrome). Gastrinoma is the second most common tumor in this syndrome following parathyroid adenoma, but its peak incidence is generally in the third decade.

VIII-9. The answer is B. (*Chap. 294*) The patient presents with nonspecific gastrointestinal symptoms, but the presence of weight loss suggests malabsorption syndrome. Patients with lactose intolerance are usually able to relate symptoms to consumption of milk-based products and also report a strong history of crampy pain and flatulence. Therefore, a lactose-free diet is unlikely to be helpful. The patient does not have nocturnal diarrhea, which is commonly a feature of steatorrhea along with floating stools. In the absence of symptoms suggesting fat malabsorption, the first test should not be fecal fat measurement. As the patient has weight loss, irritable bowel syndrome is less likely, and an increase dietary fiber is unlikely to be useful. Finally, her symptoms may be consistent with celiac disease. The widespread availability of antibodies to gliadin, endomysial, and tTG can be easily measured in peripheral blood. Antiendomysial antibody has a 90–95% sensitivity and equal specificity, making it a reasonable first test in symptomatic individuals. The presence of the antibody is not diagnostic, however, and duodenal biopsy is recommended. Duodenal biopsy will show villous atrophy, absence or reduced height of villi, cuboidal appearance of surface epithelial cells, and increased lymphocytes and plasma cells in the lamina propria. These changes regress with complete removal of gluten from the diet.

VIII-10. The answer is B. (*Chap. 294*) Short bowel syndrome is a descriptive term referring to the many clinical complications that may occur after resection of varying lengths of the small bowel. Rarely, these complications may be due to congenital abnormalities of the small bowel. Most commonly in adults, short bowel syndrome occurs in mesenteric vascular disease, primary mucosal or submucosal disease (Crohn's disease), and operations without preexisting small bowel disease such as trauma. Multiple factors contribute to diarrhea and steatorrhea including gastric acid hypersecretion, increased bile acids in the colon due to absent or decreased reabsorption in the small bowel, and lactose intolerance due to increased gastric acid secretion. Nonintestinal symptoms may include renal calcium oxalate calculi due to an increase in oxalate absorption by the large intestine with subsequent hyperoxaluria. This may be due to increased fatty acids in the colon that bind calcium, and thus calcium in the gut is not free to bind oxalate and free oxalate is absorbed in the large intestine. Increased bile acid pool size results in the generation of cholesterol gallstones from supersaturating in gallbladder bile. Gastric hypersecretion of acid is well described and thought to be due to loss of inhibition of gastric acid secretion because of absent short bowel to secrete inhibitory hormones. Coronary artery disease is not described as a complication of short bowel syndrome.

VIII-11. The answer is E. (*Chap. 294*) The patient presents with symptoms suggestive of Whipple's disease with a chronic multisystem disease often including diarrhea/steatorrhea, migratory arthralgias, weight loss, and CNS or cardiac problems. Generally the presentation is of insidious onset, and dementia is a late finding and poor prognostic sign. The disease primarily occurs in middle-aged white males. The diagnosis requires small bowel biopsy and demonstration of PAS-positive macrophages within the small bowel. Small bacilli are often present and suggest the diagnosis of Whipple's disease. Similar macrophages may be found in other affected organs, e.g., the CNS. Dilated lymphatics are present in patients with intestinal lymphangiectasia. Mononuclear cell infiltrate in the lamina propria is often demonstrated in patients with tropical sprue, and flat villi with crypt hyperplasia are the hallmark of celiac disease.

VIII-12. The answer is D. (*Chap. 294*) This patient has a stool osmolality gap (measured stool osmolality − calculated stool osmolality) of less than 50 mosmol/L, suggesting a secretory rather than an osmotic cause for diarrhea. Secretory causes of diarrhea include toxin-mediated diarrhea (cholera, enterotoxigenic *Escherichia coli*) and intestinal peptide–mediated diarrhea in which the major pathophysiology is a luminal or circulating secretagogue. The distinction between secretory diarrhea and osmotic diarrhea aids in forming a differential diagnosis. Secretory diarrhea will not decrease substantially during a fast and has a low osmolality gap. Osmotic diarrhea will generally decrease during a fast and has a high (>50 mosmol/L) osmolality gap. Celiac sprue, chronic pancreatitis, lactase deficiency, and Whipple's disease all cause an osmotic diarrhea.

VIII-13. The answer is E. (*Chaps. 294 and e37*) Cobalamin malabsorption may occur due to disease at multiple anatomic sites extending from the stomach to the ileum. In the past, the Schilling test was utilized to assess cobalamin absorption, but this test is not currently commercially available. Cobalamin is primarily present in meat, but dietary deficiency is rare except in strict vegans. Dietary cobalamin is bound in the stomach to R-binder protein that is synthesized in salivary glands and stomach. The cobalamin–R binder complex requires an acid medium. Therefore, achlorhydria of any cause may result in the inability for splitting of cobalamin from food and binding to R-binder protein. Cobalamin absorption has an absolute requirement for intrinsic factor, which allows uptake by specific receptors in the ileum. Intrinsic factor is produced and released by gastric parietal cells. Thus pernicious anemia, the autoimmune atrophy of parietal cells, is a cause of cobalamin malabsorption. Pancreatic protease enzymes lyse the cobalamin–R binder protein complex to release cobalamin in the proximal intestine where it is bound to intrinsic factor for ileal absorption. Thus a deficiency of pancreatic enzymes, such as in chronic pancreatitis, can lead to cobalamin malabsorption. Finally, cobalamin-intrinsic factor is absorbed via an intact epithelium in the ileum. Inflammation (Crohn's disease) or absence (surgical removal) of ileum will cause cobalamin malabsorption. The large intestine is not involved in cobalamin absorption; thus ulcerative colitis confined to the large intestine will not cause malabsorption.

VIII-14. The answer is D. *(Chap. 295)* The incidence of inflammatory bowel disease is highly influenced by ethnicity, location, and environmental factors. Both conditions have their highest incidence in the United Kingdom and North America, and the peak incidence has a bimodal distribution of age of presentation: 15–30 years and 60–80 years. The incidence of both ulcerative colitis and Crohn's disease is highest among persons of the Ashkenazi Jewish population. Prevalence decreases progressively in non-Jewish white, African-American, Hispanic, and Asian populations. Cigarette smoking is associated with a decreased incidence of ulcerative colitis, but may cause Crohn's disease. Oral contraceptive use is associated with a slightly higher incidence of Crohn's disease, but not ulcerative colitis. Monozygotic twins are highly concordant for Crohn's disease, but not ulcerative colitis.

VIII-15. The answer is C. *(Chap. 295)* Chronic bloody diarrhea associated with weight loss and systemic symptoms in a young person is highly suggestive of inflammatory bowel disease. Her surgical findings suggest discontinuous lesions, which is typical of Crohn's disease. Ulcerative colitis, in contrast, typically affects the rectum and proceeds caudally from there without normal mucosa until the area of inflammation terminates. The presence of strictures and fissures further supports the diagnosis of Crohn's disease, as these are not features of ulcerative colitis. Microscopically, both ulcerative colitis and Crohn's disease may have crypt abscess and, although Crohn's disease is more often transmural, full thickness disease may be present in ulcerative colitis. The hallmark of Crohn's disease is granulomas that may be present throughout the bowel wall and involve the lymph nodes, mesentery, peritoneum, liver, and pancreas. Although pathognomonic for Crohn's disease, granulomas are only found in about half of surgical resections. Flat villi are not always present in either disease and are more commonly found in isolation with celiac disease.

VIII-16. The answer is D. *(Chap. 295)* There are a number of dermatologic manifestations of inflammatory bowel disease (IBD), and each type of IBD has a particular predilection for different dermatologic conditions. This patient has pyoderma gangrenosum. Pyoderma gangrenosum can occur in up to 12% of patients with ulcerative colitis and is characterized by a lesion that begins as a pustule and progresses concentrically to surrounding normal skin. The lesions ulcerate with violaceous, heaped margins and surrounding erythema. They are typically found on the lower extremities. Often the lesions are difficult to treat and respond poorly to colectomy; similarly, pyoderma gangrenosum is not prevented by colectomy. Treatment commonly includes IV antibiotics, glucocorticoids, dapsone, infliximab, and other immunomodulatory agents. Erythema nodosum is more common in Crohn's disease, and attacks correlate with bowel symptoms. The lesions are typically multiple red hot, tender nodules measuring 1–5 cm and are found on the lower legs and arms. Psoriasis is more common in ulcerative colitis. Finally, pyoderma vegetans is a rare disorder in intertriginous areas reported to be a manifestation of inflammatory bowel disease in the skin.

VIII-17. The answer is D. *[Chap. 295, Cochrane Database Syst Rev 2007 Oct 17; (4)]* Despite being described as a clinical entity for over a century, the etiology of IBD remains cryptic. Current theory is related to an interplay between inflammatory stimuli in genetically predisposed individuals. Recent studies have identified a group of genes or polymorphisms that confer risk of IBD. Multiple microbiologic agents, including some that reside as "normal" flora, may initiate IBD by triggering an inflammatory response. Anaerobic organisms (e.g., *Bacteroides* and *Clostridia* spp.) may be responsible for the induction of inflammation. Other organisms, for unclear reasons, may have the opposite effect. These "probiotic" organisms include *Lactobacillus* spp., *Bifidobacterium* spp., *Taenia suis*, and *Saccharomyces boulardii*. *Shigella*, *Escherichia*, and *Campylobacter* spp. are known to promote inflammation. Studies of probiotic therapy in adults and children with IBD have shown potential benefit for reducing disease activity.

VIII-18. The answer is D. *(Chap. 295)* Methotrexate, azathioprine, cyclosporine, tacrolimus, and anti-tumor necrosis factor (TNF) antibody are reasonable options for patients with CD, depending on the extent of macroscopic disease. Pneumonitis is a rare but serious complication of methotrexate therapy. Primary sclerosing cholangitis is an extraintestinal manifestation of inflammatory bowel disease (IBD). Pancreatitis is an uncommon complication of azathioprine, and IBD patients treated with azathioprine are at a fourfold increased risk of developing a lymphoma. Anti-TNF antibody therapy is associated with an increased risk of tuberculosis, disseminated histoplasmosis, and a number of other infections.

VIII-19. The answer is C *(Chap. 296)* Irritable bowel syndrome is characterized by the following: recurrence of lower abdominal pain with altered bowel habits over a period of time without progressive deterioration, onset of symptoms during periods of stress or emotional upset, absence of other systemic symptoms such as fever and weight loss, and small-volume stool without evidence of blood. Warning signs that the symptoms may be due to something other than irritable bowel syndrome include presentation for the first time in old age, progressive course from the time of onset, persistent diarrhea after a 48-hour fast, and presence of nocturnal diarrhea or steatorrheal stools. Each patient, except for patient C, has "warning" symptoms that should prompt further evaluation.

VIII-20. The answer is C. *(Chap. 296)* Although this patient has signs and symptoms consistent with IBS, the differential diagnosis is large. Few tests are required for patients who have typical IBS symptoms and no alarm features. In this patient, alarm features include anemia, an elevated ESR, and evidence of WBCs in the stool. Alarm features warrant further investigation to rule out other gastrointestinal disorders such as colonic pathology including diverticular disease or inflammatory bowel disease. In this case, colonoscopy to evaluate for luminal lesions and mucosal characteristics would be the logical first step. At this point, with the warning signs, empiric therapy for IBS is premature. Reassurance, stool bulking agents, and antidepressants are all therapies to consider if a patient does indeed have IBS.

VIII-21. The answer is D. *(Chap. 296)* Up to 80% of patients with irritable bowel syndrome (IBS) also have abnormal psychiatric features; however, no single psychiatric diagnosis predominates. The mechanism is not well understood but may involve altered pain thresholds. Although these patients are hypersensitive to colonic stimuli, this does not carry over to the peripheral nervous system. Functional brain imaging shows disparate activation in, for example, the mid-cingulate cortex, but brain anatomy does not discriminate IBS patients from those without IBS. An association between a history of sexual abuse and IBS has been reported. There is no reported association with sexually transmitted diseases. Patients with IBS do not have an increased risk of autoimmunity.

VIII-22. The answer is B. *(Chap. 297)* The patient presents with classic signs of diverticulitis with fever, abdominal pain that is usually left lower quadrant, anorexia or obstipation, and leukocytosis. This most commonly occurs in older individuals. Patients may present with acute abdomen due to perforation, though this occurs in less than 25% of cases. Plain radiographs of the abdomen are seldom helpful, but may rarely show the presence of an air–fluid level in the left lower quadrant indicating a giant diverticulum with impending perforation. CT with oral contrast is the diagnostic modality of choice with the following findings: sigmoid diverticula, thickened colonic wall greater than 4 mm, and inflammation within the pericolic space with or without the collection of contrast material or fluid. Abscesses, if present, will also be demonstrated on CT. Barium enema and colonoscopy should be avoided in acute diverticulitis because the insufflation of air or contrast material may lead to perforation. Although diverticular disease may result in hematochezia, these are generally not temporally linked to diverticulitis.

VIII-23. The answer is B. *(Chap. 297)* Medical management is appropriate for many patients with uncomplicated diverticular disease. Uncomplicated disease has fever, abdominal pain, leukocytosis, and anorexia/obstipation, while complicated disease includes that with abscess formation, perforation, strictures, or fistulae. Uncomplicated disease accounts for at least 75% of cases. Medical therapy generally involves bowel rest and antibiotics, usually trimethoprim/sulfamethoxazole or ciprofloxacin and metronidazole targeting aerobic gram-negative rods and anaerobic bacteria. Patients with more than two attacks of diverticulitis were previously thought to require surgical therapy, but newer data suggest that these patients do not have an increased risk of perforation and can continue medical management. Patients with immunosuppressive therapy, chronic renal failure, or collagen vascular disease have a fivefold higher risk of perforation during recurrent attacks. Surgical therapy is indicated for surgical low-risk patients with complicated disease.

VIII-24. **The answer is B.** *(Chap. 297)* Hemorrhoids can be internal or external; however, they are normally internal and may prolapse to the external position. Hemorrhoids are staged in the following manner: stage I, enlargement with bleeding; stage II, protrusion with spontaneous reduction; stage III, protrusion requiring manual reduction; stage IV, irreducible protrusion. Stage I, which this patient has, is treated with fiber supplementation, cortisone suppositories, and/or sclerotherapy. Stage II is treated with fiber and cortisone suppositories. Stage III patients are offered the prior three therapies and banding or operative hemorrhoidectomy. Stage IV patients benefit from fiber and cortisone therapy as well as operative hemorrhoidectomy. While substantial upper GI bleeding may result in hematochezia, the absence of suggestive signs/symptoms and the consistent findings of hemorrhoids do not indicate the need for upper endoscopy.

VIII-25. **The answer is A.** *(Chap. 297)* An anorectal abscess is an abnormal fluid-containing cavity in the anorectal region. Anorectal abscess results from an infection involving the glands surrounding the anorectal canal. The disease is more common in males with a peak incidence in the third to fifth decades. Patients with diabetes, inflammatory bowel disease, or who are immunocompromised are at increased risk for this condition. Perianal pain with defecation and fever are common presenting symptoms.

VIII-26. **The answer is C.** *(Chap. 297)* This patient has symptoms (social isolation), signs (foul odor), and risk factors (multiparity) for procidentia (rectal prolapse) and fecal incontinence. Procidentia is far more common in women than men and is often associated with pelvic floor disorders. It is not uncommon for these patients to become socially withdrawn and suffer from depression because of the associated fecal incontinence. The foul odor is a result of poor perianal hygiene due to the prolapsed rectum. Although depression in the elderly is an important medical problem, it is too premature in the evaluation of this patient to initiate medical therapy for depression. Occult malignancy and thyroid abnormalities may cause fecal incontinence and depression, but a physical examination would be diagnostic and avoid costly tests. Often patients are concerned that they have a rectal mass or carcinoma. Examination after an enema often makes the prolapse apparent. Medical therapy is limited to stool bulking agents or fiber. Surgical correction is the mainstay of therapy.

VIII-27. **The answer is E.** *(Chap. 297)* Surgical therapy is indicated in all low-risk surgical patients with complicated diverticular disease. Patients with at least two episodes of diverticulitis requiring hospitalization, with disease that does not respond to medical therapy, or who develop intra-abdominal complications are considered to have complicated disease. Complicating this patient's relapse of diverticulitis is probably an enterovesicular fistula causing pneumaturia. Studies indicate that younger patients (<50 years) may experience a more aggressive form of the disease than older patients, and therefore waiting for more than two attacks before considering surgery is not recommended. Rifaximin is a poorly absorbed broad-spectrum antibiotic that, when combined with a fiber-rich diet, is associated with less frequent symptoms in patients with uncomplicated diverticular disease. Pneumaturia represents a potential surgical urgency and should not be confused with proteinuria.

VIII-28. **The answer is A.** *(Chap. 298)* Mesenteric ischemia is a relatively uncommon and highly morbid illness. Acute mesenteric ischemia is usually due to arterial embolus (usually from the heart) or from thrombosis in a diseased vascular bed. Major risk factors include age, atrial fibrillation, valvular disease, recent arterial catheterization, and recent myocardial infarction. Ischemia occurs when the intestines are inadequately perfused by the splanchnic circulation. This blood supply has extensive collateralization and can receive up to 30% of the cardiac output, making poor perfusion an uncommon event. Patients with acute mesenteric ischemia will frequently present with pain out of proportion to their initial physical examination. As ischemia persists, peritoneal signs and cardiovascular collapse will follow. Mortality is greater than 50%. While radiographic imaging can suggest ischemia, the gold standard for diagnosis is laparotomy.

VIII-29. The answer is C. *(Chap. 300)* Obstruction of the appendiceal lumen is believed to typically result in appendicitis. Although obstruction is most commonly caused by fecalith, which results from accumulation and inspissation of fecal matter around vegetable fibers, other causes have been described. These other potential causes include enlarged lymphoid follicles associated with viral infection (e.g., measles), inspissated barium, worms (e.g., pinworms, *Ascaris* and *Taenia*), and tumors such as carcinoma or carcinoid. Cholelithiasis is a common cause of acute pancreatitis.

VIII-30. The answer is E. *(Chap. 300)* Infection with *Yersinia* organisms may potentially cause acute appendicitis after obstruction occurs. High complement fixation antibody titers have been found in up to 30% of proven cases of acute appendicitis. Chronic appendicitis is quite rare, but may occur due to tuberculosis, amebiasis, and actinomycosis.

VIII-31. The answer is A. *(Chap. 300)* The patient presents with classic findings for acute appendicitis with anorexia, progressing to vague periumbilical pain, followed by localization to the right lower quadrant. Low-grade fever and leukocytosis are frequently present. Although acute appendicitis is primarily a clinical diagnosis, imaging modalities are frequently employed as the symptoms are not always classic. Plain radiographs are rarely helpful except when an opaque fecalith is found in the right lower quadrant (<5% of cases). Ultrasound may demonstrate an enlarged appendix with a thick wall, but is most useful to rule out ovarian pathology, tuboovarian abscess, or ectopic pregnancy. Recently both nonenhanced and contrasted CT have been shown be superior to ultrasound or plain radiograph in the diagnosis of acute appendicitis, with a positive predictive value of 95–97% and overall accuracy of 90–97%. Findings often include a thickened appendix with periappendiceal stranding and often the presence of a fecalith. Free air is uncommon, even in the case of a perforated appendix. Nonvisualization of the appendix on CT is associated with surgical findings of a normal appendix 98% of the time. Colonoscopy has no role in the diagnosis of acute appendicitis.

VIII-32 and VIII-33. The answers are C and D, respectively. *(Chap. 300)* The patient presents with several months of epigastric abdominal pain that is worse after eating. His symptoms are highly suggestive of peptic ulcer disease, with the worsening pain after eating suggesting a duodenal ulcer. The current presentation with acute abdomen and free air under the diaphragm diagnoses perforated viscus. Perforated gallbladder is less likely in light of the duration of symptoms and the absence of the significant systemic symptoms that often accompany this condition. As the patient is relatively young with no risk factors for mesenteric ischemia, necrotic bowel from an infarction is highly unlikely. Pancreatitis can have a similar presentation, but a pancreas cannot perforate and liberate free air. Peritonitis is most commonly associated with bacterial infection, but it can be caused by the abnormal presence of physiologic fluids, for example, gastric contents, bile, pancreatic enzymes, blood, or urine, or by foreign bodies. In this case peritonitis most likely is due to the presence of gastric juice in the peritoneal cavity after perforation of a duodenal ulcer has allowed these juices to leave the gut lumen.

VIII-34. The answer is A. *(Chap. 301)* The most common and most characteristic symptom of liver disease is fatigue. Unfortunately, it is also very nonspecific with little specific diagnostic utility. The fatigue in liver disease seems to improve in the morning and worsen throughout the day, but it can be intermittent. Jaundice is the hallmark of liver disease and is much more specific. Jaundice, however, is typically a sign of more advanced disease. Itching is also typically a symptom of more advanced disease and is more common in cholestatic causes of liver disease. Nausea often occurs in severe disease and can be accompanied by vomiting. Right upper quadrant pain is a less common symptom and indicates stretching of the liver capsule.

VIII-35. **The answer is B.** *(Chap. 301)* Women are more susceptible to the effects of alcohol on the liver. On average, drinking about two drinks daily can lead to chronic liver disease in women, whereas in men it is about three drinks daily. In individuals with alcoholic cirrhosis, the average daily alcohol intake is usually much higher, however, and heavy drinking for more than 10 years is typical before the onset of liver disease.

VIII-36. **The answer is D.** *(Chap. 302)* It is important to understand the patterns of laboratory abnormalities that indicate liver disease is present. One way to consider laboratory evaluation of liver disease is to consider three general categories of tests: tests based on excretory function of the liver, tests of biosynthetic activity of the liver, and coagulation factors. The most common tests of liver function fall under the category of tests based on the detoxification and excretory function of the liver. These include serum bilirubin, urine bilirubin, ammonia, and enzyme levels. Bilirubin can exist as a conjugated and an unconjugated form. The unconjugated form is often referred to as the indirect fraction. Elevations in the unconjugated form of bilirubin are not related to liver disease, but are most commonly seen in hemolysis and a number of benign genetic conditions such as Gilbert's syndrome. In contrast, conjugated hyperbilirubinemia almost always indicates disease of the liver or biliary tract. Conjugated bilirubin is water soluble and is excreted in the urine, but unconjugated bilirubin is not. Rather, it binds to albumin in the blood. Therefore, bilirubinuria implies liver disease as well. Among the serum enzymes, it is useful to consider those that are associated with hepatocellular injury or those that reflect cholestasis. Alanine and aspartate aminotransferases are the primary enzymes that indicate hepatocyte injury. Alkaline phosphatase is the most common enzyme elevated in cholestasis, but bone disease also causes increased alkaline phosphatase. In some cases, one needs additional information to determine if the alkaline phosphatase is liver or bone in origin. Other tests that would be elevated in cholestatic liver disease are 5′-nucleotidase and γ-glutamyl transferase. The primary test of synthetic function is measurement of serum albumin. Coagulation factors can be directly measured, but impaired production of coagulation factors in liver disease is primarily inferred from elevations in prothrombin time.

VIII-37. **The answer is A.** *(Chaps. 43 and 302)* Diagnostic paracentesis is part of the routine evaluation in a patient with ascites. Fluid should be examined for its gross appearance, protein content, cell count and differential, and albumin. Cytologic and culture studies should be performed when one suspects infection or malignancy. The serum-ascites albumin gradient (SAG) offers the best correlation with portal pressure. A high gradient (>1.1 g/dL) is characteristic of uncomplicated cirrhotic ascites and differentiates ascites caused by portal hypertension from ascites not caused by portal hypertension in more than 95% of cases. Conditions that cause a low gradient include more "exudative" processes such as infection, malignancy, and inflammatory processes. Similarly, congestive heart failure and nephrotic syndrome cause high gradients. In this patient the SAG is 1.5 g/dL, indicating a high gradient. The low number of leukocytes and polymorphonuclear cells makes bacterial or tubercular infection unlikely. Chylous ascites often is characterized by an opaque milky fluid with a triglyceride level greater than 1000 mg/dL in addition to a low SAG.

VIII-38 and VIII-39. **The answers are E and D, respectively.** *(Chap. 303)* This patient is presenting with an asymptomatic and mild elevation in unconjugated hyperbilirubinemia that has occurred during a time of increased stress, fatigue, and likely decreased caloric intake. This presentation is characteristic of Gilbert's syndrome (option E), an inherited disorder of bilirubin conjugation. In Gilbert's syndrome, there is a mutation of the *UGT1A1* gene that encodes bilirubin UDP-glucuronosyltransferase that leads to a reduction in activity on the enzyme to 10–35% of normal. This enzyme is of critical importance in the conjugation of bilirubin. Most of the time, there is no apparent jaundice, as the reduced ability to conjugate bilirubin is not reduced to a degree that leads to an elevation of bilirubin. However, during times of stress, fatigue, alcohol use, decreased caloric intake, or intercurrent illness, the enzyme can become overwhelmed, leading to a mild hyperbilirubinemia. Typical bilirubin levels are less than 4.0 mg/dL unless the individual is ill or fasting. Diagnosis usually occurs during young adulthood, and episodes are self-limited and benign. If a liver biopsy were to be performed, hepatic histology would be normal. No treatment is necessary as there are no long-term consequences of Gilbert's syndrome, and patient reassurance is recommended. Other inherited disorders of bilirubin conjugation are Crigler-Najjar syndrome types I and II. Crigler-Najjar syndrome type I is a congenital disease characterized by more dramatic elevations in bilirubin as high as 20–45 mg/dL that is first diagnosed in the neonatal period and is present throughout life. This rare disorder was once fatal in early childhood due to the development of kernicterus. However, with phototherapy, individuals are now able to survive into adulthood, although neurologic deficits are common. Crigler-Najjar syndrome type II is similar to type I, but the elevations in bilirubin are less. Kernicterus is rare. This is due to the fact that there is some residual function of the bilirubin UDP-glucoronosyltransferase enzyme (<10%), which is totally absent in type I disease. Hemolysis is another frequent cause of elevated unconjugated bilirubin. Hemolysis can be caused by many factors including medications, autoimmune disorders, and inherited disorders, among others. However, the normal hematocrit, LDH, and haptoglobin eliminate hemolysis as a possibility. Dubin-Johnson syndrome is another congenital hyperbilirubinemia. However, it is a predominantly conjugated hyperbilirubinemia caused by a defect in biliary excretion from hepatocytes. Obstructive choledocholithiasis is characterized by right upper quadrant pain that is often exacerbated by fatty meals. The absence of symptoms or elevation in other liver function tests, especially alkaline phosphatase, also makes this diagnosis unlikely.

VIII-40. **The answer is B.** (*Chap. 304*) This patient presents with acute hepatitis, which has numerous etiologies. These include viruses, toxins/drugs, autoimmune diseases, metabolic disease, alcohol, ischemia, pregnancy, and other infectious etiologies including rickettsial diseases and leptospirosis. In this clinical scenario, the patient has risk factors for hepatitis A, B, and C infection, including having had sex with men and a prior history of injection drug use. All acute viral hepatitis presents with a similar clinical pattern, although incubation periods vary after exposure. The most common initial symptoms are fatigue, anorexia, nausea, vomiting, myalgias, and headache. These symptoms precede the onset of jaundice by about 1–2 weeks. Once jaundice develops, the prodromal symptoms regress. On physical examination, there is usually obvious icterus with an enlarged and tender liver. Splenomegaly can occur. AST and ALT are elevated with peak levels that are quite variable between 400–4000 U/L, and alkaline phosphatase levels are increased to a much lesser degree. Hyperbilirubinemia (levels from 5 to 20 mg/dL) occurs with primarily increased levels of conjugated bilirubin. Thus, it is important to recognize the patterns of antibody production in the viral hepatidities. Hepatitis A is an RNA virus that presents with acute hepatitis and is transmitted by the fecal-oral route. In the acute state, the IgM would be elevated, which is not seen in this scenario. Hepatitis B virus is a DNA virus with three common antigens that are tested serologically to determine the time course of the illness. These antigens are the surface antigen, the core antigen, and the e antigen, which is a nucleocapsid protein produced from the same gene as the core antigen but is immunologically distinct. Several distinct patterns can be observed. In acute hepatitis B, the core IgM, surface antigen, and e antigens are all positive, which is what is seen in this case. At this point, the patient is highly infectious with viral shedding in body fluids, including saliva. In a late acute infection, core IgG may be positive at the same time as surface and e-antigen positivity. In chronic hepatitis B, this same pattern of serologies is seen. If a patient has a prior infection without development of chronic hepatitis, the core IgG and surface antibody is positive. However, when immunity is obtained via vaccination, only the surface antibody (SAb) is positive; the e antigen and surface antigen will be negative since the patient was never infected. The variety of antigen-antibody positivities that can result are outlined in Table VIII-40. Acute hepatitis C often is detectable with contemporary immunoassays

TABLE VIII-40 Commonly Encountered Serologic Patterns of Hepatitis B Infection

HBsAg	Anti-HBs	Anti-HBc	HBeAg	Anti-HBe	Interpretation
+	–	IgM	+	–	Acute hepatitis B, high infectivity
+	–	IgG	+	–	Chronic hepatitis B, high infectivity
+	–	IgG	–	+	1. Late acute or chronic hepatitis B, low infectivity
					2. HBeAg-negative ("precore-mutant") hepatitis B (chronic or, rarely, acute)
+	+	+	+/–	+/–	1. HBsAg of one subtype and heterotypic anti-HBs (common)
					2. Process of seroconversion from HBsAg to anti-HBs (rare)
–	–	IgM	+/–	+/–	1. Acute hepatitis B
					2. Anti-HBc "window"
–	–	IgG	–	+/–	1. Low-level hepatitis B carrier
					2. Hepatitis B in remote past
–	+	IgG	–	+/–	Recovery from hepatitis B
–	+	–	–	–	1. Immunization with HBsAg (after vaccination)
					2. Hepatitis B in the remote past (?)
					3. False positive

early in the disease when the aminotransferases are positive. Thus, a positive HCV antibody could indicate acute hepatitis C in this individual. However, given his clinical history of prior injection drug use and inability to donate blood, this likely indicates chronic hepatitis C infection. In some instances, ecstasy has been reported to cause drug-induced hepatitis, but given the viral serologies in this patient, this would be unlikely.

VIII-41. **The answer is E.** *(Chap. 304)* No treatment is recommended for acute hepatitis B in most individuals because 99% of infected individual recover without assistance. Therefore, it would not be expected that an individual would derive any particular benefit from treatment. In severe acute hepatitis B, nucleoside analogues, including lamivudine, have been used successfully, although there are no clinical trial data to support such an approach. For acute hepatitis C, however, there is a growing body of literature to support the use of interferon α therapy to prevent the development of chronic hepatitis C. In a study of 44 patients, 98% had a sustained virologic response after 3 months, and therapy was continued for a total of 24 weeks. Many experts are now recommending that pegylated interferon α plus ribavirin be used as an alternative treatment for acute hepatitis C, although clinical trial data to support this approach is also lacking. Hepatitis A is an acute and self-limited illness that does not progress to chronic liver disease. Thus, no treatment is required. Anti–hepatitis A virus immunoglobulin can be given prophylactically following a known exposure to prevent the development of disease, but it is not helpful in established disease. There is no role for oral or IV corticosteroids in the treatment of acute viral hepatitis of any etiology. It has demonstrated no clinical benefit and may increase the risk of developing chronic disease.

VIII-42. **The answer is E.** *(Chap. 304)* In most instances, patients with any form of acute viral hepatitis do not succumb to fulminant liver failure. However, pregnant women are highly susceptible to fulminant hepatic failure in the setting of acute hepatitis E infection. This RNA virus is an enteric virus that is endemic in India, Asia, Africa, the Middle East, and Central America, and is spread via contaminated water supplies. Person-to-person spread is rare. Generally, the clinical course of hepatitis E infection is mild, and the rate of fulminant hepatitis is only 1–2%. However, in pregnant women, this is as high as 10–20%. For hepatitis A and C, the rate of fulminant hepatic failure is about 0.1% or less. It is slightly higher for hepatitis B at around 0.1–1%. Hepatitis D occurs as a coinfection with hepatitis B virus. When the two viruses are acquired simultaneously, the rate of fulminant hepatitis is about 5% or less. When hepatitis D is acquired in the setting of chronic hepatitis B infection, this number rises to 20%.

VIII-43. The answer is E. *(Chap. 304)* Hepatitis A is an acute, self-limited virus that is acquired almost exclusively via the fecal-oral route. It is classically a disease of poor hygiene and overcrowding. Outbreaks have been traced to contaminated water, milk, frozen raspberries and strawberries, green onions, and shellfish. Infection occurs mostly in children and young adults. It almost invariably resolves spontaneously and results in lifelong immunity. Fulminant disease occurs in 0.1% or less of cases, and there is no chronic form (in contrast to hepatitis B and C). Diagnosis is made by demonstrating a positive IgM antibody to HAV, as described in the case for this question. An IgG antibody to HAV indicates immunity that has been obtained by previous infection or vaccination. A small proportion of patients will experience relapsing hepatitis weeks to months after a full recovery from HAV infection. This too is self-limited. There is no approved antiviral therapy for hepatitis A disease. An inactivated vaccine has decreased the incidence of the disease, and it is recommended for all U.S. children, high-risk adults, and travelers to endemic areas. Passive immunization with immune globulin is also available, and it is effective in preventing clinical disease before exposure or during the early incubation period.

VIII-44. The answer is C. *(Chap. 304)* The current hepatitis B vaccine is a recombinant vaccine consisting of yeast-derived hepatitis B surface antigen particles. A strategy of vaccinating only high-risk individuals in the United States has been shown to be ineffective, and universal vaccination against hepatitis B is now recommended. Pregnancy is *not* a contraindication to vaccination. Vaccination should ideally be performed in infancy. Routine evaluation of hepatitis serologies is not cost-effective and is not recommended. The vaccine is given in three divided IM doses at 0, 1, and 6 months.

VIII-45. The answer is A. *(Chap. 304)* A clear distinction between viral etiologies of acute hepatitis cannot be made on clinical or epidemiologic features alone. This patient is at risk for many forms of hepatitis due to his lifestyle. Given his occupation in food services, from a public health perspective it is important to make an accurate diagnosis. Serologies must be obtained to make a diagnosis. While hepatitis C virus typically does not present as an acute hepatitis, this is not absolute. Hepatitis E virus infects men and women equally and resembles hepatitis A virus in clinical presentation. This patient should be questioned regarding IV drug use, and in addition to hepatitis serologies, an HIV test should be performed.

VIII-46. The answer is C. *(Chaps. 302 and 304)* Causes of extreme elevations in serum transaminases generally fall into a few major categories, including viral infections, toxic ingestions, and vascular/hemodynamic causes. Both acute hepatitis A and hepatitis B infections may be characterized by high transaminases. Fulminant hepatic failure may occur, particularly in situations in which acute hepatitis A occurs on top of chronic hepatitis C infection, or if hepatitis B and hepatitis D are cotransmitted. Most cases of acute hepatitis A or B infection in adults are self-limited. Hepatitis C is an RNA virus that does not typically cause acute hepatitis. However, it is associated with a high probability of chronic infection. Therefore, progression to cirrhosis and hepatoma is increased in patients with chronic hepatitis C infection. Extreme transaminitis is highly unlikely with acute hepatitis C infection. Acetaminophen remains one of the major causes of fulminant hepatic failure and is managed by prompt administration of *N*-acetylcysteine. Budd-Chiari syndrome is characterized by posthepatic thrombus formation. It often presents with jaundice, painful hepatomegaly, ascites, and elevated transaminases.

VIII-47. The answer is A. *(Chap. 305)* The liver is the primary site for the metabolism of many drugs and as such is susceptible to injury related to drugs and toxins. Indeed, the most common cause of acute hepatic failure is drug-induced liver injury. In general, it is useful to think of chemical hepatotoxicity within two broad categories: direct toxic effects and idiosyncratic reactions. Drugs or toxins that cause a direct toxic effect on the liver are either poisons themselves or are metabolized to toxic substances. With agents that cause a direct toxic effect on hepatocytes, there is a predictable, dose-related pattern of injury, and the time to effect is relatively short. The most common drug or toxin causing direct hepatocyte toxicity is acetaminophen. In therapeutic doses, acetaminophen does not cause liver injury. However, in higher doses, one of the metabolites of acetaminophen, N-acetyl-p-benzoquinone-imine (NAPQI), can overwhelm the glutathione stores of the liver that are necessary to convert NAPQI to a nontoxic metabolite and lead to hepatocyte necrosis. Other medications or toxins that cause direct hepatocyte injury are carbon tetrachloride, trichloroethylene, tetracycline, and the *Amanita phalloides* mushroom. More commonly known as the deathcap mushroom, ingestion of a single mushroom can contain enough hepatotoxin to be lethal. Idiosyncratic reactions are infrequent and unpredictable. There is no dose dependency, and the timing of hepatic injury has little association with the duration of drug treatment. Many drugs produce idiosyncratic reactions, and often it is difficult to known when an idiosyncratic reaction will lead to more serious liver failure. Often, mild increases in transaminase levels will occur, but over time adaptation leads to a return of liver enzymes to normal levels. In other instances, idiosyncratic reactions can lead to fulminant hepatic failure. Although rare, serious hepatic reactions can lead to medications being removed from the market. It is now recognized that many idiosyncratic reactions are related to metabolites leading to liver injury. However, it is likely that individual genetic variations in liver metabolism are the primary cause, and these are not predictable effects of the drug given our current state of knowledge. Common medications that can lead to idiosyncratic drug reactions include halothane, isothane, isoniazid, HMG-CoA reductase inhibitors, and chlorpromazine.

VIII-48. **The answer is B.** *(Chap. 305)* Acetaminophen overdose is the most common cause of acute liver failure and drug-induced liver failure that leads to transplantation. Acetaminophen is metabolized in the liver through two pathways. The primary pathway is a phase II reaction that produces nontoxic sulfate and glucuronide metabolites. The minor pathway occurs through a phase I reaction leading to the production of N-acetyl-p-benzoquinone-imine (NAPQI). This metabolite is directly toxic to liver cells and can lead to hepatocyte necrosis. With therapeutic use of acetaminophen, glutathione in the liver rapidly converts NAPQI to a nontoxic metabolite that is excreted in the urine. However, glutathione stores can become depleted in the setting of a large acute ingestion, chronic alcoholism, or the chronic ingestion of increased acetaminophen. In addition, because alcohol upregulates the first enzyme in the metabolic pathway, NAPQI accumulates more quickly in alcoholics. Given the known hepatotoxicity of acetaminophen, the U.S. Food and Drug Administration has recommended a maximum daily dose of no more than 3.25 g, with lower doses in individuals who use alcohol chronically. Acute ingestions of 10–15 g of acetaminophen is sufficient to cause clinical evidence of liver injury, and doses higher than 25 g can lead to fatal hepatic necrosis. The course of illness with acute acetaminophen ingestion follows a predictable pattern. Nausea, vomiting, abdominal pain, and shock occur within 4–12 hours after ingestion. Liver enzymes and synthetic function are normal during this time. Within 24–48 hours, these symptoms subside and are followed by evidence of hepatic injury. Maximal levels of aminotransferases can reach more than 10,000 U/L and may not occur until 4–6 days after ingestion. These patients must be followed carefully for fulminant hepatic failure with serious complications including encephalopathy, cerebral edema, marked coagulopathy, renal failure, metabolic acidosis, electrolyte abnormalities, and refractory shock. Levels of acetaminophen are predictive of the development of hepatotoxicity. The first level should be measured no sooner than 4 hours after a known ingestion. Levels should be plotted on a nomogram that relates acetaminophen levels to the time after ingestion. If at 4 hours the acetaminophen level is greater than 300 μg/mL, significant hepatotoxicity is likely. In the setting of overdose, it may be difficult to know the exact quantity and timing of the ingestion. For the patient presenting in the clinical scenario in this question, her acetaminophen level of greater than 300 μg/mL is quite concerning for a large ingestion, and treatment should be initiated immediately. The primary treatment for acetaminophen overdose is N-acetylcysteine. N-acetylcysteine acts to replete glutathione levels in the liver and also provides a reservoir of sulfhydryl groups to bind to the toxic metabolites. The typical dose of N-acetylcysteine is 140 mg/kg given as a loading dose, followed by 70 mg/kg every 4 hours for a total of 15–20 doses. This drug can also be given by continuous infusion. Activated charcoal or cholestyramine should only be given if the patient presents within 30 minutes after ingestion. Hemodialysis will not accelerate clearance of acetaminophen and will not protect the liver. Most patients with fulminant hepatic failure develop acute renal failure, often requiring hemodialysis. If a patient survives an acetaminophen overdose, there is usually no chronic liver injury.

VIII-49. The answer is E. *(Chap. 306)* The patient in this scenario has evidence of chronic active hepatitis B virus (HBV) infection. The presence of hepatitis B e–antigen (HBeAg) is indicative of ongoing viral replication, and individuals with HBeAg positivity typically have high levels of HBV DNA on testing. The spectrum of clinical infection in chronic hepatitis B is quite variable, and often individuals are asymptomatic with elevated liver enzymes identified on testing for other reasons. Thus, the decision to treat chronic HBV infection should not be based on clinical features. Most experts recommend treatment of HBeAg-positive chronic HBV infection with HBV DNA levels above 2×10^4 IU/mL if the ALT is elevated greater than twice the upper limit of normal. At present, many treatment options are available for the treatment of HBV infection and fall broadly into two categories: nucleoside analogues and interferons. While lamivudine and interferon were the first drugs used for the treatment of chronic HBV infection, these drugs have largely been supplanted by entecavir, tenofovir, and pegylated interferon as first-line therapy. When choosing among these agents, treatment can be tailored to specific patient preferences. Pegylated interferon achieves more rapid clearance of HBeAg and does not contribute to viral mutations. However, it is associated with systemic side effects that many find intolerable and requires weekly SC injections. In contrast, the oral agents often require a longer duration of therapy, are very well tolerated, and yield a more profound suppression of HBV DNA. However, mutations can occur with the use of these medications. Combination therapy does not appear to be more effective than single-drug therapy. The patient's husband should also be screened for hepatitis B given the continued viremia.

VIII-50. The answer is E. *(Chap. 306)* Much information has been gained in recent decades about the progression and treatment of chronic hepatitis C virus (HCV) infection. Chronic hepatitis develops in about 85% of all individuals affected with HCV, and 20–25% of these individuals will progress to cirrhosis over about 20 years. Among those infected with HCV, about one-third of individuals will have normal or near-normal levels of aminotransferases, although liver biopsy demonstrates active hepatitis in as much as one-half of patients. Moreover, about 25% of individuals with normal aminotransferase levels at one point in time will develop elevations in these enzymes later, which can lead to progressive liver disease. Thus, normal aminotransferase levels at a single point in time do not definitively rule out the possibility that cirrhosis can develop. Progression to end-stage liver disease in individuals with chronic HCV hepatitis is more likely in older individuals and in those with a longer duration of infection, advanced histologic stage and grade, genotype 1 infection, more complex quasi-species diversity, concomitant other liver disease, HIV infection, and obesity. Among these factors, the best prognostic indicator for the development of progressive liver disease is liver histology. Specifically, patients who have moderate to severe inflammation or necrosis including septal or bridging fibrosis have the greatest risk of developing cirrhosis over the course of 10–20 years. Indications for therapy in those with HCV include detectable levels of HCV RNA, portal or bridging fibrosis on liver biopsy, or moderate to severe hepatitis on liver biopsy. Contraindications to treatment are age greater than 60 years, mild hepatitis on liver biopsy, and severe renal insufficiency. Standard therapy for HCV infection is pegylated interferon plus ribavirin. While genotypes 1 and 4 are less responsive to therapy than genotypes 2 and 3, the current research demonstrates a response rate of at least 40% for genotypes 1 and 4. Interestingly, even in individuals who fail to show a virologic or biochemical response, 75% will have histologic improvement on liver biopsy. The treatment course for genotypes 1 and 4 is a minimum of 48 weeks, whereas genotypes 2 and 3 can be treated for as little as 24 weeks. Once treatment has been started, a repeat HCV viral load should be assessed at 12 weeks. At this point, a 2-log drop in viral load is expected. Failure to achieve this level of response suggests that a sustained virologic response is unlikely to occur. With a drop of this magnitude, however, the likelihood of a sustained virologic response is about 66% at the end of therapy, and if the viral load is undetectable at 12 weeks, the chances of a sustained virologic response is more than 80%.

VIII-51. The answer is C. *(Chap. 306)* Three types of autoimmune hepatitis have been identified based on clinical and laboratory characteristics. Type I autoimmune hepatitis is a disorder typically seen in young women. The clinical characteristics can be variable from those of chronic hepatitis to fulminant hepatic failure, and many of the features are difficult to distinguish from other causes of chronic hepatitis. In some individuals, extrahepatic manifestations including fatigue, malaise, weight loss, anorexia, and arthralgias can be quite prominent. Liver enzymes are elevated but may not correlate with the clinical severity of disease. In more severe cases, elevations in serum bilirubin between 3 and 10 mg/dL can be seen. Hypoalbuminemia occurs in advanced disease, and hypergammaglobulinemia (>2.5 g/dL) is very common. The circulating antibody profile in autoimmune hepatitis depends to some extent on the type of hepatitis. Antinuclear antibodies are positive in a homogeneous staining pattern almost invariably in the disease, and rheumatoid factor is also common. Perinuclear antineutrophilic cytoplasmic antibody may be positive, but in an atypical fashion. Anti–smooth muscle antibodies and anti–liver/kidney microsomal antibodies are frequently seen, but these are nonspecific as other causes of chronic hepatitis can lead to positivity of these enzymes. Because of the lack of a specific autoimmune profile, the diagnostic criteria for autoimmune hepatitis incorporate a variety of clinical and laboratory features. Specific features that argue against this diagnosis include prominent alkaline phosphatase elevation, presence of mitochondrial antibodies, markers of viral hepatitis, history of hepatotoxic drugs or excess alcohol intake, and histologic evidence of bile duct injury or atypical biopsy features including excess hepatic iron, fatty infiltration, and viral inclusions. Antimitochondrial antibodies are typically seen in primary biliary cirrhosis.

VIII-52. The answer is D. *(Chap. 306)* In the course of acute hepatitis B, HBeAg positivity is common and usually transient. Persistence of HBeAg in the serum for 3 months or longer indicates an increased likelihood of development of chronic hepatitis B. In chronic hepatitis B, the presence of HBeAg in the serum indicates ongoing viral replication and increased infectivity. It is also a surrogate for inflammatory liver injury but not fibrosis. The development of antibody to HBeAg (anti-HBe) is indicative of the nonreplicative phase of HBV infection. During this phase, intact virions do not circulate and infectivity is less. Currently, quantification of HBV DNA with polymerase chain reaction allows risk stratification as fewer than 10^3 virions/μL is the approximate threshold for liver injury and infectivity.

VIII-53. The answer is C. *(Chap. 307)* This patient presents with severe acute alcoholic hepatitis. In its earliest form, alcoholic liver disease is marked by fatty infiltration of the liver. In more acute alcoholic hepatitis, there is hepatocyte injury with balloon degeneration and necrosis. Many cases of alcoholic hepatitis are asymptomatic. However, as in this case, the severe manifestations can include fever, jaundice, spider nevi, and abdominal pain that can mimic an acute abdomen in its severity. On laboratory examination, the AST is typically elevated more than the ALT, although the total transaminase levels are rarely greater than 400 U/L. Hyperbilirubinemia can be quite marked, with lesser elevation in alkaline phosphatase. Hypoalbuminemia and coagulopathy are poor prognostic indicators. A discriminate function (DF) can be calculated as (4.6 × the prolongation of prothrombin time above control) + serum bilirubin. A DF greater than 32 is associated with a poor prognosis and is an indication for the treatment of acute alcoholic hepatitis. The Model for End-Stage Liver Disease (MELD) score can also be used for prognostication in acute alcoholic hepatitis, with a score greater than 21 being an indication for treatment as well. This patient has a discriminate function of 73, indicating very severe disease and a poor prognosis. Complete abstinence from alcohol is imperative. Treatment with prednisone 40 mg daily (or prednisolone 32 mg daily) for 4 weeks should be initiated. Following the initial period, a taper should be achieved over a period of 4 weeks. Alternatively, pentoxifylline 400 mg three times daily for 4 weeks can also be used.

VIII-54. The answer is C. *(Chap. 308)* The clinical presentation is consistent with a cholestatic picture, which can present with painless jaundice and pruritus. The pruritus can be prominent and is present in 50% of individuals at the time of diagnosis. The pruritus is typically intermittent and worse in the evening. There is no other prominent associa-tion such as following hot baths or showers, which occurs in polycythemia vera. Other causes of pruritus outside of cholestasis include lymphoma and uncontrolled hypo- or hyperthyroidism. However, the laboratory studies in this patient clearly represent cholestasis with an elevation in alkaline phosphatase and bilirubin. The clinical char-acteristics are more commonly seen in primary biliary cirrhosis compared to primary sclerosis cholangitis, as the patient is a middle-aged female with positive antimito-chondrial antibodies. In contrast, primary sclerosing cholangitis is associated with positive perinuclear antineutrophil cytoplasmic antibodies in 65% of patients, and 50% of individuals with primary sclerosing cholangitis have a history of ulcerative colitis.

VIII-55. The answer is B. *(Chap. 308)* Esophageal varices develop in the setting of portal hyper-tension associated most commonly with cirrhotic liver disease. In recent years, patients with cirrhosis have been commonly screened for varices by endoscopy, as about 33% will have varices on examination. Moreover, it is estimated that one-third of individu-als with varices will develop bleeding. As this patient does not have medical care, it is unknown whether he has varices, but with the large volume of bleeding the patient has experienced, the treating physician should assume that the patient has variceal bleeding and act accordingly. The first step in the treatment of any individual with acute gas-trointestinal bleeding is to ensure appropriate large-bore IV access, preferably in a large central vein or the antecubital fossae, and begin volume resuscitation. Volume resuscita-tion should be initiated with normal saline, and blood products should be administered when available. Once volume resuscitation has been initiated, emergent consultation with GI for endoscopic evaluation should be obtained. Endoscopic treatment should include esophageal band ligation, but in the acute setting, sclerotherapy may be used to control local bleeding with band ligation occurring at a future point in time. If emergent endoscopy is not an option, placement of a Sengstaken-Blakemore or Minnesota tube to tamponade bleeding should be employed. In addition, vasoconstricting agents are used to decrease splanchnic blood flow. While vasopressin was initially the agent of choice, cardiovascular ischemia can occur with the high doses used in GI bleeding. The cur-rently preferred agents are octreotide or somatostatin by continuous infusion. Nonspe-cific beta blockers such as propranolol or nadolol are used for the primary or secondary prevention of variceal bleeding, but are not prescribed in the acute setting as these agents could worsen hypotension.

VIII-56. The answer is A. *(Chap. 308)* The cornerstone of the management of ascites is sodium restriction to less than 2 g daily. A common misconception is to institute a fluid restric-tion as well. However, this is neither effective nor necessary. With a sodium restriction to 2 g daily, most mild ascites can be managed quite well. If sodium restriction alone fails to correct ascites, then initiation of diuretics is required. Spironolactone at a dose of 100–200 mg daily is the initial diuretic used for ascites and can be titrated as high as 400–600 mg daily if tolerated. Loop diuretics can be added to spironolactone. The typical agent is furo-semide beginning at 40–80 mg daily with the maximum doses being about 120–160 mg daily. Care must be taken to avoid renal dysfunction with loop diuretics, and higher doses may not be tolerated. If ascites is refractory to these treatments, transjugular intrahepatic portosystemic shunts (TIPS) can be considered. This procedure creates a portocaval shunt be introducing an expandable metal stent from the hepatic veins through the substance of the liver into the portal veins, creating a direct portocaval shunt. Thus, TIPS decreases portal pressures to decrease ascites and the risk of variceal bleeding. However, hepatic encephalopathy typically worsens following TIPS.

VIII-57. The answer is A. *(Chap. 308)* Severe right-sided heart failure may lead to chronic liver injury and cardiac cirrhosis. Elevated venous pressure leads to congestion of the hepatic sinusoids and of the central vein and centrilobular hepatocytes. Centrilobular fibrosis develops, and fibrosis extends outward from the central vein, not the portal triads. Gross examination of the liver shows a pattern of "nutmeg liver." Although transaminases are typically mildly elevated, severe congestion, particularly associated with hypotension, may result in dramatic elevation of AST and ALT 50- to 100-fold above normal. Budd-Chiari syndrome, or occlusion of the hepatic veins or inferior vena cava, may be confused with congestive hepatopathy. However, the signs and symptoms of congestive heart failure are absent in patients with Budd-Chiari syndrome, and these patients can be easily distinguished clinically from those with heart failure. Venoocclusive disease may result from hepatic irradiation and high-dose chemotherapy in preparation for hematopoietic stem cell transplantation. It is not a typical complication of liver transplantation. Although echocardiography is a useful tool for assessing left and right ventricular function, findings may be unimpressive in patients with constrictive pericarditis. A high index of suspicion for constrictive pericarditis (e.g., prior episodes of pericarditis, mediastinal irradiation) should lead to a right-sided heart catheterization with demonstration of "square root sign," which is the limitation of right heart filling pressure in diastole that is suggestive of restrictive cardiomyopathy. Cardiac magnetic resonance imaging may also be helpful in determining which patients should proceed to cardiac surgery.

VIII-58. **The answer is B.** *(Chap. 308)* The presence of cirrhosis in an elderly woman with no prior risk factors for viral or alcoholic cirrhosis should raise the possibility of primary biliary cirrhosis (PBC). It is characterized by chronic inflammation and fibrous obliteration of intrahepatic ductules. The cause is unknown, but autoimmunity is assumed, as there is an association with other autoimmune disorders, such as autoimmune thyroiditis, CREST syndrome, and the sicca syndrome. The vast majority of patients with symptomatic disease are women. The antimitochondrial antibody test (AMA) is positive in over 90% of patients with PBC and only rarely is positive in other conditions. This makes it the most useful initial test in the diagnosis of PBC. Since there are false positives, if AMA is positive a liver biopsy is performed to confirm the diagnosis. The 24-hour urine copper collection is useful in the diagnosis of Wilson's disease. Hepatic failure from Wilson's disease typically occurs before age 50. Hemochromatosis may result in cirrhosis. It is associated with lethargy, fatigue, loss of libido, discoloration of the skin, arthralgias, diabetes, and cardiomyopathy. Ferritin levels are usually increased, and the most suggestive laboratory abnormality is an elevated transferrin saturation percentage. Although hemochromatosis is a possible diagnosis in this case, PBC is more likely in light of the clinical scenario. Although chronic hepatitis B and hepatitis C are certainly in the differential diagnosis and must be ruled out, they are unlikely because of the patient's history and lack of risk factors.

VIII-59. **The answer is D.** *(Chap. 309)* This patient presents with nonalcoholic fatty liver disease (NAFLD) that has progressed to cirrhosis. It is now commonly thought that many individuals previously identified as having cryptogenic cirrhosis had NAFLD as a cause of end-stage liver disease. With the rising prevalence of obesity in the United States and Europe, NAFLD is expected to continue to rise. At present, the prevalence of NAFLD is estimated between to be 14–20%. Of these individuals, 30–40% with nonalcoholic steatohepatitis will develop advanced fibrosis and 10–15% will develop outright cirrhosis. Most patients diagnosed with NAFLD are asymptomatic with incident note of elevated liver enzymes found on testing for other reasons. The ALT is typically slightly higher than the AST, and both enzymes are only mildly elevated. In most instances the ALT and AST are only 1.5–2 times the upper limit of normal. NAFLD often accompanies other components of the metabolic syndrome, with insulin resistance being a common link between these disorders. The diagnosis of NAFLD requires a careful history and examination to rule out other disorders. Alcohol intake should be less than 20 g/d. Comprehensive testing should include serologies for viral hepatitis, iron studies, ceruloplasmin, α_1 antitrypsin levels, and autoimmune serologies. Liver biopsy most commonly shows macrovesicular steatosis with a mixed inflammatory infiltrate in a lobular distribution. The fibrosis that occurs has a characteristic perivenular and perisinusoidal distribution. In cirrhotic patients, steatosis may not be seen, but can recur following transplant. The only known effective treatment for NAFLD is weight loss and exercise. Thiazolidinediones are currently being studied given their effects on insulin resistance. In addition, ongoing research into statins and ursodeoxycholic acid is being undertaken, but no specific medication can be recommended at this point for patients with NAFLD.

VIII-60. **The answer is C.** *(Chap. 310)* In the United States, over 6000 individuals undergo liver transplants yearly. However, the demand for organs far outpaces the supply with a waiting list of over 16,000 individuals. The most common reasons for liver transplant are alcoholic cirrhosis and chronic hepatitis C infection. When evaluating someone for liver transplantation, it is important to ensure that the patient is an appropriate candidate. For individuals with alcoholic cirrhosis, sustained abstinence and recovery need to be demonstrated, although the recidivism rate is as high as 25% after transplantation. Absolute contraindications to liver transplant include uncontrolled infection, active substance or alcohol abuse, extrahepatobiliary malignancy (excluding nonmelanoma skin cancer), metastatic malignancy to the liver, AIDS, or life-threatening or advance systemic disease. Cholangiocarcinoma almost invariably recurs following liver transplantation. Thus, it is now considered a contraindication to transplant. While primarily performed in children, living donor transplantation is increasingly being considered in adults given the poor availability of cadaveric organs. In living donor transplantation, typically the right lobe of the liver is taken from a suitable healthy donor. Currently, living donor transplantation accounts for 4% of all liver transplants. It is certainly not without risk. The average healthy donor will be medically disabled for at least 10 weeks, and the risk of death for the donor is 0.2–0.4%. Individuals receiving all forms of liver transplant have demonstrated increasing survival over the past decades. The current 5-year survival rate is more than 60%. Following transplantation, however, rejection, infection, and recurrence of primary disease can occur. For chronic hepatitis B infection, reinfection of the transplant frequently occurs, but this may be reduced to as little as 35% with post-transplantation treatment with hepatitis B immunoglobulin. For hepatitis C, reinfection is universal and is associated with the development of allograft cirrhosis in 20–30% of patients within 5 years. Autoimmune diseases can also recur in the transplanted liver, although it can be difficult to differentiate between the autoimmune disease and rejection. Wilson's disease and α_1 antitrypsin deficiency, however, do not recur following transplantation.

VIII-61. The answer is E. *(Chap. 310)* The patient has advanced cirrhosis with a high risk of mortality, as evidenced by his episode of spontaneous bacterial peritonitis. His diabetes and remote skin cancer (since it was a basal cell carcinoma, not melanoma) are not absolute contraindications for liver transplantation, but active alcohol abuse is. The other absolute contraindications to transplantation are life-threatening systemic disease, uncontrolled infections, preexisting advanced cardiac or pulmonary disease, metastatic malignancy, and life-threatening congenital malignancies. Ongoing drug or alcohol abuse is an absolute contraindication, and patients who would otherwise be suitable candidates should immediately be referred to appropriate counseling centers to achieve abstinence. Once that is achieved for an acceptable period of time, transplantation can be considered. Indeed, alcoholic cirrhosis accounts for a substantial proportion of the patients who undergo liver transplantation.

VIII-62. The answer is B. *(Chap. 311)* In the National Health and Nutrition Examination Survey, the prevalence of gallstone disease in the United States was 7.9% in men and 16.6% in women. While the disease is quite prevalent, not all patients with gallstone disease require cholecystectomy. It is estimated that 1–2% of patients with asymptomatic gallstone disease will develop complications that will require surgery yearly. Therefore, it is important to know which patients with asymptomatic gallstones require referral for surgery. The first factor to consider is whether the patient has symptoms that are caused by gallstones and whether they are frequent enough and severe enough to necessitate surgery. Commonly called biliary colic, the classic symptoms of gallstone disease are right upper quadrant pain and fullness that begins suddenly and can last as long as 5 hours. Nausea and vomiting can accompany the episode. Vague symptoms of epigastric fullness, dyspepsia, and bloating following meals should not be considered biliary colic. A second factor that would be considered in recommending a patient for cholecystectomy is whether the patient has a prior history of complications of gallstone disease such as pancreatitis or acute cholecystitis. A final factor that would lead to the recommendation for cholecystectomy is the presence of anatomical factors that would increase the likelihood of complications such as a porcelain gallbladder or congenital abnormalities of the biliary tract. Individuals with very large stones (>3 cm) would also need to be considered carefully for cholecystectomy. Ursodeoxycholic acid can be used in some instances to dissolve gallstones. It acts to decrease the cholesterol saturation of bile and also allows the dispersion of cholesterol from stones by producing a lamellar crystalline phase. It is only effective, however, in individuals with radiolucent stones measuring less than 10 mm.

VIII-63. **The answer is D.** *(Chap. 311)* A practitioner needs to have a high index of suspicion for acalculous cholecystitis in critically ill patients who develop decompensation during the course of treatment for the underlying disease and have no other apparent source of infection. Some predisposing conditions for the development of acalculous cholecystitis include serious trauma or burns, postpartum following prolonged labor, prolonged parenteral hyperalimentation, and the postoperative period following orthopedic and other major surgical procedures. The clinical manifestations of acalculous cholecystitis are identical to calculous disease, but the disease is more difficult to diagnose. Ultrasonography and CT scanning typically only show biliary sludge, but they may demonstrate large and tense gallbladders. Hepatobiliary scintigraphy often shows delayed or absent gallbladder emptying. Successful management relies on accurate and early diagnosis. In critically ill patients, a percutaneous cholecystostomy may be the safest immediate procedure to decompress an infected gallbladder. Once the patient is stabilized, early elective cholecystectomy should be considered. Metronidazole to provide anaerobic coverage should be added, but this would not elucidate or adequately treat the underlying condition.

VIII-64. **The answer is C.** *(Chap. 311)* Gallstones are very common, particularly in Western countries. Cholesterol stones are responsible for 80% of cases of cholelithiasis; pigment stones account for the remaining 20%. Cholesterol is essentially water insoluble. Stone formation occurs in the setting of factors that upset cholesterol balance. Obesity, cholesterol-rich diets, high-calorie diets, and certain medications affect the biliary secretion of cholesterol. Intrinsic genetic mutations in certain populations may affect the processing and secretion of cholesterol in the liver. Pregnancy results in both an increase in cholesterol saturation during the third trimester and changes in gallbladder contractility. Pigment stones are increased in patients with chronic hemolysis, cirrhosis, Gilbert's syndrome, and disruptions in the enterohepatic circulation. Although rapid weight loss and low-calorie diets are associated with gallstones, there is no evidence that a high-protein diet confers an added risk of cholelithiasis.

VIII-65. **The answer is B.** *(Chaps. 42 and 311)* The clinical presentation is consistent with a cholestatic picture. Painless jaundice always requires an extensive workup, as many of the underlying pathologies are ominous and early detection and intervention often offers the only hope for a good outcome. The gallbladder showed no evidence of stones and the patient shows no evidence of clinical cholecystitis, and so a hepatobiliary iminodiacetic acid (HIDA) scan is not indicated. Similarly, antibiotics are not necessary at this point. The cholestatic picture without significant elevation of the transaminases on the liver function tests makes acute hepatitis unlikely. Antimitochondrial antibodies are elevated in cases of primary biliary cirrhosis (PBC), which may present in a similar fashion. However, PBC is far more common in women than in men, and the average age of onset is the fifth or sixth decade. The lack of an obvious lesion on CT scan does not rule out a source of the cholestasis in the biliary tree. Malignant causes such as cholangiocarcinoma and tumor of the ampulla of Vater, and nonmalignant causes such as sclerosing cholangitis and Caroli's disease may be detected only by direct visualization with endoscopic retrograde cholangiopancreatography (ERCP). ERCP is useful both diagnostically and therapeutically, as stenting procedures may be done to alleviate the obstruction.

VIII-66. **The answer is A.** *(Chap. 313)* The most common cause of acute pancreatitis in the United States is gallstones causing common bile duct obstruction. Although bile duct obstruction may be demonstrated on technetium HIDA scan, right upper quadrant ultrasound is preferred for ease, demonstration of gallstones in the gallbladder, and demonstration of obstructed bile duct. Alcohol is the second most common cause, followed by complications of endoscopic retrograde cholangiopancreatography (ERCP). Hypertriglyceridemia accounts for 1–4% of cases with triglyceride levels usually greater than 1000 mg/dL. Other potential causes of pancreatitis include trauma, postoperative states, drugs such as valproic acid, anti-HIV medications, estrogens, and sphincter of Oddi dysfunction. Additionally, there are a number of rare causes that have been described. The most judicious first step in evaluation is to test for gallstones and pursue more rare causes after the most common cause has been ruled out.

VIII-67. The answer is A. *(Chap. 313)* Physical examination in acute pancreatitis commonly shows an uncomfortable patient often with low-grade fever, tachycardia, and hypotension. Abdominal tenderness and muscle rigidity are often present to varying degrees. Cullen's sign is a faint blue discoloration around the umbilicus that may occur as the result of hemoperitoneum. Turner's sign is blue-red-purple or green-brown discoloration of the flanks from tissue catabolism of hemoglobin. Both of these signs indicate the presence of severe necrotizing pancreatitis.

VIII-68. The answer is E. *(Chap. 313)* The BISAP (Bedside Index of Severity in Acute Pancreatitis) score has recently replaced Ranson's criteria and APACHE II severity scores as the recommended modality to assess the severity of pancreatitis due to the cumbersome nature of the prior scores and the requirement of prior scores to collect large amounts of clinical and laboratory data over time. Furthermore, the APACHE II and Ranson's scoring mechanisms did not have acceptable positive and negative predictive values in predicting severe acute pancreatitis. The BISAP score incorporates five variables in determining severity: BUN greater than 35 mg/dL, impaired mental status, presence of SIRS, age above 60 years, and pleural effusion on radiography. The presence of three or more of these factors is associated with substantially increased risk for in-hospital mortality. Additional risk factors initially predicting severity include BMI of 30 or above and comorbid disease.

VIII-69. The answer is E. *(Chap. 313)* Several trials over the last several decades have demonstrated that there is no role for prophylactic antibiotics in the management of either interstitial or necrotizing pancreatitis. Antibiotics are recommended for only patients who appear septic at presentation while awaiting the results of culture data. If cultures are negative, antibiotics should be discontinued to decrease the risk of the development of fungal superinfection. Similarly, several drugs have been evaluated in the treatment of acute pancreatitis and found to be of no benefit. These drugs include H₂ blockers, glucagon, protease inhibitors such as aprotinin, glucocorticoids, calcitonin, nonsteroidal anti-inflammatory drugs, and lexipafant, a platelet-activating factor inhibitor. A recent meta-analysis of somatostatin, octreotide, and the antiprotease gabexate mesylate in the therapy of acute pancreatitis suggested a reduced mortality rate but no change in complications with octreotide, and no effect on mortality but reduced pancreatic damage with gabexate.

VIII-70. The answer is C. *(Chap. 313)* Persistent inflammatory changes in the pancreas may remain for weeks to months after an episode of acute pancreatitis. Similarly, there may be prolonged elevation of amylase and lipase. In this regard, persistent changes on CT or persistent pancreatic enzyme elevation should not discourage clinicians from feeding hungry patients with acute pancreatitis. Although there had been prior concern that feeding patients with pancreatitis may exacerbate pancreatic inflammation, this has not been borne out. Similarly, enteral feeding with a nasojejunal tube in patients with acute pancreatitis has been demonstrated to have fewer infectious complications than feeding with total parenteral nutrition. Because of this, nasogastric feeding is the preferred method of nutritional support in acute pancreatitis. Enteral feeding also helps to maintain the integrity of the intestinal tract in acute pancreatitis.

VIII-71. The answer is D. *(Chap. 313)* The pathophysiology of acute pancreatitis evolves in three phases. During the initial phase, pancreatic injury leads to intrapancreatic activation of digestive enzymes with subsequent autodigestion and acinar cell injury. Acinar injury is primarily attributed to activation of zymogens (proenzymes), particularly trypsinogen, by lysosomal hydrolases. Once trypsinogen is converted to trypsin, the activated trypsin further perpetuates the process by activating other zymogens to further autodigestion.

The inflammation initiated by intrapancreatic activation of zymogens leads to the second phase of acute pancreatitis, with local production of chemokines that causes activation and sequestration of neutrophils in the pancreas. Experimental evidence suggests that neutrophilic inflammation can also cause further activation of trypsinogen, leading to a cascade of increasing acinar injury. The third phase of acute pancreatitis reflects the systemic processes that are caused by release of inflammatory cytokines and activated proenzymes into the systemic circulation. This process can lead to the systemic inflammatory response syndrome with acute respiratory distress syndrome, extensive third-spacing of fluids, and multiorgan failure.

VIII-72. **The answer is D.** *(Chap. 313)* Chronic pancreatitis is a common disorder in any patient population with relapsing acute pancreatitis, especially patients with alcohol dependence, pancreas divisum, and cystic fibrosis. The disorder is notable for both endocrine and exocrine dysfunction of the pancreas. Often diabetes ensues as a result of loss of islet cell function; though insulin-dependent, it is generally not as prone to diabetic ketoacidosis or coma as are other forms of diabetes mellitus. As pancreatic enzymes are essential to fat digestion, their absence leads to fat malabsorption and steatorrhea. In addition, the fat-soluble vitamins, A, D, E, and K, are not absorbed. Vitamin A deficiency can lead to neuropathy. Vitamin B_{12}, or cobalamin, is often deficient. This deficiency is hypothesized to be due to excessive binding of cobalamin by cobalamin-binding proteins other than intrinsic factor that are normally digested by pancreatic enzymes. Replacement of pancreatic enzymes orally with meals will correct the vitamin deficiencies and steatorrhea. The incidence of pancreatic adenocarcinoma is increased in patients with chronic pancreatitis, with a 20-year cumulative incidence of 4%. Chronic abdominal pain is nearly ubiquitous in this disorder, and narcotic dependence is common. Niacin is a water-soluble vitamin, and absorption is not affected by pancreatic exocrine dysfunction.

VIII-73. **The answer is A.** *(Chap. 313)* This patient likely has chronic pancreatitis related to long-standing alcohol use, which is the most common cause of chronic pancreatitis in adults in the United States. Chronic pancreatitis can develop in individuals who consume as little as 50 g of alcohol daily (equivalent to ~30–40 ounces of beer). The patient's description of his loose stools is consistent with steatorrhea, and the recurrent bouts of abdominal pain are likely related to his pancreatitis. In most patients, abdominal pain is the most prominent symptom. However, up to 20% of individuals with chronic pancreatitis present with symptoms of maldigestion alone. The evaluation for chronic pancreatitis should allow one to characterize the pancreatitis as large- vs. small-duct disease. Large-duct disease is more common in men and is more likely to be associated with steatorrhea. In addition, large-duct disease is associated with the appearance of pancreatic calcifications and abnormal tests of pancreatic exocrine function. Women are more likely to have small-duct disease, with normal tests of pancreatic exocrine function and normal abdominal radiography. In small-duct disease, the progression to steatorrhea is rare, and the pain is responsive to treatment with pancreatic enzymes. The characteristic findings on CT and abdominal radiograph of this patient are characteristic of chronic pancreatitis, and no further workup should delay treatment with pancreatic enzymes. Treatment with pancreatic enzymes orally will improve maldigestion and lead to weight gain, but they are unlikely to fully resolve maldigestive symptoms. Narcotic dependence can frequently develop in individuals with chronic pancreatitis due to recurrent and severe bouts of pain. However, as this individual's pain is mild, it is not necessary to prescribe narcotics at this point in time. An ERCP or magnetic resonance cholangiopancreatography (MRCP) may be considered to evaluate for a possible stricture that is amenable to therapy. However, sphincterotomy is a procedure performed via ERCP that may be useful in treating pain related to chronic pancreatitis and is not indicated in the patient. Angiography to assess for ischemic bowel disease is not indicated as the patient's symptoms are not consistent with intestinal angina. Certainly, weight loss can occur in this setting, but the patient usually presents with complaints of abdominal pain after eating and pain that is out of proportion with the clinical examination. Prokinetic agents would likely only worsen the patient's malabsorptive symptoms and are not indicated.

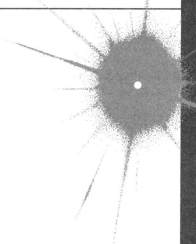

DIRECTIONS: Choose the one **best** response to each question.

IX-1. All of the following are key features of the innate immune system EXCEPT:

A. Exclusively a feature of vertebrate animals.
B. Important cells include macrophages and natural killer lymphocytes.
C. Nonrecognition of benign foreign molecules or microbes.
D. Recognition by germ line–encoded host molecules.
E. Recognition of key microbe virulence factors but not recognition of self molecules.

IX-2. A 29-year-old male with episodic abdominal pain and stress-induced edema of the lips, the tongue, and occasionally the larynx is likely to have low functional or absolute levels of which of the following proteins?

A. C1 esterase inhibitor
B. C5A (complement cascade)
C. Cyclooxygenase
D. IgE
E. T-cell receptor, α chain

IX-3. Which of the following statements best describes the function of proteins encoded by the human major histo-compatibility complex (MHC) I and II genes?

A. Activation of the complement system
B. Binding to cell surface receptors on granulocytes and macrophages to initiate phagocytosis
C. Nonspecific binding of antigen for presentation to T cells
D. Specific antigen binding in response to B-cell activation to promote neutralization and precipitation

IX-4. A 37-year-old man has recently been diagnosed with systemic hypertension. He is prescribed lisinopril as initial monotherapy. He takes this medication as prescribed for 3 days and on the third day notes that his right hand is swollen, mildly itchy, and tingling. Later that evening his lips become swollen and he has difficulty breathing. Which of the following statements accurately describes this condition?

A. His symptoms are due to direct activation of mast cells by lisinopril.
B. His symptoms are due to impaired bradykinin degradation by lisinopril.
C. His symptoms are unlikely to recur if he is switched to enalapril.
D. Peripheral blood analysis will show deficiency of C1 inhibitor.
E. Plasma IgE levels are likely to be elevated.

IX-5. A 35-year-old female comes to the local health clinic for recurrent urticarial lesions that occasionally leave a residual discoloration for the last 6 months. She also has had arthralgias. The sedimentation rate now is 85 mm/h. The procedure most likely to yield the correct diagnosis in this case would be:

A. A battery of wheal-and-flare allergy skin tests
B. Measurement of total serum IgE concentration
C. Measurement of C1 esterase inhibitor activity
D. Skin biopsy
E. Patch testing

IX-6. A 28-year-old woman seeks evaluation from her primary care doctor for recurrent episodes of hives and states that she is "allergic to cold weather." She reports that for more than 10 years she has developed areas of hives when exposed to cold temperatures, usually on her arms and legs. She has not sought evaluation previously and states that over the past several years the occurrence of the hives has become more frequent. Other than cold exposure, she can identify no other triggers for the development of hives. She has no history of asthma or atopy. She denies food intolerance. Her only medication is oral contraceptive pills, which she has taken for 5 years. She lives in a single-family home that was built 2 years ago. On examination, she develops a linear wheal after being stroked along her forearm with a tongue depressor. Upon placing her hand in cold water, her hand becomes red and swollen. In addition, there are several areas with a wheal and flare reaction on the arm above the area of cold exposure. What is the next step in the management of this patient?

A. Assess for the presence of antithyroglobulin and anti-microsomal antibodies.
B. Check C1 inhibitor levels.
C. Discontinue the oral contraceptive pills.
D. Treat with cetirizine, 10 mg daily.
E. Treat with cyproheptadine, 8 mg daily.

IX-7. A 23-year-old woman seeks evaluation for seasonal rhinitis. She reports that she develops symptoms yearly in the spring and fall. During this time, she develops rhinitis with postnasal drip and cough that disrupts her sleep. In addition, she will also have itchy and watery eyes. When the symptoms occur, she takes nonprescription loratadine, 10 mg daily, with significant improvement in her symptoms. What is the most likely allergen(s) that is/are causing this patient's symptoms?

A. Grass
B. Ragweed
C. Trees
D. A and B
E. B and C
F. All of the above

IX-8. Which of the following autoantibodies is most likely to be present in a patient with systemic lupus erythematosus?

A. Anti-dsDNA
B. Anti-RNP
C. Anti-Ro
D. Antiphospholipid
E. Antiribosomal P

IX-9. A 23-year-old woman is evaluated by her primary care physician because she is concerned that she may have systemic lupus erythematosus after hearing a public health announcement on the radio. She has no significant past medical history, and her only medication is occasional ibuprofen. She is not sexually active and works in a grocery store. She reports that she has had intermittent oral ulcers and right knee pain. Physical examination shows no evidence of alopecia, skin rash, or joint swelling/inflammation. Her blood work shows that she has a positive antinuclear antibody (ANA) at a titer of 1:40, but no other abnormalities. Which of the following statements is true?

A. Four diagnostic criteria are required to be diagnosed with systemic lupus erythematosus; this patient has three.
B. Four diagnostic criteria are required to be diagnosed with systemic lupus erythematosus; this patient has two.
C. If a urinalysis shows proteinuria, she will meet the criteria for systemic lupus erythematosus.
D. She meets the criteria for systemic lupus erythematosus because she has three criteria for the disease.
E. The demonstration of a positive ANA alone is adequate to diagnose systemic lupus erythematosus.

IX-10. A 32-year-old woman with a long-standing diagnosis of systemic lupus erythematosus is evaluated by her rheumatologist as routine follow-up. A new cardiac murmur is heard and an echocardiogram is ordered. She is feeling well, and has no fevers, weight loss, or preexisting cardiac disease. A vegetation on the mitral valve is demonstrated. Which of the following statements is true?

A. Blood cultures are unlikely to be positive.
B. Glucocorticoid therapy has been proven to lead to improvement in this condition.
C. Pericarditis is frequently present concomitantly.
D. The lesion has a low risk of embolization.
E. The patient has been surreptitiously using injection drugs.

IX-11. A 24-year-old woman is newly diagnosed with systemic lupus erythematosus. Which of the following organ system complications is she most likely to have over the course of her lifetime?

A. Cardiopulmonary
B. Cutaneous
C. Hematologic
D. Musculoskeletal
E. Renal

IX-12. A 27-year-old female with systemic lupus erythematosus (SLE) is in remission; current treatment consists of azathioprine 75 mg/d and prednisone 5 mg/d. Last year she had a life-threatening exacerbation of her disease. She now strongly desires to become pregnant. Which of the following is the least appropriate action to take?

A. Advise her that the risk of spontaneous abortion is high.
B. Warn her that exacerbations can occur in the first trimester and in the postpartum period.
C. Tell her it is unlikely that a newborn will have lupus.
D. Advise her that fetal loss rates are higher if anticardiolipin antibodies are detected in her serum.
E. Stop the prednisone just before she attempts to become pregnant.

IX-13. A 45-year-old African-American woman with systemic lupus erythematosus (SLE) presents to the emergency department with complaints of headache and fatigue. Her prior manifestations of SLE have been arthralgias, hemolytic anemia, malar rash, and mouth ulcers, and she is known to have high titers of antibodies to double-stranded DNA. She currently is taking prednisone, 5 mg daily, and hydroxychloroquine, 200 mg daily. On presentation, she is found to have a blood pressure of 190/110 mmHg with a heart rate of 98 beats/min. A urinalysis shows 25 red blood cells (RBCs) per high-power field with 2+ proteinuria. No RBC casts are identified. Her blood urea nitrogen is 88 mg/dL, and creatinine is 2.6 mg/dL (baseline 0.8 mg/dL). She has not previously had renal disease related to SLE and is not taking nonsteroidal anti-inflammatory drugs. She denies any recent illness, decreased oral intake, or diarrhea. What is the most appropriate next step in the management of this patient?

A. Initiate cyclophosphamide, 500 mg/m^2 body surface area IV, and plan to repeat monthly for 3–6 months.

B. Initiate hemodialysis.

C. Initiate high-dose steroid therapy (IV methylprednisolone, 1000 mg daily for 3 doses, followed by oral prednisone, 1 mg/kg daily) and mycophenolate mofetil, 2 g daily.

D. Initiate plasmapheresis.

E. Withhold all therapy until renal biopsy is performed.

IX-14. A 25-year-old African-American woman was has been followed in SLE clinic since her diagnosis 6 months ago. At that time she had evidence of mild joint disease, photosensitivity, malar rash, positive ANA, and anti-dsDNA. Her renal function and urinalysis were normal. She has been maintained on acetaminophen and hydroxychloroquine. She comes to the emergency department after a recent outing to the beach with friends. Over the past 2 days she's noticed a marked increase in her fatigue and morning stiffness. She also has red-tinged urine. Physical examination is notable for a skin rash in sun-exposed areas, and diffuse wrist, knee, and ankle synovial thickening. Her platelet count has fallen from normal values to 45,000 and she has new leukopenia. In addition, her serum creatinine is 2.5 and there are RBC casts on urine analysis. An emergent renal biopsy is consistent with active diffuse lupus nephritis. After receiving methylprednisolone 1 g IV for 3 days, all of the following are appropriate treatment regimens EXCEPT:

A. Prednisone 60 mg/d

B. Prednisone 60 mg/d plus azathioprine

C. Prednisone 60 mg/d plus cyclophosphamide

D. Prednisone 60 mg/d plus mycophenolate mofetil

E. Rituximab

IX-15. A 27-year-old woman is admitted to the intensive care unit after delivery of a full-term infant 3 days prior. The patient was found to have right hemiparesis and a blue left hand. Physical examination is also notable for livedo

reticularis. Her laboratories were notable for a white blood cell count of 10.2/μL, hematocrit 35%, and platelet count of 13,000/μL. Her BUN is 36 mg/dL and her creatinine is 2.3 mg/dL. Although this pregnancy was uneventful, the three prior pregnancies resulted in early losses. A peripheral smear shows no evidence of schistocytes. Which of the following laboratory studies will best confirm the underlying etiology of her presentation?

A. Anticardiolipin antibody panel

B. Antinuclear antibody

C. Doppler examination of her left arm arterial tree

D. Echocardiography

E. MRI of her brain

IX-16. A 28-year-old woman comes to the emergency department complaining of 1 day of worsening right leg pain and swelling. She drove in a car for 8 hours returning from a hiking trip 2 days ago then noticed some pain in the leg. At first she thought it was due to exertion but it has worsened over the day. Her only past medical history is related to difficulty getting pregnant with 2 prior spontaneous abortions. Her physical examination is notable for normal vital signs and heart and lung examination. Her right leg is swollen from the mid-thigh down and is tender. Doppler studies demonstrate a large deep venous thrombosis in the femoral and ileac veins extending into the pelvis. Laboratory studies on admission prior to therapy show normal electrolytes, normal white blood cell (WBC) and platelet counts, normal prothrombin time, and an activated partial thromboplastin time 3× normal. Her pregnancy test is negative. Low-molecular-weight heparin therapy is initiated in the emergency department. Subsequent therapy should include:

A. Rituximab 375 mg/m^2 per week for 4 weeks

B. Warfarin with INR goal of 2.0–3.0 for 3 months

C. Warfarin with INR goal of 2.0–3.0 for 12 months

D. Warfarin with INR goal of 2.5–3.5 for life

E. Warfarin with an INR goal of 2.5–3.5 for 12 months followed by daily aspirin for life

IX-17. Which of the following is the most frequent site of joint involvement in established rheumatoid arthritis (RA)?

A. Distal interphalangeal joint

B. Hip

C. Knee

D. Spine

E. Wrist

IX-18. In patients with established rheumatoid arthritis, all of the following pulmonary radiographic findings may be explained by their rheumatologic condition EXCEPT:

A. Bilateral interstitial infiltrates

B. Bronchiectasis

C. Lobar infiltrate

D. Solitary pulmonary nodule

E. Unilateral pleural effusion

IX-19. Which of the following is the earliest plain radiographic finding of rheumatoid arthritis?

A. Juxtaarticular osteopenia
B. No abnormality
C. Soft-tissue swelling
D. Subchondral erosions
E. Symmetric joint space loss

IX-20. Which of the following statements regarding rheumatoid arthritis is true?

A. Africans and African Americans most commonly have the class II major histocompatibility complex allele HLA-DR4.
B. Females are affected three times more often than are males, and this difference is maintained throughout life.
C. The earliest lesion in rheumatoid arthritis is an increase in the number of synovial lining cells with microvascular injury.
D. There is an association with the class II major histocompatibility complex allele HLA-B27.
E. Titers of rheumatoid factor are not predictive of the severity of rheumatoid arthritis or its extraarticular manifestations.

IX-21. A 46-year-old woman presents to your clinic with multiple complaints. She describes fatigue and general malaise over 2–3 months. Her appetite has decreased. She thinks she has unintentionally lost approximately 5.5 kg. Lately, she notes pain and stiffness in her fingers on both hands that is worse in the morning and with repetitive movement. She has a grandmother and a sister who have rheumatoid arthritis, and she is very concerned that she now has it as well. Which of her complaints represents the most common manifestation of established rheumatoid arthritis?

A. Fatigue and anorexia for more than 2 months with concomitant joint pain
B. Morning joint stiffness lasting for more than 1 hour
C. Pain in symmetric joints that is worsened with movement
D. Positive family history with two relatives with RA
E. Weight loss of more than 4.5 kg during period of active disease

IX-22. All of the following are characteristic extraarticular manifestations of rheumatoid arthritis EXCEPT:

A. Anemia
B. Cutaneous vasculitis
C. Pericarditis
D. Secondary Sjögren's syndrome
E. Thrombocytopenia

IX-23. All of the following agents have been shown to have disease-modifying antirheumatic drug (DMARD) efficacy in patients with rheumatoid arthritis EXCEPT:

A. Infliximab
B. Leflunomide
C. Methotrexate
D. Naproxen
E. Rituximab

IX-24. Which of the following is the most common clinical presentation of acute rheumatic fever (ARF)?

A. Carditis
B. Chorea
C. Erythema marginatum
D. Polyarthritis
E. Subcutaneous nodules

IX-25. A 19-year-old recent immigrant from Ethiopia comes to your clinic to establish primary care. She currently feels well. Her past medical history is notable for a recent admission to the hospital for new-onset atrial fibrillation. As a child in Ethiopia, she developed an illness that caused uncontrolled flailing of her limbs and tongue lasting approximately 1 month. She also has had three episodes of migratory large-joint arthritis during her adolescence that resolved with pills that she received from the pharmacy. She is currently taking metoprolol and warfarin and has no known drug allergies. Physical examination reveals an irregularly irregular heart beat with normal blood pressure. Her point of maximal impulse (PMI) is most prominent at the midclavicular line and is normal in size. An early diastolic rumble and a 3/6 holosystolic murmur are heard at the apex. A soft early diastolic murmur is also heard at the left third intercostal space. You refer her to a cardiologist for evaluation of valve replacement and echocardiography. What other intervention might you consider at this time?

A. Glucocorticoids
B. Daily aspirin
C. Daily doxycycline
D. Monthly penicillin G injections
E. Penicillin G injections as needed for all sore throats

IX-26. A patient with a diagnosis of scleroderma who has diffuse cutaneous involvement presents with malignant hypertension, oliguria, edema, hemolytic anemia, and renal failure. You make a diagnosis of scleroderma renal crisis (SRC). What is the recommended treatment?

A. Captopril
B. Carvedilol
C. Clonidine
D. Diltiazem
E. Nitroprusside

IX-27. A 57-year-old woman with depression and chronic migraine headaches reports several years of dry mouth and dry eyes. Her primary complaint is that she can no longer eat her favorite crackers, though she does report photosensitivity and eye burning on further questioning. She has no other associated symptoms. Examination shows dry, erythematous, sticky oral mucosa. All of the following tests are likely to be positive in this patient EXCEPT:

A. La/SS-B antibody
B. Ro/SS-A antibody
C. Schirmer's I test
D. Scl-70 antibody
E. Sialometry

IX-28. Which of the following is the most common extra-glandular manifestation of primary Sjögren's syndrome?

A. Arthralgias/arthritis
B. Lymphoma
C. Peripheral neuropathy
D. Raynaud's phenomenon
E. Vasculitis

IX-29. A 44-year-old woman presents for evaluation of dry eyes and mouth. She first noticed these symptoms more than 5 years ago and the symptoms have worsened over time. She describes her eyes as gritty feeling, as if there were sand in her eyes. Sometimes her eyes burn, and she states that it is difficult to be outside in bright sunlight. In addition, her mouth is quite dry. In her job, she is frequently asked to give business presentations and finds it increasingly difficult to complete a 30- to 60-minute presentation. She has water with her at all times. Although she reports good dental hygiene without any recent changes, her dentist has had to place fillings twice in the past 3 years for dental caries. Her only other past medical history is treated tuberculosis that she contracted while in the Peace Corps in Southeast Asia when in her 20s. She takes no medication regularly and does not smoke. Ocular examination reveals punctuate corneal ulcerations on Rose Bengal stain, and the Schirmer's test shows greater than 5 mm of wetness after 5 minutes. Her oral mucosa is dry with thick mucous secretions, and the parotid glands are enlarged bilaterally. Laboratory examination reveals positive antibodies to Ro and La (SS-A and SS-B). In addition, her chemistries reveal a sodium of 142 meq/L, potassium 2.6 meq/L, chloride 115 meq/L, and bicarbonate of 15 meq/L. What is the most likely cause of the hypokalemia and acidemia in this patient?

A. Diarrhea
B. Distal (type I) renal tubular acidosis
C. Hypoaldosteronism
D. Purging with underlying anorexia nervosa
E. Renal compensation for chronic respiratory alkalosis

IX-30. A patient with primary Sjögren's syndrome that was diagnosed 6 years ago and treated with tear replacement for symptomatic relief notes continued parotid swelling for the last 3 months. She has also noted enlarging posterior cervical lymph nodes. Evaluation shows leukopenia and low C4 complement levels. What is the most likely diagnosis?

A. Amyloidosis
B. Chronic pancreatitis
C. HIV infection
D. Lymphoma
E. Secondary Sjögren's syndrome

IX-31. The histocompatibility antigen HLA-B27 is present in what percentage of patients with ankylosing spondylitis?

A. 10%
B. 30%
C. 50%
D. 90%
E. 100%

IX-32. Which of the following is the most common extra-articular manifestation of ankylosing spondylitis?

A. Anterior uveitis
B. Aortic insufficiency
C. Inflammatory bowel disease
D. Pulmonary fibrosis
E. Third-degree heart block

IX-33. A 25-year-old man sees his primary care physician for evaluation of low back pain. The pain is severe, is worse in the morning, and is relieved with exercise and is worse with rest; in particular, nighttime sleeping is difficult. He does feel quite stiff in the morning for at least 30 minutes. An MRI of his lower back is obtained and shows active inflammation in the sacroiliac joint. On further questioning, he reports a history of unilateral eye redness treated with corticosteroids about 2 years ago. A test for HLA-B27 is positive. Which of the following is first-line therapy for his condition?

A. Infliximab
B. Naproxen
C. Prednisone
D. Rituximab
E. Tramadol

IX-34. A 27-year-old man is seen at his primary care physician's office for evaluation of painful arthritis involving the right knee that is associated with finger welling diffusely. He is otherwise healthy, but does recall a severe bout of diarrheal illness about 3–4 weeks prior that spontaneously resolved. He takes no medications and reports rare marijuana use. On review of systems, he reports painful urination. Examination shows inflammatory arthritis of the right knee, dactylitis, and normal genitourinary examination. He is diagnosed with reactive arthritis. Which of the following is the most likely etiologic agent of his diarrhea?

A. *Campylobacter jejuni*
B. *Clostridium difficile*
C. *Escherichia coli*
D. *Helicobacter pylori*
E. *Shigella flexneri*

IX-35. A 28-year-old woman undergoes evaluation for weight loss and bloody diarrhea that is ultimately diagnosed as Crohn's disease. She has been diagnosed with dactylitis and bilateral sacroiliitis within the past 6 months. She is scheduled to begin treatment with infliximab in 2 weeks for her Crohn's disease. Which of the following statements is true regarding the effect of infliximab on her arthritis?

A. Although infliximab is likely to improve her arthritic symptoms, NSAIDs should be tried first.
B. Although infliximab is very effective therapy for Crohn's disease, it will have no effect on her arthritis.
C. Her arthritis is unrelated to Crohn's disease, and because of this she should undergo a thorough evaluation for infectious causes before undergoing immunosuppressive therapy.
D. Infliximab is very effective therapy for this type of arthritis.
E. None of the above.

IX-36. Which of the following statements regarding the arthritis of Whipple's disease is true?

A. Arthritis is a rare finding in Whipple's disease.
B. Joint manifestations are usually concurrent with gastrointestinal symptoms and malabsorption.
C. Radiography frequently shows joint erosions.
D. Synovial fluid examination is unlikely to show polymorphonuclear cells.
E. None of the above.

IX-37. A 35-year-old man has severe ankylosing spondylitis that is unresponsive to NSAID therapy. Therapy with infliximab has been recommended and he is wondering about potential side effects. All of the following are common potential side effects from this medication EXCEPT:

A. Demyelinating disorders
B. Disseminated tuberculosis
C. Exacerbation of congestive heart failure
D. Hypersensitivity pneumonitis
E. Pancytopenia

IX-38. Which of the following definitions best fits the term enthesitis?

A. Alteration of joint alignment so that articulating surfaces incompletely approximate each other
B. Inflammation at the site of tendinous or ligamentous insertion into bone
C. Inflammation of the periarticular membrane lining the joint capsule
D. Inflammation of a saclike cavity near a joint that decreases friction
E. A palpable vibratory or crackling sensation elicited with joint motion

IX-39. A 35-year-old female presents to her primary care doctor complaining of diffuse body and joint pain. When asked to describe which of her joints are most affected, she answers, "All of them." There is no associated stiffness, redness, or swelling of the joints. No Raynaud's phenomenon

has been appreciated. Occasionally she notes numbness in the fingers and toes. The patient complains of chronic pain and poor sleep quality that she feels is due to her pain. She previously was seen in the clinic for chronic headaches that were felt to be tension related. She has tried taking over-the-counter ibuprofen twice daily without relief of pain. She has no other medical problems. On physical examination, the patient appears comfortable. Her joints exhibit full range of motion without evidence of inflammatory arthritis. She does have pain with palpation at bilateral suboccipital muscle insertions, at C5, at the lateral epicondyle, in the upper outer quadrant of the buttock, at the medial fat pad of the knee proximal to the joint line, and unilaterally on the second right rib. The erythrocyte sedimentation rate is 12 seconds. Antinuclear antibodies are positive at a titer of 1:40 in a speckled pattern. The patient is HLA-B27 positive. Rheumatoid factor is negative. Radiograms of the cervical spine, hips, and elbows are normal. What is the most likely diagnosis?

A. Ankylosing spondylitis
B. Disseminated gonococcal infection
C. Fibromyalgia
D. Rheumatoid arthritis
E. Systemic lupus erythematosus

IX-40. A 42-year-old male presents with complaints of a rash and joint pain. He first noticed the rash 6 months ago. It is primarily on the hands (Figure IX-40), the extensor surfaces of the elbows, and the knees, low back, and scalp. Although he complains of the appearance of these lesions, they do not itch or hurt. He has not been previously evaluated for them and has recently noticed changes in the nail beds. For the last 2 weeks, the patient has had increasingly severe pain in the distal joints of the hands and feet. His hands are so painful that he is having trouble writing and holding utensils. He denies fevers, weight loss, fatigue, cough, shortness of breath, or changes in bowel or bladder habits. Which of the following is the most likely diagnosis?

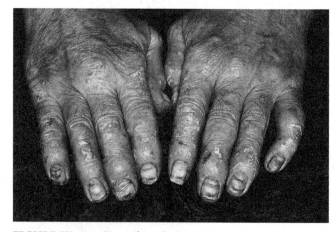

FIGURE IX-40   (See color atlas)

A. Arthritis associated with inflammatory bowel disease
B. Gout
C. Osteoarthritis
D. Psoriatic arthritis
E. Rheumatoid arthritis

IX-41. All of the following vasculitic syndromes are thought to be due to immune complex deposition EXCEPT:

A. Cryoglobulinemic vasculitis
B. Henoch-Schönlein purpura
C. Polyarteritis nodosa associated with hepatitis B
D. Serum sickness
E. Granulomatosis with polyangiitis (Wegener's)

IX-42. A 53-year-old man presents with a vasculitis syndrome. His cytoplasmic antineutrophil cytoplasmic antibodies (c-ANCA) is positive. Which of the following syndromes is he most likely to have?

A. Churg-Strauss syndrome
B. Henoch-Schönlein purpura
C. Microscopic polyangiitis
D. Ulcerative colitis
E. Granulomatosis with polyangiitis (Wegener's)

IX-43. A 40-year-old male presents to the emergency department with 2 days of low-volume hemoptysis. He reports that he has been coughing up 2–5 tablespoons of blood each day. He reports mild chest pain, low-grade fevers, and weight loss. In addition, he has had about 1 year of severe upper respiratory symptoms including frequent epistaxis and purulent discharge treated with several courses of antibiotics. Aside from mild hyperlipidemia, he is otherwise healthy. His only medications are daily aspirin and lovastatin. On physical examination he has normal vital signs, and the upper airway is notable for saddle nose deformity and clear lungs. A CT of the chest shows multiple cavitating nodules, and urinalysis shows red blood cells. Which of the following tests offers the highest diagnostic yield to make the appropriate diagnosis?

A. Deep skin biopsy
B. Percutaneous kidney biopsy
C. Pulmonary angiogram
D. Surgical lung biopsy
E. Upper airway biopsy

IX-44. An 84-year-old woman sees her primary care physician for evaluation of severe headaches. She noted these several weeks ago and they have been getting worse. Although she has not had any visual aura, she is concerned that she has been intermittently losing vision in her left eye for the last few days. She denies new weakness or numbness, but she does report jaw pain with eating. Her past medical history includes coronary artery disease requiring a bypass grafting 10 years prior, diabetes mellitus, hyperlipidemia, and mild depression. Full review of symptoms is notable for night sweats and mild low back pain that is particularly prominent in the morning. Which of the following is the next most appropriate step?

A. Aspirin 975 mg po daily
B. Measurement of erythrocyte sedimentation rate
C. Prednisone 60 mg daily
D. Referral for temporal artery biopsy
E. Referral for ultrasound of temporal artery

IX-45. A 54-year-old man is evaluated for cutaneous vasculitis and peripheral nephropathy. Because of concomitant renal dysfunction he undergoes kidney biopsy that shows glomerulonephritis. Cryoglobulins are demonstrated in the peripheral blood. Which of the following laboratory studies should be sent to determine the etiology?

A. Hepatitis B surface antigen
B. Cytoplasmic ANCA
C. Hepatitis C polymerase chain reaction (PCR)
D. HIV antibody
E. Rheumatoid factor

IX-46. A 54-year-old man is admitted for persistent lower abdominal and groin pain that began 7 months previously. Two months before his present admission, he required exploratory laparoscopy for acute abdominal pain and presumed cholecystitis. This revealed necrotic omental tissue and pericholecystitis necessitating omentectomy and cholecystectomy. However, the pain continued unchanged. He currently describes it as periumbilical and radiating into his groin and legs. It becomes worse with eating. The patient has also had episodic severe testicular pain, bowel urgency, nausea, vomiting, and diuresis. He has lost approximately 22.7 kg over the preceding 6 months. His past medical history is significant for hypertension that has recently become difficult to control.

Medications on admission include aspirin, hydrochlorothiazide, hydromorphone, lansoprazole, metoprolol, and quinapril. On physical examination, the patient appears comfortable. His blood pressure is 170/100 mmHg, his heart rate is 88 beats/min, and he is afebrile. He has normal first and second heart sounds without murmurs, and an S_4 is present. There are no carotid, renal, abdominal, or femoral bruits.

His lungs are clear to auscultation. Bowel sounds are normal. Abdominal palpation demonstrates minimal diffuse tenderness without rebound or guarding. No masses are present, and the stool is negative for occult blood. During the examination, the patient develops Raynaud's phenomenon in his right hand that persists for several minutes. His neurologic examination is intact. Admission laboratory studies reveal an erythrocyte sedimentation rate of 72 mm/h, a BUN of 17 mg/dL, and a creatinine of 0.8 mg/dL. The patient has no proteinuria or hematuria. Tests for antinuclear antibodies, anti–double-stranded-DNA antibodies, and antineutrophil cytoplasmic antibodies are negative. Liver function tests are abnormal with an AST of 89 IU/L and an ALT of 112 IU/L. Hepatitis B surface antigen and e antigen are positive. Mesenteric angiography demonstrates small, beaded aneurysms of the superior and inferior mesenteric veins. What is the most likely diagnosis?

A. Hepatocellular carcinoma
B. Ischemic colitis
C. Microscopic polyangiitis
D. Mixed cryoglobulinemia
E. Polyarteritis nodosa

IX-47. An 18-year-old man is admitted to the hospital with acute onset of crushing substernal chest pain that began abruptly 30 minutes ago. He reports the pain radiating to his neck and right arm. He has otherwise been in good health. He currently plays trumpet in his high school marching band but does not participate regularly in aerobic activities. On physical examination, he is diaphoretic and tachypneic. His blood pressure is 100/48 mmHg and heart rate is 110 beats/min. His cardiovascular examination shows a regular rhythm but is tachycardic. A II/VI holosystolic murmur is heard best at the apex and radiates to the axilla. His lungs have bilateral rales at the bases. The electrocardiogram demonstrates 4 mm of ST elevation in the anterior leads. On further questioning regarding his past medical history, he recalls having been told that he was hospitalized for some problem with his heart when he was 2 years old. His mother, who accompanies him, reports that he received aspirin and γ-globulin as treatment. Since that time, he has required intermittent follow-up with echocardiography. What is the most likely cause of this patient's acute coronary syndrome?

A. Dissection of the aortic root and left coronary ostia
B. Presence of a myocardial bridge overlying the left anterior descending artery
C. Stenosis of a coronary artery aneurysm
D. Vasospasm following cocaine ingestion
E. Vasculitis involving the left anterior descending artery

IX-48. Which of the following is required for the diagnosis of Behçet's disease?

A. Large-vessel vasculitis
B. Pathergy test
C. Recurrent oral ulceration
D. Recurrent genital ulceration
E. Uveitis

IX-49. A 25-year-old female presents with a complaint of painful mouth ulcerations. She describes these lesions as shallow ulcers that last for 1–2 weeks. The ulcers have been appearing for the last 6 months. For the last 2 days, the patient has had a painful red eye. She has had no genital ulcerations, arthritis, skin rashes, or photosensitivity. On physical examination, the patient appears well developed and in no distress. She has a temperature of 37.6°C (99.7°F), heart rate of 86 beats/min, blood pressure of 126/72 mmHg, and respiratory rate of 16 breaths/min. Examination of the oral mucosa reveals two shallow ulcers with a yellow base on the buccal mucosa. The ophthalmologic examination is consistent with anterior uveitis. The cardiopulmonary examination is normal. She has no arthritis, but medially on the right thigh there is a palpable cord in the saphenous vein. Laboratory studies reveal an erythrocyte sedimentation rate of 68 seconds. White blood cell count is 10,230/μL with a differential of 68% polymorphonuclear cells, 28% lymphocytes, and 4% monocytes. The antinuclear antibody and anti-dsDNA antibody are negative. C3 is 89 mg/dL, and C4 is 24 mg/dL. What is the most likely diagnosis?

A. Behçet's syndrome
B. Cicatricial pemphigoid
C. Discoid lupus erythematosus
D. Sjögren's syndrome
E. Systemic lupus erythematosus

IX-50. What is the best initial treatment for the patient in question IX-49?

A. Colchicine
B. Intralesional interferon α
C. Systemic glucocorticoids and azathioprine
D. Thalidomide
E. Topical glucocorticoids including ophthalmic prednisolone

IX-51. Relapsing polychondritis may be a primary disease or may be associated with other rheumatologic diseases. All of the following conditions are associated with relapsing polychondritis EXCEPT:

A. Myelodysplastic syndrome
B. Primary biliary cirrhosis
C. Scleroderma
D. Spondyloarthritides
E. Systemic lupus erythematosus

IX-52. A 47-year-old man is evaluated for 1 year of recurrent episodes of bilateral ear swelling. The ear is painful during these events, and the right ear has become floppy. He is otherwise healthy and reports no illicit habits. He works in an office and his only sport is tennis. On examination, the left ear has a beefy red color, and the pinna is tender and swollen; the earlobe appears minimally swollen but is neither red nor tender. Which of the following is the most likely explanation for this finding?

A. Behçet's syndrome
B. Cogan's syndrome
C. Hemoglobinopathy
D. Recurrent trauma
E. Relapsing polychondritis

IX-53. A 25-year-old African-American woman is evaluated for bilateral hilar lymphadenopathy found on a routine chest radiograph performed before a laparoscopic cholecystectomy. She undergoes mediastinoscopy, and multiple noncaseating granulomas are identified in her lymph nodes. All of the following may explain this finding EXCEPT:

A. Alveolar proteinosis
B. Atypical mycobacteria
C. Beryllium exposure
D. Histoplasmosis
E. Malignancy
F. Sarcoidosis

IX-54. A 34-year-old woman has a history of cutaneous sarcoidosis that has been managed with hydroxychloroquine for the last 5 years. After an episode of right flank pain and hematuria, she is diagnosed with renal calculus. Which of the following statements regarding her renal calculus is true?

A. Exogenous vitamin D and sunlight exposure in patients with sarcoidosis may exacerbate hypercalcemia and associated renal calculus.

B. Hypercalcemia is rare in sarcoidosis and is unlikely to contribute to the patient's calculus.

C. Hypercalcemia in sarcoidosis occurs through increased production of 25-dihydroxyvitamin D by the skin.

D. If she is to begin therapy with oral calcium to treat the renal stone, a 24-hour urine phosphate should be obtained before and after initiation of therapy.

E. None of the above.

IX-55. All of the following agents have been shown to improve symptoms or function in patients with sarcoidosis EXCEPT:

A. Etanercept
B. Hydroxychloroquine
C. Infliximab
D. Methotrexate
E. Prednisone

IX-56. All of the following statements regarding the clinical manifestations of sarcoidosis are true EXCEPT:

A. Cardiac involvement occurs in 25% of patients.
B. Eye involvement is typically anterior uveitis.
C. Liver involvement is typically manifest by elevation of alkaline phosphatase.
D. Lung involvement occurs in over 90% of cases.
E. Skin involvement occurs in approximately one-third of patients.

IX-57. You are seeing a 56-year-old woman for complaints of joint pain and stiffness. All of the following signs or symptoms would be indicative of inflammatory causes of arthritis EXCEPT:

A. Elevations in erythrocyte sedimentation rate
B. Fatigue, fever, or weight loss
C. Persistence for longer than 6 weeks
D. Presence of soft-tissue swelling around affected joints
E. Prolonged morning stiffness

IX-58. A 22-year-old man is seen for a shoulder injury that occurred while pitching in a baseball game. He describes feeling a snap then acute pain in the shoulder of his left arm while throwing the ball. Which of the following findings would be most concerning for a tear of one of the rotator cuff muscles?

A. Inability to hold the arm at 90° following passive abduction
B. Inability to actively raise the arm more than 90° with forward flexion
C. Pain with palpation over the bicipital groove while rotating the arm internally and externally
D. Pain with palpation while applying pressure anteriorly along the joint and rotating the arm internally and externally
E. Pain with passive abduction of the arm

IX-59. A 62-year-old white male presents with a chief complaint of right knee pain and swelling. Past medical history is significant for obesity with a body mass index (BMI) of 34 kg/m^2, diet-controlled Type 2 diabetes mellitus, and hypertension. His medications include hydrochlorothiazide and acetaminophen as needed for pain. Physical examination is remarkable for a moderately sized effusion of the right knee, with range of motion limited to 90° of flexion and 160° of extension. There is minimal warmth and no redness. He has crepitus with range of motion. With weight bearing, he has outward bowing of the legs bilaterally. A radiogram of the right knee shows osteophytes and joint space narrowing. Which of the following is the most likely finding on joint fluid examination?

A. A Gram stain showing gram-positive cocci in clusters
B. A white blood cell count of 1110/μL
C. A white blood cell count of 22,000/μL
D. Positively birefringent crystals on polarizing light microscopy
E. Negatively birefringent crystals on polarizing light microscopy

IX-60. A 62-year-old woman presents complaining of hand pain bilaterally that has been gradually progressive over the past year. She has previously worked as a seamstress in a factory making gloves for more than 35 years. You suspect osteoarthritis. All of the following factors on history or physical examination are characteristic of this diagnosis EXCEPT:

A. Evidence of bilateral swelling and warmth affecting the wrists only
B. Joint space narrowing and osteophytes at the proximal and distal interphalangeal joints on x-ray
C. Pain that becomes worse when preparing meals
D. Presence of Heberden's nodes
E. Stiffness that is worse after brief periods of rest with occasional locking of the more affecting joints

IX-61. A 73-year-old woman with a medical history of obesity and diabetes mellitus presents to your clinic complaining of right knee pain that has been progressive and is worse with walking or standing. She has taken over-the-counter nonsteroidal anti-inflammatory drugs without relief. She wants to know what is wrong with her knee and what may have caused it. X-rays are performed and reveal cartilage loss and osteophyte formation. Which of the following represents the most potent risk factor for the development of osteoarthritis?

A. Age
B. Gender
C. Genetic susceptibility
D. Obesity
E. Previous joint injury

IX-62. A 53-year-old man presents to your clinic complaining of bilateral knee pain. He states that the pain worsens with walking and is not present at rest. He has been experiencing knee pain intermittently for many months and has had no relief from over-the-counter analgesics. He has a history of hypertension and obesity. When he was in high school and college, he played football and basketball. Which of the following represents the best initial treatment strategy for this patient?

A. Avoidance of walking for several weeks
B. Light daily walking exercises
C. Low-dose, long-acting narcotics
D. Oral steroid pulse
E. Weight loss

IX-63. A 74-year-old man is seen by his primary care provider 6 weeks following an acute gout attack. He has a prior history of gout presenting similarly on two prior occasions within the past 6 months. His past medical history is significant for congestive heart failure, hypercholesterolemia, and stage III chronic kidney disease. He is taking pravastatin, aspirin, furosemide, metolazone, lisinopril, and metoprolol XL. His glomerular filtration rate is 38 mL/min, creatinine is 2.2 mg/dL, and uric acid level is 9.3 mg/dL. He is wondering if there is any therapy that might lessen his likelihood of repeated gout attacks. Which of the following medication regimens is most appropriate for the treatment of this patient?

A. Allopurinol 800 mg daily
B. Colchicine 0.6 mg bid
C. Febuxostat 40 mg daily
D. Indomethacin 25 mg twice daily
E. Probenecid 250 mg twice daily

IX-64. A 64-year-old man with congestive heart failure presents to the emergency department complaining of acute onset of severe pain in his right foot. The pain began during the night and awoke him from a deep sleep. He reports the pain to be so severe that he could not wear a shoe or sock to the hospital. His current medications are furosemide 40 mg twice daily, carvedilol 6.25 mg twice daily, candesartan 8 mg once daily, and aspirin 325 mg once daily. On examination, he is febrile to 38.5°C (101.3°F). The first toe of the right foot is erythematous and exquisitely tender to touch. There is significant swelling and effusion of the first metatarsophalangeal joint on the right foot. No other joints are affected. Which of the following findings would be expected on arthrocentesis?

A. Glucose level of less than 25 mg/dL
B. Positive Gram stain
C. Presence of strongly negatively birefringent needle-shaped crystals under polarized light microscopy
D. Presence of weakly positively birefringent rhomboidal crystals under polarized light microscopy
E. White blood cell (WBC) count greater than 100,000/μL

IX-65. A 24-year-old woman is admitted to the hospital with symptoms of fever and a swollen, painful right knee. About 3 weeks prior to the current syndrome, the patient had

systemic symptoms including fevers, chills, and migratory joint pains affecting the hands, wrists, knees, hips, and ankles. At that time, she noticed a few small papules on her upper chest and hands. These have subsequently resolved. She has no significant past medical history. She currently works as a landscape designer and does not recall any recent tick or insect bites. Her only medication is an oral contraceptive. She is unmarried and has multiple sexual partners. On physical examination, the patient has a temperature of 38.4°C (101.2°F), heart rate of 124 beats/min, respiratory rate of 24 breaths/min, and blood pressure of 102/68 mmHg. Her right knee demonstrates redness, warmth, swelling, and pain with movement. An arthrocentesis demonstrates a white blood cell count of 66,000/μL (90% neutrophils). No crystals or organisms are seen. Which of the following would be most likely to yield the correct diagnosis?

A. Bacterial cultures of the cervix
B. Bacterial cultures of the synovial fluid
C. Blood cultures
D. IgG directed against *Borrelia burgdorferi*
E. Rheumatoid factor

IX-66. A 66-year-old woman with a history of rheumatoid arthritis and frequent attacks of pseudogout in her left knee presents with night sweats and a 2-day history of left knee pain. Her medications include methotrexate 15 mg weekly, folate 1 mg daily, prednisone 5 mg daily, and ibuprofen 800 mg three times daily as needed for pain. On physical examination, her temperature is 38.6°C (101.5°F), heart rate is 110 beats/min, blood pressure is 104/78 mmHg, and oxygen saturation is 97% on room air. Her left knee is swollen, red, painful, and warm. With 5° of flexion or extension, she develops extreme pain. She has evidence of chronic joint deformity in her hands, knees, and spine. Peripheral white blood cell (WBC) count is 16,700 cells/μL with 95% neutrophils. A diagnostic tap of her left knee reveals 168,300 WBCs per μL and 99% neutrophils, and diffuse needle-shaped birefringent crystals are present. Gram stain shows rare gram-positive cocci in clusters. Management includes all of the following EXCEPT:

A. Blood cultures
B. Glucocorticoids
C. Needle aspiration of joint fluid
D. Orthopedic surgery consult
E. Vancomycin

IX-67. A 42-year-old woman is seen in her primary care doctor's office complaining of diffuse pains and fatigue. She has a difficult time localizing the pain to any particular joint or location, but reports that it affects her upper and lower extremities, neck, and hips. It is described as achy and 10 out of 10 in intensity. She feels that her joints are stiff but does not notice that it is worse in the morning. The pain has been present for the past 6 months and is increasing in intensity. She has tried both over-the-counter ibuprofen and acetaminophen without significant relief. The patient feels as if the pain is interfering with her ability to get restful sleep and is making it difficult for her to concentrate. She has missed multiple days of work as a waitress and fears that she will lose her job. There is a medical history of depression and obesity. The patient currently is taking venlafaxine sustained release 150 mg daily. She has a family history of rheumatoid arthritis in her mother. She smokes 1 pack of cigarettes daily. On physical examination vital signs are normal. Body mass index is 36 kg/m². Joint examination demonstrates no erythema, swelling, or effusions. There is diffuse pain with palpation at the insertion points of the suboccipital muscles, at the midpoint of the upper border of the trapezius muscle, along the second costochondral junction, at the lateral epicondyles, and along the medial fat pad of the knees. All of the following statements regarding the cause of this patient's diffuse pain syndrome are true EXCEPT:

A. Cognitive dysfunction, sleep disturbance, anxiety, and depression are common comorbid neuropsychological conditions.
B. Pain in this syndrome is associated with increased evoked pain sensitivity.
C. Pain in this syndrome is often localized to specific joints.
D. This syndrome is present in 2–5% of the general population, but increases in prevalence to 20% or more of patients with degenerative or inflammatory rheumatic disorders.
E. Women are nine times more likely than men to be affected by this syndrome.

IX-68. A 36-year-old woman presents to your office with diffuse pain throughout her body associated with fatigue, insomnia, and difficulty concentrating. She finds the pain difficult to localize, but reports that it is 7–8 out of 10 in intensity and is not relieved by nonsteroidal anti-inflammatory medications. She has a long-standing history of generalized anxiety disorder and is treated with sertraline 100 mg daily as well as clonazepam 1 mg twice daily. On examination, she has pain with palpation at several musculoskeletal sites. Her laboratory examination demonstrates a normal complete blood count, basic metabolic panel, erythrocyte sedimentation rate, and rheumatoid factor. You diagnose her with fibromyalgia. All of the following therapies are recommended as part of the treatment plan for fibromyalgia EXCEPT:

A. An exercise program that includes strength training, aerobic exercise, and yoga
B. Cognitive-behavioral therapy for insomnia
C. Milnacipran
D. Oxycodone
E. Pregabalin

IX-69. A 53-year-old woman presents to your clinic complaining of fatigue and generalized pain that have worsened over 2 years. She also describes irritability and poor sleep, and is concerned that she is depressed. She reveals that she was recently separated from her husband and has been stressed at work. Which of the following elements in her history and physical examination would meet American College of Rheumatology criteria for diagnosis of fibromyalgia?

A. Diffuse chronic pain and abnormal sleep
B. Diffuse pain without other etiology and evidence of major depression
C. Major depression, life stressor, chronic pain, and female gender
D. Major depression and pain on palpation at 6 of 18 tender point sites
E. Widespread chronic pain and pain on palpation at 11 of 18 tender point sites

IX-70. A 42-year-old man is found to have the following finding on a physical examination (Figure IX-70). All of the following conditions are associated with this finding EXCEPT:

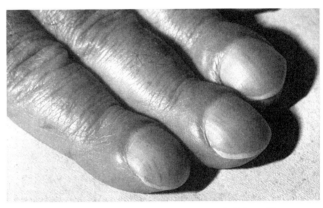

FIGURE IX-70 *(Reprinted from the Clinical Slide Collection on the Rheumatic Diseases, Copyright 1991, 1995. Used by permission of the American College of Rheumatology.)*

A. Chronic obstructive pulmonary disease
B. Cyanotic congenital heart disease
C. Cystic fibrosis
D. Hepatocellular carcinoma
E. Hyperthyroidism

IX-71. A 64-year-old woman sees her primary care physician complaining of hip pain for about 1 week. She localizes the pain to the lateral aspect of her right hip and describes it as sharp. It is worse with movement, and she finds it difficult to lie on her right side. The pain began soon after the patient planted her garden. She has a medical history of obesity, osteoarthritis of the knees, and hypertension. Her medications include losartan 50 mg daily and hydrochlorothiazide 25 mg daily. For the pain, she has taken ibuprofen 600 mg as needed with mild to moderate relief of pain. On physical examination, the patient is not febrile and her vital signs are unremarkable. On examination of the hip, pain is elicited with external rotation and resisted abduction of the hip. Direct palpation over the lateral aspect of the upper portion of the femur near the hip joint reproduces the pain. What is the most likely diagnosis in this patient?

A. Avascular necrosis of the hip
B. Iliotibial band syndrome
C. Meralgia paresthetica
D. Septic arthritis
E. Trochanteric bursitis

IX-72. A 32-year-old woman is seen in the clinic with a complaint of left knee pain. She enjoys running long distances and is currently training for a marathon. She is running on average 30–40 miles weekly. She currently is experiencing an aching pain on the lateral aspect of her left knee. There is a burning sensation that also continues up the lateral aspect of her thigh. She denies any injury to her knee, and she has not felt that it was hot or swollen. She is otherwise healthy and takes no medications other than herbal supplements. Physical examination of the knee reveals point tenderness over the lateral femoral condyle that is worse with flexing the knee. The patient is asked to lie on her right side with her right knee and hip flexed at 90°. Her left leg is extended at the hip and slowly lowered into adduction behind the bottom leg, reproducing the patient's left knee pain. All of the following treatments can be recommended for this patient EXCEPT:

A.   Assessment of the patient's running shoes to ensure a proper fit
B.   Glucocorticoid injection so as not to interfere with the patient's continued preparation for the upcoming marathon
C.   Ibuprofen 600–800 mg every 6 hours as needed for pain
D.   Referral for physical therapy
E.   Referral for surgical release if conservative therapy fails

IX-73. A 58-year-old female presents complaining of right shoulder pain. She does not recall any prior injury but notes that the shoulder has been getting progressively stiffer over the last several months. She previously had several episodes of bursitis of the right shoulder that were treated successfully with NSAIDs and steroid injections. The patient's past medical history is also significant for diabetes mellitus, for which she takes metformin and glyburide. On physical examination, the right shoulder is not warm or red but is tender to touch. Passive and active range of motion is limited in flexion, extension, and abduction. A right shoulder radiogram shows osteopenia without evidence of joint erosion or osteophytes. What is the most likely diagnosis?

A.   Adhesive capsulitis
B.   Avascular necrosis
C.   Bicipital tendinitis
D.   Osteoarthritis
E.   Rotator cuff tear

IX-74. A 32-year-old woman presents to the clinic with right thumb and wrist pain that has worsened over several weeks. She has pain when she pinches her thumb against her other fingers. Her only other history is that she is a new mother with an 8-week-old infant at home. On physical examination she has mild swelling and tenderness over the radial styloid process, and pain is elicited when she places her thumb in her palm and grasps it with her fingers. A Phalen maneuver is negative. Which condition is most likely?

A.   Carpal tunnel syndrome
B.   De Quervain's tenosynovitis
C.   Gouty arthritis of the first metacarpophalangeal joint
D.   · Palmar fasciitis
E.   Rheumatoid arthritis

ANSWERS

IX-1.   **The answer is A.** *(Chap. 314)* The innate immune system is phylogenetically the oldest form of immunologic defense system, inherited from invertebrates. This defense system uses germ line–encoded proteins to recognize pathogen-associated molecular patterns. Cells of the innate immune system include macrophages, dendritic cells, and natural killer lymphocytes. The critical components of the innate immune system include recognition by germ line–encoded host molecules, recognition of key microbe virulence factors but not recognition of self molecules, and nonrecognition of benign foreign molecules or microbes. Adaptive immunity is found only in vertebrate animals and is based on the generation of antigen receptors on T and B lymphocytes by gene rearrangements, such that individual T or B cells express unique antigen receptors on their surface capable of recognizing diverse environmental antigens.

IX-2.   **The answer is A.** *(Chap. 314)* Complement activity, which results from the sequential interaction of a large number of plasma and cell membrane proteins, plays an important role in the inflammatory response. The classic pathway of complement activation is initiated by an antibody–antigen interaction. The first complement component (C1, a complex composed of three proteins) binds to immune complexes with activation mediated by C1q. Active C1 then initiates the cleavage and concomitant activation of components C4 and C2. The activated C1 is destroyed by a plasma protease inhibitor termed C1 esterase inhibitor. This molecule also regulates clotting factor XI and kallikrein. Patients with a deficiency of C1 esterase inhibitor may develop angioedema, sometimes leading to death by asphyxia. Attacks may be precipitated by stress or trauma. In addition to low antigenic or functional levels of C1 esterase inhibitor, patients with this autosomal-dominant condition may have normal levels of C1 and C3 but low levels of C4 and C2. Danazol therapy produces a striking increase in the level of this important inhibitor and alleviates the symptoms in many patients. An acquired form of angioedema caused by a deficiency of C1 esterase inhibitor has been described in patients with autoimmune or malignant disease.

IX-3.   **The answer is C.** *(Chap. 315)* The human major histocompatibility complex genes are located on a 4-megabase region on chromosome 6. The major function of the MHC complex genes is to produce proteins that are important in developing immunologic specificity through their role in binding antigen for presentation to T cells. This process is nonspecific, and the ability of an HLA molecule to bind to a particular protein depends on the molecular fit between the amino acid sequence of a particular protein and the corresponding domain on the MHC molecule. Once a peptide has bound, the MHC-peptide complex binds to the T-cell receptor, after which the T cell must determine if an immune response should be generated. If an antigen is similar to an endogenous protein, the potential antigen will be recognized as a self-peptide and tolerance to the antigen will be continued. The MHC I and II complexes have been implicated in the development of many autoimmune diseases, which occur when T cells fail to recognize a peptide as a self-peptide and an immune response is allowed to develop. MHC I and II genes also play a major role in tissue compatibility for transplantation and are important in generating immune-mediated rejection. The other answers listed refer to functions of immunoglobulins. The variable region of the immunoglobulin is a B cell–specific response to an antigen to promote neutralization of the antigen through agglutination and precipitation. The constant region of the immunoglobulin is able to nonspecifically activate the immune system through complement activation and promotion of phagocytosis by neutrophils and macrophages.

IX-4.   **The answer is B.** *(Chap. 317)* The patient has classic symptoms of angioedema with rapid onset of facial swelling often involving the lips, frequently with preceding limb symptoms. Angioedema and urticaria are grouped by the underlying etiology. In this case, ACE inhibitor use is associated with increased levels of bradykinin that in a predisposed individual can result in angioedema. Hereditary angioedema is associated with chronically depressed levels of C1 inhibitor that is involved in the degradation of bradykinin. IgE-mediated angioedema occurs due to specific antigen sensitivity. Complement-mediated disease may be due to vasculitis, serum sickness, or reactions to blood products. Non-immunologic causes of angioedema include direct mast cell–releasing agents such as opiates and agents that alter arachidonic acid metabolism, most commonly NSAIDs. IgE levels are not elevated in bradykinin-mediated angioedema. Because of the potentially life-threatening nature of the disease, rechallenge with a second ACE inhibitor is not recommended.

IX-5.   **The answer is D.** *(Chap. 317)* Urticaria and angioedema are common disorders, affecting approximately 20% of the population. In acute urticarial angioedema, attacks of swelling are of less than 6 weeks' duration; chronic urticarial angioedema is by definition more long standing. Urticaria usually is pruritic and affects the trunk and proximal extremities. Angioedema is generally less pruritic and affects the hands, feet, genitalia, and face. This female has chronic urticaria, which probably is due to a cutaneous necrotizing vasculitis. The clues to the diagnosis are the arthralgias, the presence of residual skin discoloration, and the elevated sedimentation rate, which would be uncharacteristic of other urticarial diseases. The diagnosis can be confirmed by skin biopsy. Chronic urticaria rarely has an allergic cause; hence, allergy skin tests and measurement of total IgE levels are not helpful. Measurement of C1 esterase inhibitor activity is useful in diagnosing hereditary angioedema, a disease that is not associated with urticaria. Patch tests are used to diagnose contact dermatitis.

IX-6.   **The answer is D.** *(Chap. 317)* This patient presents with symptoms of cold urticaria, an IgE-dependent urticarial reaction to cold exposure. After exposure to cold, urticarial lesions appear in exposed areas and usually last for less than 2 hours. Histologic examination of the urticarial lesion would demonstrate mast cell degranulation with edema of the dermis and subcutaneous tissues. In experimental exposure to a cold challenge such as an ice water bath, elevated levels of histamine in venous blood may be demonstrated if assessed in the extremity exposed to a cold environment, whereas the histamine levels would be normal in a nonexposed extremity. The appearance of a linear wheal after a firm stroke is indicative of dermatographism. This condition can be seen in 1–4% of the population and is often found in individuals with cold urticaria. In general, cold urticaria is a localized process without adverse consequences. However, vascular collapse may occur if an individual is submerged in cold water. Many individuals request treatment because they are embarrassed by their condition or are symptomatic from the recurrent urticaria and pruritus. Treatment with H1 histamine receptor blockers is usually adequate for symptom control. Cyproheptadine or hydroxyzine can be added to therapy if H1 antihistamines are inadequate. In this patient, there is a clear precipitant for developing urticaria—cold exposure. Thus, no other evaluation is necessary. In the evaluation and management of chronic urticaria, the identification and elimination of precipitating factors is important. Possible etiologic factors include foods, pollens, molds, and medications. In this case the urticaria predates the use of oral contraceptive medications; thus, stopping oral contraceptives is unlikely to be helpful. Assessment of antithyroglobulin and antimicrosomal antibodies can be helpful in individuals with chronic urticaria in whom a cause is not otherwise identified. Deficiency of C1 or the presence of a C1 inhibitor presents as recurrent angioedema rather than urticaria.

IX-7.   **The answer is E.** *(Chap. 317)* Allergic rhinitis is a common problem in the United States and North America. It is estimated that about 1 in 5 individuals experiences allergic rhinitis. The incidence is greatest in childhood and adolescence, and the symptoms tend to regress with aging. Complete remissions, however, are uncommon. Many individuals experience seasonal symptoms only. These symptoms are due to pollen production by weeds, grasses, and trees that are dependent on wind currents, rather than insects, for cross-pollination. The timing of the pollination events predicts the seasonal severity of symptoms and varies little from year to year within a particular locale. Based on this pattern, one is able to predict which allergens are most likely responsible for a patient's symptoms. In the temperate regions of North America, trees pollinate in the spring, and ragweed pollinates in the fall. Grasses are responsible for seasonal allergic symptoms in the summer months. Mold allergens can have a variable pattern of symptoms, depending on climatic conditions that allow them to sporulate. Perennial rhinitis does not have a seasonal pattern and is more continually present. Allergens that cause perennial rhinitis include animal dander, dust, and cockroach-derived proteins.

IX-8.   **The answer is A.** *(Chap. 319)* Antinuclear antibodies are nearly ubiquitous in patients with systemic lupus erythematosus, with demonstration in 90% of affected patients. There are many other antibodies that can be demonstrated. The next most common antibodies are anti-dsDNA and anti-histone. Anti-dsDNA is very specific to SLE and may correlate with disease activity, nephritis, and vasculitis. Antihistone is more frequent in drug-induced SLE. Antiphospholipid antibodies can be demonstrated in about half of affected patients, while the remainder is present in less than half of SLE cases.

IX-9.   **The answer is B.** *(Chap. 319)* There are well-published, strict diagnostic criteria for systemic lupus erythematosus. They include four or more of the following criteria from Table IX-9.

TABLE IX-9   Diagnostic Criteria for Systemic Lupus Erythematosus

Malar rash	Fixed erythema, flat or raised, over the malar eminences
Discoid rash	Erythematous circular raised patches with adherent keratotic scaling and follicular plugging; atrophic scarring may occur
Photosensitivity	Exposure to ultraviolet light causes rash
Oral ulcers	Includes oral and nasopharyngeal ulcers, observed by physician
Arthritis	Nonerosive arthritis of two or more peripheral joints, with tenderness, swelling, or effusion
Serositis	Pleuritis or pericarditis documented by ECG or rub, or evidence of effusion
Renal disorder	Proteinuria >0.5 g/d or ≥3+ by dipstick or cellular casts
Neurologic disorder	Seizures or psychosis without other causes
Hematologic disorder	Hemolytic anemia or leukopenia (<4000/μL) or lymphopenia (<1500/μL) or thrombocytopenia (<100,000/μL) in the absence of offending drugs
Immunologic disorder	Anti-dsDNA, anti-Sm, and/or antiphospholipid
Antinuclear antibodies	An abnormal titer of ANA by immunofluorescence or an equivalent assay at any point in time in the absence of drugs known to induce ANAs

If 4 or more of these criteria, well documented, are present at any time in a patient's history, the diagnosis is likely to be SLE. Specificity is approximately 95%; sensitivity is approximately 75%.
Abbreviations: ANA, antinuclear antibodies; dsDNA, double-strand DNA; ECG, electrocardiography.
Source: Criteria published by EM Tan et al: *Arthritis Rheum* 25:1271, 1982; update by MC Hochberg, *Arthritis Rheum* 40:1725, 1997.

The patient described does not meet the arthritis criteria; thus her only criteria are oral ulcers and weakly positive ANA.

IX-10.   **The answer is A.** *(Chap. 319)* The patient has Libman-Sacks endocarditis associated with her SLE. This results in fibrinous endocarditis and can lead to valvular insufficiencies, most often mitral or aortic, or embolism. It is not generally found with concomitant pericarditis, though this is another common cardiac manifestation of systemic lupus erythematosus. Although glucocorticoids and anti-inflammatory therapies have no proven benefit in this condition, they are often used in conjunction with supportive care. Because Libman-Sacks endocarditis is a culture-negative endocarditis and is not thought to be due to microbial infection, blood cultures will not be positive.

IX-11.   **The answer is D.** *(Chap. 319)* Systemic lupus erythematosus is a multisystem disease with diverse organ involvement and multiple different manifestations within an organ system. The system most commonly involved is the musculoskeletal system, with 95% of patients having involvement, usually as arthralgias or myalgias. Arthritis is also common and is one of the diagnostic criteria for SLE. Cutaneous and hematologic disease occurs in approximately 80–85% of patients. Neurologic and cardiopulmonary diseases affect approximately 60% of patients, while renal and gastrointestinal diseases occur in less than 50% of cases.

IX-12.   **The answer is E.** *(Chap. 319)* Although most clinicians believe that females with SLE should not become pregnant if they have active disease or advanced renal or cardiac disease, the presence of SLE itself is not an absolute contraindication to pregnancy. The outcome of pregnancy is best for females who are in remission at the time of conception. Even in females with quiescent disease, exacerbations may occur (usually in the first trimester and the immediate postpartum period), and 25–40% of these pregnancies end in spontaneous abortion. Fetal loss rates are higher in patients with lupus anticoagulant or anticardiolipin antibodies. Flare-ups should be anticipated and vigorously treated with steroids. Steroids given throughout pregnancy usually have no adverse effects on the child. In this case, the fact that the female had a life-threatening bout of disease a year ago would argue against stopping her drugs at this time. Neonatal lupus, which is manifested by thrombocytopenia, rash, and heart block, is rare but can occur when mothers have anti-Ro antibodies.

IX-13. **The answer is C.** *(Chap. 319)* This patient is presenting with acute lupus nephritis with evidence of hematuria, proteinuria, and an acute rise in creatinine. Together with infection, nephritis is the most common cause of mortality in the first decade after diagnosis of SLE and warrants prompt immunosuppressive therapy. It is important to assess for other potentially reversible causes of acute renal insufficiency, but this patient is not otherwise acutely ill and is taking no medications that would cause renal failure. The urinalysis shows evidence of active nephritis with hematuria and proteinuria. Even in the absence of RBC casts, therapy should not be withheld to await biopsy results in someone with a known diagnosis of SLE with consistent clinical presentation and urinary findings. This patient also has other risk factors known to predict the development of lupus nephritis, including high titers of anti-dsDNA and African-American race. The mainstay of treatment for any life-threatening or organ-threatening manifestation of SLE is high-dose systemic glucocorticoids. Addition of cytotoxic or other immunosuppressive agents (cyclophosphamide, azathioprine, mycophenolate mofetil) is recommended to treat serious complications of SLE, but their effects are delayed for 3–6 weeks after initiation of therapy, whereas the effects of glucocorticoids begin within 24 hours. Thus, these agents alone should not be used to treat acute, serious manifestations of SLE. The choice of cytotoxic agent is at the discretion of the treating physician. Cyclophosphamide in combination with steroid therapy has been demonstrated to prevent the development of end-stage renal disease better than steroids alone. Likewise, mycophenolate also prevents the development of end-stage renal disease in combination with glucocorticoids, and some studies suggest that African Americans have a greater response to mycophenolate than to cyclophosphamide. Plasmapheresis is not indicated in the treatment of lupus nephritis but is useful in cases of severe hemolytic anemia or thrombotic thrombocytopenic purpura associated with SLE. This patient has no acute indication for hemodialysis and, with treatment, may recover renal function.

IX-14. **The answer is E.** *(Chap. 319)* This patient clearly has a flare of her SLE induced by ultraviolet sunlight, a common inciting factor for lupus flares. It is thought that the UV sunlight induces skin apoptosis that initiates the SLE flare. Furthermore, this patient has severe acute lupus nephritis. Aggressive therapy with high-dose methylprednisolone is life saving and gives the best chance of renal recovery. Therapy for severe lupus derives from studies of lupus nephritis. These have shown that after a "pulse" of high-dose intravenous methylprednisolone, subsequent therapy with prednisone improves renal recovery. Studies of cytotoxic agents in lupus nephritis have been conducted in combination with corticosteroid treatment. These studies have shown that cyclophosphamide, mycophenolate mofetil, and azathioprine have efficiency for induction of improvement in severely ill patients. It appears that African Americans are more likely to respond to mycophenolate. Good improvement of lupus nephritis occurs in 80% of patients receiving cyclophosphamide or mycophenolate at 1–2 years; however, many patients have flares and are more likely to progress to end-stage renal disease. The utility of biologics, including rituximab, in SLE is under vigorous investigation. Some have advocated their use in patients with refractory disease based on open-label studies. Based on this patient's first episode of lupus nephritis, there would not be an indication for rituximab at this point.

IX-15. **The answer is A.** *(Chap. 320)* The patient has multiple clinical manifestations of arterial thrombosis in her hand and brain. Combined with the likely history of placental insufficiency in the three prior pregnancies, the possibility of antiphospholipid antibody syndrome is likely. In addition, she has evidence of acute kidney injury, suggesting multisystem disease. Thrombocytopenia may be due to hemolytic anemia, but the absence of schistocytes makes it less likely that she has thrombotic thrombocytopenic purpura. Although MRI of her brain and extremity duplex may confirm the presence of thrombosis, these will not diagnose antiphospholipid antibody syndrome. An anticardiolipin antibody screening panel will look for evidence of antibodies directed against cardiolipin and β_2 glycoprotein I. Additional testing for lupus anticoagulant determined by clotting assays such as the Russell viper venom time, false-positive RPR, and the aPTT may also be useful. Antinuclear antibody is likely to be positive given the common overlap with systemic lupus erythematosus, but is nonspecific.

IX-16. **The answer is D.** *(Chap. 320)* This patient has a typical presentation of antiphospholipid syndrome (APS) with a deep venous thrombosis (DVT), history of spontaneous abortion, and isolated elevated aPTT due to a lupus anticoagulant. Additional clinical features of APS involving the arterial or venous circulation include livedo reticularis (24%), pulmonary embolism (14%), stroke (20%), transient ischemic attack (TIA) (10%), myocardial infarction (10%), migraine (20%), preeclampsia (10%), thrombocytopenia (30%), and autoimmune hemolytic anemia (10%). Laboratory criteria include demonstration of lupus anticoagulant (elevated aPTT that does not correct on mixing) in conjunction with the presence of anticardiolipin and/or anti–β_2 glycoprotein I on two occasions 3 months apart. After diagnosis of a thrombotic event due to APS, patients should receive warfarin for life with a goal INR of 2.5–3.5 alone or in combination with daily aspirin. During pregnancy patients should receive heparin plus aspirin. Patients who develop recurrent thrombosis while on effective anticoagulation may benefit from a 5-day infusion of intravenous gamma globulin or 4 weeks of rituximab therapy. The optimal therapy for patients with APS without a thrombotic event is not known; however, daily aspirin (80 mg) protects patients with SLE and antiphospholipid antibodies from thrombotic events. Warfarin for 3 months with an INR goal of 2.0–3.0 is recommended therapy for DVT with a known reversible precipitating event. Warfarin for 6–12 months with an INR goal of 2.0–3.0 is recommended therapy for first-episode idiopathic DVT.

IX-17. **The answer is E.** *(Chap. 321)* Once the disease process of rheumatoid arthritis is established, the most common joints of involvement are the wrists, metacarpophalangeal joints, and proximal interphalangeal joints. Distal interphalangeal joint involvement is rarely due to rheumatoid arthritis and more often due to coexisting osteoarthritis.

IX-18. **The answer is C.** *(Chap. 321)* There is potential involvement of multiple organ systems in RA. The most common pulmonary complication is pleural effusion that is typically exudative and presents with chest pain and dyspnea. RA is associated with a form of diffuse interstitial lung disease that may present with dyspnea and bilateral interstitial infiltrates that may be extensive enough to develop into a honeycomb pattern. Pulmonary nodules associated with RA may be solitary or multiple. They often occur in conjunction with cutaneous nodules. Bronchiectasis and respiratory bronchiolitis may also be due to RA. Many of these manifestations respond to immunosuppressive therapy. Lobar infiltrate has not been described due to RA and is more commonly due to an acute infectious etiology, often as a complication of RA immunosuppressive therapy.

IX-19. **The answer is A.** *(Chap. 321)* Joint imaging is a critical tool for both the diagnosis and monitoring of disease status in RA. Plain radiographs, because of their ready availability and ease of film comparison, are most commonly ordered. The earliest clinical sign of RA is juxtaarticular osteopenia, though this may be difficult to appreciate on newer, digitized films. Other findings include soft-tissue swelling, symmetric joint space loss, and subchondral erosions most frequently in the wrists, metacarpophalangeal, and proximal interphalangeal joints, and the metatarsophalangeal joint.

IX-20. **The answer is C.** *(Chap. 321)* The prevalence of RA is 0.8%, and females are three times more likely to be affected than males. However, as the population ages, the prevalence increases and the sex difference diminishes. RA is found throughout the world and affects people of all races. Age of onset is most commonly 35–50 years. Family studies show a clear genetic predisposition. First-degree relatives have approximately four times the expected rate of RA. Other risk factors for RA include the class II major histocompatibility antigen HLA-DR4. Approximately 70% of patients with RA have HLA-DR4. However, this association is not true in Africans or African Americans, among whom 75% do not show this allele. The role of this allele in the pathogenesis of RA remains unknown because the cause of RA is unknown. The earliest lesion in RA is microvascular injury with an increase in the number of synovial lining cells. Increased numbers of mononuclear cells are seen in the synovial lining, and this is thought to be under the control of CD4$^+$ T lymphocytes. As the inflammation continues, the articular matrix is degraded by collagenases and cathepsins produced by the inflammatory cells. Other cytokines produced by the inflammatory cells include IL-1 and TNF-α. Over time, bone and cartilage are destroyed, leading to the end-stage clinical manifestations. Rheumatoid factor (RF) is an IgM molecule directed against the Fc portion of IgG and is found in two-thirds of patients with RA. However, this molecule is found in approximately 5% of healthy persons and more than 10% of persons older than age 60. It is not known to have a role in the pathogenesis of the disease, but titers of RF are shown to be predictive of the severity of clinical manifestations or the presence of extraarticular manifestations.

IX-21. **The answer is C.** *(Chap. 321)* Rheumatoid arthritis is chronic, symmetric, inflammatory polyarthritis. In two-thirds of patients, an initial clinical presentation of fatigue, anorexia, and weakness precedes joint complaints. In established RA (i.e., in patients known to be diagnosed with this disorder), the most common manifestation is pain in affected joints that is worsened by movement. Morning stiffness of an hour or more is very common in these patients as well, but it is worth noting that this clinical finding does not allow differentiation between inflammatory and noninflammatory arthritides. Arthritic pain comes from the joint capsule itself, which is innervated and very sensitive to distention. Ten percent of patients with RA will have a first-degree relative with the disease. Weight loss is a nonspecific symptom and is not definitively associated with active disease.

IX-22. **The answer is E.** *(Chap. 321)* Anemia is common in RA and parallels the degree of inflammation as measured by C-reactive protein or ESR. Felty's syndrome, typically occurring in late-stage, poorly controlled disease, is characterized by the triad of neutropenia, splenomegaly, and rheumatoid nodules. Rheumatoid vasculitis is not common and typically occurs in long-standing disease. It is associated with hypocomplementemia. The cutaneous signs are typical of vasculitic lesions with palpable purpura, digital infarcts, livedo reticularis, and ulcers. Clinical manifestations of pericarditis occur in 10% of patients, with echocardiographic or autopsy findings in about half of those cases. Secondary Sjögren's syndrome manifest as keratoconjunctivitis sicca or xerostomia occurs in approximately 10% of patients with RA. RA also appears to increase the risk of developing B-cell lymphoma by two to four times in the general population. The risk of lymphoma appears to correlate with high levels of disease activity or the presence of Felty's syndrome. Platelet counts in RA are typically elevated in association with the acute phase response of inflammation. Immune thrombocytopenia is rare.

IX-23. **The answer is D.** *(Chap. 321)* The therapy of RA has changed dramatically in the past two decades with the development of drugs that modify the disease course of RA. Methotrexate is the DMARD of first choice for treatment of early RA. Other conventional DMARDs include hydroxychloroquine, sulfasalazine, and leflunomide. Leflunomide, an inhibitor of pyrimidine synthesis, is efficacious as a single agent or in combination with methotrexate. Hydroxychloroquine and sulfasalazine are typically reserved for mild disease. The biologic DMARDs have dramatically improved the treatment of RA in the past decade. There are currently five anti-TNF agents, including infliximab, approved for use in patients with RA. Rituximab, an anti-CD20 antibody, is approved for refractory RA in combination with methotrexate. It is more efficacious in seropositive than seronegative patients. Other biologics approved for use in RA include anakinra (IL-1 receptor antagonist), abatacept (CD28/CD80/86 antagonist), and tocilizumab (IL-6 antagonist). Nonsteroidal anti-inflammatory drugs, including Naprosyn (naproxen), were formally utilized as core RA therapy; however, they are now utilized as adjunctive treatment for symptom management.

IX-24. **The answer is D.** *(Chap. 322)* Acute rheumatic fever (ARF) is almost universally due to group A streptococcal disease at the present time, though virtually all streptococcal disease may be capable of precipitating rheumatic fever. Although skin infections may be associated with rheumatic fever, far and away the most common presentation is with preceding pharyngitis. There is a latent period of approximately 3 weeks from an episode of sore throat to presentation of ARF. The most common manifestations are fever and polyarthritis, with polyarthritis being present in 60–75% of cases. Carditis may also be present, though somewhat less frequently in 50–60% of cases. Chorea and indolent carditis may have a subacute presentation. Chorea is present in 2–30% of affected individuals, while erythema marginatum and subcutaneous nodules are rare. Sixty percent of patients with ARF progress to rheumatic heart disease, with the endocardium, pericardium, and myocardium all potentially involved. All patients with ARF should receive antibiotics sufficient to treat the precipitating group A streptococcal infection.

IX-25.   **The answer is D.** *(Chap. 322)* This patient has a history very suggestive of recurrent bouts of ARF with evidence of mitral regurgitation, mitral stenosis, and aortic regurgitation on physical examination. This and the presence of atrial fibrillation imply severe rheumatic heart disease. Risk factors for this condition include poverty and crowded living conditions. As a result, ARF is considerably more common in the developing world. Daily aspirin is the treatment of choice for the migratory large-joint arthritis and fever that are common manifestations of ARF. Practitioners sometimes use steroids during acute bouts of carditis to quell inflammation, though this remains a controversial practice and has no role between flares of ARF. Secondary prophylaxis with either daily oral penicillin or, preferably, monthly IM injections is considered the best method to prevent further episodes of ARF, and therefore prevent further valvular damage. Primary prophylaxis with penicillin on an as-needed basis is equally effective for preventing further bouts of carditis. However, most episodes of sore throat are too minor for patients to present to a physician. Therefore, secondary prophylaxis is considered preferable in patients who already have severe valvular disease. Doxycycline is not a first-line agent for group A *Streptococcus*, the pathogen that incites ARF.

IX-26.   **The answer is A.** *(Chap. 323)* The prognosis for patients with scleroderma renal disease is poor. In SRC patients prompt treatment with an ACE inhibitor may reverse acute renal failure. In recent studies the initiation of ACE inhibitor therapy resulted in 61% of patients having some degree of renal recovery and not needing chronic dialysis support. The survival rate is estimated to be 80–85% at 8 years. Among patients who needed dialysis, when treated with ACE inhibitors, over 50% were able to discontinue dialysis after 3–18 months. Therefore, ACE inhibitors should be used even if the patient requires dialysis support.

IX-27.   **The answer is D.** *(Chap. 324)* The patient presented with classic symptoms for Sjögren's syndrome including dry mouth and eyes. This condition may be primary, as in this case, or secondary in association with another connective tissue disease such as scleroderma or rheumatoid arthritis. Many autoantibodies may be demonstrated in the serum of patients with Sjögren's including antibodies to Ro/SS-A or La/SS-b. Sialometry will demonstrate decreased production of saliva, and MRI or MR sialography of the major salivary glands is used also. Ocular involvement with decreased tear production is demonstrated by the Schirmer's I test. Scl-70 antibody is associated with scleroderma and should not be positive in primary Sjögren's syndrome.

IX-28.   **The answer is A.** *(Chap. 324)* Although Sjögren's syndrome most commonly affects the eyes and mouth, there are a number of common extraglandular sites of involvement. The most common is arthritis or arthralgias that complicated up to 60% of cases. Raynaud's phenomenon is the second most common extraglandular site. Lung involvement and vasculitis are found in less than 20% of patients. Lymphoma, though a concerning and highly morbid complication, is relatively rare, affecting only 6% of patients with Sjögren's syndrome.

IX-29.   **The answer is B.** *(Chap. 324)* The patient in this vignette is presenting with severely dry eyes and mouth in the presence of autoantibodies to Ro and La (SS-A and SS-B, extractable nuclear and cytoplasmic antigens) consistent with the diagnosis of Sjögren's syndrome. This autoimmune disorder is associated with the lymphocytic infiltration of exocrine glands that results in decreased tear and saliva production as the most prominent symptoms. Sjögren's syndrome affects women nine times more frequently than men and usually presents in middle age. Other autoimmune diseases often have associated xerostomia and dry eyes (secondary Sjögren's syndrome). High titers of antibodies to Ro and La are associated with longer disease duration, salivary gland enlargement, and the development of extraglandular involvement, especially cutaneous vasculitis and demyelinating syndromes. One-third of patients with Sjögren's syndrome have extraglandular involvement of the disease, most commonly in the lungs and kidneys. In this patient with acidemia and hypokalemia, the possibility of renal disease due to Sjögren's syndrome should be considered. Interstitial nephritis is a common manifestation of Sjögren's syndrome in the kidneys. Distal (type I) renal tubular acidosis is also frequent, occurring in 25% of individuals with Sjögren's syndrome. Diagnosis could be confirmed by obtaining urine electrolytes to demonstrate a positive urine anion gap. Renal biopsy is not necessary. Treatment does not require immunosuppression as the acidemia can be treated with bicarbonate replacement. Diarrhea could cause similar electrolyte abnormalities with a non–anion gap acidosis, but the patient would be symptomatic. Furthermore, gastrointestinal symptoms do not commonly occur in Sjögren's syndrome. Hypoaldosteronism is associated with a type IV renal tubular acidosis that results in hyperkalemia and a non–anion gap acidosis. Renal compensation for respiratory alkalosis should not result in hypokalemia. Purging in anorexia nervosa could result in hypokalemia and increased risk of dental caries, but it would be associated with metabolic alkalosis rather than acidosis.

IX-30.   **The answer is D.** *(Chap. 324)* Lymphoma is well known to develop specifically in the late stage of Sjögren's syndrome. Common manifestations of this malignant condition include persistent parotid gland enlargement, purpura, leukopenia, cryoglobulinemia, and low C4 complement levels. Most of the lymphomas are extranodal, marginal zone B cell, and low grade. Low-grade lymphomas may be detected incidentally during a labial biopsy. Mortality is higher in patients with concurrent B symptoms (fevers, night sweats, and weight loss), a lymph node mass greater than 7 cm, and a high or intermediate histologic grade.

IX-31.   **The answer is D.** *(Chap. 325)* Ankylosing spondylitis is closely correlated with the presence of the histocompatibility antigen HLA-B27. In North American whites, the prevalence of B27 is 7%, but in patients with ankylosing spondylitis it is 90%. Not all persons with B27 develop ankylosing spondylitis; the disease is only present in 1–6% of B27-positive individuals.

IX-32.   **The answer is A.** *(Chap. 325)* Although the most serious spine complication of ankylosing spondylitis is fracture, there are a number of important extraarticular manifestations. Anterior uveitis is the most common, occurring in 40% of patients with ankylosing spondylitis. Inflammatory bowel disease has been reported to be frequently present. Less common complications include aortic insufficiency, third-degree heart block, pulmonary nodules and upper lobe fibrosis, cardiac dysfunction, retroperitoneal fibrosis, prostatitis, and amyloidosis.

IX-33.   **The answer is B.** *(Chap. 325)* Nonsteroidal anti-inflammatory drugs are the first line of pharmacologic therapy for ankylosing spondylitis, of which this patient has a classic presentation. These agents have been shown to reduce pain and tenderness and increase mobility. There is even some evidence that they slow disease progression. Given their proven efficacy, tolerability, and safety, they remain first-line therapy. Anti–TNF-α agents have been reported to have dramatic effects in ankylosing spondylitis, with infliximab, etanercept, adalimumab, and golimumab having published reports of success. Because of their potential side effects, including serious infections, hypersensitivity reactions, and others, these agents should be reserved for patients who fail therapy with NSAIDs.

IX-34.   **The answer is E.** *(Chap. 325)* Reactive arthritis refers to an acute, nonpurulent arthritis that occurs after an infection elsewhere in the body. Often presenting with lower joint inflammatory arthritis occurring 1–4 weeks after a diarrheal episode, reactive arthritis may also include uveitis or conjunctivitis, dactylitis, urogenital lesions, and characteristic mucocutaneous lesions such as keratoderma blennorrhagica. The most common organism associated with reactive arthritis is *Shigella* species, although *Yersinia*, *Chlamydia*, and, to a much lesser extent, *Salmonella* and *Campylobacter* have been described.

IX-35. **The answer is D.** *(Chap. 325)* The patient has a spondyloarthritic syndrome with enthesitis and sacroiliitis associated with inflammatory bowel disease. This is a common association called enteropathic arthritis. Generally, enteropathic arthritis responds well to suppression of gastrointestinal disease using anti–TNF-α agents such as infliximab. Other treatments for inflammatory bowel disease are also effective in the resolution of arthritis, such as glucocorticoids and sulfasalazine. NSAIDs may be helpful, but there is significant concern for the precipitation of flares of inflammatory bowel disease and precipitation of ulcers.

IX-36. **The answer is E.** *(Chap. 325)* Whipple's disease is a rare chronic bacterial infection of the gastrointestinal tract most commonly affecting middle-aged men. Arthritis is a common early manifestation of the disease, with arthritis predating gastrointestinal symptoms by 5 years or more. Large and small joints may be affected and sacroiliitis is common. Arthritis is often migratory and lasts several days with spontaneous recovery. Synovial fluid is generally inflammatory. Radiographs rarely show joint erosions, though sacroiliitis may be demonstrated. Diagnosis is often made by PCR amplification of genetic material from *Tropheryma whippelii* in biopsied material, most commonly the gut.

IX-37. **The answer is D.** *(Chap. 325)* Although anti–TNF-α drugs such as infliximab are potent and relatively safe, several types of side effects are not rare. These include serious infections such as disseminated tuberculosis, fungal (histoplasmosis, aspergillus, pneumocystis) and bacterial (legionella, pneumococcus) infections, hematologic disorders such as pancytopenia, demyelinating disorders, systemic lupus erythematosus-related autoantibodies, and potential risk of lymphoma. Additionally, clinical features such as exacerbation of congestive heart failure, hypersensitivity infusion or injection site reactions, and severe liver disease have been described. There are some isolated reports of hypersensitivity pneumonitis, but these are confounded by coadministration of known pulmonary toxic agents.

IX-38. **The answer is B.** *(Chap. 325)* Enthesopathy or enthesitis is the term used to describe inflammation at the site of tendinous or ligamentous insertion into bone. This type of inflammation is seen most frequently in patients with seronegative spondyloarthropathies and various infections, especially viral infections. The other definitions apply to other terms used in the orthopedic and rheumatic examination. Subluxation is the alteration of joint alignment so that articulating surfaces incompletely approximate each other. Synovitis refers to the inflammation of the periarticular membrane lining the joint capsule. Inflammation of a saclike cavity near a joint that decreases friction is the definition of bursitis. Finally, crepitus is a palpable vibratory or crackling sensation elicited with joint motion.

IX-39. **The answer is C.** *(Chap. 325)* This patient complains of symptoms consistent with a diagnosis of fibromyalgia. Patients with fibromyalgia frequently complain of diffuse body pain, stiffness, paresthesias, disturbed sleep, easy fatigability, and headache. The prevalence of fibromyalgia is approximately 3.4% of females and 0.5% of males. This disorder is thought to represent a disturbance of pain perception. Disturbed sleep with a loss of stage 4 sleep has been implicated as a factor in the pathogenesis of the disease. Serotonin levels in the cerebrospinal fluid have also commonly been seen and may play a role in the pathogenesis. A diagnosis of fibromyalgia is based on the American College of Rheumatology criteria, which combine symptoms and physical examination. The patient must exhibit diffuse pain in all areas of the body with tenderness to palpation at 11 of 18 designated tender point sites. These sites include the occiput, trapezius, cervical spine, lateral epicondyles, supraspinatus muscle, second rib, gluteus, greater trochanter, and knee. Digital palpation should be performed with a moderate degree of pressure. Examination of the joints shows no evidence of inflammatory arthropathy. There are no laboratory tests that are specific for the diagnosis. Positive antinuclear antibodies may be seen, but at the same frequency as in the normal population. HLA-B27 is found in 7% of the white population, but only 1–6% of people with HLA-B27 will develop ankylosing spondylitis. Radiograms are normal in these patients.

IX-40. **The answer is D.** *(Chap. 325)* This patient shows the typical features of psoriatic arthritis. Five to ten percent of patients with psoriasis will develop an arthritis associated with the rash. In 60–70% of cases, the rash precedes the diagnosis. However, another 15–20% of patients will have joint complaints as the presenting symptom of their psoriasis. The disease typically begins in the fourth or fifth decade of life. Psoriatic arthritis has varied joint presentations with five commonly described patterns of joint involvement: (1) arthritis of the distal interphalangeal (DIP) joints, (2) asymmetric oligoarthritis, (3) symmetric polyarthritis similar to RA, (4) axial involvement, and (5) arthritis mutilans with the typical "pencil in cup" deformity seen on hand radiography. Erosive joint disease ultimately develops in almost all these patients, and most of them become disabled. Nail changes are prominent in 90% of patients with psoriatic arthritis. Changes that are frequently seen include pitting, horizontal ridging, onycholysis, yellowish discoloration of the nail margins, and dystrophic hyperkeratosis. The diagnosis of psoriatic arthritis is primarily clinical. Thus, in patients with joint symptoms that precede the onset of rash, the diagnosis is frequently missed until dermatologic or nail changes develop. A family history of psoriasis is important to ascertain in any patient with an undiagnosed inflammatory polyarthropathy. The differential diagnosis of DIP arthritis is short; only osteoarthritis and gout are commonly seen in these joints. Radiography may show typical changes, particularly in patients with arthritis mutilans. Treatment is directed at both the rash and the joint disease simultaneously. Anti–TNF-α therapy has recently been shown to be helpful for both the dermatologic and joint manifestations of disease. Other treatments include methotrexate, sulfasalazine, cyclosporine, retinoic acid derivatives, and psoralen plus ultraviolet light.

IX-41. **The answer is E.** *(Chap. 326)* Although the molecular pathology of most vasculitic syndromes is poorly understood, the deposition of immune complexes is commonly thought to play an important role in vasculitis associated with Henoch-Schönlein purpura, cryoglobulinemic vasculitis associated with hepatitis C, serum sickness and cutaneous vasculitic syndromes, and polyarteritis nodosa–like vasculitis associated with hepatitis B. Granulomatosis with polyangiitis (Wegener's), Churg-Strauss, and microscopic polyangiitis are thought to be due to production of antineutrophilic antibodies. Pathogenic T lymphocyte responses are also implicated in giant cell arteritis, Takayasu's arteritis, granulomatosis with polyangiitis (Wegener's), and Churg-Strauss syndrome.

IX-42. **The answer is E.** *(Chap. 326)* ANCAs are antibodies directed at proteins in the cytoplasmic granules of neutrophils and monocytes. cANCA, or cytoplasmic ANCA, is directed against proteinase-3, a proteinase present in neutrophil azurophilic granules. More than 90% of patients with granulomatosis with polyangiitis (Wegener's) will be cANCA positive. Perinuclear ANCA or pANCA refers to a more localized perinuclear staining pattern and antibodies are most commonly directed against myeloperoxidase, though other antigens have been described. pANCA has been reported in variable percentages in microscopic polyangiitis, Churg-Strauss syndrome, and granulomatosis with polyangiitis (Wegener's) and its variants. Additionally, pANCA staining that is not due to antimyeloperoxidase antibodies has been described in a number of other conditions including rheumatic and nonrheumatic autoimmune disease and inflammatory bowel disease.

IX-43. **The answer is D.** *(Chap. 326)* The patient presents with classic symptoms for granulomatosis with polyangiitis (Wegener's), also known as granulomatosis with polyangiitis. The average age of diagnosis is 40 years and there is a male predominance. Upper respiratory symptoms often predate lung or renal findings and may even present with septal perforation. The diagnosis is made by demonstration of necrotizing granulomatous vasculitis on biopsy. Pulmonary tissue offers the highest yield. Biopsy of the upper airway usually shows the granulomatous inflammation but infrequently shows vasculitis. Renal biopsy may show the presence of pauci-immune glomerulonephritis.

IX-44. **The answer is C.** *(Chap. 326)* The patient has a classic presentation for giant cell arteritis with associated polymyalgia rheumatica including headache, jaw claudication, and visual disturbances. Her age makes this diagnosis highly likely as well. The diagnosis is confirmed by temporal artery biopsy; however, in the presence of visual symptoms, initiation of therapy should not be delayed pending a biopsy, as the biopsy may be positive even after approximately 14 days of glucocorticoid therapy. Delay in therapy risks irreversible visual loss. Additionally, a dramatic response to therapy may lend further support to the diagnosis. The primary therapy is prednisone at 40–60 mg daily for 1 month with gradual tapering. Although erythrocyte sedimentation rate is nearly universally elevated, it is not specific for the diagnosis. Temporal artery ultrasound may be suggestive but is not diagnostic.

IX-45. **The answer is C.** *(Chap. 326)* The most common manifestations of cryoglobulinemic vasculitis are cutaneous vasculitis, arthritis, peripheral neuropathy, and glomerulonephritis. The demonstration of circulating cryoprecipitates is a critical component of the diagnosis, and often rheumatoid factor can be found as well. Because hepatitis C infection is present in the vast majority of patients with cryoglobulinemic vasculitis, infection should be sought in all patients with this clinical syndrome.

IX-46. **The answer is E.** *(Chap. 326)* This patient has polyarteritis nodosa associated with hepatitis B infection. Polyarteritis nodosa (PAN) is a small- and medium-vessel vasculitis that classically involves the muscular mesenteric and renal arteries. Pulmonary arteries are spared. Classic PAN is a rare disease, but its exact prevalence is unknown because reported cases frequently also include other vasculitides such as microscopic polyangiitis. Prior to the Chapel Hill Consensus Conference of 1992, microscopic polyangiitis and PAN were considered as the same disease, but it has been recognized that these are two separate diseases with different serologic markers and vascular predilection. Clinical manifestations of PAN are commonly vague, and often patients have been ill for several months prior to diagnosis. Symptoms include fatigue, weight loss, abdominal pain, headache, and hypertension. The pathologic lesion of PAN is necrotizing inflammation of the small- and medium-sized muscular arteries, and diagnosis relies on demonstration of this lesion on biopsy. However, in the absence of easily obtainable tissue, the presence of multiple aneurysmal dilatations on mesenteric angiogram is highly suggestive of PAN in the appropriate clinical setting. There are no serologic tests that are diagnostic of PAN. It is rare to have positive antibodies to pANCA or cANCA in PAN. Interestingly, 30% of cases of PAN are associated with active hepatitis B infection, as in this patient, and it is thought that circulating immune complexes may play a role in the pathogenesis of this disease. Unlike PAN, microscopic polyangiitis (MPA) involves venules and capillaries in addition to small arteries. The histopathologic lesion of MPA is a necrotizing vasculitis that is pauci immune with minimal deposition of immune complexes. Typical presenting features are rapidly progressive glomerulonephritis and pulmonary hemorrhage, which are distinctly uncommon features of PAN. Antimyeloperoxidase antibodies (pANCA) are frequently present. Mixed cryoglobulinemia is a small-vessel vasculitis most often associated with hepatitis C infection. Skin involvement with leukocytoclastic vasculitis and palpable purpura are the most common presenting features. Proliferative glomerulonephritis is present in 20–60% of individuals and is the most common cause of morbidity. Ischemic colitis typically presents with abdominal pain out of proportion to the examination as in this case, but the mesenteric angiogram would show atherosclerotic narrowing rather than aneurysmal dilatation. Hepatocellular carcinoma is not associated with vasculitis and typically presents with vague abdominal pain and obstructive jaundice.

IX-47. **The answer is C.** *(Chap. 326; JW Newberger et al: Circulation 110:2747, 2004.)* The most likely cause of the acute coronary syndrome in this patient is thrombosis of a coronary artery aneurysm in an individual with a past history of Kawasaki disease. Kawasaki disease is an acute multisystem disease that primarily presents in children less than 5 years of age. The clinical manifestations in childhood are nonsuppurative cervical lymphadenitis; desquamation of the fingertips; and erythema of the oral cavity, lips, and palms. Approximately 25% of cases are associated with coronary artery aneurysms that occur late in illness in the convalescent stage. Early treatment (within 7–10 days of onset) with IV immunoglobulin and high-dose aspirin decreases the risk of developing coronary aneurysms to about 5%. Even if coronary artery aneurysms develop, most regress over the course of the first year if the size is smaller than 6 mm. Aneurysms larger than

8 mm, however, are unlikely to regress. Complications of persistent coronary artery aneurysms include rupture, thrombosis and recanalization, and stenosis at the outflow area. Dissection of the aortic root and coronary ostia is a common cause of death in Marfan's syndrome and can also be seen with aortitis due to Takayasu's arteritis. In this patient, there is no history of hypertension, limb ischemia, or systemic symptoms that would suggest an active vasculitis. In addition, there are no other ischemic symptoms that would be expected in Takayasu's arteritis. Myocardial bridging overlying a coronary artery is seen frequently at autopsy but is an unusual cause of ischemia. The possibility of cocaine use as a cause of myocardial ischemia in a young individual must be considered, but given the clinical history it is a less likely cause of ischemia in this case.

IX-48. **The answer is C.** *(Chap. 327)* Recurrent oral ulceration is required for the diagnosis of Behçet's disease. The ulcers may be single or multiple, are shallowly based with a yellow necrotic base, and are painful. They are generally small, less than 10 mm in diameter. The diagnosis of Behçet's also requires two of the following: recurrent genital ulceration, eye lesions, skin lesions, and pathergy test. Nonspecific skin inflammatory reactivity to any scratches or intradermal saline injection (pathergy test) is common and specific.

IX-49 and IX-50. **The answers are A and C, respectively.** *(Chap. 327)* Behçet's syndrome is a multisystem disorder of uncertain cause that is marked by oral and genital ulcerations and ocular involvement. This disorder affects males and females equally and is more common in persons of Mediterranean, Middle Eastern, and Far Eastern descent. Approximately 50% of these persons have circulating autoantibodies to human oral mucosa. The clinical features are quite varied. The presence of recurrent aphthous ulcerations is essential for the diagnosis. Most of these patients have primarily oral ulcerations, although genital ulcerations are more specific for the diagnosis. The ulcers are generally painful, can be shallow or deep, and last for 1–2 weeks. Other skin involvement may occur, including folliculitis, erythema nodosum, and vasculitis. Eye involvement is the most dreaded complication because it may progress rapidly to blindness. It often presents as panuveitis, iritis, retinal vessel occlusion, or optic neuritis. This patient also presents with superficial venous thrombosis. Superficial and deep venous thromboses are present in one-fourth of these patients. Neurologic involvement occurs in up to 10%. Laboratory findings are nonspecific with elevations in the erythrocyte sedimentation rate and the white blood cell count. Treatment varies with the extent of the disease. Patients with mucous membrane involvement alone may respond to topical steroids. In more serious or refractory cases, thalidomide is effective. Other options for mucocutaneous disease include colchicines and intralesional interferon α. Ophthalmologic or neurologic involvement requires systemic glucocorticoids and azathioprine or cyclosporine. Life span is usually normal unless neurologic disease is present. Ophthalmic disease frequently progresses to blindness.

IX-51. **The answer is C.** *(Chap. 328)* Relapsing polychondritis is a disease of unknown cause characterized by inflammation of the cartilage predominantly in the ears, nose, and laryngotracheobronchial tree. Although it may be a primary disorder, relapsing polychondritis is often associated with a number of other conditions including systemic vasculitis, systemic lupus erythematosus, Sjögren's syndrome, spondyloarthritides, Behçet's disease, inflammatory bowel disease, primary biliary cirrhosis, and myelodysplastic syndrome. It is not associated with scleroderma, which causes distinct skin changes that are typically not inflammatory and are not associated with cartilaginous inflammatory disease.

IX-52. **The answer is E.** *(Chap. 328)* Relapsing polychondritis most often presents with recurrent painful swelling of the ear. Although other cartilaginous sites may be involved such as the nose and the tracheobronchial tree, these are less frequent. Episodes of ear involvement may result in floppy ears. Typically the pinna is affected while the earlobe is spared, as there is no cartilage in the lobe. Cogan's syndrome is a rare vasculitic syndrome involving hearing loss, but cartilage inflammation is not a feature. Recurrent trauma or irritation is a consideration but the history is not suggestive, and would be less likely to be bilateral and accompanied by inflammatory findings and a relatively spared ear lobe.

IX-53. The answer is A. *(Chap. 329)* The finding of noncaseating granulomas is highly suggestive of sarcoidosis, but not confirmatory. To make a specific diagnosis, two or more organs must be affected; however, a suggestive radiograph and positive biopsy are often adequate. Prior to a definitive diagnosis, however, other conditions that may cause noncaseating granulomas should be ruled out. These include beryllium exposure, often in workers in the nuclear industry; atypical mycobacterial infection; and fungal infection such as histoplasmosis. Many malignancies, including testes, and a number of lymphomas may have granulomas, particularly in reactive areas near tumor deposits. Adequate tissue sampling must be ensured to rule out malignancy. Pulmonary alveolar proteinosis is a disease characterized by PAS-positive protein deposits in the alveolar spaces. It is not typically associated with acute or chronic inflammation in the absence of secondary infection.

IX-54. The answer is A. *(Chap. 329)* Hypercalcemia and/or hypercalciuria occurs in approximately 10% of patients with sarcoidosis and is thought to be due to increased production of 1, 25-dihydroxyvitamin D by the granuloma itself, with resultant increased gut calcium absorption. Sun and exogenous vitamin D can exacerbate the problem. Because of this, renal calculi are relatively common. If a patient with sarcoidosis is to begin therapy with calcium supplementation, 24-hour urine for calcium excretion should be performed before and after initiation of therapy. Often small doses of glucocorticoids are adequate to control this problem.

IX-55. The answer is A. *(Chap. 329)* The treatment of sarcoidosis depends on whether it is in the acute or chronic form. In many cases, acute disease without abnormalities of neurologic, cardiac, ocular, or metabolic systems may not require therapy. The mainstay of systemic therapy remains to be glucocorticoids. In the chronic form, treatment is dependent on the response to corticosteroids and the tolerability of tapering to low doses (<10 mg/d). Hydroxychloroquine has been shown to be effective in skin disease due to sarcoidosis. Methotrexate works in approximately two-thirds of patients, regardless of disease manifestations. Azathioprine is another cytotoxic agent that is often used in chronic disease, although the evidence in support of this therapy is mostly retrospective. Prospective studies of etanercept and infliximab in patients have shown that etanercept has a limited role as a steroid-sparing agent. In contrast, infliximab, when added to a regimen including prednisone and a cytotoxic agent, improved lung function. The difference in responses to these anti-TNF agents may have to do with the difference in mechanism (receptor antagonism vs. antibody).

IX-56. The answer is A. *(Chap. 329)* Sarcoidosis is often discovered on routine chest radiograph by the presence of bilateral hilar adenopathy, often in asymptomatic patients. The Scadding method of scoring the standard chest radiograph is still utilized despite CT being more sensitive. Stage 1 is hilar adenopathy (+/– right paratracheal adenopathy) alone; stage 2 is adenopathy plus parenchymal infiltrates; stage 3 is parenchymal infiltrates alone; and stage 4 is fibrosis. When parenchymal disease is present, the upper lobes often predominate in contrast to most other lung disorders. Skin involvement includes erythema nodosum, maculopapular lesions, hyper- and hypopigmentation, keloid formation, subcutaneous nodules, and lupus pernio. Erythema nodosum is usually seen in the acute form of sarcoidosis and often portends a positive prognosis. Liver involvement is difficult to assess. Granulomas may be seen in over 50% of liver biopsies in patients with sarcoidosis, but approximately 20% have evidence by laboratory studies. The typical pattern is an elevation of alkaline phosphatase typical of all forms of granulomatous hepatitis. There may be some accompanying elevation of transaminases. Eye disease is most commonly anterior uveitis, although posterior (retinal and pars planitis) involvement may occur. There is a marked racial difference in eye involvement due to sarcoidosis. In Japan, over 70% of patients have eye disease, whereas in the United States the prevalence is about 30% (with it being more common in African Americans than white Americans). Cardiac involvement varies dramatically by race. In the United States and Europe, less than 5% of patients develop cardiac disease, whereas in Japan the prevalence is over 25%. There is no difference between whites and African Americans. Cardiac manifestations are conduction and systolic dysfunction due to granulomatous inflammation and infiltration.

IX-57. **The answer is C.** *(Chap. 331)* Inflammatory arthritis can have a variety of causes, either acute or chronic, and affect single or multiple joints. Acute causes of inflammatory arthritis most commonly include infectious etiologies (*Neisseria gonorrhoeae*, septic arthritis, Lyme disease) and crystal-induced arthropathies (gout, pseudogout). Chronic inflammatory arthritis is more likely to be related to autoimmune diseases such as rheumatoid arthritis, reactive arthritis, or psoriatic arthritis. A frequent feature of inflammatory arthritis is the presence of morning stiffness. The stiffness of inflammatory arthritis is more severe after a prolonged rest period, which is why it is characteristically worse in the morning. The stiffness can persist as long as an hour or more, is quite severe, and improves with movement. In contrast, noninflammatory arthritis such as osteoarthritis is more typically associated with stiffness that occurs after a brief rest, lasts less than 60 minutes, and worsens with increased activity. Individuals with inflammatory arthritis also frequently have associated systemic symptoms such as fatigue, fever, rash, or weight loss. On physical examination, one should observe the affected joints for signs of inflammation including redness, swelling, warmth, and pain with movement. Nonspecific laboratory evidence of inflammation is often present, including elevation of erythrocyte sedimentation rate, C-reactive protein, and platelet count, anemia of chronic disease or hypoalbuminemia.

IX-58. **The answer is A.** *(Chap. 331)* Rotator cuff tendinitis or tear is a common cause of shoulder pain. The rotator cuff is formed by the tendons of four muscles that attach to the humerus. These muscles are responsible for stabilizing the humerus within the glenohumeral joint and are important in lifting and rotating the arm, especially in abduction. The muscles that comprise the rotator cuff are the supraspinatus, infraspinatus, teres minor, and subscapularis muscles. In young individuals, it is uncommon to have a complete tear of the rotator cuff unless there is trauma. In most cases, rotator cuff tendinitis is the more common cause of pain due to rotator cuff injuries. Rotator cuff tendinitis is demonstrated by pain with active, but not passive, abduction of the arm. Other symptoms of rotator cuff tendinitis include pain over the lateral deltoid muscle, night pain, and the impingement sign. The impingement sign is positive if pain is elicited with forward flexion of the arm at less than 180°. However, individuals who engage in activities that cause repetitive stress to the rotator cuff can develop tears in the tendons that would require surgery. Examples of such activities include baseball, rowing, and tennis. To evaluate for a tear of the rotator cuff, the arm is passively abducted and the individual is asked to maintain the arm in abduction. The test is positive if the individual is not able to maintain the arm at 90° of abduction. Pain with palpation over the bicipital groove is a sign of bicipital tendinitis. Pain with palpation anteriorly when the arm is rotated internally and externally is a sign of problems within the glenohumeral joint.

IX-59. **The answer is B.** *(Chap. 331)* This patient has degenerative arthritis. His obesity predisposes him to degenerative joint disease that will be worse in the large weight-bearing joints. The physical examination findings of decreased range of motion, crepitus, and varus deformity that is exacerbated on weight bearing are consistent with this diagnosis. The radiogram of the knee demonstrates narrowing of the joint space with osteophyte formation. Occasional effusions may be seen, especially after overuse injuries. The joint fluid analysis in patients with degenerative disease reveals a clear, viscous fluid with a white blood cell count less than 2000/μL. Positively birefringent crystals on polarizing light microscopy will be seen in pseudogout that most commonly affects the knee, whereas negatively birefringent crystals are characteristic of gout. Joint fluid in these inflammatory conditions would generally have a white blood cell count of less than 50,000/μL and is yellow and turbid in character. Septic arthritis presents with fevers and a very warm and tender joint. The joint fluid can have the appearance of frank pus and is opaque. The white blood cell count is usually higher than 50,000/μL and can have a positive Gram stain for organisms.

IX-60. **The answer is A.** *(Chap. 332)* Osteoarthritis (OA) is one of the most common causes of disability among older adults and is more common among women than men. OA characteristically affects some joints but spares others. The joints in the hands most commonly affected by OA are the distal and proximal interphalangeal joints and the base of the thumb. It is uncommon for OA to affect the wrist. In addition, OA also is more common in the hips, knees, and cervical and lumbosacral spine. The pain that occurs in OA occurs during or just after joint use, gradually resolving with rest. Thus, the pain of OA in the hands would be expected to be worse while preparing meals (option C) or sewing. The stiffness of OA is not prominent in the mornings as is common in inflammatory arthritis. Rather, stiffness in OA is most marked following brief periods of rest. It can also be associated with the gel phenomenon in which a joint can lock following brief rest periods. On physical examination of the hands of an individual with OA, one may note the presence of bony swellings of the distal and proximal interphalangeal joints. These are known as Heberden's and Bouchard's nodes, respectively. No blood tests are routinely required for the evaluation of OA when the history and physical examination are consistent with the diagnosis. If radiographs are performed, one would expect joint space narrowing due to loss of cartilage. In addition, osteophytes and bony enlargement can be seen. Findings of joint swelling, warmth, and erythema are more common in inflammatory causes of arthritis, and furthermore, it would be unlikely for OA to affect only the wrists.

IX-61. **The answer is A.** (*Chap. 332*) Osteoarthritis (OA) represents joint failure in which pathologic changes have occurred in all structures of the affected joint. The central pathology in OA is articular cartilage loss. The components leading to the development of OA can be separated into those that contribute to joint loading and those that increase joint vulnerability. The most potent risk factor for OA is aging, which affects joint vulnerability. Radiographic evidence of OA is rare in individuals younger than 40; however, more than 50% of individuals older than 70 will have changes of OA. A young joint has in place protective mechanisms that allow it to tolerate excessive loading without lasting damage. Specifically, the cartilage of younger joints is more responsive to dynamic loading, whereas older cartilage fails to respond, leading to breakdown of the cartilage matrix. Women are more susceptible to OA than men, especially after the sixth decade, but the relationship is not as strong as with aging and OA. Joint injury is a strong predictor of the future development of osteoarthritis. Obesity is a well-recognized risk factor in hip and knee arthritis likely due to increased loading forces. Obesity appears to play a role in OA of the hand as well, suggesting that obesity has both a mechanical and metabolic mechanism of action. The genetics of OA are not well understood. Inherited polymorphisms appear to play a role in hand and hip OA but not as much in other joints.

IX-62. **The answer is E.** (*Chap. 332*) This patient presents with symptoms suggestive of OA. OA is primarily a disease that is mechanically driven, and nonpharmacologic therapy should be a first-line treatment for disease that is mild or intermittent. Avoiding activities that cause pain and overload the joint, strengthening and conditioning the adjacent muscle groups, and supporting or unloading the joint with a brace or crutch are all examples of fundamental treatments aimed at reversing the pathophysiology of OA. In this patient, weight loss should be the primary goal of therapy. Each pound of weight increases loading across a weight-bearing joint three- to six-fold. This patient would benefit from a daily minimal-weight-bearing exercise regimen combined with nutritional goals aimed at slow, consistent weight loss. Avoidance of walking is impractical; a cane or supportive device to lessen the joint load can be offered. Steroids and narcotics are not indicated in this case.

IX-63. **The answer is C.** (*Chap. 333*) This individual has had three recent acute gout attacks and has risk factors for recurrence including chronic kidney disease and the need for diuretic therapy. In this setting, he demonstrates elevation of his uric acid levels. When considering initiation of hypouricemic therapy, one should consider the number of attacks, the serum uric acid levels outside of an acute attack, and the patient's willingness to commit to lifelong therapy. In addition, individuals with uric acid stones or tophaceous gout should also receive hypouricemic therapy. Current agents that are commonly used to treat hyperuricemia include uricosuric agents and xanthine oxidase inhibitors. Probenecid is the most commonly used uricosuric agent. It is started at a dose of 250 mg twice daily, but can be titrated as high as 3 g daily. However, it is generally not effective when the serum creatinine is greater than 2.0 mg/dL. Benzbromarone is a uricosuric agent that is more effective in individuals with renal failure, but it is not available in the United States. The medication most commonly prescribed in individuals with recurrent gout is allopurinol. This xanthine oxidase inhibitor lowers serum uric acid levels in overproducers, but has multiple associated toxicities including toxic epidermal necrolysis, bone marrow suppression, and renal failure. The initial starting dose is typically 300 mg daily and can be increased to as high as 800 mg daily. However, caution must be taken in individuals with renal failure. Febuxostat is a newer chemically unrelated xanthine oxidase inhibitor. It has been demonstrated to lower uric acid levels as effectively as allopurinol. The initial dose of febuxostat is 40–80 mg daily, and dose adjustment is not required in mild to moderate renal failure. Colchicine is a microtubule stabilizer that decreases inflammation in acute gout attacks. It does not affect levels of uric acid. However, it is commonly used as adjunctive therapy in individuals to prevent gout flares that occur as uric acid levels decline. Indomethacin is a nonsteroidal anti-inflammatory agent that is commonly used in acute gout flares. It does not have a role in the treatment of hyperuricemia or outside of the acute gout attack. Caution should be taken in using nonsteroidal anti-inflammatory drugs in individuals with renal insufficiency.

IX-64. **The answer is C.** (*Chap. 333*) Acute gouty arthritis is frequently seen in individuals on diuretic therapy. Diuretics result in hyperuricemia through enhanced urate reabsorption in the proximal tubule of the kidney in the setting of volume depletion. Hyperuricemia remains asymptomatic in many individuals but may manifest as acute gout. Acute gout is an intensely inflammatory arthritis that frequently begins at night. While any joint may be affected, the initial presentation of gout is often in the great toe at the metatarsophalangeal joint. There is associated joint swelling, effusion, erythema, and exquisite tenderness. A typical patient will complain that the pain is so great that he or she is unable to wear socks or allow sheets or blankets to cover the toes. Arthrocentesis will reveal an inflammatory cloudy-appearing fluid. The diagnosis of gout is confirmed by the demonstration of monosodium urate crystals seen both extracellularly and intracellularly within neutrophils. Monosodium urate crystals appear strongly negatively birefringent under polarized light microscopy and have a typical needle- and rod-shaped appearance. The WBC count is usually below 50,000/μL with values above 100,000/μL being more likely to be associated with a septic arthritis. Likewise, very low glucose levels and a positive Gram stain are not manifestations of acute gout but are common in septic arthritis. Calcium pyrophosphate dihydrate crystals appear as weakly positively birefringent rhomboidal crystals and are seen in pseudogout.

IX-65. **The answer is A.** (*Chap. 334*) This patient presents with a history consistent with a true septic arthritis due to gonococcal infection. Although gonococcal infection has generally declined in incidence in the past several decades, *Neisseria gonorrhoeae* is responsible for about 70% of acute infectious arthritis in individuals younger than 40 years. Women are two to three times more likely to develop disseminated gonococcal infection than men, likely related to the fact that asymptomatic cervical infection is more common in women. Women appear to be at greatest risk for disseminated gonococcal infection during menses or pregnancy. Disseminated gonococcal infection presents with fevers, chills, migratory arthritis and tenosynovitis, and a papular rash on the trunk and the extensor surfaces of the distal extremities. The rash can progress to hemorrhagic pustules. The joint symptoms and rash are thought to represent immune-complex deposition. In disseminated gonococcal infection, the synovial fluid from inflamed joints usually contains only 10,000–20,000 leukocytes/μL. In this setting, synovial cultures are negative and blood cultures are positive less than 45% of the time.

In this patient, there is evidence of a true septic arthritis with involvement of a single joint and a high leukocyte count (>50,000/μL). Septic arthritis due to *N. gonorrhoeae* is less common than disseminated gonococcal infection but always follows this syndrome. In the clinical scenario presented, the symptoms of fevers, chills, migratory arthralgias, and rash occurred 3 weeks prior to presentation with monoarticular septic arthritis. Blood cultures are almost always negative, and synovial fluid cultures are positive less than 40% of the time. The diagnostic procedure of choice is a culture of a potentially infected mucosal site, including the cervix, urethra, or pharynx.

Individuals with Lyme disease who are untreated frequently develop joint symptoms. Most commonly, this presents as waxing and waning episodes of mono- or oligoarthritis. Ten percent of individuals can develop an inflammatory erosive arthritis that leads to destructive disease of the joint if untreated. This patient's symptoms are not consistent with Lyme arthritis and testing for *Borrelia burgdorferi* is not indicated. Likewise, this patient presents with findings of monoarticular arthritis, which is not consistent with rheumatoid arthritis, and a rheumatoid factor is not indicated.

IX-66. **The answer is B.** (*Chap. 334*) Although the crystals suggest that the patient may have active pseudogout, the more important acute medical problem is septic arthritis. This is highly probable based on the joint leukocyte count above 100,000/μL, high percentage of PMNs, and positive Gram stain. Crystal-induced, rheumatoid, and other noninfectious causes of arthritis typically have WBC counts in the 30,000–50,000/μL range. WBC counts in indolent infections such as fungal or mycobacterial arthritis are commonly in the 10,000–30,000/μL range. The bacteria of septic arthritis usually enter the joint via hematogenous spread through synovial capillaries. Patients with rheumatoid arthritis are at high risk of a septic arthritis due to *Staphylococcus aureus* because of chronic inflammation and glucocorticoid therapy. The concurrent presence of pseudogout does not preclude the diagnosis of septic arthritis. In adults, the most common bacterial pathogens are *Neisseria gonorrhoeae* and *S. aureus*. Antibiotics, prompt surgical evaluation for drainage, and blood cultures to rule out bacteremia are all indicated. Prompt local and systemic treatment of infection can prevent the destruction of cartilage, joint instability, or deformity. Direct instillation of antibiotics into the joint fluid is not necessary. If the smear shows no organisms, a third-generation cephalosporin is reasonable empirical therapy. In the presence of gram-positive cocci in clusters, antistaphylococcal therapy should be instituted based on the community prevalence of methicillin resistance or recent hospitalization (which would favor empirical vancomycin). Typically, acute flairs of pseudogout can be addressed with glucocorticoids. However, this could portend a higher risk in the context of infection. Nonsteroidal anti-inflammatory agents might be a possibility depending on the patient's renal function and gastrointestinal history.

IX-67. **The answer is C.** (*Chap. 335*) This patient presents with a characteristic history for fibromyalgia, a diffuse pain syndrome associated with increased sensitivity to evoked pain. The underlying pathophysiology of pain in fibromyalgia is felt to be related to altered pain processing in the central nervous system. Epidemiologically, women are affected nine times more frequently than men. The worldwide prevalence of fibromyalgia is 2–3%, but in primary care practices it is as high as 5–10%. The disorder is even more common in patients with degenerative or inflammatory rheumatic disorders, with a prevalence of 20% or higher. The most common presenting complaint is diffuse pain that is difficult to localize. Pain is both above and below the waist and affects the extremities as well as the axial skeleton. However, it does not localize to a specific joint. The pain is noted to be severe in intensity, difficult to ignore, and interferes with daily functioning. While this patient demonstrates pain at several tender points, the American College of Rheumatology no longer includes tender point assessment in the diagnostic criteria for fibromyalgia. Rather, the new criteria focus on clinical symptoms of widespread pain and neuropsychological symptoms that have been present for at least 3 months. Some of the neuropsychological conditions that are frequently observed in fibromyalgia include sleep disturbance, impaired cognitive functioning, fatigue, stiffness, anxiety, and depression. The lifetime prevalence of mood disorders in patients with fibromyalgia is 80%. Sleep disturbances can include difficulty falling asleep, difficulty staying asleep, and nonrestorative sleep, among others.

IX-68. **The answer is D.** (*Chap. 335*) Fibromyalgia is a common disorder affecting 2–5% of the population. It presents as a diffuse pain syndrome with associated neuropsychological symptoms including depression, anxiety, fatigue, cognitive dysfunction, and disturbed sleep. Treatment for fibromyalgia should include a combination of non-pharmacologic and pharmacologic approaches. Patient education regarding the disease is important to provide a framework for understanding symptoms. The focus of treatment should not be on eliminating pain, but rather improving function and quality of life. Physical conditioning is an important part of improving function and should include a multifaceted exercise program with aerobic exercise, strength training, and exercises that incorporate relaxation techniques such as yoga or Tai Chi. Cognitive behavioral therapy can be useful in improving sleep disturbance and also in decreasing illness behaviors.

Pharmacologic therapy in fibromyalgia is targeted at the afferent and efferent pain pathways. The two most common categories of medications for fibromyalgia are antidepressants and anticonvulsants. Amitriptyline, duloxetine, and milnacipran have all been used with some efficacy in fibromyalgia. Duloxetine and milnacipran have been approved by the U.S. Food and Drug Administration for the treatment of fibromyalgia. The anticonvulsants that are predominantly used in fibromyalgia are those that are ligands of the α-2-δ subunit of voltage-gated calcium channels. These include gabapentin and pregabalin, which are also FDA approved for treatment of fibromyalgia.

Anti-inflammatory medications and glucocorticoids are not effective in fibromyalgia. However, if there is a comorbid triggering condition such as rheumatoid arthritis, appropriate therapy directed at the underlying disorder is critical to controlling symptoms of fibromyalgia as well. Opioid analgesics such as oxycodone should be avoided. They have no efficacy in treating fibromyalgia and may induce hyperalgesia that can worsen both pain and function.

IX-69.   **The answer is A.** *(Chap. 335)* Fibromyalgia is characterized by chronic widespread musculoskeletal pain, stiffness, paresthesia, disturbed sleep, and easy fatigability. It occurs in a 9:1 female-to-male ratio. It is not confined to any particular region, ethnicity, or climate. While the pathogenesis is not clear, there are associations with disturbed sleep and abnormal pain perception. Fibromyalgia is diagnosed by the presence of widespread pain, a history of widespread musculoskeletal pain that has been present for more than 3 months, and the presence of neuropsychological dysfunction (fatigue, waking unrefreshed, or cognitive symptoms). In the prior diagnostic criteria, it was required to demonstrate pain on palpation at 11 of 18 tender point sites. However, this was abandoned in the updated criteria because it was felt that strict application of a threshold of pain could lead to under-diagnosis of the disorder. Besides pain on palpation, the neurologic and musculoskeletal examinations are normal in patients with fibromyalgia. Psychiatric illnesses, particularly depression and anxiety disorders, are common comorbidities in these patients but do not help satisfy any diagnostic criteria.

IX-70.   **The answer is A.** *(Chap. 336)* The finding shown in Figure IX-70 is characteristic of clubbing. Clubbing occurs in the distal portions of the digits and is characterized by widening of the fingertips, convexity of the nail contour, and loss of the normal 15° angle between the proximal nail and cuticle. Clinically, it sometimes can be difficult to ascertain whether clubbing is present. One approach to the diagnosis of clubbing is to measure the diameter of the finger at the base of the nail and at the tip of the finger in all 10 fingers. For each finger, a ratio between the base of the nail and the tip of the finger is determined. If the sum of all 10 fingers is greater than 1, then clubbing is felt to be present. A simpler approach is to have an individual place the dorsal surfaces of the distal fourth digits from each hand together. In a normal individual, there should be a diamond shaped space between the digits. When an individual has clubbing, this space is obliterated.

Clubbing most commonly occurs in advanced lung disease, especially bronchiectasis, cystic fibrosis, and interstitial lung diseases like sarcoidosis or idiopathic pulmonary fibrosis. Clubbing was originally described in individuals with empyema and can occur in chronic lung infections, including lung abscess, tuberculosis, or fungal infections. Pulmonary vascular lesions and lung cancer also are associated with clubbing. However, chronic obstructive pulmonary disease does not cause clubbing.

The causes of clubbing are not limited, however, to the pulmonary system alone. Clubbing can be a benign familial condition and is also associated with a variety of other disorders. This includes cyanotic congenital heart disease, subacute bacterial endocarditis, Crohn's disease, ulcerative colitis, celiac disease, and cancer of the esophagus, liver, small bowel, and large bowel. In untreated hyperthyroidism clubbing can occur in association with periostitis in a condition called thyroid acropachy. While these numerous clinical associations have been described for many centuries, the cause of clubbing remains unknown.

IX-71.   **The answer is E.** *(Chap. 337)* Trochanteric bursitis is a common cause of hip pain and results from inflammation within the bursa that surrounds the insertion of the gluteus medius onto the greater trochanter of the femur. Bursae lie throughout the body with the purpose of facilitating movement of tendons and muscles over bony prominences. Bursitis has many causes including overuse, trauma, systemic disease, or infection. Trochanteric bursitis typically presents with acute or subacute hip pain with a varying quality. The pain localizes to the lateral aspect of the hip and upper thigh. Direct palpation over the posterior aspect of the greater trochanter reproduces the pain, and often sleeping on the affected side is painful. Pain is also elicited with external rotation and resisted abduction of the hip. Treatment of trochanteric bursitis includes the use of nonsteroidal anti-inflammatory medications and avoidance of overuse. If the pain persists, steroid injection into the affected bursa may be beneficial.

Other causes of hip pain include osteoarthritis, avascular necrosis, meralgia paresthetica, septic arthritis, occult hip fracture, and referred pain from lumbar spine disease. In patients with true disorders of the hip joint such as osteoarthritis, avascular necrosis, and occult hip fracture, the pain is most commonly localized to the groin area. Meralgia paresthetica (lateral femoral nerve entrapment syndrome) causes a neuropathic pain in the upper outer thigh with symptoms ranging from tingling sensations to a burning pain. When degenerative spinal disease is the cause of referred hip pain, there is typically back pain as well. In addition, palpation over the lateral joint would not reproduce the pain. Iliotibial band syndrome causes lateral knee pain but not hip pain.

IX-72.   **The answer is B.** *(Chap. 337)* The iliotibial band is comprised of thick connective tissue that runs along the outer thigh from the ilium to the fibula. When this band becomes tightened or inflamed, pain most commonly occurs where the band passes over the lateral femoral condyle of the knee, leading to a burning or aching pain in this area that can radiate toward the outer thigh. This overuse injury is most often seen in runners and can be caused by improperly fitted shoes, running on uneven surfaces, and excessive running. It is also more common in individuals with a varus alignment of the knee (bowlegged). Treatment of iliotibial band syndrome includes rest, NSAIDs, physical therapy, and addressing risk factors such as poorly fitted shoes or running on uneven surfaces. Glucocorticoid injection at the lateral femoral condyle may alleviate pain, but running must strictly be avoided for 2 weeks following injection. In refractory cases, surgical release of the iliotibial band may be beneficial.

IX-73.   **The answer is A.** *(Chap. 337)* Adhesive capsulitis is characterized by pain and restricted motion of the shoulder. Usually this occurs in the absence of intrinsic shoulder disease, including osteoarthritis and avascular necrosis. It is, however, more common in patients who have had bursitis or tendinitis previously, as well as patients with other systemic illnesses, such as chronic pulmonary disease, ischemic heart disease, and diabetes mellitus. The etiology is not clear, but adhesive capsulitis appears to develop in the setting of prolonged immobility. Reflex sympathetic dystrophy may also occur in the setting of adhesive capsulitis. Clinically, this disorder is more commonly seen in females over age 50. Pain and stiffness develop over the course of months to years. On physical examination, the affected joint is tender to palpation, with a restricted range of motion. The gold standard for diagnosis is arthrography with limitation of the amount of injectable contrast to less than 15 mL. In most patients, adhesive capsulitis will regress spontaneously within 1–3 years. NSAIDs, glucocorticoid injections, physical therapy, and early mobilization of the arm are useful therapies.

IX-74. **The answer is B.** *(Chap. 331)* Inflammation of the abductor pollicis longus and the extensor pollicis brevis at the radial styloid process tendon sheath is known as De Quervain's tenosynovitis. Repetitive twisting of the wrist can lead to this condition. Pain occurs when grasping with the thumb and can extend radially along the wrist to the radial styloid process. Mothers often develop this tenosynovitis by holding their babies with the thumb outstretched. The Finkelstein sign is positive in De Quervain's tenosynovitis. It is positive if the patient develops pain by placing the thumb in the palm, closing the fingers around the thumb and deviating the wrist in the ulnar direction. Management of De Quervain's tenosynovitis includes nonsteroidal anti-inflammatory drugs and splinting. Glucocorticoid injections can be effective. A Phalen maneuver is used to diagnose carpal tunnel syndrome and does not elicit pain. The wrists are flexed for 60 seconds to compress the median nerve to elicit numbness, burning, or tingling. Gouty arthritis will present as an acutely inflamed joint with crystal-laden fluid. Rheumatoid arthritis is a systemic illness with characteristic joint synovitis and radiographic features.

SECTION X
Endocrinology and Metabolism

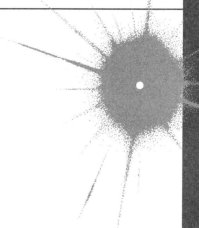

QUESTIONS

DIRECTIONS: Choose the **one best** response to each question.

X-1. All of the following represent examples of hypothalamic-pituitary negative feedback EXCEPT:

A. Cortisol on the CRH-ACTH axis
B. Gonadal steroids on the GnRH-LH/FSH axis
C. IGF-1 on the growth hormone–releasing hormone (GHRH)-GH axis
D. Renin-angiotensin-aldosterone axis
E. Thyroid hormones on TRH-TSH axis

X-2. Endocrine dysfunction can be separated into glandular hyperfunction or hypofunction, or hormone resistance. Which of the following diseases is due to hormone resistance?

A. Graves' disease
B. Hashimoto's thyroiditis
C. Pheochromocytoma
D. Sheehan's syndrome
E. Type 2 diabetes mellitus

X-3. Secretion of gonadotropin-releasing hormone (GnRH) normally stimulates the release of luteinizing hormone (LH) and follicle-stimulating hormone (FSH), which promote the production and release of testosterone and estrogen. Which mechanism best explains how long-acting gonadotropin-releasing hormone agonists (e.g., leuprolide) decrease testosterone levels in the management of prostate cancer?

A. GnRH agonists also promote the production of sex hormone–binding globulin, which decreases the availability of testosterone.
B. Negative feedback loop between GnRH and LH/FSH.
C. Sensitivity of LH and FSH to pulse frequency of GnRH.
D. Translocation of the cytoplasmic nuclear receptor into the nucleus with constitutive activation of GnRH.

X-4. The mineralocorticoid receptor in the renal tubule is responsible for the sodium retention and potassium wasting that is seen in mineralocorticoid excess states such as aldosterone-secreting tumors. However, states of glucocorticoid excess (e.g., Cushing's syndrome) can also present with sodium retention and hypokalemia. What characteristic of the mineralocorticoid-glucocorticoid pathways explains this finding?

A. Higher affinity of the mineralocorticoid receptor for glucocorticoids
B. Oversaturation of the glucocorticoid degradation pathway in states of glucocorticoid excess
C. Similar, but distinct, DNA-binding sites producing the same metabolic effect
D. Upregulation of the mineralocorticoid-binding protein in states of glucocorticoid excess

X-5. All of the following hormones are produced by the anterior pituitary EXCEPT:

A. Adrenocorticotropic hormone
B. Growth hormone
C. Oxytocin
D. Prolactin
E. Thyroid-stimulating hormone

X-6. A 22-year-old woman who is otherwise healthy undergoes an uneventful vaginal delivery of a full-term infant. One day postpartum she complains of visual changes and severe headache. Two hours after these complaints, she is found unresponsive and profoundly hypotensive. She is intubated and placed on mechanical ventilation. Her blood pressure is 68/28 mmHg, heart rate is regular at 148 beats/min, and oxygen saturation is 95% on FiO_2 0.40. Physical exam is unremarkable. Her laboratories are notable for glucose of 49 mg/dL and normal hematocrit and white blood cell count. Which of the following is most likely to reverse her hypotension?

A. Activated drotrecogin alfa
B. Hydrocortisone
C. Piperacillin/tazobactam
D. T_4
E. Transfusion of packed red blood cells

X-7. A 45-year-old man reports to his primary care physician that his wife has noted coarsening of his facial features over several years. In addition, he reports low libido and decreased energy. Physical examination shows frontal bossing and enlarged hands. An MRI confirms that he has a pituitary mass. Which of the following screening tests should be ordered to diagnose the cause of the mass?

A. 24-hour urinary free cortisol
B. ACTH assay
C. Growth hormone level
D. Serum IGF-1 level
E. Serum prolactin level

X-8. All of the following are potential causes of hyperprolactinemia EXCEPT:

A. Cirrhosis
B. Hirsutism
C. Nipple stimulation
D. Opiate abuse
E. Rathke's cyst

X-9. A 28-year-old woman presents to her primary care physician's office with 1 year of amenorrhea. She reports mild galactorrhea and headaches. Although she is sexually active, a urine pregnancy test is negative. Serum prolactin level is elevated and she is subsequently diagnosed with a microscopic prolactinoma. Which of the following represents the primary goal of bromocriptine therapy for her condition?

A. Control of hyperprolactinemia
B. Reduction in tumor size
C. Resolution of galactorrhea
D. Restoration of menses and fertility
E. All of the above

X-10. A 58-year-old man undergoes severe head trauma and develops pituitary insufficiency. After recovery, he is placed on thyroid hormone, testosterone, glucocorticoids, and vasopressin. On a routine visit he questions his

primary care physician regarding potential growth hormone deficiency. All of the following are potential signs or symptoms of growth hormone deficiency EXCEPT:

A. Abnormal lipid profile
B. Atherosclerosis
C. Increased bone mineral density
D. Increased waist:hip ratio
E. Left ventricular dysfunction

X-11. A 75-year-old man presents with development of abdominal obesity, proximal myopathy, and skin hyperpigmentation. His laboratory evaluation shows a hypokalemic metabolic alkalosis. Cushing's syndrome is suspected. Which of the following statements regarding this syndrome is true?

A. Basal ACTH level is likely to be low.
B. Circulating corticotropin-releasing hormone is likely to be elevated.
C. Pituitary MRI will visualize all ACTH-secreting tumors.
D. Referral for urgent performance of inferior petrosal venous sampling is indicated.
E. Serum potassium level below 3.3 mmol/L is suggestive of ectopic ACTH production.

X-12. A 23-year-old college student is followed in the student health center for medical management of panhypopituitarism after resection of craniopharyngioma as a child. She reports moderate compliance with her medications but feels generally well. A TSH is checked and is below the limits of detection of the assay. Which of the following is the next most appropriate action?

A. Decrease levothyroxine dose to half of current dose.
B. Do nothing.
C. Order free T_4 level.
D. Order MRI of her brain.
E. Order thyroid uptake scan.

X-13. A 23-year-old woman presents to the clinic complaining of months of weight gain, fatigue, amenorrhea, and worsening acne. She cannot precisely identify when her symptoms began, but she reports that without a change in her diet she has noted a 12.3-kg weight gain over the past 6 months. She has been amenorrheic for several months. On examination she is noted to have truncal obesity with bilateral purplish striae across both flanks. Cushing's syndrome is suspected. Which of the following tests should be used to make the diagnosis?

A. 24-hour urine free cortisol
B. Basal adrenocorticotropic hormone (ACTH)
C. Corticotropin-releasing hormone (CRH) level at 8 a.m.
D. Inferior petrosal venous sampling
E. Overnight 1-mg dexamethasone suppression test

X-14. A patient visited a local emergency room 1 week ago with a headache. She received a head MRI, which did not reveal a cause for her symptoms, but the final report states,

"An empty sella is noted. Advise clinical correlation." The patient was discharged from the emergency department with instructions to follow up with her primary care physician as soon as possible. Her headache has resolved, and the patient has no complaints; however, she comes to your office 1 day later very concerned about this unexpected MRI finding. What should be the next step in her management?

A. Diagnose her with subclinical panhypopituitarism, and initiate low-dose hormone replacement.
B. Reassure her and follow laboratory results closely.
C. Reassure her and repeat MRI in 6 months.
D. This may represent early endocrine malignancy—whole-body positron emission tomography/CT is indicated.
E. This MRI finding likely represents the presence of a benign adenoma—refer to neurosurgery for resection.

X-15. A 31-year-old woman is admitted to the hospital after an appendectomy for acute appendicitis. The surgery is uncomplicated, but postoperatively she is noted to make copious urine (6 L/d) and complain of severe thirst. On the third postoperative day, her BUN and creatinine are noted to be elevated. On further questioning, she reports a long history of extreme thirst, urinary frequency, and occasional episodes of enuresis that she was too embarrassed to bring to the attention of a health care practitioner. Aside from oral contraceptives, she takes no medications and reports no past medical history. Which of the following is the most appropriate first step to confirm her diagnosis?

A. 24-hour urine volume and osmolarity measurement
B. Fasting morning plasma osmolarity
C. Fluid deprivation test
D. MRI of the brain
E. Plasma ADH level

X-16. A 63-year-old man is admitted to the hospital to begin induction chemotherapy for acute myelomonocytic leukemia (AML-M4). He is afebrile and has been feeling well other than fatigue and bruising. His physical examination is notable for normal vital signs and no focal findings other than three 1- × 2-cm subcutaneous nodules that had previously been demonstrated to be cutaneous spread of AML-M4. On the night of admission, the patient's wife calls for assistance because her husband's mental status is altered. He is confused and somnolent. You notice that there are four urinals filled with urine by his bed. His wife reports that for the last 6 hours he has been urinating frequently and has been drinking water constantly. However, over the last hour, despite urinating frequently, he has not been able to drink water due to somnolence. Laboratory studies are notable for an absolute neutrophil count of 400, a platelet count of 35,000, and a serum sodium of 155. Which of the following therapies should be administered immediately?

A. All-*trans* retinoic acid (ATRA)
B. Desmopressin
C. Hydrochlorothiazide
D. Hydrocortisone
E. Lithium

X-17. Which of the following is the most common cause of preventable mental deficiency in the world?

A. Beriberi disease
B. Cretinism
C. Folate deficiency
D. Scurvy
E. Vitamin A deficiency

X-18. Which of the following proteins is the primary source of bound T_4 in the plasma?

A. Albumin
B. Gamma globulins
C. Transthyretin
D. Thyroid peroxidase
E. Thyroxine-binding globulin

X-19. All of the following are associated with increased levels of total T_4 in the plasma with a normal free T_4 EXCEPT:

A. Cirrhosis
B. Pregnancy
C. Sick-euthyroid syndrome
D. Familial dysalbuminemic hyperthyroxinemia
E. Familial excess thyroid-binding globulin

X-20. Which of the following is the most common cause of hypothyroidism worldwide?

A. Graves' disease
B. Hashimoto's thyroiditis
C. Iatrogenic hypothyroidism
D. Iodine deficiency
E. Radiation exposure

X-21. A 75-year-old woman is diagnosed with hypothyroidism. She has long-standing coronary artery disease and is wondering about the potential consequences for her cardiovascular system. Which of the following statements is true regarding the interaction of hypothyroidism and the cardiovascular system?

A. Myocardial contractility is increased with hypothyroidism.
B. A reduced stroke volume is found with hypothyroidism.
C. Pericardial effusions are a rare manifestation of hypothyroidism.
D. Reduced peripheral resistance is found in hypothyroidism and may be accompanied by hypotension.
E. Blood flow is diverted toward the skin in hypothyroidism.

X-22. A 38-year-old mother of three presents to her primary care office with complaints of fatigue. She feels that her energy level has been low for the past 3 months. She was previously healthy and was taking no medications. She does report that she has gained about 5 kg and has severe constipation, for which she has been taking a number of laxatives. A TSH is elevated at 25 mU/L. Free T_4 is low. She is wondering why she has hypothyroidism. Which of the following tests is most likely to diagnose the etiology?

A. Antithyroglobulin antibody
B. Antithyroid peroxidase antibody
C. Radioiodine uptake scan
D. Serum thyroglobulin level
E. Thyroid ultrasound

X-23. A 54-year-old woman with long-standing hypothyroidism is seen in her primary care physician's office for a routine evaluation. She reports feeling fatigued and somewhat constipated. Since her last visit, her other medical conditions, which include hypercholesterolemia and systemic hypertension, are stable. She was diagnosed with uterine fibroids and started on iron recently. Her other medications include levothyroxine, atorvastatin, and hydrochlorothiazide. A TSH is checked and it is elevated to 15 mU/L. Which of the following is the most likely reason for her elevated TSH?

A. Celiac disease
B. Colon cancer
C. Medication noncompliance
D. Poor absorption of levothyroxine due to ferrous sulfate
E. TSH-secreting pituitary adenoma

X-24. An 87-year-old woman is admitted to the intensive care unit with depressed level of consciousness, hypothermia, sinus bradycardia, hypotension, and hypoglycemia. She was previously healthy with the exception of hypothyroidism and systemic hypertension. Her family recently checked in on her and found that she was not taking any of her medications because of financial difficulties. There is no evidence of infection on exam, urine microscopy, or chest radiograph. Her serum chemistries are notable for mild hyponatremia and a glucose of 48. TSH is above 100 mU/L. All of the following statements regarding this condition are true EXCEPT:

A. External warming is a critical feature of therapy in patients with a temperature above 34°C (93.2°F).
B. Hypotonic intravenous solutions should be avoided.
C. IV levothyroxine should be administered with IV glucocorticoids.
D. Sedation should be avoided if possible.
E. This condition occurs almost exclusively in the elderly and often is precipitated by an unrelated medical illness.

X-25. A 29-year-old woman is evaluated for anxiety, palpitations, and diarrhea and is found to have Graves' disease. Before she begins therapy for her thyroid condition, she has an episode of acute chest pain and presents to the emergency department. Although a CT angiogram is ordered, the radiologist calls to notify the treating physician that this is potentially dangerous. Which of the following best explains the radiologist's recommendation?

A. Iodinated contrast exposure in patients with Graves' disease may exacerbate hyperthyroidism.
B. Pulmonary embolism is exceedingly rare in Graves' disease.
C. Radiation exposure in patients with hyperthyroidism is associated with increased risk of subsequent malignancy.
D. Tachycardia with Graves' disease limits the image quality of CT angiography and will not allow accurate assessment of pulmonary embolism.
E. The radiologist was mistaken; CT angiography is safe in Graves' disease.

X-26. What percentage of patients with hyperthyroidism and atrial fibrillation convert to sinus rhythm after treatment of thyroid state alone?

A. 20%
B. 30%
C. 50%
D. 70%
E. 90%

X-27. Which of the following statements best describes Graves' ophthalmopathy?

A. Although a cosmetic problem, Graves' ophthalmopathy is rarely associated with major ocular complications.
B. Diplopia may occur from periorbital muscle swelling.
C. It is never found without concomitant hyperthyroidism.
D. The most serious complication is corneal abrasion.
E. Unilateral disease is not found.

X-28. Which of the following is the most important mechanism of action of propylthiouracil in the treatment of Graves' disease?

A. Impaired production of transthyretin
B. Inhibition of production of thyroid-stimulating immunoglobulins
C. Inhibition of the function of thyroid peroxidase
D. Reduced peripheral conversion of T_4 to T_3
E. Reversal of iodine organification

X-29. A 44-year-old male is involved in a motor vehicle collision. He sustains multiple injuries to the face, chest, and pelvis. He is unresponsive in the field and is intubated for airway protection. An intravenous line is placed. The patient is admitted to the intensive care unit (ICU) with multiple orthopedic injuries. He is stabilized medically and on hospital day 2 undergoes successful open reduction and internal fixation of the right femur and right humerus. After his return to the ICU, you review his laboratory values. TSH is 0.3 mU/L, and the total T_4 level is normal. T_3 is 0.6 μg/dL. What is the most appropriate next management step?

A. Initiation of levothyroxine
B. Initiation of prednisone
C. Observation
D. Radioiodine uptake scan
E. Thyroid ultrasound

X-30. A 29-year-old woman presents to your clinic complaining of difficulty swallowing, sore throat, and tender swelling in her neck. She has also noted fevers intermittently over the past week. Several weeks prior to her current symptoms she experienced symptoms of an upper respiratory tract infection. She has no past medical history. On physical examination, she is noted to have a small goiter that is painful to the touch. Her oropharynx is clear. Laboratory studies are sent and reveal a white blood cell count of 14,100 cells/μL with a normal differential, erythrocyte sedimentation rate (ESR) of 53 mm/h, and a thyroid-stimulating hormone (TSH) of 21 μIU/mL. Thyroid antibodies are negative. What is the most likely diagnosis?

A. Autoimmune hypothyroidism
B. Cat-scratch fever
C. Graves' disease
D. Ludwig's angina
E. Subacute thyroiditis

X-31. What is the most appropriate treatment for the patient described in question X-30?

A. Iodine ablation of the thyroid
B. Large doses of aspirin
C. Local radiation therapy
D. No treatment necessary
E. Propylthiouracil

X-32. Which of the following is consistent with a diagnosis of subacute thyroiditis?

A. A 38-year-old female with a 2-week history of a painful thyroid, elevated T_4, elevated T_3, low TSH, and an elevated radioactive iodine uptake scan
B. A 42-year-old male with a history of a painful thyroid 4 months ago, fatigue, malaise, low free T_4, low T_3, and elevated TSH
C. A 31-year-old female with a painless enlarged thyroid, low TSH, elevated T_4, elevated free T_4, and an elevated radioiodine uptake scan
D. A 50-year-old male with a painful thyroid, slightly elevated T_4, normal TSH, and an ultrasound showing a mass

X-33. A healthy 53-year-old man comes to your office for an annual physical examination. He has no complaints and has no significant medical history. He is taking an over-the-counter multivitamin and no other medicines. On physical examination he is noted to have a nontender thyroid nodule. His thyroid-stimulating hormone (TSH) level is checked and is found to be low. What is the next step in his evaluation?

A. Close follow-up and measure TSH in 6 months
B. Fine-needle aspiration
C. Low-dose thyroid replacement
D. Positron emission tomography followed by surgery
E. Radionuclide thyroid scan

X-34. A patient has neurosurgery for a pituitary tumor that requires resection of the gland. Which of the following functions of the adrenal gland will be preserved in this patient immediately postoperatively?

A. Morning peak of plasma cortisol level
B. Release of cortisol in response to stress
C. Sodium retention in response to hypovolemia
D. None of the above

X-35. Which of the following is the most common cause of Cushing's syndrome?

A. ACTH-producing pituitary adenoma
B. Adrenocortical adenoma
C. Adrenocortical carcinoma
D. Ectopic ACTH secretion
E. McCune-Albright syndrome

X-36. All of the following are features of Conn's syndrome EXCEPT:

A. Alkalosis
B. Hyperkalemia
C. Muscle cramps
D. Normal serum sodium
E. Severe systemic hypertension

X-37. All of the following statements regarding asymptomatic adrenal masses (incidentalomas) are true EXCEPT:

A. All patients with incidentalomas should be screened for pheochromocytoma.
B. Fine-needle aspiration may distinguish between benign and malignant primary adrenal tumors.
C. In patients with a history of malignancy, the likelihood that the mass is a metastasis is approximately 50%.
D. The majority of adrenal incidentalomas are non-secretory.
E. The vast majority of adrenal incidentalomas are benign.

X-38. A 43-year-old man with episodic, severe hypertension is referred for evaluation of possible secondary causes of hypertension. He reports feeling well generally, except for episodes of anxiety, palpitations, and tachycardia with elevation in his blood pressure during these episodes. Exercise often brings on these events. The patient also has mild depression and is presently taking sertraline, labetalol, amlodipine, and lisinopril to control his blood pressure. Urine 24-hour total metanephrines are ordered and show an elevation of 1.5 times the upper limit of normal. Which of the following is the next most appropriate step?

A. Hold labetalol for 1 week and repeat testing.
B. Hold sertraline for 1 week and repeat testing.
C. Immediately refer for surgical evaluation.
D. Measure 24-hour urine vanillylmandelic acid level.
E. Send for MRI of the abdomen.

X-39. A 45-year-old man is diagnosed with pheochromocytoma after presentation with confusion, marked hypertension to 250/140 mmHg, tachycardia, headaches, and flushing. His fractionated plasma metanephrines show a normetanephrine level of 560 pg/mL and a metanephrine level of 198 pg/mL (normal values: normetanephrine: 18–111 pg/mL; metanephrine: 12–60 pg/mL). CT scanning of the abdomen with IV contrast demonstrates a 3-cm mass in the right adrenal gland. A brain MRI with gadolinium shows edema of the white matter near the parietooccipital junction consistent with reversible posterior leukoencephalopathy. You are asked to consult regarding management. Which of the following statements is true regarding management of pheochromocytoma is this individual?

A. Beta-blockade is absolutely contraindicated for tachycardia even after adequate alpha-blockade has been attained.
B. Immediate surgical removal of the mass is indicated, because the patient presented with hypertensive crisis with encephalopathy.
C. Salt and fluid intake should be restricted to prevent further exacerbation of the patient's hypertension.
D. Treatment with phenoxybenzamine should be started at a high dose (20–30 mg three times daily) to rapidly control blood pressure, and surgery can be undertaken within 24–48 hours.
E. Treatment with IV phentolamine is indicated for treatment of the hypertensive crisis. Phenoxybenzamine should be started at a low dose and titrated to the maximum tolerated dose over 2–3 weeks. Surgery should not be planned until the blood pressure is consistently below 160/100 mmHg.

X-40. Which of the following ethnic populations in the United States has the highest risk of diabetes mellitus?

A. Asian American
B. Hispanic
C. Non-Hispanic black
D. Non-Hispanic white

X-41. Which of the following defines **normal** glucose tolerance?

A. Fasting plasma glucose below 100 mg/dL
B. Fasting plasma glucose below 126 mg/dL following an oral glucose challenge
C. Hemoglobin A1C below 5.6% and fasting plasma glucose below 140 mg/dL
D. Hemoglobin A1C below 6.0%
E. Fasting plasma glucose below 100 mg/dL, plasma glucose below 140 mg/dL following an oral glucose challenge, and hemoglobin A1C below 5.6%

X-42. A 37-year-old woman with obesity presents to the clinic for a routine health evaluation. She reports that over the last year she has had two yeast infections treated with over-the-counter remedies and frequently feels thirsty. She does report waking up at night to urinate. Which of the following studies is the most appropriate first test in evaluating the patient for diabetes mellitus?

A. Hemoglobin A1C
B. Oral glucose tolerance test
C. Plasma C-peptide level
D. Plasma insulin level
E. Random plasma glucose level

X-43. All of the following are risk factors for type 2 diabetes mellitus EXCEPT:

A. BMI above 25 kg/m^2
B. Delivery of a baby more than 3.5 kg
C. HDL level below 35 mg/dL
D. Hemoglobin A1C 5.7–6.4%
E. Systemic hypertension

X-44. A 27-year-old woman with mild obesity is seen in her primary care office for increased thirst and polyuria. Diabetes mellitus is suspected, and a random plasma glucose of 211 mg/d confirms this diagnosis. Which of the following tests will strongly indicate that she has type 1 diabetes mellitus?

A. Anti–GAD-65 antibody.
B. Peroxisome proliferator-activated receptor γ-2 polymorphism testing.
C. Plasma insulin level.
D. Testing for HLA-DR3.
E. There is no laboratory test indicating type 1 diabetes mellitus.

X-45. In patients with impaired fasting glucose, all of the following interventions have been proven to decrease progression to type 2 diabetes mellitus EXCEPT:

A. Diet modification
B. Exercise
C. Glyburide
D. Metformin

X-46. A patient is evaluated in the emergency department for complications of diabetes mellitus with an episode of life stressors. All of the following laboratory tests are consistent with the diagnosis of diabetic ketoacidosis EXCEPT:

A. Arterial pH 7.1
B. Glucose 550 mg/dL
C. Markedly positive plasma ketones
D. Normal serum potassium
E. Plasma osmolality 380 mosm/mL

X-47. All of the following are consistent with nonproliferative diabetic retinopathy EXCEPT:

A. Blot hemorrhages
B. Cotton-wool spots
C. Neovascularization
D. Occurs in first or second decade of diabetes mellitus
E. Retinal vascular microaneurysms

X-48. A 68-year-old man with poorly controlled type 2 diabetes mellitus is admitted to the hospital with an ulcer on the lateral surface of his right lower extremity that has been painful and appears purulent. He has had 3 days of fever. All of the following interventions are recommended to improve wound healing in a patient with a diabetic wound EXCEPT:

A. Appropriate use of antibiotics
B. Debridement
C. Hyperbaric oxygen
D. Off-loading
E. Revascularization

X-49. Pick the correct combination of onset of action and duration of action for the following insulins:

A. Aspart: 1 hour, 6 hours
B. Detemir: 2 hours, 12 hours
C. Lispro: 0.5 hour, 2 hours
D. NPH: 2 hours, 14 hours
E. Regular: 0.25 hour, 6 hours

X-50. A 54-year-old woman is diagnosed with type 2 diabetes mellitus after a routine follow-up for impaired fasting glucose showed that her hemoglobin A1C is now 7.6%. She has attempted to lose weight and to exercise with no improvement in her hemoglobin A1C, and drug therapy is now recommended. She has mild systemic hypertension that is well controlled and no other medical conditions. Which of the following is the most appropriate first-line therapy?

A. Acarbose
B. Exenatide
C. Glyburide
D. Metformin
E. Sitagliptin

X-51. The Diabetes Control and Complications Trial (DCCT) provided definitive proof that reduction in chronic hyperglycemia:

A. Improves microvascular complications in type 1 diabetes mellitus
B. Improves macrovascular complications in type 1 diabetes mellitus
C. Improves microvascular complications in type 2 diabetes mellitus
D. Improves macrovascular complications in type 2 diabetes mellitus
E. Improves both microvascular and macrovascular complications in type 2 diabetes mellitus

X-52. A patient is seen in the clinic for follow-up of type 2 diabetes mellitus. Her hemoglobin A1C has been poorly controlled at 9.4% recently. The patient can be counseled to expect all the following improvements with improved glycemic control EXCEPT:

A. Decreased microalbuminuria
B. Decreased risk of nephropathy
C. Decreased risk of neuropathy
D. Decreased risk of peripheral vascular disease
E. Decreased risk of retinopathy

X-53. A 21-year-old female with a history of type 1 diabetes mellitus is brought to the emergency department with nausea, vomiting, lethargy, and dehydration. Her mother notes that she stopped taking insulin 1 day before presentation. She is lethargic, has dry mucous membranes, and is obtunded. Blood pressure is 80/40 mmHg, and heart rate is 112 beats/min. Heart sounds are normal. Lungs are clear. The abdomen is soft, and there is no organomegaly. She is responsive and oriented × 3 but diffusely weak. Serum sodium is 126 meq/L, potassium is 4.3 meq/L, magnesium is 1.2 meq/L, blood urea nitrogen is 76 mg/dL, creatinine is 2.2 mg/dL, bicarbonate is 10 meq/L, and chloride is 88 meq/L. Serum glucose is 720 mg/dL. All of the following are appropriate management steps EXCEPT:

A. 3% sodium solution
B. Arterial blood gas
C. Intravenous insulin
D. Intravenous potassium
E. Intravenous fluids

X-54. Which of the following studies is the most sensitive for detecting diabetic nephropathy?

A. Creatinine clearance
B. Glucose tolerance test
C. Serum creatinine level
D. Ultrasonography
E. Urine albumin

X-55. Alteration in which of the following substance levels is the first defense against hypoglycemia?

A. Cortisol
B. Epinephrine
C. Glucagon
D. Insulin
E. Insulin-like growth factor

X-56. A 25-year-old health care worker is seen for evaluation of recurrent hypoglycemia. She has had several episodes at work over the past year in which she feels shaky, anxious, and sweaty, and when she measures her finger stick glucose, it is 40–55 mg/dL. She drinks orange juice and feels better. These episodes have not happened outside the work environment. Aside from oral contraceptives, she takes no medications and is otherwise healthy. Which of the following tests is most likely to demonstrate the underlying cause of her hypoglycemia?

A. Measurement of insulin-like growth factor 1
B. Measurement of fasting insulin and glucose levels
C. Measurement of fasting insulin, glucose, and C-peptide levels
D. Measurement of insulin, glucose, and C-peptide levels during a symptomatic episode
E. Measurement of plasma cortisol

X-57. All of the following statements regarding hypoglycemia in diabetes mellitus are true EXCEPT:

A. Individuals with type 2 diabetes mellitus experience less hypoglycemia than those with type 1 diabetes mellitus.

B. From 2–4% of deaths in type 1 diabetes mellitus are directly attributable to hypoglycemia.

C. Recurrent episodes of hypoglycemia predispose to the development of autonomic failure with defective glucose counterregulation and hypoglycemia unawareness.

D. The average person with type 1 diabetes mellitus has two episodes of symptomatic hypoglycemia weekly.

E. Thiazolidinediones and metformin cause hypoglycemia more frequently than sulfonylureas.

X-58. A 58-year-old man is seen in his primary care physician's office for evaluation of bilateral breast enlargement. This has been present for several months and is accompanied by mild pain in both breasts. He reports no other symptoms. His other medical conditions include coronary artery disease with a history of congestive heart failure, atrial fibrillation, obesity, and type 2 diabetes mellitus. His current medications include lisinopril, spironolactone, furosemide, insulin, and digoxin. He denies illicit drug use and has fathered three children. Examination confirms bilateral breast enlargement with palpable glandular tissue that measures 2 cm bilaterally. Which of the following statements regarding his gynecomastia is true?

A. He should be referred for mammography to rule out breast cancer.

B. His gynecomastia is most likely due to obesity with adipose tissue present in the breast.

C. Serum testosterone, LH, and FSH should be measured to evaluate for androgen insensitivity.

D. Spironolactone should be discontinued and exam followed for regression.

E. Liver function testing should be performed to screen for cirrhosis.

X-59. All the following drugs may interfere with testicular function EXCEPT:

A. Cyclophosphamide

B. Ketoconazole

C. Metoprolol

D. Prednisone

E. Spironolactone

X-60. Clinical signs and findings of the presence of ovulation include all of the following EXCEPT:

A. Detection of urinary LH surge

B. Estrogen peak during secretory phase of menstrual cycle

C. Increase in basal body temperature more than 0.5°F in the second half of the menstrual cycle

D. Presence of *mittelschmerz*

E. Progesterone level above 5 ng/mL 7 days before expected menses

X-61. A couple has been married for 5 years and has attempted to conceive a child for the last 12 months. Despite regular intercourse they have not achieved pregnancy. They are both 32 years of age and have no medical problems. Neither partner is taking medications. Which of the following is the most likely cause of their infertility?

A. Endometriosis

B. Male causes

C. Ovulatory dysfunction

D. Tubal defect

E. Unexplained

X-62. A couple seeks advice regarding infertility. The female partner is 35 years old. She has never been pregnant and took oral contraceptive pills from age 20 until age 34. It is now 16 months since she discontinued her oral contraceptives. She is having menstrual cycles approximately once every 35 days, but occasionally will go as long as 60 days between cycles. Most months, she develops breast tenderness about 2–3 weeks after the start of her menstrual cycle. When she was in college, she was treated for *Neisseria gonorrhoeae* that was diagnosed when she presented to the student health center with a fever and pelvic pain. She otherwise has no medical history. She works about 60 hours weekly as a corporate attorney and exercises daily. She drinks coffee daily and alcohol on social occasions only. Her body mass index (BMI) is 19.8 kg/m². Her husband, who is 39 years old, accompanies her to the evaluation. He also has never had children. He was married previously from the ages of 24–28. He and his prior wife attempted to conceive for about 15 months, but were unsuccessful. At that time, he was smoking marijuana on a daily basis and attributed their lack of success to his drug use. He has now been completely free of drugs for 9 years. He suffers from hypertension and is treated with lisinopril 10 mg daily. He is not obese (BMI, 23.7 kg/m²). They request evaluation for their infertility and help with conception. Which of the following statements is true in regard to their infertility and likelihood of success in conception?

A. Determination of ovulation is not necessary in the female partner as most of her cycles occur regularly, and she develops breast tenderness midcycle, which is indicative of ovulation.

B. Lisinopril should be discontinued immediately because of the risk of birth defects associated with its use.

C. The female partner should be assessed for tubal patency by a hysterosalpingogram. If significant scarring is found, in vitro fertilization should be strongly considered to decrease the risk of ectopic pregnancy.

D. The prolonged use of oral contraceptives for more than 10 years has increased the risk of anovulation and infertility.

E. The use of marijuana by the male partner is directly toxic to sperm motility, and this is the likely cause of their infertility.

X-63. Which of the following forms of contraception have theoretical efficacy of more than 90%?

A. Condoms
B. Intrauterine devices
C. Oral contraceptives
D. Spermicides
E. All of the above

X-64. A 30-year-old male, the father of three children, has had progressive breast enlargement during the last 6 months. He does not use any drugs. Laboratory evaluation reveals that both LH and testosterone are low. Further evaluation of this patient should include which of the following?

A. 24-hour urine collection for the measurement of 17 ketosteroids
B. Blood sampling for serum glutamic-oxaloacetic transaminase (SGOT) and serum alkaline phosphatase and bilirubin levels
C. Breast biopsy
D. Karyotype analysis to exclude Klinefelter's syndrome
E. Measurement of estradiol and human chorionic gonadotropin (hCG) levels

X-65. The Women's Health Initiative study investigated hormonal therapy in postmenopausal women. The study was stopped early due to increased risk of which of the following diseases in the estrogen-only arm?

A. Deep venous thrombosis
B. Endometrial cancer
C. Myocardial infarction
D. Osteoporosis
E. Stroke

X-66. A 37-year-old man is evaluated for infertility. He and his wife have been attempting to conceive a child for the past 2 years without success. He initially saw an infertility specialist, but was referred to endocrinology after sperm analysis showed no sperm. He is otherwise healthy and only takes a multivitamin. On physical examination his vital signs are normal. He is tall and has small testes, gynecomastia, and minimal facial and axillary hair. Chromosomal analysis confirms Klinefelter's syndrome. Which of the following statements is true?

A. Androgen supplementation is of little use in this condition.
B. He is not at increased risk for breast tumors.
C. Increased plasma concentrations of estrogen are present.
D. Most cases are diagnosed prepuberty.
E. Plasma concentrations of FSH and LH are decreased in this condition.

X-67. A 17-year-old woman is evaluated in your office for primary amenorrhea. She feels as if she has not entered puberty in that she has never had a menstrual period and has sparse axillary and pubic hair growth. On examination, she is noted to be 150 cm tall. She has a low hairline and slight webbing of her neck. Her follicle-stimulating

hormone level is 75 mIU/mL, luteinizing hormone is 20 mIU/mL, and estradiol level is 2 pg/mL. You suspect Turner's syndrome. All of the following tests are indicated in this individual EXCEPT:

A. Buccal smear for nuclear heterochromatin (Barr body)
B. Echocardiogram
C. Karyotype analysis
D. Renal ultrasound
E. Thyroid-stimulating hormone (TSH)

X-68. A 35-year-old man is seen in the emergency department for evaluation of epigastric pain, diarrhea, and reflux. He reports frequent similar episodes and has undergone multiple endoscopies. In each case he was told that he has a duodenal ulcer. He has become quite frustrated because he was told that ulcers are usually due to a bacteria that can be treated, but he does not have *Helicobacter pylori* present on any of his ulcer biopsies. His current medications are high-dose omeprazole and oxycodone/acetaminophen. He is admitted to the hospital for pain control. Which of the following is the most appropriate next step in his diagnostic evaluation?

A. CT scan of the abdomen.
B. Discontinue omeprazole for 1 week and measure plasma gastrin level.
C. Gastric pH measurement.
D. Plasma gastrin level.
E. Screen for parathyroid hyperplasia.

X-69. A 48-year-old female is undergoing evaluation for flushing and diarrhea. Physical examination is normal except for nodular hepatomegaly. A CT scan of the abdomen demonstrates multiple nodules in both lobes of the liver consistent with metastases in the liver and a 2-cm mass in the ileum. The 24-hour urinary 5-HIAA excretion is markedly elevated. All the following treatments are appropriate EXCEPT:

A. Diphenhydramine
B. Interferon α
C. Octreotide
D. Ondansetron
E. Phenoxybenzamine

X-70. While undergoing a physical examination during medical student clinical skills, the patient in question X-69 develops severe flushing, wheezing, nausea, and lightheadedness. Vital signs are notable for a blood pressure of 70/30 mmHg and a heart rate of 135 beats/min. Which of the following is the most appropriate therapy?

A. Albuterol
B. Atropine
C. Epinephrine
D. Hydrocortisone
E. Octreotide

X-71. A 49-year-old male is brought to the hospital by his family because of confusion and dehydration. The family reports that for the last 3 weeks he has had persistent copious, watery diarrhea that has not abated with the use of over-the-counter medications. The diarrhea has been unrelated to food intake and has persisted during fasting. The stool does not appear fatty and is not malodorous. The patient works as an attorney, is a vegetarian, and has not traveled recently. No one in the household has had similar symptoms. Before the onset of diarrhea, he had mild anorexia and a 5-lb weight loss. Since the diarrhea began, he has lost at least 5 kg. The physical examination is notable for blood pressure of 100/70 mmHg, heart rate of 110 beats/min, and temperature of 36.8°C (98.2°F). Other than poor skin turgor, confusion, and diffuse muscle weakness, the physical examination is unremarkable. Laboratory studies are notable for a normal complete blood count and the following chemistry results:

Na$^+$	146 meq/L
K$^+$	3.0 meq/L
Cl$^-$	96 meq/L
HCO$_3^-$	36 meq/L
BUN	32 mg/dL
Creatinine	1.2 mg/dL

A 24-hour stool collection yields 3 L of tea-colored stool. Stool sodium is 50 meq/L, potassium is 25 meq/L, and stool osmolality is 170 mosmol/L. Which of the following diagnostic tests is most likely to yield the correct diagnosis?

A. Serum cortisol
B. Serum TSH
C. Serum VIP
D. Urinary 5-HIAA
E. Urinary metanephrine

X-72. An 18-year-old girl is evaluated at her primary care physician's office for a routine physical. She is presently healthy. Her family history is notable for a father and two aunts with MEN 1, and the patient has undergone genetic testing and carries the *MEN 1 gene*. Which of the following is the first and most common presentation for individuals with this genetic mutation?

A. Peptic ulcer disease
B. Hypercalcemia
C. Hypoglycemia
D. Amenorrhea
E. Uncontrolled systemic hypertension

X-73. A 35-year-old male is referred to your clinic for evaluation of hypercalcemia noted during a health insurance medical screening. He has noted some fatigue, malaise, and a 4-lb weight loss over the last 2 months. He also has noted constipation and "heartburn." He is occasionally nauseated after large meals and has water brash and a sour taste in his mouth. The patient denies vomiting, dysphagia, or odynophagia. He also notes decreased libido and

a depressed mood. Vital signs are unremarkable. Physical examination is notable for a clear oropharynx, no evidence of a thyroid mass, and no lymphadenopathy. Jugular venous pressure is normal. Heart sounds are regular with no murmurs or gallops. The chest is clear. The abdomen is soft with some mild epigastric tenderness. There is no rebound or organomegaly. Stool is guaiac positive. Neurologic examination is nonfocal. Laboratory values are notable for a normal complete blood count. Calcium is 11.2 mg/dL, phosphate is 2.1 mg/dL, and magnesium is 1.8 meq/dL. Albumin is 3.7 g/dL, and total protein is 7.0 g/dL. TSH is 3 μIU/mL, prolactin is 250 μg/L, testosterone is 620 ng/dL, and serum insulin-like growth factor 1 (IGF-1) is normal. Serum intact parathyroid hormone level is 135 pg/dL. In light of the patient's abdominal discomfort and heme-positive stool, you perform an abdominal computed tomography (CT) scan that shows a lesion measuring 2 × 2 cm in the head of the pancreas. What is the diagnosis?

A. Multiple endocrine neoplasia (MEN) type 1
B. MEN type 2a
C. MEN type 2b
D. Polyglandular autoimmune syndrome
E. Von-Hippel Lindau (VHL) syndrome

X-74. A 55-year-old male is admitted to the intensive care unit with fever and cough. He was well until 1 week before admission, when he noted progressive shortness of breath, cough, and productive sputum. On the day of admission the patient's wife noted him to be lethargic. Emergency response found the patient unresponsive. He was intubated in the field and brought to the emergency department. His medications include insulin. The past medical history is notable for alcohol abuse and diabetes mellitus. Temperature is 38.9°C (102°F), blood pressure is 76/40 mmHg, and oxygen saturation is 86% on room air. On examination, the patient is intubated on mechanical ventilation. Jugular venous pressure is normal. There are decreased breath sounds at the right lung base with egophony. Heart sounds are normal. The abdomen is soft. There is no peripheral edema. Chest radiography shows a right lower lobe infiltrate with a moderate pleural effusion. An electrocardiogram is normal. Sputum Gram stain shows gram-positive diplococci. White blood cell count is 23 × 10^3/μL, with 70% polymorphonuclear cells and 6% bands. Blood urea nitrogen is 80 mg/dL, and creatinine is 3.1 mg/dL. Plasma glucose is 425 mg/dL. He is started on broad-spectrum antibiotics, intravenous fluids, omeprazole, and an insulin drip. A nasogastric tube is inserted, and tube feedings are started. On hospital day 2, his creatinine improves to 1.6 mg/dL. However, plasma phosphate is 1.0 mg/dL (0.3 mmol/L) and calcium is 8.8 mg/dL. All of following are causes of hypophosphatemia in this patient EXCEPT:

A. Alcoholism
B. Insulin
C. Malnutrition
D. Renal failure
E. Sepsis

X-75. In the patient in question X-74, what is the most appropriate approach to correcting the hypophosphatemia?

A. Administer IV calcium gluconate 1 g followed by infusion of IV phosphate at a rate of 8 mmol/h for 6 hours.

B. Administer IV phosphate alone at a rate of 2 mmol/h for 6 hours.

C. Administer IV phosphate alone at a rate of 8 mmol/h for 6 hours.

D. Continue close observation as redistribution of phosphate is expected to normalize over the course of the next 24–48 hours.

E. Initiate oral phosphate replacement at a dose of 1500 mg/d.

X-76. A 35-year-old woman is admitted to the hospital at 37 weeks' gestation following a seizure associated with an elevated blood pressure to 190/96 mmHg. She is treated acutely with magnesium sulfate intravenously for eclampsia and is starting on a continuous magnesium sulfate infusion at 1 g/h, which will be continued for 24 hours following her seizure. An emergency caesarian section is planned. Serum magnesium levels will be measured every 6 hours. What magnesium level would be worrisome for the development of central nervous system depression, respiratory muscle paralysis, and cardiac arrhythmias?

A. 0.5 mmol/L

B. 1.0 mmol/L

C. 2.5 mmol/L

D. 3.0 mmol/L

E. 5.0 mmol/L

X-77. You are caring for a 72-year-old man who has been living in a nursing home for the past 3 years. He has severe chronic obstructive pulmonary disease and requires continuous oxygen at 3 L/min. He also previously had a stroke, which has left him with a right hemiparesis. His current medications include aspirin, losartan, hydrochlorothiazide, fluticasone/salmeterol, tiotropium, and albuterol. His body mass index is 18.5 kg/m^2. You are concerned that he may have vitamin D deficiency. Which of the following is the best test to determine if vitamin D deficiency is present?

A. 1,25-hydroxy vitamin D

B. 25-hydroxy vitamin D

C. Alkaline phosphatase

D. Parathyroid hormone

E. Serum total and ionized calcium levels

X-78. A 42-year-old man presents to the emergency department with acute-onset right-sided flank pain. He describes the pain as 10 out of 10 in severity radiating to the groin. He has had one episode of hematuria. A noncontrast CT scan confirms the presence of a right-sided renal stone that is currently located in the distal ureter. He has a past medical history of pulmonary sarcoidosis that is not currently treated. This was diagnosed by bronchoscopic biopsy showing noncaseating granulomas. His chest radiograph shows bilateral hilar adenopathy. His serum calcium level is 12.6 mg/dL. What is the mechanism of hypercalcemia in this patient?

A. Increased activation of 25-hydroxy vitamin D to 1,25-hydroxy vitamin D by macrophages within granulomas

B. Increased activation of 25-hydroxy vitamin D to 1,25-hydroxy vitamin D by the kidney

C. Increased activation of vitamin D to 25-hydroxy vitamin D by macrophages within granulomas

D. Missed diagnosis of lymphoma with subsequent bone marrow invasion and resorption of bone through local destruction

E. Production of parathyroid hormone–related peptide by macrophages within granulomas

X-79. A 52-year-old man has end-stage kidney disease from long-standing hypertension and diabetes mellitus. He has been managed with hemodialysis for the past 8 years. Throughout this time, he has been poorly compliant with his medications and hemodialysis schedule, frequently missing one session weekly. He is now complaining of bone pain and dyspnea. His oxygen saturation is noted to be 92% on room air, and his chest radiograph shows hazy bilateral infiltrates. Chest CT shows ground-glass infiltrates bilaterally. His laboratory data include calcium of 12.3 mg/dL, phosphate of 8.1 mg/dL, and parathyroid hormone of 110 pg/mL. Which of the following would be the best approach to the treatment of the patient's current clinical condition?

A. Calcitriol 0.5 μg intravenously with hemodialysis with sevelamer three times daily

B. Calcitriol 0.5 μg orally daily with sevelamer 1600 mg three times daily

C. More aggressive hemodialysis to achieve optimal fluid and electrolyte balance

D. Parathyroidectomy

E. Sevelamer 1600 mg three times daily

X-80. A 54-year-old woman undergoes total thyroidectomy for follicular carcinoma of the thyroid. About 6 hours after surgery, the patient complains of tingling around her mouth. She subsequently develops a pins-and-needles sensation in the fingers and toes. The nurse calls the physician to the bedside to evaluate the patient after she has severe hand cramps when her blood pressure is taken. Upon evaluation, the patient is still complaining of intermittent cramping of her hands. Since surgery, she has received morphine sulfate 2 mg for pain and Compazine 5 mg for nausea. She has had no change in her vital signs and is afebrile. Tapping on the inferior portion of the zygomatic arch 2 cm anterior to the ear produces twitching at the corner of the mouth. An electrocardiogram (ECG) shows a QT interval of 575 milliseconds. What is the next step in the evaluation and treatment of this patient?

A. Administration of benztropine 2 mg IV

B. Administration of calcium gluconate 2 g IV

C. Administration of magnesium sulphate 4 g IV

D. Measurement of calcium, magnesium, phosphate, and potassium levels

E. Measurement of forced vital capacity

X-81. A 68-year-old woman with stage IIIB squamous cell carcinoma of the lung is admitted to the hospital because of altered mental status and dehydration. Upon admission, she is found to have a calcium level of 19.6 mg/dL and phosphate of 1.8 mg/dL. Concomitant measurement of parathyroid hormone was 0.1 pg/mL (normal 10–65 pg/mL), and a screen for parathyroid hormone–related peptide was positive. Over the first 24 hours, the patient receives 4 L of normal saline with furosemide diuresis. The next morning, the patient's calcium is 17.6 mg/dL and phosphate is 2.2 mg/dL. She continues to have delirium. What is the best approach for ongoing treatment of this patient's hypercalcemia?

A. Continue therapy with large-volume fluid administration and forced diuresis with furosemide.
B. Continue therapy with large-volume fluid administration, but stop furosemide and treat with hydrochlorothiazide.
C. Initiate therapy with calcitonin alone.
D. Initiate therapy with pamidronate alone.
E. Initiate therapy with calcitonin and pamidronate.

X-82. A 60-year-old woman is referred to your office for evaluation of hypercalcemia of 12.9 mg/dL. This was found incidentally on a chemistry panel that was drawn during a hospitalization for cervical spondylosis. Despite fluid administration in the hospital, her serum calcium at discharge was 11.8 mg/dL. The patient is asymptomatic. She is otherwise in good health and has had her recommended age-appropriate cancer screening. She denies constipation or bone pain and is now 8 weeks out from her spinal surgery. Today, her serum calcium level is 12.4 mg/dL, and phosphate is 2.3 mg/dL. Her hematocrit and all other chemistries including creatinine were normal. What is the most likely diagnosis?

A. Breast cancer
B. Hyperparathyroidism
C. Hyperthyroidism
D. Multiple myeloma
E. Vitamin D intoxication

X-83. All of the following are actions of parathyroid hormone EXCEPT:

A. Direct stimulation of osteoblasts to increase bone formation
B. Direct stimulation of osteoclasts to increase bone resorption
C. Increased reabsorption of calcium from the distal tubule of the kidney
D. Inhibition of phosphate reabsorption in the proximal tubule of the kidney
E. Stimulation of renal 1-α-hydroxylase to produce 1,25-hydroxycholecalciferol

X-84. Which of the following statements regarding the epidemiology of osteoporosis and bone fractures is correct?

A. For every 5-year period after age 70, the incidence of hip fractures increases by 25%.
B. Fractures of the distal radius increase in frequency before age 50 and plateau by age 60 with only a modest age-related increase.
C. Most women meet the diagnostic criteria for osteoporosis between the ages of 60 and 70.
D. The risk of hip fracture is equal when white women are compared to black women.
E. Women outnumber men with osteoporosis at a ratio of about 10 to 1.

X-85. A 50-year-old woman presents to your office to inquire about her risk of fracture related to osteoporosis. She has a positive family history of osteoporosis in her mother, but her mother never experienced any hip or vertebral fractures. The patient herself has also not experienced any fractures. She is white and has a 20 pack-year history of tobacco, quitting 10 years prior. At the age of 37, she had a total hysterectomy with bilateral salpingo-oophorectomy for endometriosis. She is lactose intolerant and does not consume dairy products. She currently takes calcium carbonate 500 mg daily. Her weight is 52 kg. All of the following are risk factors for an osteoporotic fracture in this woman EXCEPT:

A. Early menopause
B. Female sex
C. History of cigarette smoking
D. Low body weight
E. Low calcium intake

X-86. All of the following diseases are associated with an increased risk of osteoporosis EXCEPT:

A. Anorexia nervosa
B. Chronic obstructive pulmonary disease
C. Congestive heart failure
D. Malabsorption syndromes
E. Hyperparathyroidism

X-87. A 54-year-old woman is referred to the endocrinology clinic for evaluation of osteoporosis after a recent examination for back pain revealed a compression fracture of the T_4 vertebral body. She is perimenopausal with irregular menstrual periods and frequent hot flashes. She does not smoke. She otherwise is well and healthy. Her weight is 70 kg and height is 168 cm. She has lost 5 cm from her maximum height. A bone mineral density scan shows a T-score of –3.5 SD and a Z-score of –2.5 SD. All of the following tests are indicated for the evaluation of osteoporosis in this patient EXCEPT:

A. 24-hour urine calcium
B. Follicle-stimulating hormone and luteinizing hormone levels
C. Serum calcium
D. Thyroid-stimulating hormone
E. Vitamin D levels (25-hydroxyvitamin D)

X-88. A 45-year-old white woman seeks advice from her primary care physician regarding her risk for osteoporosis and the need for bone density screening. She is a lifelong nonsmoker and drinks alcohol only socially. She has a history of moderate-persistent asthma since age 12. She is currently on fluticasone, 44 mg/puff twice daily, with good control currently. She last required oral prednisone therapy about 6 months ago when she had influenza that was complicated by an asthma flare. She took prednisone for a total of 14 days. She has had three pregnancies and two live births at ages 39 and 41. She currently has irregular periods occurring approximately every 42 days. Her follicle-stimulating hormone level is 25 mIU/L and 17β-estradiol level is 115 pg/mL on day 12 of her menstrual cycle. Her mother and maternal aunt both have been diagnosed with osteoporosis. Her mother also has rheumatoid arthritis and requires prednisone therapy, 5 mg daily. Her mother developed a compression fracture of the lumbar spine at age 68. On physical examination, the patient appears well and healthy. Her height is 168 cm. Her weight is 66.4 kg. The chest, cardiac, abdominal, muscular, and neurologic examinations are normal. What do you tell the patient about the need for bone density screening?

A. As she is currently perimenopausal, she should have a bone density screen every other year until she completes menopause and then have bone densitometry measured yearly thereafter.
B. Because of her family history, she should initiate bone density screening yearly beginning now.
C. Bone densitometry screening is not recommended until after completion of menopause.
D. Delayed childbearing until the fourth and fifth decade decreases her risk of developing osteoporosis so bone densitometry is not recommended.
E. Her use of low-dose inhaled glucocorticoids increases her risk of osteoporosis threefold, and she should undergo yearly bone density screening.

X-89. What is the definition of osteoporosis by dual-energy x-ray absorptiometry testing (bone densitometry)?

A. A patient with a bone density less than the mean of age-, race-, and gender-matched controls
B. A patient with a bone density less than 1.0 standard deviation (SD) below the mean of race- and gender-matched controls
C. A patient with a bone density less than 1.0 SD below the mean of age-, race-, and gender-matched controls
D. A patient with a bone density less than 2.5 SD below the mean of race- and gender-matched controls
E. A patient with a bone density less than 2.5 SD below the mean of age-, race-, and gender-matched controls

X-90. A 66-year-old Asian woman seeks treatment for osteoporosis. She fell and fractured her right hip, requiring a surgical intervention 3 months ago. She was told while hospitalized that she had osteoporosis but had not previously been evaluated for this. During the hospitalization, she developed a deep venous thrombosis (DVT) with pulmonary embolus, for which she is currently taking warfarin. She completed menopause at age 52. She is a former smoker, quitting about 6 years ago. She has always been thin, and her current body mass index (BMI) is 19.2 kg/m^2. Her laboratory studies show

calcium of 8.7 mg/dL, phosphate of 3 mg/dL, creatinine of 0.8 mg/dL, and 25-hydroxyvitamin D levels of 18 ng/mL (normal >30 ng/mL). A dual-energy x-ray absorptiometry scan of bone mineral density has a T-score of –3.0. What is the best initial therapy for this patient?

A. Calcitonin 200 IU intranasally daily
B. Calcium carbonate 1200 mg and vitamin D 400 IU daily
C. Ethinyl estradiol 5 μg and medroxyprogesterone acetate 625 mg daily
D. Raloxifene 60 mg daily
E. Risedronate 35 mg once weekly, and calcium carbonate 1200 mg and vitamin D 400 IU daily

X-91. A 52-year-old man is found to have an elevated alkaline phosphatase level during routine blood chemistry testing prior to obtaining life insurance after changing jobs. He has a history of hypertension and hyperlipidemia. He previously had a cholecystectomy for gallstone disease. His current medications include losartan 25 mg daily, hydrochlorothiazide 25 mg daily, and rosuvastatin 20 mg daily. He is physically active and has a body mass index of 25.2 kg/m^2. His only complaint is low back pain that has been more severe recently. He has had no further evaluation for his back pain. His physical examination is normal. His liver is 10 cm to percussion. It is palpable with deep inspiration at the right costal margin. It is noted to be smooth. Murphy's sign is negative. There is no warmth or tenderness to palpation over the vertebral bodies of the lumbosacral spine. Laboratory evaluation reveals an alkaline phosphatase level of 468 U/L, alanine aminotransferase level of 22 U/L, aspartate aminotransferase level of 32 U/L, total bilirubin of 1.0 mg/dL, calcium of 9.4 mg/dL, phosphate 3.2 mg/dL, and γ-glutamyl transferase level of 20 U/L. What is the most likely diagnosis?

A. Adverse reaction to rosuvastatin
B. Paget's disease
C. Primary biliary cirrhosis
D. Retained common bile duct stone
E. Vertebral osteomyelitis

X-92. Which of the following tests is most likely to lead to the diagnosis of the patient in question X-91?

A. Magnetic resonance cholangiopancreatography
B. Magnetic resonance imaging of the lumbosacral spine
C. Plain radiographs of the lumbosacral spine
D. Right upper quadrant ultrasound
E. Serum osteocalcin

X-93. Which of the following biochemical tests is most likely to be within the normal range in a healthy, active individual with Paget's disease?

A. Serum alkaline phosphatase
B. Serum C-telopeptide
C. Serum calcium
D. Serum N-telopeptide
E. Serum osteocalcin

X-94. A 67-year-old woman presents to the clinic after a fall on the ice a week ago. She visited the local emergency department immediately after the fall, where hip radiographs were performed and were negative for fracture or dislocation. They did reveal fusion of the sacroiliac joints and coarse trabeculations in the ilium, consistent with Paget's disease. A comprehensive metabolic panel was also sent at that visit and is remarkable for an alkaline phosphatase of 257 U/L, with normal serum calcium and phosphate levels. She was discharged with analgesics and told to follow up with her primary care doctor for further management of her radiographic findings. She is recovering from her fall and denies any long-standing pain or immobility of her hip joints. She states that her father suffered from a bone disease that caused him headaches and hearing loss near the end of his life. She is very concerned about the radiographs and wants to know what they mean. Which of the following is the best treatment strategy at this point?

A. Initiate physical therapy and non–weight bearing exercises to strengthen the hip.
B. Initiate therapy with vitamin D and calcium.
C. Initiate therapy with an oral bisphosphonate.
D. Initiate therapy with prednisone 1 mg/kg, tapering over 6 months.
E. No treatment is required as she is asymptomatic.

X-95. A 32-year-old man is evaluated at a routine clinic visit for coronary risk factors. He is healthy and reports no tobacco use, his systemic blood pressure is normal, and he does not have diabetes. His family history is notable for high cholesterol in his mother and maternal grandparents. Physical examination shows tendon xanthomas. A fasting cholesterol is notable for a low-density lipoprotein cholesterol (LDL-C) of 387 mg/dL. Which of the following is the most likely genetic disorder affecting this individual?

A. Autosomal dominant hypercholesterolemia
B. Familial defective apoB-100
C. Familial hepatic lipase deficiency
D. Familial hypercholesterolemia
E. Lipoprotein lipase deficiency

X-96. All of the following are potential causes of elevated LDL EXCEPT:

A. Anorexia nervosa
B. Cirrhosis
C. Hypothyroidism
D. Nephrotic syndrome
E. Thiazide diuretics

X-97. A 16-year-old male is brought to your clinic by his parents due to concern about his weight. He has not seen a physician for many years. He states that he has gained weight due to inactivity and that he is less active because of exertional chest pain. He takes no medications. He was adopted and his parents do not know the medical history of his biological parents. Physical examination is notable for stage 1 hypertension and body mass index

of 30 kg/m². He has xanthomas on his hands, heels, and buttocks. Laboratory testing shows a low-density lipoprotein (LDL) of 210 mg/dL, creatinine of 0.7 mg/dL, total bilirubin of 3.1 mg/dL, haptoglobin below 6 mg/dL, and a glycosylated hemoglobin of 6.7%. You suspect a hereditary lipoproteinemia due to the clinical and laboratory findings. Which test would be diagnostic of the primary lipoprotein disorder in this patient?

A. Congo red staining of xanthoma biopsy
B. CT scan of the liver
C. Family pedigree analysis
D. Gas chromatography
E. LDL receptor function in skin biopsy

X-98. Your 60-year-old patient with a monoclonal gammopathy of unclear significance presents for a follow-up visit and to review recent laboratory data. His creatinine is newly elevated to 2.0 mg/dL, potassium is 3.7 mg/dL, calcium is 12.2 mg/dL, low-density lipoprotein (LDL) is 202 mg/dL, and triglycerides are 209 mg/dL. On further questioning he reports 3 months of swelling around the eyes and "foamy" urine. On examination, he has anasarca. Concerned for multiple myeloma and nephrotic syndrome, you order a urine protein/creatinine ratio, which returns at 14:1. Which treatment option would be most appropriate to treat his lipid abnormalities?

A. Cholesterol ester transfer protein inhibitor
B. Dietary management
C. HMG-CoA reductase inhibitors
D. Lipid apheresis
E. Niacin and fibrates

X-99. A 40-year-old man is evaluated as part of an executive physical examination. He has read about different screening procedures on the Internet and is interested in being screened for hemochromatosis. He is otherwise healthy and takes only a daily multivitamin. Which of the following tests is the most appropriate first step to screen for this disorder?

A. Genetic testing for C282Y mutation.
B. HFE activity assay.
C. Liver MRI.
D. Screening for hemochromatosis is not cost-effective and not advised.
E. Transferrin saturation, serum iron, and serum ferritin.

X-100. A 55-year-old white male with a history of diabetes presents to your office with complaints of generalized weakness, weight loss, nonspecific diffuse abdominal pain, and erectile dysfunction. The patient has a past history of hypercholesterolemia and takes atorvastatin. The examination is significant for hepatomegaly without tenderness, testicular atrophy, and gynecomastia. Skin examination shows a diffuse slate-gray hue that is slightly more pronounced on the face and neck. Joint examination shows mild swelling of the second and third metacarpophalangeal joints on the right hand. Which of the following studies is most likely to lead to the correct diagnosis?

A. Anti–smooth muscle antibody
B. Ceruloplasmin
C. Hepatic ultrasound with Doppler imaging
D. Hepatitis B surface antibody
E. *HFE* gene mutation screen

X-101. A 28-year-old man is evaluated for recurrent abdominal pain. He reports that over the last 5 years he has had bouts of severe abdominal pain that is diffuse with distention and not accompanied by vomiting or diarrhea. The pain is not crampy and occurs approximately four to five times per year. One of these episodes was accompanied by hallucinations. He is otherwise healthy, reports engaging in weight lifting, and admits to occasionally using anabolic steroids. During several prior episodes he visited the emergency department and underwent extensive testing including abdominal CT scan with IV and oral contrast. No cause was identified and the symptoms spontaneously resolved after about a day. Which of the following is the next most appropriate step in his evaluation?

A. Endoscopy and colonoscopy
B. Measurement of plasma gastrin level during attack
C. Measurement of urine porphyrobilinogen during attack
D. Prescription of hyoscyamine
E. Referral to psychiatry

X-102. A 58-year-old man is evaluated as part of a life insurance physical examination. He reports feeling well and is without complaints. His past medical history is notable for mild hyperlipidemia and an episode of appendicitis several years ago. He exercises about twice a week playing tennis and does not smoke. His only medication is atorvastatin. On physical examination he is mildly obese, but vital signs and the remainder of the examination are normal. Laboratories are drawn and are normal, with the exception of a uric acid level of 12 mg/dL. Which of the following statements regarding this finding is true?

A. Allopurinol should be prescribed.
B. Careful evaluation for features of insulin resistance should be undertaken.
C. He is at an increased risk of uric acid nephrolithiasis.
D. Most patients with hyperuricemia produce more uric acid than the general population.
E. Over 10 years, most patients with hyperuricemia will develop gout.

X-103. All of the following are associated with hyperuricemia EXCEPT:

A. Cardiovascular disease
B. Gouty arthritis
C. Nephrolithiasis
D. Peripheral neuropathy
E. Urate nephropathy

X-104. A 28-year-old woman seeks counseling before getting pregnant. She had a brother who died at age 9 of Lesch-Nyhan syndrome, and she is a known carrier of the genetic defect. She has no significant past medical history, and her husband has no significant family history. Which of the following statements is true?

A. Her children have no risk of disease since she is not symptomatic.
B. Her husband should be screened for carrying the genetic defect of Lesch-Nyhan syndrome.
C. If she has a daughter, the child has a 50% chance of being a carrier.
D. If she has an affected son, starting him on allopurinol from birth will prevent clinical manifestations of disease.
E. She should start taking allopurinol to decrease her risk of gout and urate nephropathy.

X-105. A 28-year-old man is admitted to the intensive care unit with fulminant hepatic failure and hemolysis. On further questioning, his family reports that he has been diagnosed with depression for 5 years and been told that his liver is "damaged." He is taking an antidepressant and occasional ibuprofen, but no other medications. Physical examination is notable for ascites and altered mental status with dystonia. Abdominal CT scan shows no biliary obstruction, but a cirrhotic liver. Which of the following findings would be most likely to confirm the underlying diagnosis?

A. 24-hour urine level of iron
B. Brain MRI showing damage to the basal ganglia
C. Genotype for HFE mutation
D. Schistocytes on peripheral blood smear
E. Slit-lamp ocular examination showing Kayser-Fleischer rings

X-106. Which of the following is the most appropriate initial treatment for the patient in question X-105?

A. Cholestyramine
B. D-penicillamine
C. Liver transplantation
D. Trientine
E. Zinc

X-107. Which of the following is true of Wilson's disease?

A. Early diagnosis is crucial as highly effective therapy is available.
B. It is inherited in an autosomal dominant pattern.
C. Serum copper levels are usually two to three times above normal.
D. The frequency of disease in the general population is approximately 1%.
E. The liver and pancreas are the most commonly affected organs.

X-108. A 19-year-old girl is evaluated by her primary care physician for recurrent long bone fractures. She has fractured her femur twice and her humerus three times. She has not had an abnormal number of falls and reports also having easy bruising. Aside from these repeated orthopedic injuries, she is otherwise healthy. Physical examination shows mildly disfigured bones; small, amber-yellowish teeth; and bluish-colored sclera. Osteogenesis imperfecta is suspected. Which of the following statements is true regarding this condition?

A. A mutation in type 1 procollagen likely is present in this patient.
B. Bone biopsy is needed for definitive diagnosis.
C. Bisphosphonates have shown long-term success in preventing long bone fractures in this condition.
D. Fractures in females tend to increase after puberty.
E. Increased bone mineral density may be demonstrated on x-ray absorptiometry.

X-109. More than 90% of patients with Marfan's syndrome have mutations in which gene?

A. *BMPR2*
B. *COL1A1*
C. *Fibrillin*
D. *TGFβ*
E. *Type IV collagen*

X-110. A 21-year-old woman comes to the clinic on the advice of her yoga instructor. She recently began classes to increase her activity level and her instructor told her that her joints seemed incredibly flexible, particularly given her inexperience. During the Scorpion exercise, she was able to extend well beyond her classmates. The patient reports good health and a mostly sedentary lifestyle. Throughout her life, she's been able to perform feats of joint laxity. Her physical examination is notable only for velvety skin and flexible joints. She is able to hyperextend her wrists at least 90°. Which of the following statements regarding this patient is true?

A. She is at risk of aortic dissection or rupture in the next 20 years.
B. She is at risk of hip dislocation in the next 20 years.
C. She is at risk of uterine rupture during pregnancy.
D. She likely has a mutation in the elastin gene.
E. She likely has a mutation of the fibrillin gene.

ANSWERS

X-1. **The answer is D.** *(Chap. 338)* Feedback control may be either positive or negative. The primary means of hormone control within the endocrine system is negative feedback. For example, when a steroid hormone level is sensed to be low by the hypothalamus a releasing hormone is released, which effects the release of a stimulatory hormone from the pituitary, and the target gland secretes the steroid hormone and plasma levels rise. The hypothalamus then senses this and decreases the release of the releasing hormone. This is employed by the endocrine system to control levels of thyroid hormone, cortisol, gonadal steroids, and growth hormone. The renin-angiotensin-aldosterone axis is independent of the pituitary and hypothalamus and involves the liver, lungs, and kidney.

X-2. **The answer is E.** *(Chap. 338)* Hormone resistance may be due to receptor mutations or signaling pathway mutations, or, most commonly, postreceptor alterations. Type 2 diabetes mellitus and leptin resistance are examples of postreceptor alterations resulting in hormone resistance. Pheochromocytoma and Graves' disease are examples of organ hyperfunction, Hashimoto's thyroiditis and Sheehan's syndrome are diseases of organ hypofunction. In the case of Sheehan's syndrome, the affected organ is the pituitary gland.

X-3. **The answer is C.** *(Chap. 338)* Intermittent pulses of GnRH are necessary to maintain pituitary sensitivity to the hormone. Continuous exposure to GnRH causes pituitary gonadotrope desensitization, which ultimately leads to decreased levels of testosterone. The relationship between GnRH and LH/FSH is a positive feedback loop where GnRH causes secretion of LH and FSH. Receptor translocation from the cytoplasm into the nucleus occurs with certain hormones (e.g., glucocorticoid); however, this receptor phenomenon is not specific to any regulatory mechanism. GnRH does not promote the production of sex hormone–binding globulin. Moreover, although binding globulins can decrease the amount of bound hormone measured in the serum, abnormal levels of binding globulins usually do not have any clinical significance because the free hormone levels usually increase.

X-4.   **The answer is B.** *(Chap. 338)* With few exceptions, hormone binding is highly specific for a single type of nuclear receptor. The mineralocorticoid-glucocorticoid hormones are a notable exception because the mineralocorticoid receptor also has a high, but not greater, affinity for glucocorticoid. An enzyme (11 β-hydroxysteroid dehydrogenase) located in renal tubules inactivates glucocorticoid, allowing selective responses to mineralocorticoid. When there is glucocorticoid excess, the enzyme becomes oversaturated and glucocorticoid can exhibit mineralocorticoid effects. This effect is in contrast to the estrogen receptor, where different compounds confer unique transcription machinery. Mineralocorticoid hormones do not have serum-binding proteins. Examples of hormones that circulate with serum-binding proteins are T_4, T_3, cortisol, estrogen, and growth hormone. Most binding protein abnormalities have little clinical consequence because the free concentrations of the hormone often remain normal.

X-5.   **The answer is C.** *(Chap. 339)* Hormones produced by the anterior pituitary include adrenocorticotropic hormone, thyroid-stimulating hormone, luteinizing hormone, follicle-stimulating hormone, prolactin, and growth hormone. The posterior pituitary produces vasopressin and oxytocin. The anterior and posterior pituitary has a separate vascular supply, and the posterior pituitary is directly innervated by the hypothalamic neurons via the pituitary stalk, thus making it susceptible to shear stress–associated dysfunction. Hypothalamic control of anterior pituitary function is through secreted hormones; thus it is less susceptible to traumatic injury.

X-6.   **The answer is B.** *(Chap. 339)* The patient has evidence of Sheehan's syndrome postpartum. In this syndrome, the hyperplastic pituitary postpartum is at increased risk for hemorrhage and/or infarction. This leads to bilateral visual changes, headache, and meningeal signs. Ophthalmoplegia may be observed. In severe cases, cardiovascular collapse and altered levels of consciousness may be observed. Laboratory evaluation commonly shows hypoglycemia. Pituitary CT or MRI may show signs of sellar hemorrhage if present. Involvement of all pituitary hormones may be seen, though the most acute finding is often hypoglycemia and hypotension from the failure of adrenocorticotropic hormone. The hypoglycemia and hypotension present in this case suggest failure of the glucocorticoid system; thus treatment with a corticosteroid is indicated. There is no evidence of sepsis; thus antibiotics and drotrecogin alfa are not indicated. With a normal hematocrit and no reported evidence of massive hemorrhage, packed red cell transfusion is unlikely to be helpful. Although thyroid-stimulating hormone production is undoubtedly low in this patient, the most immediate concern is replacement of glucocorticoid.

X-7.   **The answer is D.** *(Chap. 339)* Functional pituitary adenoma presentations include acromegaly, as in this patient, prolactinomas, and Cushing's syndrome. Hypersecretion of growth hormone underlies this syndrome in patients with pituitary masses, though ectopic production of growth hormone, particularly by tumors, has been reported. Because growth hormone is secreted in a highly pulsatile fashion, obtaining random serum levels is not reliable. Thus, the downstream mediator of systemic effects of growth hormone, IGF-1, is measured to screen for growth hormone excess. IGF-1 is made by the liver in response to growth hormone stimulation. An oral glucose tolerance test with growth hormone obtained at 0, 30, and 60 minutes may also be used to screen for acromegaly, as normal persons should suppress growth hormone to this challenge. Serum prolactin level is useful to screen for prolactinomas; 24-hour urinary free cortisol and ACTH assay are useful screens for Cushing's disease.

X-8.   **The answer is B.** *(Chap. 339)* Hyperprolactinemia is the most common pituitary hormone hypersecretion syndrome in both men and women. Although pituitary adenoma is a frequent cause, there are several physiologic, medication-related, and potentially reversible etiologies. Prolactin is normally elevated during pregnancy and lactation, though levels should fall to normal within 6 months of cessation of breastfeeding. Nipple stimulation, sleep, and stress may all increase prolactin levels. Systemic disorders such as chronic renal failure and cirrhosis may also cause elevated prolactin levels. Prolactin levels are also typically elevated after generalized seizures, which may be useful in the evaluation of pseudoseizures. Drug-induced hypersecretion is associated with dopamine receptor blockers, dopamine synthesis inhibitors, opiates, H_2 antagonists, imipramines, selective serotonin reuptake inhibitors, and calcium channel blockers. Hypothalamic-pituitary stalk damage may also cause hyperprolactinemia. Rathke's cysts, which are benign intra-sellar lesions, may produce endocrinologic abnormalities similar to pituitary adenomas.

X-9.   **The answer is E.** *(Chap. 339)* Tumors arising from the lactotrope cells of the pituitary account for half of all functioning pituitary tumors and most commonly affect women. The most common presentations are amenorrhea, infertility, and/or galactorrhea. Micro-adenomas rarely progress to become macroadenomas. For symptomatic disease, the primary goals of therapy are control of hyperprolactinemia, reduction of tumor size, restoration of menses and fertility, and resolution of galactorrhea. Usually oral dopamine agonists, such as carbergoline and bromocriptine, are used for this purpose.

X-10.   **The answer is C.** *(Chap. 339)* Adult growth hormone deficiency is usually caused by hypothalamic or pituitary damage. Because growth hormone is no longer important for achieving stature, the presentation is different from childhood growth hormone deficiency. Although growth hormone has direct tissue effects, it primarily acts through increasing secretion of IGF-1, which in turn stimulates lipolysis, increases circulating fatty acids, reduces omental fat mass, and enhances lean body mass. Thus, deficiency of growth hormone causes the opposite effects. In addition, hypertension, left ventricular dysfunction, and increased plasma fibrinogen levels may also be present with deficient growth hormone. Reduced, not increased, bone mineral density may also occur in adults with growth hormone deficiency.

X-11.   **The answer is E.** *(Chap. 339)* The patient has a clinical presentation consistent with Cushing's syndrome. Although many cases of inappropriate elevation of ACTH are due to pituitary tumors, a substantial proportion are due to ectopic ACTH secretion. Clues to this diagnosis include a rapid onset of hypercortisolism features associated with skin hyperpigmentation and severe myopathy. Additionally, hypertension, hypokalemic metabolic alkalosis, glucose intolerance, and edema are more prominent in ectopic ACTH secretion than in pituitary tumors. Serum potassium below 3.3 mmol/L is present in 70% of ectopic ACTH cases, but in less than 10% of pituitary-dependent Cushing's syndrome. ACTH levels will be high, as this is the underlying cause of both types of Cushing's syndrome. Corticotropin-releasing hormone is rarely the cause of Cushing's syndrome. Unfortunately, MRI of the pituitary gland will not visualize lesions less than 2 mm; thus occasional sampling of the inferior petrosal veins is required, but this is not indicated in the case presented at this time in the evaluation.

X-12.   **The answer is C.** *(Chap. 339)* The patient has panhypopituitarism and is unable to make TSH; thus her plasma TSH level will always be low, regardless of the adequacy of her T_4 replacement. A free T_4 level will allow the determination of whether her plasma level is in the normal range of thyroid hormone. This, coupled with her symptoms, will aid in the determination of proper levothyroxine dosing. There is no evidence of recurrent disease clinically; thus MRI is not useful. She is unlikely to have primary thyroid disease, and T_4 level is unknown presently, so thyroid uptake scan is not indicated at this time.

X-13.   **The answer is A.** *(Chap. 339)* The diagnosis of Cushing's syndrome relies on documentation of endogenous hypercortisolism. Of the list of choices, the most cost-effective and precise test is the 24-hour urine free cortisol. Failure to suppress plasma morning cortisol after overnight suppression with 1 mg dexamethasone is an alternative. Most ACTH-secreting pituitary adenomas are less than 5 mm in diameter, and approximately half are not detected even with sensitive MRI. Further, because incidental microadenomas are common in the pituitary, the presence of a small pituitary abnormality on MRI may not establish the source of ACTH production. Basal plasma ACTH levels are used to distinguish between ACTH-independent (adrenal or exogenous glucocorticoid) and ACTH-dependent (pituitary, ectopic ACTH) sources of hypercortisolism. Mean basal ACTH levels are higher in patients with ectopic ACTH production than in patients with pituitary ACTH adenomas. There is significant overlap in ACTH levels, however, and this test should not be used as an initial diagnostic test. Rarely, patients have Cushing's syndrome and elevated ACTH due to a CRH-releasing tumor. In this case, CRH levels are elevated. Inferior petrosal venous sampling can be used to identify a pituitary source of ACTH secretion when imaging modalities do not reveal a source.

X-14.   **The answer is B.** (*Chap. 339*) The identification of an empty sella is often the result of an incidental MRI finding. Typically these patients will have normal pituitary function and should be reassured. It is likely that the surrounding rim of pituitary tissue is functioning normally. An empty sella may signal the insidious onset of hypopituitarism, and laboratory results should be followed closely. Unless her clinical situation changes, repeat MRI is not indicated. Endocrine malignancy is unlikely, and surgery is not part of the management of an empty sella.

X-15.   **The answer is A.** (*Chap. 340*) The patient has a classic presentation for a patient with idiopathic diabetes insipidus with long-standing urinary frequency, thirst, enuresis, and nocturia. Patients may also report mild fatigue from frequent nocturnal awakenings. Diabetes insipidus may be nephrogenic or central, though this case presentation is not specific for either etiology. Diabetes insipidus is confirmed by measurement of 24-hour urine volume, which is more than 50 mg/kg per day (3500 mL in a 70-kg male), and urine osmolarity of greater than 300 mosmol/L. In order to differentiate central from nephrogenic diabetes insipidus, history may be useful in determining prior head trauma, neurosurgery, or granulomatous disease that may damage the neurohypophysis, or may suggest a medication such as lithium known to cause nephrogenic diabetes insipidus. The fluid deprivation test, in which a patient is deprived of fluid and hourly urine output; body weight; plasma osmolarity and/or sodium concentration; and urine osmolarity are measured. If fluid deprivation confirms persistent elevation of urine osmolarity, then severe diabetes insipidus is again confirmed. Desmopressin can be administered at this point and if the electrolyte, urinary, and clinical variables are corrected, central disease is confirmed. In nephrogenic diabetes insipidus, there is minimal response to ADH, as the primary defect is in the kidney. MRI of the brain is not useful until after central disease is confirmed.

X-16.   **The answer is B.** (*Chap. 340*) This patient presents with acute central diabetes insipidus (DI) in the context of AMML. MRI will most likely demonstrate a chloroma (myeloid tumor often seen in AMML) in the posterior pituitary, particularly given his history of other extra–bone marrow tumor nodules. The urine is dilute due to the ADH deficiency leading to hypernatremia. The altered mental status is likely due to the hypernatremia, which typically develops in central DI as water intake cannot keep up with urine output, which can exceed 5 L/d. Immediate replacement of ADH in the form of desmopressin will confirm the diagnosis of central DI if urine output drops and will provide symptomatic relief. Desmopressin may be administered nasally or intravenously with rapid onset of action. Hydrochlorothiazide is used in nephrogenic DI to increase proximal sodium and water reabsorption. ATRA is used to treat acute promyelocytic leukemia, not AMML. Hydrocortisone would be the therapy of choice for acute Addisonian crisis, not central DI. Lithium is a well-known cause of nephrogenic DI.

X-17.   **The answer is B.** (*Chap. 341*) Nutritional and maternal iodine deficiencies are common in many parts of the developing world and, when severe, can result in cretinism. Cretinism is characterized by mental and growth retardation but is preventable by administration of iodine and/or thyroid hormone early in life. Concomitant selenium deficiency can contribute to the neurologic manifestations. Iodine supplementation of bread, salt, and other foods has markedly decreased the rates of this disease. Beriberi disease is a nervous system ailment caused by a thiamine deficiency in the diet. Scurvy is due to vitamin C deficiency.

Folate deficiency in pregnant women is associated with an increased risk preterm labor and a number of congenital malformations, most notably involving the neural tube. Folate supplementation can lower the risk of spina bifida, anencephaly, congenital heart disease, cleft lips, and limb deformities. Vitamin A deficiency is a common cause of blindness in the developing world.

X-18.   **The answer is E.** *(Chap. 341)* T_4 is secreted from the thyroid gland in approximately 20-fold greater quantities than T_3. Both hormones are bound to plasma proteins including albumin, transthyretin, and thyroxine-binding protein. Thyroxine-binding protein has a high affinity for T_4; thus despite its low concentration it carries 80% of the plasma hormone. It is followed by albumin and then transthyretin. Pregnant women may be euthyroid with elevated levels of total T_4 because of the increase in thyroid-binding globulin. T_3 is less protein bound than T_4. Unbound hormone is thought to be biologically available to tissues, and normalization of the unbound fraction is the primary goal of homeostatic mechanisms. Measurement of free T_4 is biologically more relevant than total T_4. Thyroid peroxidase is an enzyme within the thyroid involved in the organification of iodine.

X-19.   **The answer is C.** *(Chap. 341)* There are a number of conditions associated with normal thyroid function, but hyperthyroxinemia. Although some of these are associated with clinical hyperthyroidism, many simply have elevated levels of total T_4 and normal conversion to T_3 and thus are clinically normal. Anything that increases liver production of thyroid-binding globulin will produce elevated total T_4 levels and normal free T_4 and T_3 levels. In this category are pregnancy, estrogen-containing oral contraceptives, cirrhosis, and familial excess thyroid-binding globulin production. Familial dysalbuminemic hyperthyroxinemia results in an albumin mutation and increased T_4 with normal free T_4 and T_3 levels. Sick-euthyroid syndrome occurs during acute medical and psychiatric illness. In this syndrome, there is transiently increased unbound T_4 and decreased TSH. Total T_4 and T_3 may be decreased, particularly later in the course of disease.

X-20.   **The answer is D.** *(Chap. 341)* Iodine deficiency remains the most common cause of hypothyroidism worldwide. It is present at relatively high levels even in the developed world including Europe. In areas of iodine sufficiency, autoimmune disease (Hashimoto's thyroiditis) and iatrogenic hypothyroidism (treatment of hyperthyroidism) are the most common causes.

X-21.   **The answer is B.** *(Chap. 341)* There are a number of important effects of thyroid hormone (or its absence) on the cardiovascular system. Importantly, hypothyroidism is associated with bradycardia and reduced myocardial contractility, and thereby reduced stroke volume. Increased peripheral resistance may be accompanied by systemic hypertension, particularly diastolic hypertension in hypothyroidism. Pericardial effusions are found in up to 30% of patients with hypothyroidism, though they rarely cause decreased cardiac function. Finally, in hypothyroid patients, blood flow is directed away from the skin and thus produces cool extremities.

X-22.   **The answer is B.** *(Chap. 341)* The most common cause of hypothyroidism in the United States is autoimmune thyroiditis, as it is an iodine-replete area. Although earlier in the disease, a radioiodine uptake scan may have shown diffusely increased uptake from lymphocytic infiltration, at this point in the disease when the infiltrate is "burned out" there is likely to be little found on the scan. Likewise, a thyroid ultrasound would only be useful for presumed multinodular goiter. Antithyroid peroxidase antibodies are commonly found in patients with autoimmune thyroiditis, while antithyroglobulin antibodies are found less commonly. Antithyroglobulin antibodies are also found in other thyroid disorders (Graves' disease, thyrotoxicosis) as well as systemic autoimmune diseases (SLEs). Thyroglobulin is released from the thyroid in all types of thyrotoxicosis with the exception of factitious disease. This patient, however, was hypothyroid, and thus serum thyroglobulin levels are unlikely to be helpful.

X-23. **The answer is D.** *(Chap. 341)* An increase in TSH in a patient with hypothyroidism that was previously stable in dosing for many years suggests either a failure of taking the medication, difficulty with absorption from bowel disease, or medication interaction or drug-drug interaction affecting clearance. Patients with normal body weight taking more than 200 μg of levothyroxine per day who have elevated TSH strongly suggests noncompliance. Such patients should be encouraged to take two tablets at one time on the day they remember, to attempt to reach the weekly target dose; the long drug half-life makes this practice safe. Other causes of increased thyroxine requirements include malabsorption, such as with celiac disease or small bowel surgery, estrogen therapy, and drugs that interfere with T_4 absorption (e.g., ferrous sulfate and cholestyramine) or clearance, such as lovastatin, amiodarone, carbamazepine, and phenytoin.

X-24. **The answer is A.** *(Chap. 341)* The patient has myxedema coma. This condition of profound hypothyroidism most commonly occurs in the elderly, and often a precipitating condition may be identified such as myocardial infarction or infection. Clinical manifestations include altered level of consciousness, bradycardia, and hypothermia. Management includes repletion of thyroid hormone through IV levothyroxine, but also supplementation of glucocorticoids because there is impaired adrenal reserve in severe hypothyroidism. Care must be taken with rewarming as it may precipitate cardiovascular collapse. Therefore, external warming is indicated only if the temperature is below 30°C. Hypertonic saline and glucose may be used if hyponatremia or hypoglycemia is severe; however, hypotonic solutions should be avoided as they may worsen fluid retention. Because the metabolism of many substances is markedly reduced, sedation should be avoided or minimized. Similarly, blood levels of drugs should be monitored when available.

X-25. **The answer is A.** *(Chap. 341)* Patients with Graves' disease produce thyroid-stimulating immunoglobulins. They subsequently produce higher levels of T_4 compared with the normal population. As a result, many patients with Graves' disease are mildly iodine deficient, and T_4 production is somewhat limited by the availability of iodine. Exposure to iodinated contrast thus reverses iodine deficiency and may precipitate worsening hyperthyroidism. Additionally, the reversal of mild iodine deficiency may make I-125 therapy for Graves' disease less successful because thyroid iodine uptake is lessened in the iodine-replete state.

X-26. **The answer is C.** *(Chap. 341)* Hyperthyroidism is associated with a number of cardiovascular complications including tachycardia, palpitations, high cardiac output with bounding pulse, widened pulse pressure, and aortic systolic murmur. This may lead to worsened angina in predisposed patients. Atrial fibrillation is more common in patients greater than 50 years of age, and treatment of thyroid state alone will lead to the reversal of atrial fibrillation in half of patients, suggesting underlying cardiac disorder in the remainder of unconverted patients.

X-27. **The answer is B.** *(Chap. 341)* Although lid retraction can occur in any type of hyperthyroidism, Graves' disease is associated with specific eye signs that are thought to be due to the interaction of autoantibodies with periorbital muscles. The onset of Graves' ophthalmopathy may occur before or after hyperthyroidism, and rarely may not be associated with hyperthyroidism at all, but simply the effects of the presence of autoantibodies on the periorbital muscles. Subtle features are eye grittiness, discomfort, and excess tearing. Proptosis occurs in one-third of patients and may result in corneal abrasion if there is a failure of closure of the eyelids, particularly during sleep. The most serious manifestation is compression of the optic nerve at the apex of the orbit, which can lead to papilledema and permanent vision loss if left untreated.

X-28. **The answer is C.** *(Chap. 341)* The main antithyroid drugs used in the treatment of Graves' disease are propylthiouracil, carbimazole, and the active metabolite of carbimazole, methimazole. All act to inhibit the function of thyroid peroxidase. While propylthiouracil also reduces the peripheral conversion of T_4 to T_3, this is not its major mechanism of action and is not responsible for the majority of the drug's utility in the therapy of Graves' disease.

X-29. **The answer is C.** *(Chap. 341)* Sick-euthyroid syndrome can occur in the setting of any acute, severe illness. Abnormalities in the levels of circulating TSH and thyroid hormone are thought to result from the release of cytokines in response to severe stress. Multiple abnormalities may occur. The most common hormone pattern is a decrease in total and unbound T_3 levels as peripheral conversion of T_4 to T_3 is impaired. Teleologically, the fall in T_3, the most active thyroid hormone, is thought to limit catabolism in starved or ill patients. TSH levels may vary dramatically, from 0.1 to above 20 mU/L, depending on when they are measured during the course of illness. Very sick patients may have a decrease in T_4 levels. This patient undoubtedly has abnormal thyroid function tests as a result of his injuries from the motor vehicle accident. There is no indication for obtaining further imaging in this case. Steroids have no role. The most appropriate management consists of simple observation. Over the course of weeks to months, as the patient recovers, thyroid function will return to normal.

X-30 and X-31. **The answers are E and B, respectively.** *(Chap. 341)* Subacute thyroiditis, also known as de Quervain's thyroiditis, granulomatous thyroiditis, or viral thyroiditis, is a multiphase illness that occurs three times more frequently in women than men. Multiple viruses have been implicated, but none have been definitively identified as the trigger for subacute thyroiditis. The diagnosis can be overlooked in patients as the symptoms mimic pharyngitis, and it frequently has a similarly benign course. In this patient, Graves' disease is unlikely given her elevated TSH and negative antibody panel. Autoimmune hypothyroidism should be considered; however, the tempo of her illness, the tenderness of the thyroid on examination, and her preceding viral illness make this diagnosis less likely. Ludwig's angina is a potentially life-threatening bacterial infection of the retropharyngeal and submandibular spaces, often caused by preceding dental infection. Cat-scratch fever is a usually benign illness that presents with lymphadenopathy, fever, and malaise. It is caused by *Bartonella henselae* and is frequently transmitted from cat scratches that penetrate the epidermis. It will not cause an elevated TSH. Subacute thyroiditis can present with hypothyroidism, thyrotoxicosis, or neither. In the first phase of the disease, thyroid inflammation leads to follicle destruction and release of thyroid hormone. Thyrotoxicosis ensues. In the second phase, the thyroid is depleted of hormone and hypothyroidism results. A recovery phase typically follows in which decreased inflammation allows the follicles to heal and regenerate hormone.

X-32. **The answer is B.** *(Chap. 341)* Subacute thyroiditis, also known as de Quervain's thyroiditis, granulomatous thyroiditis, and viral thyroiditis, is characterized clinically by fever, constitutional symptoms, and a painful, enlarged thyroid. The etiology is thought to be a viral infection. The peak incidence is between 30 and 50 years of age, and women are affected more frequently than men. The symptoms depend on the phase of the illness. During the initial phase of follicular destruction, there is a release of thyroglobulin and thyroid hormones. As a result, there is increased circulating T_4 and T_3, with concomitant suppression of TSH. Symptoms of thyrotoxicosis predominate at this point. Radioiodine uptake is low or undetectable. After several weeks, thyroid hormone is depleted and a phase of hypothyroidism ensues, with low unbound T_4 levels and moderate elevations of TSH. Radioiodine uptake returns to normal. Finally, after 4–6 months, thyroid hormone and TSH levels return to normal as the disease subsides. Patient A is consistent with the thyrotoxic phase of subacute thyroiditis except for the increased radioiodine uptake scan. Patient C is more consistent with Graves' disease with suppression of TSH, an elevated uptake scan, and elevated thyroid hormones as a result of stimulating immunoglobulin. Patient D is consistent with a neoplasm. Patient E is consistent with central hypothyroidism.

X-33. **The answer is E.** *(Chap. 341)* Thyroid nodules are found in 5% of patients. Nodules are more common with age, in women, and in iodine-deficient areas. Given their prevalence, the cost of screening, and the generally benign course of most nodules, the choice and order of screening tests have been very contentious. A small percentage of incidentally discovered nodules will represent thyroid cancer, however. A TSH should be the first test to check after detection of a thyroid nodule. A majority of patients will have normal thyroid function tests. In the case of a normal TSH, fine-needle aspiration or ultrasound-guided biopsy can be pursued. If the TSH is low, a radionuclide scan should be performed to determine if the nodule is the source of thyroid hyperfunction (a "hot" nodule). In this case, this is the best course of action. "Hot" nodules can be treated medically, resected, or ablated with radioactive iodine. "Cold" nodules should be further evaluated with a fine-needle aspiration. Four percent of nodules undergoing biopsy are malignant, 10% are suspicious for malignancy, and 86% are indeterminate or benign.

X-34. **The answer is C.** *(Chap. 342)* The adrenal gland has three major functions: glucocorticoid synthesis, aldosterone synthesis, and androgen precursor synthesis. Glucocorticoid synthesis is controlled by the pituitary secretion of ACTH. The primary stimulus for aldosterone synthesis is the renin-angiotensin-aldosterone system, which is independent of the pituitary. Thus, morning cortisol secretion and release of cortisol in response to stress are regulated by the pituitary gland, while regulation of sodium retention and potassium excretion by aldosterone is independent of the pituitary and would be preserved in this patient.

X-35. **The answer is A.** *(Chap. 342)* Cushing's syndrome is a constellation of features that result from chronic exposure to elevated levels of cortisol from any etiology. Although the most common etiology is ACTH-producing pituitary adenoma, which accounts for 75% of Cushing's syndrome, 15% is due to ectopic ACTH syndromes such as bronchial or pancreatic tumors, small cell lung cancer, and others. ACTH-independent Cushing's syndrome is much more rare. Adrenocortical adenoma underlies 5–10% of cases, and adrenocortical carcinoma is present in 1% of Cushing's cases. McCune-Albright syndrome is a genetic cause of bone abnormalities, skin lesions (cafe au lait), and premature puberty, particularly in girls. Interestingly, it is caused by a sporadic in utero mutation, not an inherited disorder, and thus will not be passed onto progeny.

X-36. **The answer is B.** *(Chap. 342)* Conn's syndrome refers to an aldosterone-producing adrenal adenoma. Although it accounts for 40% of hyperaldosterone states, bilateral micronodular adrenal hyperplasia is more common. Other causes of hyperaldosteronism are substantially more rare, accounting for less than 1% of disease. The hallmark of Conn's syndrome is hypertension with hypokalemia. Because aldosterone stimulates sodium retention and potassium excretion, all patients should be hypokalemic at presentation. Serum sodium is usually normal because of concurrent fluid retention. Hypokalemia may be associated with muscle weakness, proximal myopathy, or even paralysis. Hypokalemia may be exacerbated by thiazide diuretics. Additional features include metabolic alkalosis that may contribute to muscle cramps and tetany.

X-37. **The answer is B.** *(Chap. 342)* Incidental adrenal masses are often discovered during radiographic testing for another condition and are found in approximately 6% of adult subjects at autopsy. Fifty percent of patients with a history of malignancy and a newly discovered adrenal mass will actually have an adrenal metastasis. Fine-needle aspiration of a suspected metastatic malignancy will often be diagnostic. In the absence of a suspected nonadrenal malignancy, most adrenal incidentalomas are benign. Primary adrenal malignancies are uncommon (<0.01%), and fine-needle aspiration is not useful to distinguish between benign and malignant primary adrenal tumors. Although 90% of these masses are nonsecretory, patients with an incidentaloma should be screened for pheochromocytoma and hypercortisolism with plasma free metanephrines and an overnight dexamethasone suppression test, respectively. When radiographic features suggest a benign neoplasm (<3 cm), scanning should be repeated in 3–6 months. When masses are larger than 6 cm, surgical removal (if more likely to be primary adrenal malignancy) or fine-needle aspiration (if more likely to be metastatic malignancy) is preferred.

X-38. **The answer is A.** *(Chap. 343)* When the diagnosis of pheochromocytoma is entertained the first step is measurement of catecholamines and/or metanephrines. This can be achieved by urinary tests for vanillylmandelic acid, catecholamines, fractionated metanephrines, or total metanephrines. Total metanephrines have a high sensitivity and therefore are frequently used. A value of three times the upper limit of normal is highly suggestive of pheochromocytoma. Borderline elevations, as this patient had, are likely to be false positives. The next most appropriate step is to remove potentially confounding dietary or drug exposures, if possible, and repeat the test. Likely culprit drugs include levodopa, sympathomimetics, diuretics, tricyclic antidepressants, and alpha and beta blockers (labetalol in this case). Sertraline is an SSRI antidepressant, not a tricyclic. Alternatively, a clonidine suppression test may be ordered.

X-39.   **The answer is E.** (Chap. 343) Complete removal of the pheochromocytoma is the only therapy that leads to a long-term cure, although 90% of tumors are benign. However, preoperative control of hypertension is necessary to prevent surgical complications and lower mortality. This patient is presenting with encephalopathy in a hypertensive crisis. The hypertension should be managed initially with IV medications to lower the mean arterial pressure by approximately 20% over the initial 24-hour period. Medications that can be used for hypertensive crisis in pheochromocytoma include nitroprusside, nicardipine, and phentolamine. Once the acute hypertensive crisis has resolved, transition to oral α-adrenergic blockers is indicated. Phenoxybenzamine is the most commonly used drug and is started at low doses (5–10 mg three times daily) and titrated to the maximum tolerated dose (usually 20–30 mg daily). Once alpha blockers have been initiated, beta blockade can safely be utilized and is particularly indicated for ongoing tachycardia. Liberal salt and fluid intake helps expand plasma volume and treat orthostatic hypotension. Once blood pressure is maintained below 160/100 mmHg with moderate orthostasis, it is safe to proceed to surgery. If blood pressure remains elevated despite treatment with alpha blockade, addition of calcium channel blockers, angiotensin receptor blockers, or angiotensin-converting enzyme inhibitors should be considered. Diuretics should be avoided, as they will exacerbate orthostasis.

X-40.   **The answer is C.** (Chap. 344) The risk of both type 1 and type 2 diabetes mellitus is rising in all populations, but the risk of type 2 diabetes is rising at a substantially faster rate. In the United States, the age-adjusted prevalence of diabetes mellitus is 7.1% in non-Hispanic whites, 7.5% in Asian Americans, 11.8% in Hispanics, and 12.6% in non-Hispanic blacks. Comparable data are not available for individuals belonging to American Indian, Alaska Native, or Pacific Islander populations, but the prevalence is thought to be even higher than in the non-Hispanic black population.

X-41.   **The answer is E.** (Chap. 344) Glucose tolerance is classified into three categories: normal glucose tolerance, impaired glucose homeostasis, and diabetes mellitus. Normal glucose tolerance is defined by the following: fasting plasma glucose below 100 mg/dL, plasma glucose below 140 mg/dL following an oral glucose challenge, and hemoglobin A1C less than 5.6%. Abnormal glucose homeostasis is defined as fasting plasma glucose 100–125 mmol/dL or plasma glucose 140–199 following oral glucose tolerance test or hemoglobin A1C of 5.7–6.4%. Actual diabetes mellitus is defined by either a fasting plasma glucose above 126 mg/dL, glucose of 200 mg/dL after oral glucose tolerance test, or hemoglobin A1C of 6.5% or above.

X-42.   **The answer is E.** (Chap. 344) Because the patient has symptoms, she is not being screened for diabetes mellitus. For screening, the fasting plasma glucose or hemoglobin A1C is recommended. Because the patient has symptoms, a random plasma glucose of greater than 200 mg/dL is adequate to diagnose diabetes mellitus. Other criteria include fasting plasma glucose above 126 mg/dL or hemoglobin A1C above 6.4% or 2-hour plasma glucose above 200 during an oral glucose tolerance test. C peptide is a useful tool to determine if the normal cleavage of insulin from its precursor is occurring. A normal C-peptide level with hypoglycemia suggests surreptitious insulin use, and a low C-peptide with hyperglycemia suggests pancreatic failure.

X-43.   **The answer is B.** (Chap. 344) Risk factors for type 2 diabetes mellitus include family history of diabetes mellitus, including parent or sibling, BMI greater than 25 kg/m², physical inactivity, race/ethnicity, previously identified impaired fasting glucose or hemoglobin

A1C 5.7–6.4%, systemic hypertension, history of gestational diabetes or delivery of a baby greater than 4 kg, HDL less than 35 mmol/L and/or triglyceride level greater than 250 mg/dL, polycystic ovarian disease or acanthosis nigricans, and history of cardiovascular disease.

X-44.   **The answer is A.** *(Chap. 344)* Type 1 diabetes mellitus often has a more severe presentation with diabetic ketoacidosis and often presents in younger individuals compared with type 2 diabetes; however, there are some cases where the distinction of type 1 from type 2 is not straightforward. There is HLA-DR3 localization preferences for type 1 diabetes; several haplotypes are present in 40% of children with type 1 diabetes mellitus, but it is still the minority. Immunologic destruction of the beta cell is the primary cause of disease in type 1 diabetes, and islet cell antibodies are commonly present. GAD, insulin, IA/ICA-512, and ZnT-8 are the most common targets. Commercially available assays for GAD-65 autoantibodies are widely available and can demonstrate antibodies in more than 85% of individuals with recent-onset type 1 diabetes. These autoantibodies are infrequently present in type 2 diabetes; mellitus at 5–10%. There may be some residual insulin in the plasma in early type 1 diabetes; thus this will not distinguish the two conditions reliably. Polymorphisms of the peroxisome proliferator-activated receptor γ-2 have been described in type 2 diabetes mellitus, but cannot distinguish the two conditions.

X-45.   **The answer is C.** *(Chap. 344)* Type 2 diabetes mellitus is preceded by a period of impaired fasting glucose or impaired glucose tolerance, and a number of agents and interventions have been studied in this period to prevent progression to frank diabetes mellitus. The Diabetes Prevention Program demonstrated that intensive lifestyle changes including diet and exercise prevented or delayed the development of diabetes mellitus by 58% compared to placebo. Metformin was used in the same study and prevented the development of diabetes by 31%. Other drug therapies have been studied and showed delayed progression including alpha-glucosidase inhibitors, thiazolidinediones, and orlistat, though none are approved for this purpose, and the American Diabetes Association recommends only metformin for therapy in impaired glucose tolerance. Sulfonylureas, such as glyburide, stimulate glucose secretion and have not been shown to delay progression to type 2 diabetes.

X-46.   **The answer is E.** *(Chap. 344)* Diabetic ketoacidosis and hyperglycemic hyperosmolar state exist on a spectrum, with diabetic ketoacidosis being more common in patients with type 1 diabetes mellitus, but it does occur with some frequency in patients with type 2 diabetes. Both conditions include hyperglycemia, dehydration, absolute or relative insulin deficiency, and acid-base abnormalities. Ketosis is more common in diabetic ketoacidosis. In diabetic ketoacidosis, glucose normally ranges from 250 to 600 mg/dL, while it is frequently 600–1200 mg/dL in the hyperglycemic hyperosmolar state. Sodium is often mildly depressed in ketoacidosis and is preserved in the hyperosmolar state. Potassium is normal to elevated in diabetic ketoacidosis and normal in hyperglycemic hyperosmolar patients. Magnesium, chloride, and phosphate are normal in both conditions. Creatinine may be slightly elevated in diabetic ketoacidosis, but is often moderately elevated in the hyperglycemic hyperosmolar state. Plasma ketones may be slightly positive in hyperosmolar patients, but are always strongly positive in diabetic ketoacidosis. Because hyperosmolarity is the hallmark of hyperglycemic hyperosmolar patients, they have an osmolarity of 330–380 mosm/mL, while patients with diabetic ketoacidosis have a plasma osmolarity ranging from 300 to 320 mosm/mL. Serum bicarbonate is markedly depressed in diabetic ketoacidosis and normal or slightly depressed in the hyperosmolar state. Arterial pH is depressed at less than 7.3 in ketoacidosis and more than 7.3 in the hyperosmolar state. Finally, the anion gap is wide in diabetic ketoacidosis and normal to slightly elevated in the hyperglycemic hyperosmolar state.

X-47.   **The answer is C.** *(Chap. 344)* Diabetic retinopathy is the leading cause of blindness in adults aged 20–74 years in the United States. Blindness is the result of macular edema and progressive retinopathy, which can be divided into nonproliferative and proliferative retinopathy. Nonproliferative retinopathy tends to occur in the first and early second decades after diagnosis and is characterized by retinal vascular microaneurysms, blot hemorrhages, and cotton-wool spots. Neovascularization is the hallmark of proliferative retinopathy and occurs in response to retinal hypoxemia. Newly formed vessels occur in the retina and, because they are fragile, rupture easily and cause vitreous hemorrhage, fibrosis, and ultimately retinal detachment.

X-48. **The answer is C.** *(Chap. 344)* Diabetic ulcers represent a major source of morbidity and even mortality in patients with diabetes mellitus. Although a number of interventions have been tried, only six interventions are recommended by the American Diabetes Association for demonstrated efficacy in the management of diabetic foot wounds: (1) off-loading, (2) debridement, (3) wound dressings, (4) appropriate use of antibiotics, (5) revascularization, and (6) limited amputation. Hyperbaric oxygen therapy has been used and is widely promoted through marketing, but rigorous proof of efficacy is lacking.

X-49. **The answer is D.** *(Chap. 344)* Insulin preparations can be divided into short-acting and long-acting insulins. The short-acting insulins include regular and new preparations including aspart, glulisine, and lispro. Regular insulin has an onset of action of 0.5–1 hour and is effective for 4–6 hours. The other three short-acting insulins have an onset of action of less than 0.25 hours and are effective for 3–4 hours. Long-acting insulins include detemir, glargine, and NPH. Detemir and glargine have an onset of action of 1–4 hours and last up to 24 hours, while NPH has an onset of action of 1–4 hours and is effective for 10–16 hours. These insulins have a number of combination preparations that take advantage of the different durations of onset and action to provide optimal efficacy and compliance.

X-50. **The answer is D.** *(Chap. 344)* First-line oral therapy for patients with type 2 diabetes mellitus is metformin. It is contraindicated in patients with GFR less than 60 mL/min, any form of acidosis, congestive heart failure, liver disease, or severe hypoxemia, but is well tolerated in most individuals. Insulin secretagogues, biguanides, alpha-glucosidase inhibitors, thiazolidinediones, GLP-1 agonists, DPP-IV inhibitors, and insulin have all been approved as monotherapy for type 2 diabetes. Because of extensive clinical experience with metformin, favorable side effect profile, and relatively low cost, it is the recommended first-line agent. It has additional benefits of promotion of mild weight loss, lower insulin levels, and mild improvements in lipid profile. Sulfonylureas such as glyburide, GLP-1 agonists such as exenatide, and insulin dipeptidyl peptidase-4 inhibitors such as sitagliptin may be appropriate as combination therapy, but are not considered first-line therapy for most patients.

X-51. **The answer is A.** *(Chap. 344)* The Diabetes Control and Complications Trial (DCCT) found definitive proof that a reduction in chronic hyperglycemia can prevent many of the complications of type 1 diabetes mellitus (DM). This multicenter randomized trial enrolled over 1400 patients with type 1 DM to either intensive or conventional diabetes management and prospectively evaluated the development of retinopathy, nephropathy, and neuropathy. The intensive group received multiple administrations of insulin daily along with education and psychological counseling. The intensive group achieved a mean hemoglobin A1C of 7.3% versus 9.1% in the conventional group. Improvement in glycemic control resulted in a 47% reduction in retinopathy, a 54% reduction in nephropathy, and a 60% reduction in neuropathy. There was a nonsignificant trend toward improvement in macrovascular complications. The results of the DCCT showed that individuals in the intensive group would attain up to 7 more years of intact vision and up to 5 more years free from lower limb amputation. Later, the United Kingdom Prospective Diabetes Study (UKPDS) studied over 5000 individuals with type 2 DM. Individuals receiving intensive glycemic control had a reduction in microvascular events but no significant change in macrovascular complications. These two trials were pivotal in showing a benefit of glycemic control in reducing microvascular complications in patients with type 1 and type 2 DM, respectively. Another result from the UKPDS was that strict blood pressure control resulted in an improvement in macrovascular complications.

X-52. **The answer is D.** *(Chap. 344)* Tight glycemic control with a hemoglobin A1C of 7% or less has been shown in the Diabetes Control and Complications Trial (DCCT) in type 1 diabetic patients and the United Kingdom Prospective Diabetes Study (UKPDS) in type 2 diabetic patients to lead to improvements in microvascular disease. Notably, a decreased incidence of neuropathy, retinopathy, microalbuminuria, and nephropathy was shown in individuals with tight glycemic control. Interestingly, glycemic control had no effect on macrovascular outcomes. Instead, it was blood pressure control to at least moderate goals (142/88 mmHg) in the UKPDS that resulted in a decreased incidence of macrovascular outcomes, namely, DM-related death, stroke, and heart failure. Improved blood pressure control also resulted in improved microvascular outcomes.

X-53. **The answer is A.** *(Chap. 344)* Diabetic ketoacidosis is an acute complication of diabetes mellitus. It results from a relative or absolute deficiency of insulin combined with a counterregulatory hormone excess. In particular, a decrease in the ratio of insulin to glucagons promotes gluconeogenesis, glycogenolysis, and the formation of ketone bodies in the liver. Ketosis results from an increase in the release of free fatty acids from adipocytes, with a resultant shift toward ketone body synthesis in the liver. This is mediated by the relationship between insulin and the enzyme carnitine palmitoyltransferase I. At physiologic pH, ketone bodies exist as ketoacids, which are neutralized by bicarbonate. As bicarbonate stores are depleted, acidosis develops. Clinically, these patients have nausea, vomiting, and abdominal pain. They are dehydrated and may be hypotensive. Lethargy and severe central nervous system depression may occur. The treatment focuses on replacement of the body's insulin, which will result in cessation of the formation of ketoacids and improvement of the acidotic state. Assessment of the level of acidosis may be done with an arterial blood gas. These patients have an anion gap acidosis and often a concomitant metabolic alkalosis resulting from volume depletion. Volume resuscitation with intravenous fluids is critical. Many electrolyte abnormalities may occur. Patients are total-body sodium, potassium, and magnesium depleted. As a result of the acidosis, intracellular potassium may shift out of cells and cause a normal or even elevated potassium level. However, with improvement in the acidosis, the serum potassium rapidly falls. Therefore, potassium repletion is critical despite the presence of a "normal" level. Because of the osmolar effects of glucose, fluid is drawn into the intravascular space. This results in a drop in the measured serum sodium. There is a drop of 1.6 meq/L in serum sodium for each rise of 100 mg/dL in serum glucose. In this case, the serum sodium will improve with hydration alone. The use of 3% saline is not indicated because the patient has no neurologic deficits, and the expectation is for rapid resolution with IV fluids alone.

X-54. **The answer is E.** *(Chap. 344; Nathan, N Engl J Med 328:1676–1685, 1993.)* Nephropathy is a leading cause of death in diabetic patients. Diabetic nephropathy may be functionally silent for 10–15 years. Clinically detectable diabetic nephropathy begins with the development of microalbuminuria (30–300 mg of albumin per 24 hours). The glomerular filtration rate actually may be elevated at this stage. Only after the passage of additional time will the proteinuria be overt enough (0.5 g/L) to be detectable on standard urine dipsticks. Microalbuminuria precedes nephropathy in patients with both non–insulin-dependent and insulin-dependent diabetes. An increase in kidney size also may accompany the initial hyperfiltration stage. Once the proteinuria becomes significant enough to be detected by dipstick, a steady decline in renal function occurs, with the glomerular filtration rate falling an average of 1 mL/min per month. Therefore, azotemia begins about 12 years after the diagnosis of diabetes. Hypertension clearly is an exacerbating factor for diabetic nephropathy.

X-55. **The answer is D.** *(Chap. 345)* Maintenance of euglycemia involves a number of systems to lower elevated blood glucose, but also to restore normal levels when hypoglycemia is present or impending. Decreased insulin secretion is the primary glucose regulator factor and its secretion is inhibited with a plasma glucose of 80–85 mg/dL. Glucagon secretion is the second defense against hypoglycemia, secreted at a glucose of 65–70 mg/dL. Epinephrine and cortisol secretion are third and are released at a glucose of 65–70 mg/dL. Finally, symptoms develop with a glucose of 50–55 mg/dL that will lead the patient to find a source of food, and decreased cognition occurs with glucose less than 50 mg/dL.

X-56. **The answer is D.** *(Chap. 345)* The patient presents with recurrent episodes of hypoglycemia that meet Whipple's triad of symptoms, documented low glucose at the time of symptoms, and reversal of symptoms upon administration of glucose. The differential starts with measuring insulin levels during hypoglycemia. The levels must be obtained during an episode to be interpretable. If insulin is elevated, it suggests either endogenous hyperproduction from an insulin-secreting tumor or exogenous administration causing factitious hypoglycemia. Because C peptide is cleaved from native proinsulin to make the secreted product, it will be high in the case of endogenous hyperinsulinemia and low during an episode of factitious hypoglycemia. Surreptitious ingestion of sulfonylurea could cause hypoglycemia along with high insulin and C-peptide levels since the drugs stimulate pancreatic insulin secretion. In this case, a sulfonylurea drug screen would be indicated. Red flags in this case that point to surreptitious insulin use include the patient being a health care worker and the presence of symptoms only at work. Other groups in which this is common is relatives of patients with diabetes and patients with a history of other factitious disorders. It is possible that she has an insulin-secreting beta-cell tumor, but this is much less likely, and symptoms would be present during times other than work. Evaluation is aimed at demonstrating that pancreatic insulin secretion is suppressed during the episode of hypoglycemia. Although a failure of counterregulatory hormones can produce hypoglycemia, this is a very rare cause of hypoglycemia, and evaluation should be aimed at this only after surreptitious use is ruled out.

X-57. **The answer is E.** *(Chap. 345)* The most common cause of hypoglycemia is related to the treatment of diabetes mellitus. Individuals with type 1 diabetes mellitus (T1DM) have more symptomatic hypoglycemia than individuals with type 2 diabetes mellitus (T2DM). On average, those with T1DM experience two episodes of symptomatic hypoglycemia weekly, and at least once yearly, individuals with T1DM will have a severe episode of hypoglycemia that is at least temporarily disabling. It is estimated that 2–4% of individuals with T1DM will die from hypoglycemia. In addition, recurrent episodes of hypoglycemia in T1DM contribute to the development of hypoglycemia-associated autonomic failure. Clinically, this is manifested as hypoglycemia unawareness and defective glucose counterregulation, with lack of glucagon and epinephrine secretion as glucose levels fall. Individuals with T2DM are less likely to develop hypoglycemia. Medications that are associated with hypoglycemia in T2DM are insulin and insulin secretagogues, such as sulfonylureas. Metformin, thiazolidinediones, α-glucosidase inhibitors, glucagon-like peptide-1 receptor agonists, and dipeptidyl peptidase-IV inhibitors do not cause hypoglycemia.

X-58. **The answer is D.** *(Chap. 346)* Gynecomastia is a relatively common complaint in men and may be caused by either obesity with adipose tissue expansion in the breast or by an increased estrogen/androgen ratio in which there is true glandular enlargement, as in this case. If the breast is unilaterally enlarged or if it is hard or fixed to underlying tissue, mammography is indicated. Alternatively, if cirrhosis or a causative drug is present, these may be adequate explanations, particularly when gynecomastia develops later in life in previously fertile men. If the breast tissue is greater than 4 cm or there is evidence of very small testes and no causative drugs or liver disease, a search for alterations in serum testosterone, LH, FSH estradiol, and hCG levels should be undertaken. An androgen deficiency or resistance syndrome may be present or an hCG-secreting tumor may be found. In this case, spironolactone is the likely culprit, and it may be stopped or switched to eplerenone and gynecomastia reassessed.

X-59. **The answer is C.** *(Chap. 346)* Many drugs may interfere with testicular function through a variety of mechanisms. Cyclophosphamide damages the seminiferous tubules in a dose- and time-dependent fashion and causes azoospermia within a few weeks of initiation. This effect is reversible in approximately half of these patients. Ketoconazole inhibits testosterone synthesis. Spironolactone causes a blockade of androgen action, which may also cause gynecomastia. Glucocorticoids lead to hypogonadism predominantly through inhibition of hypothalamic-pituitary function. Sexual dysfunction has been described as a side effect of therapy with beta blockers. However, there is no evidence of an effect on testicular function. Most reports of sexual dysfunction were in patients receiving older beta blockers such as propranolol and timolol.

X-60.   **The answer is B.** *(Chap. 347)* Women who have regular monthly bleeding cycles that do not vary by more than 4 days generally have ovulatory cycles, but several other indicators suggest that ovulation is likely. These include the presence of *mittelschmerz*, which is described as midcycle pelvic discomfort that is thought to be caused by rapid expansion of the dominant follicle at the time of ovulation or premenstrual symptoms such as breast tenderness, bloating, and food cravings. Additional objective parameters suggest the presence of ovulation including a progesterone level greater than 5 ng/mL 7 days before expected menses, an increase in basal body temperature more than 0.5°F in the second half of the menstrual cycle, and detection of urinary LH surge. Estrogen levels are elevated at the time of ovulation and during the secretory phase of the menstrual cycle, but are not useful in detection of ovulation.

X-61.   **The answer is C.** *(Chap. 347)* Infertility, defined as the inability to conceive after 12 months of unprotected intercourse, is a common problem in the United States with estimates of 15% of couples affected. Initial evaluation should include an evaluation of current menstrual history, counseling regarding the appropriate timing of intercourse, and education regarding modifiable risk factors such as drug use, alcohol intake, smoking, caffeine, and obesity. Male factors are at root of approximately 25% of cases of infertility, unexplained infertility is found in 17% of cases, and female causes underlie 58% of infertility. Among the female causes, the most common is amenorrhea/ovulatory dysfunction, which is present in 46% of cases. This is most frequently due to hypothalamic or pituitary cases or polycystic ovary syndrome. Tubal defects and endometriosis are less common.

X-62.   **The answer is C.** *(Chap. 347)* Evaluation of infertility should include evaluation of common male and female factors that could be contributing. Abnormalities of menstrual function are the most common cause of female infertility, and initial evaluation of infertility should include evaluation of ovulation and assessment of tubal and uterine patency. The female partner reports an episode of gonococcal infection with symptoms of pelvic inflammatory disease, which would increase her risk of infertility due to tubal scarring and occlusion. A hysterosalpingogram is indicated. If there is evidence of tubal abnormalities, many experts recommend in vitro fertilization for conception, as these women are at increased risk of ectopic pregnancy if conception occurs. The female partner reports some irregularity of her menses, suggesting anovulatory cycles, and thus evidence of ovulation should be determined by assessing hormonal levels. There is no evidence that prolonged use of oral contraceptives affects fertility adversely (A Farrow, et al: *Hum Reprod* 17: 2754, 2002). Angiotensin-converting enzyme inhibitors, including lisinopril, are known teratogens when taken by women but have no effects on chromosomal abnormalities in men. Recent marijuana use may be associated with increased risk of infertility, and in vitro studies of human sperm exposed to a cannabinoid derivative showed decreased motility (LB Whan, et al: *Fertil Steril* 85: 653, 2006). However, no studies have shown long-term decreased fertility in men who previously used marijuana.

X-63.   **The answer is E.** *(Chap. 347)* All of the choices have a theoretical efficacy in preventing pregnancy of more than 90%. However, the actual effectiveness can vary widely. Spermicides have the greatest failure rate of 21%. Barrier methods (condoms, cervical cap, diaphragm) have an actual efficacy between 82% and 88%. Oral contraceptives and intrauterine devices perform similarly, with 97% efficacy in preventing pregnancy in clinical practice.

X-64.   **The answer is E.** *(Chap. 347)* Pathologic gynecomastia develops when the effective testosterone-to-estrogen ratio is decreased owing to diminished testosterone production (as in primary testicular failure) or increased estrogen production. The latter may arise from direct estradiol secretion by a testis stimulated by LH or hCG, or from an increase in peripheral aromatization of precursor steroids, most notably androstenedione. Elevated androstenedione levels may result from increased secretion by an adrenal tumor (leading to an elevated level of urinary 17-ketosteroids) or decreased hepatic clearance in patients with chronic liver disease. A variety of drugs, including diethylstilbestrol, heroin, digitalis, spironolactone, cimetidine, isoniazid, and tricyclic antidepressants, also can cause gynecomastia. In this patient, the history of paternity and the otherwise normal physical examination indicate that a karyotype is unnecessary, and the bilateral breast enlargement essentially excludes the presence of carcinoma and thus the need for biopsy. The presence of a low LH and testosterone suggests either estrogen or hCG production. Because of the normal testicular examination, a primary testicular tumor is not suspected. Carcinoma of the lung and germ cell tumors both can produce hCG, causing gynecomastia.

X-65. **The answer is E.** *(Chap. 348)* The Women's Health Initiative was the largest study of hormone therapy to date including 27,000 postmenopausal women aged 50–79 for an average of 5–7 years. This trial was stopped early because of an unfavorable risk-to-benefit ratio in the estrogen-progestin arm and an increased risk of stroke that was not offset by lower coronary heart disease in the estrogen-only arm. Endometrial cancer risk was higher in patients with estrogen only and uterus. Use of progesterone eliminates this risk. Unopposed estrogen was associated with increased risk of stroke that far outweighed the decreased risk of coronary heart disease. Estrogen-progestin together was associated with an increased risk of coronary heart disease. Osteoporosis risk was decreased in both estrogen and estrogen-progestin groups. Venous thromboembolism risk was higher in both treatment groups as well. These therapies do reduce important menopausal symptoms such as hot flashes and vaginal drying. This seminal study caused a dramatic reevaluation of the use of estrogen/progesterone in postmenopausal women to reduce cardiovascular risk.

X-66. **The answer is C.** *(Chap. 349)* Klinefelter's syndrome is a chromosomal disorder with 47,XXY. Because the primary feature of this disorder is gonadal failure, low testosterone is present and thus increased LH and FSH are produced in an attempt to increase testosterone production in the feedback loop of sex hormones. Increased estrogen is often produced because of chronic Leydig cell stimulation by LH and because of aromatization of androstenedione by adipose tissue. The lower testosterone:estrogen ratio results in mild feminization with gynecomastia. Features of low testosterone are small testes and "eunuchoid" proportions with long legs and incomplete virilization. Biopsy of the testes, though rarely performed, shows hyalinization of the seminiferous tubules and azoospermia. Although severe cases are diagnosed prepubertally with small testes and impaired androgenization, approximately 75% of cases are not diagnosed and the frequency in the general population is 1/1000. Patients with Klinefelter's syndrome are at increased risk of breast tumors, thromboembolic disease, learning difficulties, obesity, diabetes mellitus, and varicose veins.

X-67. **The answer is A.** *(Chap. 349)* Turner's syndrome most frequently results from a 45,X karyotype, but mosaicism (45,X/46,XX) also can result in this disorder. Clinically, Turner's syndrome manifests as short stature and primary amenorrhea if presenting in young adulthood. In addition, chronic lymphedema of the hands and feet, nuchal folds, a low hairline, and high arched palate are also common features. To diagnose Turner's syndrome, karyotype analysis should be performed. A Barr body results from inactivation of one of the X chromosomes in women and is not seen in males. In Turner's syndrome, the Barr body should be absent, but only 50% of individuals with Turner's syndrome have the 45,X karyotype. Thus, the diagnosis could be missed in those with mosaicism or other structural abnormalities of the X chromosome.

Multiple comorbid conditions are found in individuals with Turner's syndrome, and appropriate screening is recommended. Congenital heart defects affect 30% of women with Turner's syndrome, including bicuspid aortic valve, coarctation of the aorta, and aortic root dilatation. An echocardiogram should be performed, and the individual should be assessed with blood pressures in the arms and legs. Hypertension can also be associated with structural abnormalities of the kidney and urinary tract, most commonly horseshoe kidney. A renal ultrasound is also recommended. Autoimmune thyroid disease affects 15–30% of women with Turner's syndrome and should be assessed by screening TSH. Other comorbidities that may occur include sensorineural hearing loss, elevated liver function enzymes, osteoporosis, and celiac disease.

X-68. **The answer is B.** *(Chap. 350)* The patient presents with recurrent peptic ulcers without evidence of *H. pylori* infection. The diagnosis of Zollinger-Ellison syndrome should be obtained. Additional features that suggest nonclassic idiopathic ulcer disease include the presence of diarrhea, which is commonly present in Zollinger-Ellison syndrome, but not idiopathic ulcers. The diagnosis is commonly made through measurement of plasma gastrin levels, which should be markedly elevated, but common use of proton pump inhibitors (PPIs) that potently suppress gastric acid secretion confound this measurement. Because PPI use suppresses gastric acid production, gastrin rises. Thus PPI use should be discontinued for 1 week prior to measurement of gastrin in plasma. Often this requires collaboration with gastroenterologists to ensure safety and potentially offer alternative pharmacology during this time. Once hypergastrinemia is confirmed, the presence of low gastric pH must be confirmed, as the most common cause of elevated gastrin is achlorhydria due to pernicious anemia. Imaging of the abdomen is indicated after demonstration of hypergastrinemia. Finally, although Zollinger-Ellison syndrome may be associated with multiple endocrine neoplasia type 1, which often has parathyroid hyperplasia or adenoma, this is less likely than isolated Zollinger-Ellison syndrome.

X-69 and X-70. **The answers are E and E, respectively.** *(Chap. 350)* In patients with a nonmetastatic carcinoid, surgery is the only potentially curative therapy. The extent of surgical resection depends on the size of the primary tumor because the risk of metastasis is related to the size of the tumor. Symptomatic treatment is aimed at decreasing the amount and effect of circulating substances. Drugs that inhibit the serotonin 5-HT$_1$ and 5-HT$_2$ receptors (methysergide, cyproheptadine, ketanserin) may control diarrhea but not flushing. 5-HT$_3$ receptor antagonists (ondansetron, tropisetron, alosetron) control nausea and diarrhea in up to 100% of these patients and may alleviate flushing. A combination of histamine H$_1$ and H$_2$ receptor antagonists may control flushing, particularly in patients with foregut carcinoid tumors. Somatostatin analogues (octreotide, lanreotide) are the most effective and widely used agents to control the symptoms of carcinoid syndrome, decreasing urinary 5-HIAA excretion and symptoms in 70–80% of patients. Interferon α, alone or combined with hepatic artery embolization, controls flushing and diarrhea in 40–85% of these patients. Phenoxybenzamine is an α$_1$-adrenergic receptor blocker that is used in the treatment of pheochromocytoma.

Carcinoid crisis is a life-threatening complication of carcinoid syndrome. It is most common in patients with intense symptoms from foregut tumors or markedly high levels of urinary 5-HIAA. The crisis may be provoked by surgery, stress, anesthesia, chemotherapy, or physical trauma to the tumor (biopsy or, in this case, physical compression of liver lesions). These patients develop severe typical symptoms plus systemic symptoms such as hypotension and hypertension with tachycardia. Synthetic analogues of somatostatin (octreotide, lanreotide) are the treatment of choice for carcinoid crisis. They are also effective in preventing crises when administered before a known inciting event. Octreotide 150–250 μg subcutaneously every 6–8 hours should be started 24–48 hours before a procedure that is likely to precipitate a carcinoid crisis.

X-71. **The answer is C.** *(Chap. 350)* This patient presents with the classic findings of a VIPoma, including large-volume watery diarrhea, hypokalemia, dehydration, and hypochlorhydria (WDHA, or Verner-Morrison syndrome). Abdominal pain is unusual. The presence of a secretory diarrhea is confirmed by a stool osmolal gap [2(stool Na + stool K) – (stool osmolality)] below 35 and persistence during fasting. In osmotic or laxative-induced diarrhea, the stool osmolal gap is over 100. In adults, over 80% of VIPomas are solitary pancreatic masses that usually are larger than 3 cm at diagnosis. Metastases to the liver are common and preclude curative surgical resection. The differential diagnosis includes gastrinoma, laxative abuse, carcinoid syndrome, and systemic mastocytosis. Diagnosis requires the demonstration of large-volume secretory diarrhea (>700 mL/d) and elevated serum VIP. CT scan of the abdomen will often demonstrate the pancreatic mass and liver metastases.

X-72. **The answer is B.** *(Chap. 351)* Multiple endocrine neoplasia syndrome is defined as a disorder with neoplasms affecting two or more hormonal tissues in several members of the family. The most common of these is MEN 1, which is caused by the gene coding the nuclear protein called Menin. MEN 1 is associated with tumors or hyperplasia of the parathyroid, pancreas, pituitary, adrenal cortex, and foregut, and/or subcutaneous or visceral lipomas. The most common and earliest manifestation is hyperparathyroidism with symptomatic hypercalcemia. This most commonly occurs in the late teenage years and 93–100% of mutation carriers develop this complication. Gastrinomas, insulinomas, and prolactinomas are less common and tend to occur in patients in their 20s, 30s, and 40s. Pheochromocytoma may occur in MEN 1, but is more commonly found in MEN 2A or von Hippel-Lindau syndrome.

X-73. **The answer is A.** *(Chap. 351)* This patient's clinical scenario is most consistent with MEN 1, or the "3 Ps": parathyroid, pituitary, and pancreas. MEN 1 is an autosomal dominant genetic syndrome characterized by neoplasia of the parathyroid, pituitary, and pancreatic islet cells. Hyperparathyroidism is the most common manifestation of MEN 1. The neoplastic changes affect multiple parathyroid glands, making surgical care difficult. Pancreatic islet cell neoplasia is the second most common manifestation of MEN 1. Increased pancreatic islet cell hormones include pancreatic polypeptide, gastrin, insulin, vasoactive intestinal peptide, glucagons, and somatostatin. Pancreatic tumors may be multicentric, and up to 30% are malignant, with the liver being the first site of metastases. The symptoms depend on the type of hormone secreted. The Zollinger-Ellison syndrome (ZES) causes elevations of gastrin, resulting in an ulcer diathesis. Conservative therapy is often unsuccessful. Insulinoma results in documented hypoglycemia with elevated insulin and C-peptide levels. Glucagonoma results in hyperglycemia, skin rash, anorexia, glossitis, and diarrhea. Elevations in vasoactive intestinal peptide result in profuse watery diarrhea. Pituitary tumors occur in up to half of patients with MEN 1. Prolactinomas are the most common. The multicentricity of the tumors makes resection difficult. Growth hormone–secreting tumors are the next most common, with ACTH- and corticotropin-releasing hormone (CRH)-secreting tumors being more rare. Carcinoid tumors may also occur in the thymus, lung, stomach, and duodenum.

X-74 and X-75. **The answers are D and C, respectively.** *(Chap. 352)* Hypophosphatemia results from one of three mechanisms: inadequate intestinal phosphate absorption, excessive renal phosphate excretion, and rapid redistribution of phosphate from the extracellular space into bone or soft tissue. Inadequate intestinal absorption is rare since antacids containing aluminum hydroxide are no longer commonly prescribed. Malnutrition from fasting or starvation may result in depletion of phosphate. This is also commonly seen in alcoholism. In hospitalized patients, redistribution is the main cause. Insulin promotes phosphate entry into cells along with glucose. When nutrition is initiated, refeeding further increases redistribution of phosphate into cells and is more pronounced when IV glucose is used alone. Sepsis may cause destruction of cells and metabolic acidosis, resulting in a net shift of phosphate from the extracellular space into cells. Renal failure is associated with hyperphosphatemia, not hypophosphatemia, and initial prerenal azotemia, such as in this presentation, can obscure underlying phosphate depletion.

The approach to treating hypophosphatemia should take into account several factors, including the likelihood (and magnitude) of underlying phosphate depletion, renal function, serum calcium levels, and the concurrent administration of parenteral glucose. In addition, the treating physician should assess the patient for complications of hypophosphatemia, which can include neuromuscular weakness, cardiac dysfunction, hemolysis, and platelet dysfunction. Severe hypophosphatemia generally occurs when the serum concentration falls below 2 mg/dL (<0.75 mmol/L). This becomes particularly dangerous when there is underlying chronic phosphate depletion. However, there is no simple formula to determine the body's phosphate needs from measurement of the serum phosphate levels because most phosphate is intracellular. It is generally recommended to use oral phosphate repletion when the serum phosphate levels are greater than 1.5–2.5 mg/dL (0.5–0.8 mmol/L). The dose of oral phosphate is 750–2000 mg daily of elemental phosphate given in divided doses. More severe hypophosphatemia as in the case presented requires intravenous repletion. Intravenous phosphate repletion is given as neutral mixtures of sodium and potassium phosphate salts at doses of 0.2–0.8 mmol/kg given over 6 hours. Table X-75 outlines the total dose and recommended infusion rates for a range of phosphate levels. In this patient with a level of 1.0 mg/dL, the recommended infusion rate is 8 mmol/h over 6 hours for a total dose of 48 mmol. Until the underlying hypophosphatemia is corrected, one should measure phosphate and calcium levels every 6 hours. The infusion should be stopped if the calcium phosphate product rises to higher than 50 to decrease the risk of heterotopic calcification. Alternatively, if hypocalcemia is present coincident with the hypophosphatemia, it is important to correct the calcium prior to administering phosphate.

TABLE X-75   Intravenous Therapy for Hypophosphatemia

Consider

Likely severity of underlying phosphate depletion

Concurrent parenteral glucose administration

Presence of neuromuscular, cardiopulmonary, or hematologic complications of hypophosphatemia

Renal function [reduce dose by 50% if serum creatinine >220 μmol/L (>2.5 mg/dL)]

Serum calcium level (correct hypocalcemia first; reduce dose by 50% in hypercalcemia)

Guidelines

Serum Phosphorus, mM (mg/dL)	Rate of Infusion, mmol/h	Duration, h	Total Administered, mmol
<0.8 (<2.5)	2	6	12
<0.5 (<1.5)	4	6	24
<0.3 (<1)	8	6	48

Notes: Rates shown are calculated for a 70-kg person. Levels of serum calcium and phosphorus must be measured every 6–12 hours during therapy. Infusions can be repeated to achieve stable serum phosphorus levels above 0.8 mmol/L (>2.5 mg/dL). Most formulations available in the United States provide 3 mmol/mL of sodium or potassium phosphate.

X-76.   **The answer is E.** *(Chap. 352)* Magnesium sulfate is first-line therapy for seizures associated with eclampsia of pregnancy. A pregnant woman presenting with seizures and hypertension is initially treated with a bolus of magnesium sulfate at a dose of approximately 4 g followed by a continuous infusion at 1 g/h. While definitive treatment of eclampsia is delivery of the baby, ongoing therapy with magnesium sulfate for 24 hours following the last seizure is recommended. Patients should be monitored throughout the infusion for signs of hypermagnesemia, and levels should be measured at least every 6 hours. The usual magnesium concentration is 0.7–1 mmol/L (1.5–2 meq/L), and the desired level for treatment of preeclampsia is usually 1.7–3.5 mmol/L, although signs and symptoms of hypermagnesemia can develop with levels of 2 mmol/L or higher. The initial signs of hypermagnesemia include prolongation of the QRS complex, depression of deep tendon reflexes, and hypotension that is refractory to vasopressors. At concentrations greater than 4 mmol/L, nausea, lethargy, and weakness can appear and progress to paralysis and respiratory failure. The symptoms become increasingly severe, and asystole occurs when levels approach 10 mmol/L.

X-77.   **The answer is B.** *(Chap. 352)* Vitamin D deficiency is highly prevalent in the United States and is most common in older individuals who are hospitalized or institutionalized. Vitamin D deficiency can occur as a result of inadequate dietary intake, decreased production in the skin, decreased intestinal absorption, accelerated losses, or impaired vitamin D activation in the liver or kidney. Clinically, vitamin D deficiency in older individuals is most often silent. Often practitioners fail to consider vitamin D deficiency until a patient has been diagnosed with osteoporosis or suffered a fracture. However, some individuals can experience diffuse muscle and bone pain. When assessing vitamin D levels, the appropriate test is 25-hydroxy vitamin D [25(OH)D] levels. Optimal 25(OH)D levels are greater than 80 nmol/L (32 ng/mL); however, an individual is not considered deficient until the level is less than 37 nmol/L (15 ng/mL). When the 25(OH)D level falls below this level, parathyroid hormone (PTH) may rise, and it is also associated with a lower bone density. Vitamin D deficiency leads to decreased intestinal absorption of calcium with resultant hypocalcemia and secondary hyperparathyroidism. In response to this, there is higher bone turnover, which can be associated with an increase in alkaline phosphatase levels. In addition, elevated PTH stimulates renal conversion of 25-hydroxy vitamin D to 1,25-hydroxy vitamin D, the activated form of vitamin D. Thus, even in the face of severe vitamin D deficiency, the activated 1,25(OH)D levels may be normal and do not accurately reflect vitamin D stores. Thus, 1,25(OH)D should not be used to make a diagnosis of vitamin D deficiency. While vitamin D deficiency may be associated with abnormalities in PTH, alkaline phosphatase, and calcium levels, these biochemical abnormalities are seen in many other diseases and are neither sensitive nor specific for the diagnosis of vitamin D deficiency.

X-78.   **The answer is A.** *(Chap. 353)* Granulomatous disorders including sarcoidosis, tuberculosis, and fungal infections can be associated with hypercalcemia-caused increased synthesis of 1,25-hydroxy vitamin D by macrophages within the granulomas. This process bypasses the normal feedback mechanisms, and elevated levels of both 25-hydroxy and 1,25-hydroxy vitamin can be seen. This does not normally occur as 1,25-hydroxy-vitamin D levels are normally tightly controlled through feedback mechanisms on renal 1-hydroxylase, the primary producer of activated vitamin D in normal circumstances. In addition, the normal feedback provided by parathyroid hormone concentrations is also bypassed and the PTH level may be low.

X-79.   **The answer is D.** *(Chap. 353)* This patient demonstrates evidence of tertiary hyperparathyroidism, with inappropriate elevations in parathyroid hormone despite increases in calcium and phosphate. In addition, the patient is demonstrating clinical evidence of disease including bony pain and ectopic calcification. Tertiary hyperparathyroidism most commonly develops in individuals with long-standing renal failure who have been nonadherent to therapy. In this case scenario, the hypoxemia and ground-glass infiltrates on chest CT represent ectopic calcification of the lungs. This can be difficult to identify with typical imaging, and a technetium-99 bone scan will show increased uptake in the lungs. Treatment of tertiary hyperparathyroidism with severe clinical manifestations requires parathyroidectomy.

X-80.   **The answer is B.** *(Chap. 353)* Hypocalcemia can be a life-threatening consequence of thyroidectomy if the parathyroid glands are inadvertently removed during the surgery, as the four parathyroid glands are located immediately posterior to the thyroid gland. This is an infrequent occurrence currently as the parathyroid glands can be better identified both before and during surgery. However, hypoparathyroidism may occur even if the parathyroid glands are not removed by thyroidectomy due to devascularization or trauma to the parathyroid glands. Hypocalcemia following removal of the parathyroid glands may begin any time during the first 24–72 hours, and monitoring of serial calcium levels is recommended for the first 72 hours. The earliest symptoms of hypocalcemia are typically circumoral paresthesias and paresthesias with a "pins-and-needles" sensation in the fingers and toes. The development of carpal spasms upon inflation of the blood pressure cuff is a classic sign of hypocalcemia and is known as Trousseau sign. Chvostek sign is the other classic sign of hypocalcemia and is elicited by tapping the facial nerve in the preauricular area causing spasm of the facial muscles. A prolongation of the QT interval on ECG suggests life-threatening hypocalcemia that may progress to fatal arrhythmia, and treatment should not be delayed for serum testing to occur in a patient with a known cause of hypocalcemia. Immediate treatment with IV calcium should be initiated. Maintenance therapy with calcitriol and vitamin D is necessary for ongoing treatment of acquired hypoparathyroidism. Alternatively, surgeons may implant parathyroid tissue into the soft tissue of the forearm, if it is thought that the parathyroid glands will be removed. Hypomagnesemia can cause hypocalcemia by suppressing parathyroid hormone release despite the presence of hypocalcemia. However, in this patient, hypomagnesemia is not suspected after thyroidectomy, and magnesium administration is not indicated. Benztropine is a centrally acting anticholinergic medication that is used in the treatment of dystonic reactions that can occur after taking centrally acting antiemetic medications with dopaminergic activity, such as metoclopramide or Compazine. Dystonic reactions involve focal spasms of the face, neck, and extremities. While this patient has taken a medication (morphine) that can cause a dystonic reaction, the spasms that she is experiencing are more consistent with tetanic contractions of hypocalcemia than dystonic reactions. Finally, measurement of forced vital capacity is most commonly used as a measurement of disease severity in myasthenia gravis or Guillain-Barré syndrome. Muscle weakness is a typical presenting feature but not paresthesias.

X-81.   **The answer is E.** *(Chap. 353)* Malignancy can cause hypercalcemia by several different mechanisms, including metastasis to bone, cytokine stimulation of bone turnover, and production of a protein structurally similar to parathyroid hormone by the tumor. This protein is called parathyroid hormone–related peptide (PTHrp) and acts at the same receptors as parathyroid hormone (PTH). Squamous cell carcinoma of the lung is the most common tumor associated with the production of PTHrp. Serum calcium levels can become quite high in malignancy because of unregulated production of PTHrp that is outside of the negative feedback control that normally results in the setting of hypercalcemia. PTH hormone levels should be quite low or undetectable in this setting. When hypercalcemia is severe (>15 mg/dL), symptoms frequently include dehydration and altered mental status. The electrocardiogram may show a shortened QTc interval. Initial therapy includes large-volume fluid administration to reverse the dehydration that results from hypercalciuria. In addition, furosemide is added to promote further calciuria. If the calcium remains elevated, as in this patient, additional measures should be undertaken to decrease the serum calcium. Calcitonin has a rapid onset of action with a decrease in serum calcium seen within hours. However, tachyphylaxis develops, and the duration of benefit is limited. Pamidronate is a bisphosphonate that is useful for the hypercalcemia of malignancy. It decreases serum calcium by preventing bone resorption and release of calcium from the bone. After IV administration, the onset of action of pamidronate is 1–2 days with a duration of action of at least 2 weeks. Thus, in this patient with ongoing severe symptomatic hypercalcemia, addition of both calcitonin and pamidronate is the best treatment. The patient should continue to receive IV fluids and furosemide. The addition of a thiazide diuretic is contraindicated because thiazides cause increased calcium resorption in the kidney and would worsen hypercalcemia.

X-82.   **The answer is B.** *(Chap. 353)* Hyperparathyroidism is the most common cause of hypercalcemia and is the most likely cause in an adult who is asymptomatic. Cancer is the second most common cause of hypercalcemia but usually is associated with symptomatic hypercalcemia. In addition, there are frequently symptoms from the malignancy itself that dominate the clinical picture. Primary hyperparathyroidism results from autonomous secretion of parathyroid hormone (PTH) that is no longer regulated by serum calcium levels, usually related to the development of parathyroid adenomas. Most patients are asymptomatic or have minimal symptoms at the time of diagnosis. When present, symptoms include recurrent nephrolithiasis, peptic ulcers, dehydration, constipation, and altered mental status. Laboratory studies show elevated serum calcium with decreased serum phosphate. Diagnosis can be confirmed with measurement of parathyroid hormone levels. Surgical removal of autonomous adenomas is generally curative, but not all patients need to be treated surgically. It is recommended that individuals below age 50 undergo primary surgical resection. However, in those above 50 years, a cautious approach with frequent laboratory monitoring is often used. Surgery can then be undertaken if a patient develops symptomatic or worsening hypercalcemia or complications such as osteopenia. Breast cancer is a frequent cause of hypercalcemia because of metastatic disease to the bone. In this patient who has received routine mammography as part of age-appropriate cancer screening and is asymptomatic, this would be unlikely. Multiple myeloma is another malignancy frequently associated with hypercalcemia that is thought to be due to the production of cytokines and humoral mediators by the tumor. Multiple myeloma should not present with isolated hypercalcemia and is associated with anemia and elevations in creatinine.

Approximately 20% of individuals with hyperthyroidism develop hypercalcemia related to increased bone turnover. This patient exhibits no signs or symptoms of hyperthyroidism, making the diagnosis unlikely. Vitamin D intoxication is a rare cause of hypercalcemia. An individual must ingest 40–100 times the recommended daily amount in order to develop hypercalcemia. Because vitamin D acts to increase both calcium and phosphate absorption from the intestine, serum levels of both minerals would be elevated, which is not seen in this case.

X-83. **The answer is B.** *(Chap. 353)* Parathyroid hormone (PTH) is produced by the four small parathyroid glands that lie posterior to the thyroid gland and is the primary hormone responsible for regulating serum calcium and phosphate balance. PTH secretion is tightly regulated with negative feedback to the parathyroid glands by serum calcium and vitamin D levels. PTH primarily affects serum calcium and phosphate levels through its action in the bone and the kidney. In the bone, PTH increases bone remodeling through its actions on the osteoblasts and osteoclasts. It directly stimulates osteoblasts to increase bone formation, and this action of PTH has been utilized in the treatment of osteoporosis. Its action on osteoclasts, however, is indirect and likely is mediated through its actions on the osteoblasts. The osteoclast has no receptors for PTH. It has been hypothesized that cytokines produced by osteoblasts are responsible for increased osteoclastic activity that is seen after PTH administration, as PTH fails to have an effect on osteoclasts in the absence of osteoblasts. The net effect of PTH on the bone is to increase bone remodeling. Ultimately, this leads to an increase in serum calcium, an effect that can be seen within hours of drug administration. In the kidney, PTH acts to increase calcium reabsorption while increasing phosphate excretion. At the proximal tubule, PTH acts to decrease phosphate transport, thus facilitating its excretion. Calcium reabsorption is increased by the action of PTH on the distal tubule. A final action of PTH in the kidney is to increase the production of 1,25-hydroxycholecalciferol, the activated form of vitamin D, through stimulation of 1-α-hydroxylase. Activated vitamin D then helps to increase calcium levels by increasing intestinal absorption of both calcium and phosphate.

X-84. **The answer is B.** *(Chap. 354)* Osteoporosis refers to a chronic condition characterized by decreased bone strength and frequently manifests as vertebral and hip fractures. In the Unites States, about 8 million women have osteoporosis compared to about 2 million men, for a ratio between men and women of 4 to 1. An additional 18 million individuals are estimated to have osteopenia. The risk of osteoporosis increases with advancing age and rapidly worsens following menopause in women. Most women meet the diagnostic criteria for osteoporosis between the ages of 70 and 80. White women have an increased risk for osteoporosis when compared to African-American women.

The epidemiology for bone fractures follows the epidemiology for osteoporosis. Fractures of the distal radius (Colles' fracture) increases up to age 50 and plateaus by age 60, and there is only a modest increase in risk thereafter. This is contrasted with the risk of hip fractures. Incidence rates for hip fractures double every 5 years after the age of 70. This change in fracture pattern is not entirely due to osteoporosis, but is also related to the fact that fewer falls in the elderly occur onto an outstretched arm and are more likely to occur directly onto the hip. Black women experience hip fractures at approximately half the rate as white women. The mortality rate in the year following a hip fracture is 5–20%. Vertebral fractures are also common manifestations of osteoporosis. While most are found incidentally on chest radiograph, severe cases can lead to height loss, pulmonary restriction, and respiratory morbidity.

X-85. **The answer is C.** *(Chap. 354)* There are multiple risks for osteoporotic bone fractures that can be either modifiable or nonmodifiable. These are outlined in Table X-85. Nonmodifiable risk factors include a previous history of fracture as an adult, female sex, white race, dementia, advanced age, and history of fracture (but not osteoporosis) in a first-degree relative. Risk factors that are potentially modifiable include body weight less than 58 kg (127 lb), low calcium intake, alcoholism, impaired eyesight, recurrent falls, inadequate physical activity, poor health, and estrogen deficiency including menopause prior to age 45 or prolonged premenstrual amenorrhea. Current cigarette smoking is a risk factor for osteoporosis-related fracture while a prior history of cigarette use is not.

TABLE X-85   Risk Factors for Osteoporosis Fracture

Nonmodifiable	Estrogen deficiency
Personal history of fracture as an adult	Early menopause (<45 years) or bilateral ovariectomy
History of fracture in first-degree relative	Prolonged premenstrual amenorrhea (>1 year)
Female sex	Low calcium intake
Advanced age	Alcoholism
White race	Impaired eyesight despite adequate correction
Dementia	
Potentially modifiable	**Recurrent falls**
Current cigarette smoking	Inadequate physical activity
Low body weight [<58 kg (127 lb)]	Poor health/frailty

X-86.   **The answer is C.** *(Chap. 354)* A variety of diseases in adults increase the risk of osteoporosis. First, diseases that lead to estrogen deficiency or hypogonadism can lead to osteoporosis. This would include Turner's syndrome, Klinefelter's syndrome, and hyperprolactinemia, among others. A wide range of endocrine disorders can also lead to abnormal bone metabolism, especially hyperparathyroidism and thyrotoxicosis. Poor nutrition and gastrointestinal disorders increase the likelihood of developing osteoporosis. Anorexia nervosa causes both hypogonadism and poor nutritional status. Malabsorption syndromes lead to decreased intake of calcium and vitamin D, which are essential to good bone health. Chronic obstructive pulmonary disease also has a high prevalence of osteoporosis, which is may be related to a chronic inflammatory state with high bone turnover that is exacerbated by frequent corticosteroid use, frequent vitamin D deficiency, and low activity states. Other broad categories of disease that can lead to osteoporosis include rheumatologic disorders, hematologic malignancies, and some inherited disorders such as osteogenesis imperfecta, Marfan's syndrome, and porphyria, among many others. It is well known that immobilization, pregnancy, and lactation can lead to osteoporosis as well.

X-87.   **The answer is B.** *(Chap. 354)* Osteoporosis is a common disease affecting 8 million women and 2 million men in the United States. It is most common in postmenopausal women, but the incidence is also increasing in men. Estrogen loss probably causes bone loss by activation of bone remodeling sites and exaggeration of the imbalance between bone formation and resorption. Osteoporosis is diagnosed by bone mineral density scan. Dual-energy x-ray absorptiometry (DXA) is the most accurate test for measuring bone mineral density. Clinical determinations of bone density are most commonly measured at the lumbar spine and hip. In the DXA technique, two x-ray energies are used to measure the area of the mineralized tissues and compared to gender- and race-matched normative values. The T-score compares an individual's results to a young population, whereas the Z-score compares the individual's results to an age-matched population. Osteoporosis is diagnosed when the T-score is –2.5 SD in the lumbar spine, femoral neck, or total hip. An evaluation for secondary causes of osteoporosis should be considered in individuals presenting with osteoporotic fractures at a young age and those who have very low Z-scores. Initial evaluation should include serum and 24-hour urine calcium levels, renal function panel, hepatic function panel, serum phosphorous level, and vitamin D levels. Other endocrine abnormalities including hyperthyroidism and hyperparathyroidism should be evaluated, and urinary cortisol levels should be checked if there is a clinical suspicion for Cushing's syndrome. Follicle-stimulating hormone and luteinizing hormone levels would be elevated but are not useful in this individual, as she presents with a known perimenopausal state.

X-88.   **The answer is C.** *(Chap. 354)* Determination of when to initiate screening for osteoporosis with bone densitometry testing can be complicated by multiple factors. In general, most women do not require screening for osteoporosis until after completion of menopause unless there have been unexplained fractures or other risk factors that would suggest osteoporosis.

There is no benefit to initiating screening for osteoporosis in the perimenopausal period. Indeed most expert recommendations do not recommend routine screening for osteoporosis until age 65 or older unless risk factors are present. Risk factors for osteoporosis include advanced age, current cigarette smoking, low body weight (<57.7 kg), family history of hip fracture, and long-term glucocorticoid use. Inhaled glucocorticoids may cause increased loss of bone density, but as this patient is on a low dose of inhaled fluticasone and is not estrogen deficient, bone mineral densitometry cannot be recommended at this time. The risk of osteoporosis related to inhaled glucocorticoids is not well defined, but most studies suggest that the risk is relatively low. Delaying childbearing until the fourth and fifth decade does increase the risk of osteoporosis but does not cause early onset of osteoporosis prior to completion of menopause. The patient's family history of menopause likewise does not require early screening for osteoporosis.

X-89.   **The answer is D.** *(Chap. 354)* Osteoporosis is defined as a reduction of bone mass or density or the presence of a fragility fracture. Operationally, the World Health Organization (WHO) defines osteoporosis as a bone density more than 2.5 SD less than the mean for young healthy adults of the same race and sex. Dual-energy x-ray absorptiometry (DXA) is the most widely used study to determine bone density. Bone density is expressed as a T-score, that is, the SD below the mean of young adults of the same race and gender. A T-score higher than 2.5 characterizes osteoporosis, and a T-score less than 1 identifies patients at risk of osteoporosis. The Z-score compares individuals with those in an age-, race-, and gender-matched population.

X-90.   **The answer is E.** *(Chap. 354)* Multiple treatment choices are available to prevent fractures and reverse bone loss in osteoporosis, and the side-effect profiles should be carefully considered when making the appropriate choice for this patient. Risedronate belongs to a family of drugs called bisphosphonates. Bisphosphonates act to inhibit osteoclast activity to decrease bone resorption and increase bone mass. Alendronate, risedronate, and ibandronate are approved for the treatment of postmenopausal osteoporosis, and alendronate and risedronate are also approved for the treatment of steroid-induced osteoporosis and osteoporosis in men. In clinical trials, risedronate decreases the risk of hip and vertebral fracture in women with osteoporosis by about 40% over 3 years. However, risedronate is not effective in decreasing hip fracture in women over the age of 80 without proven osteoporosis. The major side effect of bisphosphonate compounds taken orally is esophagitis. These drugs should be taken with a full glass of water, and the patient should remain upright for 30 minutes after taking the drug. There is also some concern about increased risk of osteonecrosis of the jaw in individuals treated with high doses of IV bisphosphonates or treated with oral therapy for prolonged periods, but in this patient with severe osteoporosis and a recent fracture, the benefits outweigh potential risks. Estrogens are also effective in preventing and treating osteoporosis. Epidemiologic data indicate that women taking estrogen have a 50% decreased risk of hip fracture. Raloxifene is a selective estrogen receptor modulator (SERM). The effect of raloxifene on bone density is somewhat less than that of estrogen, but it does decrease the risk of vertebral fracture by 30–50%. However, both drugs are contraindicated in this patient because of the recent occurrence of venous thromboembolic disease. Both estrogen and SERMs increase the risk of DVT and pulmonary embolus several-fold. If estrogen is to be used, it should be used in combination with a progestin compound in women with an intact uterus to decrease the risk of uterine cancer associated with unopposed estrogen stimulation. Both calcium and vitamin D supplementation are recommended as supplemental therapy, but given the degree of osteoporosis are inadequate alone. Calcitonin is available as an intranasal spray and produces small increases in bone density, but it has no proven effectiveness on the prevention of fractures.

X-91 and X-92.   **The answers are B and C, respectively.** *(Chap. 355)* The most likely diagnosis in this case is Paget's disease. A normal level of γ-glutamyl transferase localizes the cause of the elevated alkaline phosphatase to the bone. Thus, diseases of the liver and biliary tree are excluded. While both vertebral osteomyelitis and Paget's disease could cause elevations in alkaline phosphatase, the patient has no symptoms of systemic illness that one would typically expect with vertebral osteomyelitis. Paget's disease is a common dysplasia of the bone associated with localized bone remodeling that can affect numerous discreet areas of the skeleton. This disorder is relatively common. In autopsy series, Paget's lesions can be demonstrated in about 3% of individuals older than 40 years of age, although clinical manifestations of the disease are far less common. Diagnosis is most often made in individuals with asymptomatic elevations of alkaline phosphatase or through characteristic radiographic changes in individuals who underwent biochemical or radiographic testing for other reasons. In symptomatic individuals, localized pain is most commonly seen. The bones most often affected include the femur, skull, pelvis, vertebral bodies, and tibia, and the specific symptoms depend on the location of the Paget's lesion. When the vertebral bodies are involved, back pain can result from enlarged vertebrae, compression fractures of the spine, and spinal stenosis. In rare instances, spinal cord compression can occur. In this scenario, it is possible that the patient's back pain is due to undiagnosed Paget's disease. Diagnosis is typically made based on typical findings on radiographs and biochemical testing. Radiographs may demonstrate the enlargement or expansion of an entire bone, cortical thickening, coarsening of the trabecular markings, and both lytic and sclerotic changes. Characteristic findings of the vertebrae include cortical thickening of the superior and inferior endplates, creating a "picture frame" vertebra. If a vertebra is diffusely enlarged, the radiodensity created is known as an "ivory vertebra." An elevation in alkaline phosphatase is the classic finding in Paget's disease and is the test of choice for both diagnosis and assessing response to therapy. Serum osteocalcin, a marker of bone formation, is not always elevated in Paget's for unknown reasons and is not recommended for either diagnosis or response to therapy. Serum or urine N-telopeptide or C-telopeptide are also bone resorption markers and are elevated in active Paget's disease. These markers decrease more rapidly in response to therapy than alkaline phosphatase. Serum calcium and phosphate levels are normal in Paget's disease unless a patient becomes immobilized.

X-93.   **The answer is C.** (*Chap. 355*) Paget's disease of the bone is associated with localized bone dysplasia that can occur in numerous discreet areas of bone. Pathologically, the disease is initiated by overactivity of osteoclasts leading to high bone turnover and subsequent increase in osteoblastic activity, resulting in both lytic and sclerotic lesions in bone. Biochemically, there is typically evidence of high bone turnover, with an elevation in alkaline phosphatase being the characteristic biochemical abnormality that is used for both diagnosis of Paget's disease as well as response to treatment. Other markers of high bone resorption are the C- and N-telopeptides, which are typically elevated in both the serum and urine. These proteins decline more rapidly in response to therapy than alkaline phosphatase. Serum osteocalcin is also a marker of high bone turnover, and it may be elevated or normal in those with Paget's disease. However, serum calcium is always normal in those with Paget's disease unless the person becomes immobilized.

X-94.   **The answer is C.** (*Chap. 355*) Despite her lack of symptoms this patient has enough evidence to diagnose her with Paget's disease. Her radiographs show characteristic changes of active disease in the pelvis, which is one of the most common areas for Paget's disease to present. Her elevated alkaline phosphatase provides further evidence of active bone turnover. The normal serum calcium and phosphate levels are characteristic for Paget's disease. Management of asymptomatic Paget's disease has changed since effective treatments have become available. Treatment should be initiated in all symptomatic patients and in asymptomatic patients who have evidence of active disease (high alkaline phosphatase or urine hydroxyproline) or disease adjacent to weight-bearing structures, vertebrae, or the skull. Second-generation oral bisphosphonates such as tiludronate, alendronate, and risedronate are excellent choices due to their ability to decrease bone turnover. The major side effect from these agents is esophageal ulceration and reflux. They should be taken in the morning, on an empty stomach, and sitting upright to minimize the risk of reflux. Duration of use depends on the clinical response; typically 3–6 months are needed to see the alkaline phosphatase begin to normalize. Intravenous zoledronate and pamidronate are adequate alternatives to oral bisphosphonates. While their IV administration avoids the risk of reflux, there is a potential of developing a flulike syndrome within 24 hours of use. The presence of this side effect does not require drug discontinuation. The same time to response can be expected from these agents.

X-95. **The answer is D.** *(Chap. 356)* Mutation of the LDL receptor results in hypercholesterolemia. This mutation may be homozygous or heterozygous and occurs in approximately 1/500 people in its heterozygous form. Homozygous disease is more severe, with the development of symptomatic coronary atherosclerosis in childhood, while heterozygous patients have hypercholesterolemia from birth, and disease recognition is usually not until adulthood when patients are found to have tendon xanthomas or coronary artery disease. In patients with heterozygous disease, there is generally a family history on at least one side of the family. In familial hypercholesterolemia, there is an elevation of LDL-C between 200 and 400 mg/dL without alterations in chylomicrons or VLDL. Familial defective apoB-100 has a similar presentation but is less common (1/1000). Autosomal dominant history may be present in this family to suggest autosomal dominant hypercholesterolemia; however, this condition is quite rare (<1/1,000,000) and therefore much less likely. Familial hepatic lipase deficiency and lipoprotein lipase deficiency are associated with increased chylomicrons, not LDL-C, and present with eruptive xanthomas, hepatosplenomegaly, and pancreatitis. These conditions occur rarely (<1/1,000,000).

X-96. **The answer is B.** *(Chap. 356)* There are many secondary forms of elevated LDL that warrant consideration in a patient found to have abnormal LDL. These include hypothyroidism, nephritic syndrome, cholestasis, acute intermittent porphyria, anorexia nervosa, hepatoma, and drugs such as thiazides, cyclosporine, and Tegretol. Cirrhosis is associated with reduced LDL because of inadequate production. Malabsorption, malnutrition, Gaucher's disease, chronic infectious disease, hyperthyroidism, and niacin toxicity are all similarly associated with reduced LDL.

X-97. **The answer is D.** *(Chap. 356)* This patient has signs and symptoms of familial hypercholesterolemia (FH) with elevated plasma LDL, normal triglycerides, tendon xanthomas, and premature coronary artery disease. FH is an autosomal codominant lipoprotein disorder that is the most common of these syndromes caused by a single gene disorder. It has a higher prevalence in Afrikaners, Christian Lebanese, and French Canadians. There is no definitive diagnostic test for FH. It may be diagnosed with a skin biopsy that shows reduced LDL receptor activity in cultured fibroblasts (although there is considerable overlap with normals). FH is predominantly a clinical diagnosis, although molecular diagnostics are being developed. Hemolysis is not a feature of FH. Sitosterolemia is distinguished from FH by episodes of hemolysis. It is a rare autosomal recessive disorder that causes a marked increase in the dietary absorption of plant sterols. Hemolysis is due to incorporation of plant sterols into the red blood cell membrane. Sitosterolemia is confirmed by demonstrating an increase in the plasma levels of sitosterol using gas chromatography. CT scanning of the liver does not sufficiently differentiate between the hyperlipoproteinemias. Many of the primary lipoproteinemias, including sitosterolemia, are inherited in an autosomal recessive pattern, and thus a pedigree analysis would not be likely to isolate the disorder.

X-98. **The answer is C.** *(Chap. 356)* This patient has nephrotic syndrome, which is likely a result of multiple myeloma. The hyperlipidemia of nephrotic syndrome appears to be due to a combination of increased hepatic production and decreased clearance of very low-density lipoproteins, with increased LDL production. It is usually mixed but can manifest as hypercholesterolemia or hypertriglyceridemia. Effective treatment of the underlying renal disease normalizes the lipid profile. Of the choices presented, HMG-CoA reductase inhibitors would be the most effective to reduce this patient's LDL. Dietary management is an important component of lifestyle modification but seldom results in a greater than 10% fall in LDL. Niacin and fibrates would be indicated if the triglycerides were higher, but the LDL is the more important lipid abnormality to address at this time. Lipid apheresis is reserved for patients who cannot tolerate the lipid-lowering drugs or who have a genetic lipid disorder refractory to medication. Cholesterol ester transfer protein inhibitors have been shown to raise high-density lipoprotein levels, and their role in the treatment of lipoproteinemias is still under investigation.

X-99. **The answer is C.** *(Chap. 357)* Hereditary hemochromatosis is a common genetic condition, with 1 in 10 people of northern European ancestry being heterozygotes and 0.3–0.5% being homozygotes. The recessive condition occurs from a mutation in the gene *HFE,* which is involved in iron metabolism. Clinical manifestations include initially iron overload (as measured biochemically) without symptoms, then later iron overload with symptoms. Initial symptoms often include lethargy, arthralgia, change in skin color, loss of libido, and diabetes mellitus. Cirrhosis, cardiac arrhythmias, and infiltrative cardiomyopathy are later manifestations. Because the clinical manifestations of the disease can be prevented with iron chelation and the mutation is so common, some have advocated for screening the population for evidence of iron overload. Although routine screening is still controversial, recent studies indicate that it is highly effective for primary care physicians to screen subjects using serum iron, transferrin saturation, and serum ferritin levels. This will detect anemia and iron deficiency as well. Liver biopsy or MRI may demonstrate later findings of increased iron deposition and/or cirrhosis, but these are more costly and possibly invasive or risky, and are not recommended for screening. Genetic testing is also not recommended as a first step, though it is indicated if evidence of iron overload is found on serum iron studies, as described in this case. There is no HFE activity assay currently available.

X-100. **The answer is E.** *(Chap. 357)* This patient presents with the classic finding of diffuse organ iron infiltration due to hemochromatosis. The iron accumulation in the pancreas, testes, liver, joints, and skin explain his findings. Hemochromatosis is a common disorder of iron storage in which inappropriate increases in intestinal iron absorption result in excessive deposition in multiple organs but predominantly in the liver. There are two forms: hereditary hemochromatosis, in which the majority of cases are associated with mutations of the *HFE* gene, and secondary iron overload, which usually is associated with iron-loading anemias such as thalassemia and sideroblastic anemia. In this case, without a history of prior hematologic disease, the most likely diagnosis is hereditary hemochromatosis. Serum ferritin testing and plasma iron studies can be very suggestive of the diagnosis, with the ferritin often greater than 500 μg/L and transferrin saturation of 50–100%. However, these tests are not conclusive, and further testing is still required for the diagnosis. Although liver biopsy and evaluation for iron deposition or a hepatic iron index (μg/g dry weight)/56 × age > 2 is the definitive diagnosis, genetic testing is widely available today, and because of the high prevalence of *HFE* gene mutations associated with hereditary hemochromatosis, it is recommended for diagnostic evaluation. If the genetic testing is inconclusive, the invasive liver biopsy evaluation may be indicated. Anti–smooth muscle antibody testing is useful for the evaluation of autoimmune hepatitis and is indicated in any case of cryptogenic cirrhosis. Plasma ceruloplasmin is the initial study in the evaluation of Wilson's disease, and is also a cause of occult liver disease. However, Wilson's disease would not be likely to be associated with the pancreatic, joint, and skin findings. If chronic hepatitis B is suspected, a viral load or surface antigen test would be indicated. Hepatitis B surface antibody is useful to demonstrate resolved hepatitis B or prior vaccination. Hepatic ultrasound is useful in the evaluation of acute and chronic liver disease to demonstrate portal flow or vascular occlusion. It may be useful in the physiologic evaluation of this patient but would have little diagnostic value.

X-101. **The answer is C.** *(Chap. 358)* The patient has a classic presentation for acute intermittent porphyria, a disorder of hepatic (not bone marrow) heme synthesis. This is generally autosomal dominant and is widespread, especially in Scandinavia and Great Britain. Although disease presentation and penetrance is highly variable, it is most commonly associated with attacks of abdominal pain and neurologic symptoms that develop after puberty. Often a precipitating cause of symptomatic episodes can be identified such as steroid hormone use, oral contraceptives, systemic illness, reduced caloric intake, and many other medications. This diagnosis should be considered in any individual with recurrent abdominal pain, especially when accompanied by neuropsychiatric complaints. The abdominal symptoms are often more prominent, sometimes including vomiting, diarrhea, and ileus. Neurologic findings may include peripheral neuropathy, sensory changes, and seizures. The diagnosis is made by measurement of urine porphyrobilinogens (PBG) during a spot urine taken during an attack. During an attack, the precursors of heme synthesis build up. Urine aminolevulinic acid (ALA) is also almost uniformly elevated during these attacks.

The porphobilinogen level will drop in the recovery phase and be normal between attacks. Therapy for acute attack is with carbohydrate loading, narcotic pain control, anxiolysis, and IV hemin, which repletes the end product in heme synthesis.

X-102. **The answer is B.** *(Chap. 359)* Hyperuricemia is a common finding, affecting approximately 5% of the general population and 25% of hospitalized individuals. Increased levels of plasma uric acid may be due to overproduction of uric acid (as in the presence of tumor) or underexcretion of uric acid, which is by far the most common mechanism. Because hyperuricemia is so common and most patients with this condition never develop a complication, asymptomatic hyperuricemia is not an indication for treatment. Patients with hyperuricemia are not known to be at increased risk for uric acid nephrolithiasis. Recently, the metabolic syndrome (central obesity, insulin resistance, dyslipidemia, and hypertension) has been linked to hyperuricemia. Hyperinsulinemia results in reduced renal excretion of uric acid and sodium; thus hyperuricemia may be an early indicatory of type 2 diabetes mellitus.

X-103. **The answer is D.** *(Chap. 359)* Although most patients with hyperuricemia never develop any complications, several have been recognized. The most common complication is gouty arthritis, which depends on the duration and severity of hyperuricemia. Several renal diseases have been described in association with hyperuricemia including urate nephropathy, in which monosodium urate crystals deposit in the renal interstitium; uric acid nephropathy, in which large amounts of uric acid crystals deposit in the renal collecting ducts, pelvis, and ureters; and nephrolithiasis. Cardiovascular disease and renal disease are associated with hyperuricemia, but lowering uric acid levels is not shown to change these specific outcomes. There is no association between hyperuricemia and peripheral neuropathy.

X-104. **The answer is C.** *(Chap. 353)* Lesch-Nyhan syndrome is characterized by the complete absence of the enzyme hypoxanthine phosphoribosyltransferase (HPRT), a component of purine metabolism that is related to purine recycling into guanosine monophosphate and inosine monophosphate. Hyperuricemia develops from urate overproduction. The gene for HPRT is located on the X chromosome, so Lesch-Nyhan disease is transmitted as an X-linked disorder. Homozygous males have the disease, and heterozygous carrier females are asymptomatic. Therefore, the daughter of a carrier has a 50% chance of being a carrier and a son has a 50% chance of having the disease. Carrier females do not have an increased risk of gout or urate nephropathy. Lesch-Nyhan syndrome is characterized by hyperuricemia, gouty arthritis, nephrolithiasis, self-mutilative behavior, choreoathetosis, and mental retardation. Treatment of affected patients with allopurinol will eliminate or prevent the problems related to hyperuricemia but will not have any beneficial effect on the behavioral or neurologic manifestations. Since it is an X-linked disorder, screening the husband has no value.

X-105 and X-106. **The answers are E and D, respectively.** *(Chap. 360)* The patient presents with liver disease, hemolysis, and psychiatric illness, which suggests the presence of Wilson's disease. Wilson's disease is an autosomal recessive disorder caused by mutations in the ATP7B gene, a copper-transporting ATP-asa. As a result of this mutation, patients store abnormally high levels of copper in their liver initially, but later in other organs such as the brain. While liver dysfunction is a hallmark of the disease, it may have several presentations: acute hepatitis, cirrhosis, or hepatic decompensation, as in this case. Hemolysis may complicate acute decompensation because of the massive release of copper from the liver into the blood leading to hemolysis. Accumulation of copper in the basal ganglia results in Parkinson-like syndromes. Up to 50% of patients with Wilson's disease will have Kayser-Fleischer rings on ocular slit-lamp examination. These brownish rings surrounding the cornea are due to copper deposition within the cornea and are diagnostic when found. Twenty-four–hour urinary copper levels are universally elevated in this disease and are the primary diagnostic modality when Kayser-Fleischer rings are absent. Liver biopsy can also be used to confirm increased copper content. Although MRI will show basal ganglia damage, it is not specific for Wilson's disease. *HFE* mutation is present in hemochromatosis, which this patient does not have. Urine iron levels are not indicated.

Therapy for Wilson's disease is dependent on degree of disease at the time of presentation. Patients with mild hepatitis may be treated with zinc, which blocks the intestinal absorption of copper and results in a negative copper balance, and also induces hepatic metallothionein synthesis, which sequesters additional toxic copper. Trientine serves as a copper chelator and is used for more severe liver dysfunction, or neurologic or psychiatric disease. Zinc should not be used acutely in hepatic decompensation because zinc may be chelated instead of copper. Liver transplantation is appropriate for patients who have failed the initial therapy.

X-107. **The answer is A.** (*Chap. 360*) Wilson's disease is an autosomal recessive disorder caused by mutations in the *ATP7B* gene, which leads to copper accumulation and toxicity. The *ATP7B* gene encodes a membrane-bound copper-transporting ATPase. Deficiency of this protein leads to decreased biliary copper excretion and resultant buildup of copper in the tissues. The two most affected organs are the liver and the brain. Patients may present with hepatitis, cirrhosis, hepatic failure, movement disorders, or psychiatric disorders. Serum copper levels are usually lower than normal due to low blood ceruloplasmin, which usually binds serum copper. About 1% of the population are carriers of an *ATP7B* mutation; the disease is present in 1 in 30,000–40,000 people. The disease is close to 100% penetrant and requires treatment in almost all cases. DNA haplotype analysis can be used to genotype siblings of an affected patient. Patients are treated with zinc, which induces a negative copper balance by blocking intestinal absorption; trientine, which acts as a potent copper chelator; or both. Severe hepatic decompensation may require liver transplantation.

X-108. **The answer is A.** (*Chap. 363*) Osteogenesis imperfecta is a heritable disorder of connective tissue in which there is a severe decrease of bone mass that makes bone brittle and prone to fracture. The disease is often inherited in an autosomal dominant fashion. There are several subtypes, with type 1 being the most mild and likely to present in adulthood. Most of the other subtypes present in early childhood and may be lethal. In type 1 osteogenesis imperfecta, mutations in the type 1 procollagen gene are present in 90% of cases. Type 1 disease may present in adulthood, where abnormalities of teeth color and shape are common in addition to the characteristic blue sclera. Fractures tend to decrease after puberty in both sexes, but may increase in women at the time of pregnancy and after menopause. Decreased bone mineral density is demonstrated in a variety of imaging techniques including x-ray absorptiometry and plain radiographs. Bone biopsy is not required for diagnosis and may cause morbidity. The diagnosis is usually clinical with the characteristic physical examination findings, history of fractures, and often a positive family history. Although bisphosphonates are well tolerated and often used for severe disease where they may decrease bone pain, their long-term effects and safety in osteogenesis imperfecta are unknown.

X-109. **The answer is C.** (*Chap. 363*) Marfan's syndrome is an autosomal dominant syndrome characterized by skeletal changes including long, thin extremities; loose joints; lens dislocation with reduced vision; and aortic aneurysms. The incidence is high, affecting 1 in 3000–5000 live births in most racial and ethnic groups. More than 90% of Marfan's syndrome patients have mutations in the *fibrillin-1* gene. Although Marfan's syndrome is rarely associated with mutations in *TGFβ*, recent work has highlighted the close interaction between fibrillin mutation and alterations in TGFβ signaling, offering new therapeutic potential. *BMPR2* mutation is associated with heritable pulmonary arterial hypertension. *COL1A1* mutation is found in Ehlers-Danlos syndrome and osteogenesis imperfecta. *Type IV collagen* mutations have been described in Alport's syndrome.

X-110. **The answer is B.** (*Chap. 363*) This patient has Ehlers-Danlos syndrome (EDS), most likely type 2. There are over 10 types of EDS that vary clinically, biochemically, and genetically. Classic EDS has a severe (type 1) form that usually presents in childhood, and the milder type 2 form. These are characterized by joint hypermobility and velvety skin that scars easily and is hyperextensible. Patients with classic EDS are at risk of joint dislocation, including the hips and other large joints. Extreme joint extension in yoga is likely not advisable. Many patients with classic EDS benefit from braces or joint surgery for stabilization. The most dangerous form of EDS is the vascular or type 4 form. These patients have more skin than joint changes and are at risk of major vascular events or rupture of hollow organs (esophagus or bowel). Pregnant women with type 4 EDS are at risk of uterine rupture during pregnancy. Because of the overlapping clinical features, many patients and families cannot be given a firm type diagnosis of EDS. The diagnosis of EDS remains clinical because of the great phenotype-genotype variability. Genetic tests are most useful in familial cases of type 4 EDS because of the high risk of complications. Patients with Marfan's syndrome who have mutations of the fibrillin gene are also at risk of aortic dissection or rupture. Mutations of the elastin gene are associated with supravalvular aortic stenosis and cutis laxa.

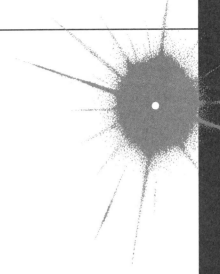

SECTION XI
Neurologic Disorders

QUESTIONS

DIRECTIONS: Choose the **one best** response to each question.

XI-1. All of the following neurologic conditions have a mechanistic association with abnormalities of ion channel function EXCEPT:

A. Epilepsy
B. Lambert-Eaton syndrome
C. Migraine
D. Parkinson's disease
E. Spinocerebellar ataxia

XI-2. All of the following neurologic diseases are matched correctly with the neurotransmitter system that is dysfunctional EXCEPT:

A. Lambert-Eaton syndrome: acetylcholine
B. Myasthenia gravis: acetylcholine
C. Orthostatic tachycardia syndrome: serotonin
D. Parkinson's disease: dopamine
E. Stiff-person syndrome: GABA

XI-3. During a neurologic examination, you ask a patient to stand with both arms fully extended and parallel to the ground with his eyes closed for 10 seconds. What is the name of this test?

A. Babinski sign
B. Dysdiadochokinesis
C. Lhermitte symptom
D. Pronator drift
E. Romberg sign

XI-4. This sign is considered positive if there is flexion at the elbows or forearms, or if there is pronation of the forearms. A positive test is a sign of:

A. Abnormal sensation
B. Early dementia
C. Localized brainstem disease
D. Potential weakness
E. Underlying cerebellar dysfunction

XI-5. A 55-year-old woman with known metastatic breast cancer presents to the emergency department complaining of new-onset weakness and numbness. The symptoms involve both arms and legs. She also has developed urinary incontinence over the past 24 hours. On physical examination, strength is 3/5 in the lower extremities and 4/5 in the upper extremities. Anal sphincter tone is decreased. Babinski sign is positive. Sensation is decreased in the extremities, but not in the face. Cranial nerves are symmetric and intact, and mental status is normal. Based on this information, what is the most likely site of the lesion causing the patient's symptoms?

A. Brainstem
B. Cerebrum
C. Cervical spinal cord
D. Lumbar spinal cord
E. Neuromuscular junction

XI-6. A 54-year-old woman presents to the emergency department complaining of the abrupt onset of what she describes as the worst headache of her life. You are concerned about the possibility of subarachnoid hemorrhage. What is the most appropriate initial test for diagnosis?

A. Cerebral angiography
B. CT of the head with IV contrast
C. CT of the head without IV contrast
D. Lumbar puncture
E. Transcranial Doppler ultrasound

XI-7. A 74-year-old woman has a recent diagnosis of small cell lung cancer. She is now complaining of headaches, and her family has noticed confusion as well. Metastatic disease to the brain is suspected. A mass lesion on magnetic resonance imaging (MRI) is demonstrated in the right parietal lobe. Which MRI technique would best identify the extent of the edema surrounding the lesion?

A. MR angiography
B. FLAIR
C. T1-weighted
D. T2-weighted
E. B and D

XI-8. Which of the following is a possible complication of administration of gadolinium to a patient with chronic kidney disease?

A. Acute renal failure
B. Hyperthyroidism
C. Hypocalcemia
D. Lactic acidosis
E. Nephrogenic systemic sclerosis

XI-9. In a patient with coma, an EEG showing triphasic waves is most suggestive of which of the following clinical disorders?

A. Brain abscess
B. Herpes simplex encephalitis
C. Locked-in syndrome
D. Metabolic encephalopathy
E. Nonconvulsive status epilepticus

XI-10. An 18-year-old man seeks evaluation at his university health center for increasing episodes of sudden onset smelling of burning kerosene. These episodes had occurred every few months during high school and he never told anyone. However, since starting college, he notes an increasing frequency, often when sleep deprived. The episodes typically start without warning and he'll smell a distinct kerosene smell no matter the environment. The episodes last about 3–5 minutes and stop spontaneously. He has never lost consciousness. During the episodes, he can communicate with friends. An EEG during an episode shows abnormal discharges distinctly localized to an area of the frontal lobe. Which of the following is the most accurate classification of his seizure disorder?

A. Focal seizures with dyscognitive features
B. Focal seizures without dyscognitive features
C. Generalized seizure
D. Myoclonic seizures
E. Typical absence seizure

XI-11. On the neurologic consultation service, you are asked to evaluate a patient with mesial temporal lobe epilepsy syndrome. The patient has a history of intractable focal seizures that rarely generalize. Her seizures often begin with an aura and commonly manifest as behavioral arrests, complex automatisms, and unilateral posturing. MRI findings include small temporal lobes and a small hippocampus with increased signal on T2-weighted sequences. Which of these additional historic factors is also likely to be present in this patient?

A. History of febrile seizures
B. Hypothyroidism
C. Neurofibromas
D. Recurring genital ulcers
E. Type 2 diabetes mellitus

XI-12. You have just admitted a young man with a prior history of seizure disorder who was witnessed to have a seizure. His family's description suggests a focal seizure involving the left hand that spread to involve the entire arm. He did not lose consciousness. He was brought in 2 hours after symptom onset and is currently awake, alert, and oriented. He has not had any further seizures but has been unable to move his left hand since his seizure. His electrolytes and complete blood count are within normal limits. A noncontrast CT scan of his head is unremarkable. On examination, sensation is intact in the affected limb, but his strength is 0 out of 5 in the musculature of the left hand. What is the best course of action at this time?

A. Cerebral angiogram
B. Lumbar puncture
C. Magnetic resonance angiogram
D. Psychiatric evaluation
E. Reassess in a few hours

XI-13. A 37-year-old man is witnessed by his family to have a generalized tonic-clonic seizure at a party. He does not have a known seizure disorder. There is no history of head trauma, stroke, or tumor. The patient is unemployed, married, and takes no medication. Physical examination shows no skin abnormalities and no stigmata of chronic liver or renal disease. The patient is postictal. His neck is difficult to maneuver due to stiffness. His white blood cell count is 19,000/μL, hematocrit 36%, and platelets 200,000/μL. Glucose is 102 mg/dL, sodium 136 meq/dL, calcium 9.5 mg/dL, magnesium 2.2 mg/dL, SGOT 18 U/L, blood urea nitrogen 7 mg/dL, and creatinine 0.8 mg/dL. Urine toxicology screen is positive for cocaine metabolites. Which next step is most appropriate in this patient's management?

A. Electroencephalogram (EEG)
B. IV loading with antiepileptic medication
C. Lumbar puncture
D. Magnetic resonance imaging
E. Substance abuse counseling

XI-14. All of the following statements regarding epilepsy are true EXCEPT:

    A.   The incidence of suicide is higher in epileptic patients than it is in the general population.

    B.   Mortality is no different in patients with epilepsy than it is in age-matched controls.

    C.   A majority of patients with epilepsy that is completely controlled with medication eventually will be able to discontinue therapy and remain seizure-free.

    D.   Surgery for mesial temporal lobe epilepsy (MTLE) decreases the number of seizures in over 70% of patients.

    E.   Tricyclic antidepressants lower the seizure threshold and may precipitate seizures.

XI-15. A 20-year-old woman is brought to the emergency department after a witnessed generalized tonic-clonic seizure. She has no identifying information, and her past medical history is unknown. What is the most likely cause of her seizure?

    A.   Amyloid angiopathy

    B.   Fever

    C.   Genetic disorder

    D.   Illicit drug use

    E.   Uremia

XI-16. A 36-year-old man is brought to the emergency department because of a seizure. His family reports he has a history of seizure disorder but stopped his medications a month ago due to financial issues. He had a brief seizure at home that stopped within a few minutes. However, 15 minutes later he began seizing again and the tonic-clonic activity has persisted for 30 minutes. On physical examination he is afebrile, hypertensive, and actively seizing. All of the following are potential therapies for his condition EXCEPT:

    A.   Carbamazepine

    B.   Fosphenytoin

    C.   Lorazepam

    D.   Phenobarbital

    E.   Valproate

XI-17. The most common cause of a cerebral embolism is:

    A.   Atrial fibrillation

    B.   Cardiac prosthetic valves

    C.   Dilated cardiomyopathy

    D.   Endocarditis

    E.   Rheumatic heart disease

XI-18. A 54-year-old male is referred to your clinic for evaluation of atrial fibrillation. He first noted the irregular heartbeat 2 weeks ago and presented to his primary care physician. He denies chest pain, shortness of breath, nausea, or gastrointestinal symptoms. Past medical history is unremarkable. There is no history of hypertension, diabetes, or tobacco use. His medications include metoprolol. The examination is notable for a blood pressure of 126/74 mmHg and a pulse of 64 beats/min. The jugular venous pressure is not elevated. His heart is irregularly irregular,

with normal S_1 and S_2. The lungs are clear, and there is no peripheral edema. An echocardiogram shows a left atrial size of 3.6 cm. Left ventricular ejection fraction is 60%. There are no valvular or structural abnormalities. Which of the following statements regarding his atrial fibrillation and stroke risk is true?

    A.   He requires no antiplatelet therapy or anticoagulation because the risk of embolism is low.

    B.   Lifetime vitamin K antagonist therapy is indicated for atrial fibrillation in this situation to reduce the risk of stroke.

    C.   He should be admitted to the hospital for IV heparin and undergo electrical cardioversion; afterward there is no need for anticoagulation.

    D.   His risk of an embolic stroke is less than 1%, and he should take a daily aspirin.

    E.   He should be started on SC low-molecular-weight heparin and transitioned to warfarin.

XI-19. All the following have been shown to reduce the risk of atherothrombotic stroke in primary or secondary prevention EXCEPT:

    A.   Aspirin

    B.   Blood pressure control

    C.   Clopidogrel

    D.   Statin therapy

    E.   Warfarin

XI-20. A 57-year-old man is brought to the emergency department after falling while playing tennis and developing garbled speech. He has a past history of hypertension and hypercholesterolemia. His medications include atorvastatin and enalapril. On physical examination, his blood pressure is 210/115 mmHg with heart rate 105 beats/min, respirations 28 breaths/min, temperature 37°C (98.6°F), and oxygen saturation 94% on room air. He is alert but aphasic with upper and lower left extremity hemiparesis. He is able to move his right side normally. Based on the results of immediate imaging, all of the following are potential therapeutic considerations for his condition EXCEPT:

    A.   Anticoagulation

    B.   Blood pressure lowering

    C.   Hypothermia protocol

    D.   Intracerebral stent placement

    E.   IV thrombolysis

XI-21. Which of the following statements regarding Alzheimer's disease is true?

    A.   Delusions are uncommon.

    B.   It accounts for over half of the cases of significant memory loss in patients over 70 years of age.

    C.   It typically presents with rapid (<6 months) significant memory loss.

    D.   Less than 5% of patients present with nonmemory complaints.

    E.   Pathologically, the most notable abnormalities are in the cerebellar regions.

XI-22. All of the following medications have been shown to have potential efficacy in the treatment of Alzheimer's disease EXCEPT:

A. Donepezil
B. Galantamine
C. Memantine
D. Oxybutynin
E. Rivastigmine

XI-23. A 72-year-old right-handed male with a history of atrial fibrillation and chronic alcoholism is evaluated for dementia. His son gives a history of a stepwise decline in the patient's function over the last 5 years with the accumulation of mild focal neurologic deficits. On examination he is found to have a pseudobulbar affect, mildly increased muscle tone, and brisk deep-tendon reflexes in the right upper extremity and an extensor plantar response on the left. The history and examination are most consistent with which of the following?

A. Alzheimer's disease
B. Binswanger's disease
C. Creutzfeldt-Jakob disease
D. Multi-infarct dementia
E. Vitamin B$_{12}$ deficiency

XI-24. A 49-year-old woman presents for a second opinion regarding symptoms of tremors, difficulty with ambulation, and periodic flushing. Her symptoms originally began approximately 3 years ago. At that time, she was hospitalized for a syncopal episode, after which she was told to increase her salt intake. Since then, she has had progressive motor difficulties including bilateral tremors and a stiff, slow gait. She also has had several more episodes of syncope. She states that she knows when these syncopal events will occur because she feels faint and weak. She has never had an injury from syncope. A final recent symptom has been periodic flushing and sweating. A neurologist previously diagnosed her with Parkinson's disease and prescribed therapy with ropinirole. Despite increasing doses, she does not feel improved, but rather has recently noticed uncontrollable movements that she describes as tics of her face. Her only other medical history is recent recurrent urinary tract infections. Her medications are ropinirole 24 mg daily and nitrofurantoin 100 mg daily. She reports no history of drug use. On physical examination, her blood pressure is 130/70 mmHg with a heart rate of 78 beats/min while sitting. Upon standing, her blood pressure drops to 90/50 mmHg with a heart rate of 110 beats/min. Her ocular movements are full and intact. She has recurrent motor movements of the right side of her face. Her neurologic examination shows increased muscle tone in the lower extremities with bilateral 4-Hz tremor. Deep tendon reflexes are brisk and 3+ in upper and lower extremities. Three beats of myoclonus are present at the ankles bilaterally. She walks with a spastic gait. Strength is normal. What is the most likely diagnosis?

A. Corticobasal degeneration
B. Diffuse Lewy body dementia
C. Drug-induced Parkinson's disease
D. Multiple system atrophy with parkinsonian features
E. Parkinson's disease with inadequate treatment

XI-25. A 65-year-old man presents to your office complaining of a tremor and progressive gait abnormalities. He states that he first noticed a slowing of his gait approximately 6 months ago. He has difficulty rising to a standing position and states that he shuffles when he walks. In addition, he states that his right hand shakes more so than his left, and he is right handed. He believes it to be worse when not moving but states there are times when he spills his morning coffee because of the tremors. He has retired but states he is not able to play tennis and golf any longer because of his motor symptoms. He denies syncope or presyncope, difficulty swallowing, changes to his voice, or memory difficulties. His past medical history is significant for hypertension and hypercholesterolemia. His medications are hydrochlorothiazide 25 mg daily, ezetimibe 10 mg daily, and lovastatin 40 mg daily. He drinks a glass of wine with dinner daily and is a lifelong nonsmoker. On physical examination, he has masked facies. His gait shows decreased arm swing with slow shuffling steps. He turns en bloc. A pill-rolling tremor is present on the right side. There is cogwheel rigidity bilaterally. Eye movements are full and intact. There is no orthostatic hypotension. A brain MRI with gadolinium shows no evidence of mass lesions, hydrocephalus, or vascular disease. You diagnose the patient with Parkinson's disease. The patient asks about his prognosis and likelihood of disability. Which of the following is correct about the clinical course and treatment of Parkinson's disease?

A. Early initiation of therapy with levodopa predisposes an individual to a higher likelihood of dyskinesias early in the disease.
B. Early therapy with bilateral deep-brain stimulation of the subthalamic nuclei slows the progression of Parkinson's disease.
C. Initial treatment with a dopamine agonist such as pramipexole is likely to be effective in controlling his motor symptoms for 1–3 years before the addition of levodopa or another agent is necessary.
D. Levodopa should be started immediately to prevent the development of disabling rigidity.
E. MAO inhibitors are contraindicated once the diagnosis of Parkinson's disease is established.

XI-26. All of the following statements regarding restless legs syndrome (RLS) are true EXCEPT:

A. Dopamine antagonists are effective therapy.
B. Most patients develop symptoms before the age of 30 years old.
C. RLS may cause sleep disorder and daytime hypersomnolence.
D. RLS is more common in Asians than in the general U.S. population.
E. Symptoms may involve the upper extremity.

XI-27. A 63-year-old man seeks medical attention because of progressive weakness of the left foot and lower leg over the last 6 months. The progression has been gradual, and he only noticed it initially because of cramping and tripping while playing squash. He denies back pain. His only medication is atorvastatin. On physical examination, vital signs are normal and the only abnormalities are on neurologic examination. His left leg strength is notably diminished in the hip flexors, hip adductors, quadriceps, and calf muscles. There is atrophy of the quadriceps and calf. His ankle and knee reflexes are increased on the left. He has subtle weakness on the right quadriceps. There are no sensory abnormalities in light touch, pinprick, temperature, or proprioception. There are occasional fasciculations of the abdominal muscles. Before diagnosing the patient with amyotrophic lateral sclerosis (ALS), all of the following alternative diagnoses should be ruled out EXCEPT:

A. Cervical spondylosis
B. Foramen magnum tumor
C. Lead poisoning
D. Multifocal motor neuropathy with conduction block
E. Vitamin C deficiency

XI-28. A 42-year-old woman seeks medical attention for a 5- to 6-week history of marked fatigue that is affecting her work. She reports that she has felt some general fatigue but her symptoms are most notable when she starts moving around during the day. She has taken her pulse and it feels fast to her. She reports no loss of consciousness, but does say that she feels lightheaded and has blurred vision after arising. Sitting or lying down improves the symptoms. She has no notable past medical history and takes no medications other than a calcium/vitamin supplement. On physical examination, her supine heart rate is 90 beats/min with blood pressure of 110/70 mmHg. Upon standing her heart rate increases to 130 beats/min and is regular, and her blood pressure standing is 115/75 mmHg. She reports lightheadedness during the episode. An ECG while symptomatic shows sinus tachycardia without any conduction abnormalities. Which of the following is the most likely diagnosis?

A. Addison's disease
B. Autoimmune autonomic neuropathy
C. Diabetic neuropathy
D. Multisystem atrophy
E. Postural orthostatic tachycardia syndrome

XI-29. A 45-year-old male complains of severe right arm pain. He gives a history of having slipped on the ice and severely contusing his right shoulder approximately 6 months ago. Soon thereafter, he developed sharp, knifelike pain in the right arm and forearm that lasted for a few months. There was some arm swelling and warmth. He was evaluated in an urgent care setting. There were no radiographic abnormalities and he was not treated. Since the injury, the pain and swelling have persisted. Physical examination reveals a right arm that is more moist and hairy than the left arm. There is no specific weakness or sensory change. However, the right arm is clearly more edematous than the left, and the skin appears shiny and cool. The patient's pain most likely is due to:

A. Acromioclavicular separation
B. Brachial plexus injury
C. Cervical radiculopathy
D. Complex regional pain syndrome
E. Subclavian vein thrombosis

XI-30. Which of the following criteria suggests the diagnosis of trigeminal neuralgia?

A. Deep-seated, steady facial pain
B. Elevated erythrocyte sedimentation rate (ESR)
C. Objective signs of sensory loss on physical examination
D. Response to gabapentin therapy
E. None of the above

XI-31. A 72-year-old woman presents with recurrent episodes of incapacitating facial pain lasting from second to minutes and then dissipating. The episodes occur usually twice per day, usually without warning, but are also occasionally provoked by brushing of her teeth. On physical examination, she appears well with normal vital signs. Detailed cranial nerve examination reveals no sensory or motor abnormalities. The remainder of her neurologic examination is normal. What is the next step in her management?

A. Brain MRI
B. Brain MRI plus carbamazepine therapy
C. Carbamazepine therapy
D. Glucocorticoid therapy
E. Referral to Otolaryngology for surgical cure

XI-32. A 72-year-old female presents with brief, intermittent excruciating episodes of lancinating pain in the lips, gums, and cheek. Touching the lips or moving the tongue can initiate these intense spasms of pain. The results of a physical examination are normal. MRI of the head is also normal. The most likely cause of this patient's pain is:

A. Acoustic neuroma
B. Amyotrophic lateral sclerosis
C. Meningioma
D. Trigeminal neuralgia
E. Facial nerve palsy

XI-33. A 33-year-old woman presents with rapidly worsening pain at the top of the back over the last 3 days. The pain is not relieved by lying down or by wearing a soft neck collar. She notes that the pain is much worse with movement and has woken her from sleep. The pain is severe and is impeding her daily activities. She denies any arm pain or weakness. There is no history of prior back or neck pain, trauma, or arthritis. She works as a postal delivery agent and her only physical activity is walking. She is monogamous with her husband and has no illicit activities. Her family history is notable for an aunt and mother with breast cancer. Her MRI is shown in Figure XI-33. Which is the most likely diagnosis?

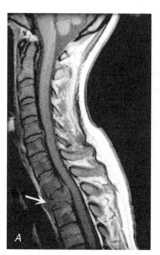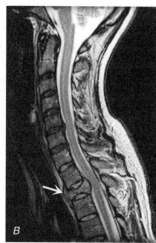

FIGURE XI-33

A. Cervical spondylosis
B. Hematomyelia
C. Metastatic breast cancer
D. Spinal epidural abscess
E. Spinal epidural hematoma

XI-34. A 34-year-old female complains of lower extremity weakness for the last 3 days. She has noted progressive weakness in the lower extremities with loss of sensation "below the belly button" and incontinence. She had had some low-grade fevers for the last week. She denies recent travel. Past medical history is unremarkable. Physical examination is notable for a sensory level at the level of the umbilicus. The lower extremities show +3/5 strength bilaterally proximally and distally. Reflexes, cerebellar examination, and mental status are normal. All of the following are appropriate steps in evaluating this patient EXCEPT:

A. Antinuclear antibodies
B. Electromyography
C. Lumbar puncture
D. MRI of the spine
E. Viral serologies

XI-35. Which of the following statements about syringomyelia is true?

A. More than half the cases are associated with Chiari malformations.
B. Symptoms typically begin in middle age.
C. Vibration and position sensation are usually diminished.
D. Syrinx cavities are always congenital.
E. Neurosurgical decompression is usually effective in relieving the symptoms.

XI-36. A 17-year-old adolescent is seen in the clinic several weeks after he suffered a concussion during a high-school football game. At the time of the event, paramedics reported that he experienced no loss of consciousness but was confused for a period of about 10 minutes. Head imaging was normal. He describes a generalized headache that is present all the time since his trauma, and he occasionally feels dizzy. His mother is concerned that he is having a hard time concentrating in school and seems depressed to her lately; she describes him as being very energetic prior to his concussion. The patient's physical examination is entirely normal except for a somewhat flattened affect. Which of the following statements regarding his condition is true?

A. He has an excellent prognosis.
B. He meets the criteria for postconcussive syndrome and should improve over 1–2 months.
C. He should avoid contact sports for 2 weeks.
D. He is most likely malingering.
E. Low-dose narcotics should be started for headache.

XI-37. A 68-year-old man is brought to the clinic by his wife for evaluation. She has noticed that over past 2–3 months her husband has had increasingly slowed thinking and a change in his personality in that he has become very withdrawn. His only complaint is a mild but persistent, diffuse headache. There is no history of head trauma, prior neurologic or psychiatric disease, or family history of dementia. Physical examination is only notable for a moderate cognitive deficit with a mini-mental examination of 19/30. His head CT is shown in Figure XI-37. What is the most likely diagnosis?

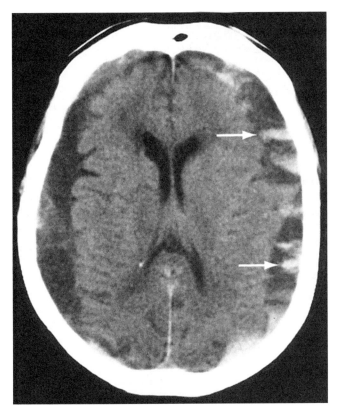

FIGURE XI-37

A. Acute epidural hematoma
B. Acute subarachnoid hemorrhage
C. Alzheimer's disease
D. Chronic subdural hematomas
E. Normal-pressure hydrocephalus

XI-38. A 76-year-old nursing home resident is brought to the local emergency department after falling out of bed. The fall was not witnessed; however, she was suspected to have hit her head. She is not responsive to verbal or light tactile stimuli. At baseline she is able to converse but is frequently disoriented to place and time. She has a medical history that includes stable coronary disease, mild emphysema, and multi-infarct dementia. Immediately after triage she is taken for a CT scan of the head. Which of the following is true regarding head injury and hematomas?

A. More than 80% of patients with subdural hematomas will experience a lucid interval prior to loss of consciousness.
B. Epidural hematomas generally arise from venous sources.
C. Epidural hematomas are common among the elderly with minor head trauma.
D. Most patients presenting with epidural hematomas are unconscious.
E. Subdural hematomas lead to rapid increases in intracranial pressure and can require arterial ligation.

XI-39. A 49-year-old man is admitted to the hospital with a seizure. He does not have a history of seizures and he currently takes no medications. He has AIDS and is not under any care at this time. His physical examination is most notable for small, shoddy lymphadenopathy in the cervical region. A head CT shows a ring-enhancing lesion in the right temporal lobe, with edema but no mass effect. A lumbar puncture shows no white or red blood cells, and the Gram stain is negative. His serum *Toxoplasma* IgG is positive. He is treated with pyrimethamine, sulfadiazine, and levetiracetam. After 2 weeks of therapy the central nervous system (CNS) lesion has not changed in size and he has not had any more seizures. All microbiologic cultures and viral studies, including Epstein-Barr virus DNA from the cerebrospinal fluid, are negative. What is the best course of action for this patient at this time?

A. Continue treatment for CNS toxoplasmosis.
B. Dexamethasone.
C. IV acyclovir.
D. Stereotactic brain biopsy.
E. Whole-brain radiation therapy.

XI-40. A young man with a history of a low-grade astrocytoma comes into your office complaining of weight gain and low energy. He is status post resection of his low-grade astrocytoma and had a course of whole-brain radiation therapy (WBRT) 1 year ago. A laboratory workup reveals a decreased morning cortisol level of 1.9 μg/dL. In addition to depressed adrenocorticotropic hormone (ACTH) function, which of the following hormones is most sensitive to damage from whole-brain radiation therapy?

A. Growth hormone
B. Follicle-stimulating hormone
C. Prolactin
D. Thyroid-stimulating hormone

XI-41. A 37-year-old woman with a history of 6 months of worsening headache is admitted to the hospital after a tonic-clonic seizure that occurred at work. The seizure lasted a short time and terminated spontaneously. On examination her vital signs are normal, she is somnolent but awake, and there are no focal abnormalities. Her initial CT scan showed no acute hemorrhage but was abnormal. An MRI is obtained and is shown in Figure XI-41. What is the most likely diagnosis in this patient?

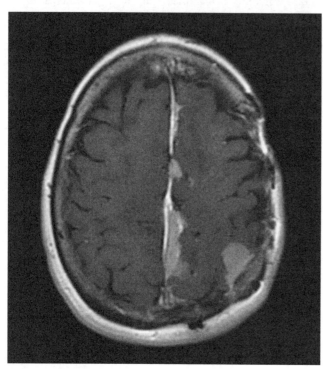

FIGURE XI-41

A. Brain abscess
B. Glioblastoma
C. Low-grade astrocytoma
D. Meningioma
E. Oligodendroglioma

XI-42. All of the following are frequent initial symptoms of multiple sclerosis EXCEPT:

A. Optic neuritis
B. Paresthesias
C. Sensory loss
D. Visual loss
E. Weakness

XI-43. Which of the following is the most common clinical classification of multiple sclerosis?

A. Autoimmune autonomic neuropathy
B. Primary progressive
C. Progressive relapsing
D. Relapsing/remitting
E. Secondary progressive

XI-44. Lumbar puncture should be preceded by CT or MRI in all of the following subsets of patients suspected of having meningitis EXCEPT those with:

A. Depressed consciousness
B. Focal neurologic abnormality
C. Known central nervous system (CNS) mass lesion
D. Positive Kernig's sign
E. Recent head trauma

XI-45. A 78-year-old man with diabetes mellitus presents with fever, headache, and altered sensorium. On physical exam his temperature is 40.2°C (104.4°F), heart rate is 103 beats/min, and blood pressure is 84/52 mmHg. His neck is stiff and he has photophobia. His cerebrospinal fluid (CSF) examination shows 2100 cells/μL, with 100% neutrophils, glucose 10 mg/dL, and protein 78 mg/dL. CSF Gram stain is negative. In addition to empiric antibacterial antibiotics, initial therapy should include which of the following?

A. Acyclovir
B. Dexamethasone after antibiotics
C. Dexamethasone prior to antibiotics
D. IV γ globulin
E. Valacyclovir

XI-46. Which of the following groups of patients should receive empirical antibiotic therapy that includes coverage of *Listeria monocytogenes* in cases of presumed meningitis?

A. Immunocompromised patients
B. Elderly patients
C. Infants
D. All of the above

XI-47. Which of the following medicines has been most commonly implicated in the development of noninfectious chronic meningitis?

A. Acetaminophen
B. Acyclovir
C. β-lactam antibiotics
D. Ibuprofen
E. Phenobarbital

XI-48. Variant Creutzfeldt-Jakob disease (vCJD) has been diagnosed in which of the following populations?

A. Family members with well-defined germ-line mutations leading to autosomal dominant inheritance of a fatal neurodegenerative disease
B. New Guinea natives practicing cannibalism
C. Patients accidentally inoculated with infected material during surgical procedures
D. Worldwide, in sporadic cases, mostly during the fifth and sixth decades of life
E. Young adults in Europe thought to have been exposed to tainted beef products

XI-49. The presence of startle myoclonus in a 60-year-old man with rapidly progressive deficits in cortical dysfunction is which of the following?

A. Neither sensitive nor specific for Creutzfeldt-Jacob disease (CJD) but does represent grounds to explore further for this condition with an electroencephalogram (EEG)

B. Neither sensitive nor specific for CJD but does represent grounds to explore further for this condition with an EEG and brain MRI

C. Sensitive but not specific for CJD and is not enough to prompt a further workup for this condition unless other clinical criteria are met

D. Specific but not sensitive for CJD and should therefore prompt immediate referral for brain biopsy to confirm the diagnosis

E. Virtually diagnostic for CJD, and further workup including EEG, brain MRI, and perhaps brain biopsy serves only a prognostic purpose

XI-50. A 24-year-old man presents for evaluation of footdrop. He has noted that for the last several months, he has had difficulty picking his feet up to walk up stairs and over thresholds. His right leg is more affected than his left leg. He has not noted any sensory changes. He has several family members with similar complaints. His exam is notable for distal leg weakness with reduced sensation to light touch in both lower extremities. Knee and ankle jerk reflexes are unobtainable. Calves are reduced in size bilaterally. Upper extremity examination is normal. Which of the following is the most likely diagnosis?

A. Charcot-Marie-Tooth syndrome
B. Fabry disease
C. Guillain-Barré syndrome
D. Hereditary neuralgic amyotrophy
E. Hereditary sensory and autonomic neuropathy

XI-51. A 57-year-old immigrant from Vietnam is evaluated by his primary caregiver for dysesthesias that have been present in his hands and feet for the past several weeks. He also reports some difficulty walking. His past medical history is notable for hypertriglyceridemia, tobacco abuse, and a recently discovered positive PPD with sputum that is smear-negative for *Mycobacterium tuberculosis*. His medications include niacin, aspirin, and isoniazid. Which of the following is likely to reverse his symptoms?

A. Cobalamin
B. Levothyroxine
C. Neurontin
D. Pregabalin
E. Pyridoxine

XI-52. A 52-year-old woman with long-standing, poorly controlled type 2 diabetes mellitus is evaluated for a sensation of numbness in her fingers and toes, as if she is wearing gloves and socks all the time. She also reports tingling and burning in the same location, but no weakness. Her symptoms have been intermittently present for

the last several months. After a thorough evaluation, nerve biopsy is obtained and demonstrates axonal degeneration, endothelial hyperplasia, and perivascular inflammation. Which of the following statements regarding this condition is true?

A. Autonomic neuropathy is rarely seen in combination with sensory neuropathy.

B. The presence of retinopathy or nephropathy does not portend increased risk for diabetic neuropathy.

C. This is the most common cause of peripheral neuropathy in developed countries.

D. Tight glucose control from now on will reverse her neuropathy.

E. None of the above is true.

XI-53. All the following cause primarily a sensory neuropathy EXCEPT:

A. Acromegaly
B. Critical illness
C. HIV infection
D. Hypothyroidism
E. Vitamin B_{12} deficiency

XI-54. A 50-year-old male complains of weakness and numbness in the hands for the last month. He describes paresthesias in the thumb and the index and middle fingers. The symptoms are worse at night. He also describes decreased grip strength bilaterally. He works as a mechanical engineer. The patient denies fevers, chills, or weight loss. The examination is notable for atrophy of the thenar eminences bilaterally and decreased sensation in a median nerve distribution. You consider the diagnosis of carpal tunnel syndrome. All the following are causes of carpal tunnel syndrome EXCEPT:

A. Amyloidosis
B. Chronic lymphocytic leukemia
C. Diabetes mellitus
D. Hypothyroidism
E. Rheumatoid arthritis

XI-55. A 27-year-old woman is diagnosed with Guillain-Barré syndrome after presenting with flaccid paralysis and sensory disturbance several weeks after a diarrheal illness. Which of the following bacteria have been implicated in cases of Guillain-Barré syndrome?

A. *Bartonella henselae*
B. *Campylobacter jejuni*
C. *Escherichia coli*
D. *Proteus mirabilis*
E. *Tropheryma whippelii*

XI-56. A 34-year-old female complains of weakness and double vision for the last 3 weeks. She has also noted a change in her speech, and her friends tell her that she is "more nasal." She has noticed decreased exercise tolerance and difficulty lifting objects and getting out of a chair. The patient denies pain. The symptoms are worse at the end of the day and with repeated muscle use. You suspect myasthenia gravis. All the following are useful in the diagnosis of myasthenia gravis EXCEPT:

A. Acetylcholine receptor (AChR) antibodies
B. Edrophonium
C. Electrodiagnostic testing
D. Muscle-specific kinase (MuSK) antibodies
E. Voltage-gated calcium channel antibodies

XI-57. A 38-year-old female patient with facial and ocular weakness has just been diagnosed with myasthenia gravis. You intend to initiate therapy with anticholinesterase medications and glucocorticoids. All of the following tests are necessary before instituting this therapy EXCEPT:

A. MRI of mediastinum
B. Purified protein derivative skin test
C. Lumbar puncture
D. Pulmonary function tests
E. Thyroid-stimulating hormone

XI-58. All of the following lipid-lowering agents are associated with muscle toxicity EXCEPT:

A. Atorvastatin.
B. Ezetimibe.
C. Gemfibrozil.
D. Niacin.
E. All of the above are associated with muscle toxicity.

XI-59. All of the following endocrine conditions are associated with myopathy EXCEPT:

A. Hypothyroidism.
B. Hyperparathyroidism.
C. Hyperthyroidism.
D. Acromegaly.
E. All of the above are associated with myopathy.

XI-60. A 34-year-old woman seeks evaluation for weakness. She has noted tripping when walking, particularly in her left foot, for the past 2 years. She recently also began to drop things, once allowing a full cup of coffee to spill onto her legs. In this setting, she also feels as if the appearance of her face has changed over the course of many years, stating that she feels as if her face is becoming more hollow and elongated, although she hasn't lost any weight recently. She has not seen a physician in many years and has no past medical history. Her only medications are a multivitamin and calcium with vitamin D. Her family history is significant for similar symptoms of weakness in her brother who is 2 years older. Her mother, who is 58 years old, was diagnosed with mild weakness after her brother was evaluated, but is not symptomatic. On physical examination, the patient's face appears long

and narrow with wasting of the temporalis and masseter muscles. Her speech is mildly dysarthric, and the palate is high and arched. Strength is 4/5 in the intrinsic muscles of the hand, wrist extensors, and ankle dorsiflexors. After testing handgrip strength, you notice that there is a delayed relaxation of the muscles of the hand. What is the most likely diagnosis?

A. Acid maltase deficiency (Pompe's disease)
B. Becker muscular dystrophy
C. Duchenne muscular dystrophy
D. Myotonic dystrophy
E. Nemaline myopathy

XI-61. An elevation in which of the following serum enzymes is the most *sensitive* indicator of myositis?

A. Aldolase
B. Creatinine kinase
C. Glutamic-oxaloacetic transaminase
D. Glutamate pyruvate transaminase
E. Lactate dehydrogenase

XI-62. A 64-year-old woman is evaluated for weakness. For several weeks she has had difficulty brushing her teeth and combing her hair. She has also noted a rash on her face. Examination is notable for a heliotrope rash and proximal muscle weakness. Serum creatine kinase (CK) is elevated and she is diagnosed with dermatomyositis. After evaluation by a rheumatologist, she is found to have anti-Jo-1 antibodies. She is also likely to have which of the following findings?

A. Ankylosing spondylitis
B. Inflammatory bowel disease
C. Interstitial lung disease
D. Primary biliary cirrhosis
E. Psoriasis

XI-63. A 63-year-old woman is evaluated for a rash on her eyes and fatigue for 1 month. She reports difficulty with arm and leg strength and constant fatigue, but no fevers or sweats. She also notes that she has a red discoloration around her eyes. She has hypothyroidism but is otherwise well. On examination she has a heliotrope rash and proximal muscle weakness. A diagnosis of dermatomyositis is made after demonstration of elevated serum creatinine kinase and confirmatory EMGs. Which of the following studies should be performed as well to look for associated conditions?

A. Mammogram
B. Serum antinuclear antibody measurement
C. Stool examination for ova and parasites
D. Thyroid-stimulating immunoglobulins
E. Titers of antibodies to varicella zoster

XI-64. You are seeing your patient with polymyositis for follow-up. He has been taking prednisone at high doses for 2 months, and you initiated mycophenolate mofetil at the last clinic visit for a steroid-sparing effect. He began a steroid taper 2 weeks ago. His symptoms were predominantly in the lower extremities and face, and he has improved considerably. He no longer needs a cane and his voice has returned to normal. Laboratory data show a creatine kinase (CK) of 1300 U/L, which is unchanged from 2 months ago. What is the most appropriate next step in this patient's management?

A. Continue current management.
B. Continue high-dose steroids with no taper.
C. Switch mycophenolate to methotrexate.
D. Repeat muscle biopsy.

XI-65. A 45-year-old woman who is 6 months post–liver transplant is admitted to the hospital after two grand mal seizures in the last 45 minutes. For the last day she has complained about headache and confusion. Her medications include diltiazem, cyclosporine, prednisone, and mycophenolate mofetil. She is now awake but somnolent. Her vital signs are normal except a blood pressure of 150/90 mmHg. There is bilateral afferent pupillary defect, and she reports she cannot see out of either eye. Hearing is intact. There is no nuchal rigidity. Her cyclosporine level is therapeutic. The FLAIR image of her MRI is shown in Figure XI-65. Which of the following is the most likely diagnosis?

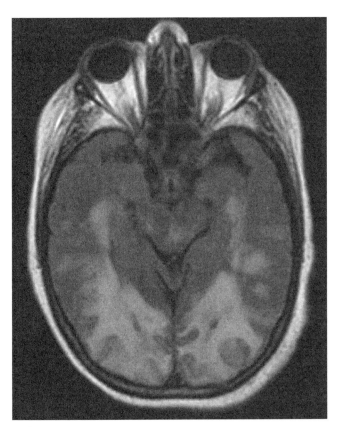

FIGURE XI-65

A. Acoustic neuroma
B. Calcineurin-inhibitor toxicity
C. Panhypopituitarism
D. Streptococcal meningitis
E. Tuberculous meningitis

XI-66. A 77-year-old man undergoes coronary artery bypass grafting for refractory angina and three-vessel disease. Prior to surgery he still worked as a classics professor at a university teaching a renowned course on Dante's "Inferno." One month after surgery, his cardiac status is normal and his exercise tolerance is better than presurgery. However, his wife reports that he seems depressed and is often confused. His short-term memory is poor and he exhibits no enthusiasm for teaching. He has no fever or night sweats. Current medications include lovastatin and lisinopril. His physical examination is normal except for poor performance on serial 7 subtraction and only recalling 1 or 3 objects at 15 minutes. Which of the following is the most likely diagnosis?

A. Multiple sclerosis
B. Post–cardiac bypass brain injury
C. Streptococcal meningitis
D. Variant Creutzfeldt-Jacob disease
E. West Nile virus encephalitis

XI-67. A 24-year-old man is recovering from ARDS due to severe influenza A infection. During his complicated 3-week course of respiratory failure, he was placed on high-frequency ventilation and prone positioning necessitating paralysis and heavy sedation. Passive splints were placed on his upper and lower extremities. He is now extubated and awake, requiring only nasal oxygen. While starting his physical therapy, it is noted that he has right footdrop and numbness on the lateral leg. Additional examination reveals a unilateral right motor defect in foot dorsiflexion with intact inversion. There is sensory loss of the lateral aspect of the leg below the knee extending to the dorsum of the foot. The rest of the neurologic examination of the right leg and foot appears normal. Which of the following is the most likely etiology of his defects?

A. Cauda equina syndrome
B. Femoral nerve injury
C. L4 radiculopathy
D. L5 radiculopathy
E. Peroneal nerve injury

XI-68. In the CDC diagnostic criteria for chronic fatigue syndrome, in addition to clearly delineated findings of fatigue, all of the following symptoms or findings must be concurrently present for at least 6 months EXCEPT:

A. Delusional disorder
B. Impaired memory or concentration
C. Muscle pain
D. Sore throat
E. Tender cervical or axillary lymph nodes

XI-69. Which of the following is a beneficial therapy for chronic fatigue syndrome?

A. Bupropion
B. Cognitive behavioral therapy
C. Doxycycline
D. Fluoxetine
E. Olanzapine

XI-70. A 26-year-old woman presents to the emergency department complaining of shortness of breath and chest pain. These symptoms began abruptly and became progressively worse over 10 minutes, prompting her to call 911. Over this same period, the patient describes feeling her heart pounding and states that she felt like she was dying. She feels lightheaded and dizzy. It is currently about 20 minutes since the onset of symptoms and the severity has abated, although she continues to feel not back to her baseline. She denies any immediate precipitating cause, although she has been under increased stress as her mother has been hospitalized recently with advanced breast cancer. She does not take any medications and has no medical history. She denies tobacco, alcohol, or drug use. On initial examination, she appears somewhat anxious and diaphoretic. Her initial vital signs show a heart rate of 108 beats/min, blood pressure 122/68 mmHg, and respiratory rate 20 breaths/min. She is afebrile. Her examination is normal. Her arterial blood gas shows a pH of 7.52, $PaCO_2$ of 28 mmHg, and PaO_2 of 116 mmHg. The ECG is normal as is a chest radiograph. What is the next best step in the management of this patient?

A. Initiate therapy with alprazolam 0.5 mg four times daily.
B. Initiate therapy with fluoxetine 20 mg daily.
C. Perform a CT pulmonary angiogram.
D. Reassure the patient and suggest medical and/or psychological therapy if symptoms recur on a frequent basis.
E. Refer for cognitive behavioral therapy.

XI-71. All of the following antidepressant medications are correctly paired with their class of medication EXCEPT:

A. Duloxetine—Selective serotonin reuptake inhibitor
B. Fluoxetine—Selective serotonin reuptake inhibitor
C. Nortriptyline—Tricyclic antidepressant
D. Phenelzine—Monoamine oxidase inhibitor
E. Venlafaxine—Mixed norepinephrine/serotonin reuptake inhibitor and receptor blocker

XI-72. A 42-year-old woman seeks your advice regarding symptoms concerning for post-traumatic stress disorder. She was the victim of a home invasion 6 months previously where she was robbed and beaten by a man at gunpoint. She thought she was going to die and was hospitalized with multiple blunt force injuries including a broken nose and zygomatic arch. She now states that she is unable to be alone in her home and frequently awakens with dreams of the event. She is irritable with her husband and children and cries frequently. She has worsening insomnia and often stays awake most of the night watching out her window because she is afraid her assailant will return. She has begun drinking a bottle of wine nightly to help her fall asleep, although she notes that this has worsened her nightmares in the early morning hours. You concur that post-traumatic stress disorder is likely. What treatment do you recommend for this patient?

A. Avoidance of alcohol
B. Cognitive behavioral therapy
C. Paroxetine 20 mg daily
D. Trazodone 50 mg nightly
E. All of the above

XI-73. A 36-year-old man is being treated with venlafaxine 150 mg twice daily for major depression. He has currently been on the medication for 4 months. After 2 months, his symptoms were inadequately controlled, necessitating an increase in the dose of venlafaxine from 75 mg twice daily. He has had one prior episode of major depression when he was 25. At that time, he was treated with fluoxetine 80 mg daily for 12 months, but found the sexual side effects difficult to tolerate. He asks when he can safely discontinue his medication. What is your advice to the patient?

A. He should continue on the medication indefinitely as his depression is likely to recur.
B. The current medication should be continued for a minimum of 6–9 months following control of his symptoms.
C. The medication can be discontinued safely if he establishes a relationship with a psychotherapist who will monitor his progress and symptoms.
D. The medication can be discontinued safely now as his symptoms are well controlled.
E. The medication should be switched to fluoxetine to complete 12 months of therapy, as this was previously effective for him.

XI-74. Which of the following will lead to a faster rate of absorption of alcohol from the gut into the blood?

A. Coadministration with a carbonated beverage
B. Concentration of alcohol of more than 20% by volume
C. Concurrent intake of a high-carbohydrate meal
D. Concurrent intake of a high-fat meal
E. Concurrent intake of a high-protein meal

XI-75. Which of the following best reflects the effect of alcohol on neurotransmitters in the brain?

A. Decreases dopamine activity
B. Decreases serotonin activity
C. Increases γ-aminobutyric acid activity
D. Stimulates muscarinic acetylcholine receptors
E. Stimulates N-methyl-D-aspartate excitatory glutamate receptors

XI-76. In an individual without any prior history of alcohol intake, what serum concentration of ethanol (in grams per deciliter) would likely result in death?

A. 0.02
B. 0.08
C. 0.28
D. 0.40
E. 0.60

XI-77. All of the following statements regarding the epidemiology and genetics of alcoholism are true EXCEPT:

A. Among individuals who have demonstrated alcohol abuse, about 10% will develop true alcohol dependence.

B. Approximately 60% of the risk for alcohol abuse disorders is attributed to genetics.

C. Children of alcoholics have a 10-fold higher risk of alcohol abuse and dependence.

D. The presence of a mutation of aldehyde dehydrogenase that results in intense flushing with alcohol consumption confers a decreased risk of alcohol dependence.

E. The lifetime risk of alcohol dependence in most Western countries is about 10–15% for men and 5–8% for women.

XI-78. A 42-year-old man with alcohol dependence is admitted to the hospital for acute pancreatitis. Upon admission, he has an abdominal CT scan that shows edema without necrosis or hemorrhage of the pancreas. He is treated with IV fluids with dextrose, multivitamins, thiamine 50 mg daily, pain control, and bowel rest. He typically drinks 24 12-ounce beers daily. Forty-eight hours after admission, you are called because the patient is febrile and combative with the nursing staff. His vital signs demonstrate a heart rate of 132 beats/min, blood pressure of 184/96 mmHg, respiratory rate of 32 breaths/min, temperature of 38.7°C (101.7°F), and oxygen saturation of 94% on room air. He is agitated, diaphoretic, and pacing his room. He is oriented to person only. His neurologic examination appears nonfocal, although he does not cooperate. He is tremulous. What is the next step in the management of this patient?

A. Administer a bolus of 1 L of normal saline and thiamine 100 mg IV.

B. Administer diazepam 10–20 mg IV followed by bolus doses of 5–10 mg as needed until the patient is calm but able to be aroused.

C. Perform an emergent head CT.

D. Perform two peripheral blood cultures and begin treatment with imipenem 1 g IV every 8 hours.

E. Place the patient in four-point restraints and treat with haloperidol 5 mg IV.

XI-79. A 48-year-old woman is recovering from alcohol dependence and requests medication to help prevent relapse. She has a medical history of stroke occurring during a hypertensive crisis. Which of the following medications could be considered?

A. Acamprosate

B. Disulfiram

C. Naltrexone

D. A and C

E. All of the above

XI-80. What is the most common initial illicit drug of abuse among U.S. adolescents?

A. Benzodiazepines

B. Heroin

C. Marijuana

D. Methamphetamines

E. Prescription narcotics

XI-81. A 32-year-old woman is admitted to the hospital for drainage and treatment of a soft tissue abscess of her left forearm. She uses IV heroin on a daily basis, often spending $100 or more per day on drugs. Upon admission, she has a 4 × 2-cm fluctuant mass in the left forearm associated with fevers to 39.3°C (102.7°F) and tachycardia. The abscess is drained and packed, and the patient is initiated on therapy with IV clindamycin. About 10 hours after admission, you are called to the patient's bedside for a change in the patient's condition. You are suspecting narcotic withdrawal. All of the following symptoms are consistent with this diagnosis EXCEPT:

A. Hyperthermia

B. Hypotension

C. Piloerection

D. Sweating

E. Vomiting

XI-82. A 24-year-old man is brought to the emergency department by emergency medical services (EMS) about 2 hours after an intentional overdose of sustained-release oxycodone that was taken in conjunction with alcohol. Upon arrival at the scene, emergency medical technicians found an empty bottle of sustained-release oxycodone tablets with a dose of 20 mg. It is unknown how many pills the patient ingested, but the prescription was written for 60 tablets. The patient was unresponsive with a respiratory rate of 4 breaths/min, blood pressure of 80/56 mmHg, heart rate of 65 beats/min, and oxygen saturation of 86% on room air. The patient was intubated in the field and naloxone 2 mg IM was administered. He is currently intubated and unresponsive without spontaneous respiration above the set ventilator rate. His blood pressure is 82/50 mmHg and heart rate is 70 beats/min. Which of the following is most appropriate at the present time in the evaluation and treatment of this patient?

A. Activated charcoal

B. IV saline bolus 1 L followed by repeated 500–1000 mL boluses to maintain adequate blood pressure

C. Naloxone continuous infusion at a rate of 0.4 mg/h

D. Urine drug screen, acetaminophen levels, and blood alcohol content

E. All of the above

XI-83. Which of the following statements is TRUE with regard to the chronic effects of marijuana use?

A. Chronic use of marijuana is associated with low testosterone levels.
B. Chronic use of marijuana is the primary cause of amotivational syndrome.
C. Marijuana use is associated with an increased risk of psychotic symptoms in individuals with a past history of schizophrenia.
D. Physical and psychological tolerance does not develop in chronic users of marijuana.
E. There is no withdrawal syndrome associated with cessation of marijuana use.

XI-84. All of the following malignancies are associated with cigarette smoking EXCEPT:

A. Acute myeloid leukemia
B. Bladder
C. Cervix
D. Pancreas
E. Postmenopausal breast cancer

XI-85. A 42-year-old woman seeks advice from you regarding smoking cessation. She began smoking at age 15. On average, she has smoked about 1.5 packs of tobacco daily and is currently smoking 1 pack daily. She was able to successfully quit for a period of 8 months when she was pregnant with her child at the age of 28, but quickly began smoking again shortly after the baby's birth. Her past medical history is significant for depression, but she is not currently on any medication. She does admit to ongoing symptoms of depression that contribute to her perceived need for ongoing cigarette use. Which of the following would you recommend for this patient?

A. Bupropion titrated to a dose of 150 mg twice daily
B. Bupropion titrated to a dose of 150 mg twice daily in combination with nicotine replacement therapy
C. In-office counseling alone with a negotiated quit date
D. Varenicline titrated to a dose of 1 mg twice daily
E. Varenicline titrated to a dose of 1 mg twice daily in combination with nicotine replacement therapy

XI-86. What percentage of cigarette smokers will die prematurely if they are unable to quit?

A. 2%
B. 10%
C. 25%
D. 40%
E. 70%

XI-87. You are counseling your patient on the need to quit smoking cigarettes. She has been smoking for over two decades and wants to quit in order to avoid the harmful physical effects of smoking. Wanting to take "baby steps," she has switched to low-tar, low-nicotine cigarettes. Which of the following statements is TRUE about the potential benefit of switching to these low-yield cigarettes?

A. Fewer smoking-drug interactions are found among smokers of low-yield cigarettes.
B. Most smokers inhale the same amount of nicotine and tar even if they switch to low-yield cigarettes.
C. Smokers of low-yield cigarettes tend to inhale less deeply and smoke fewer cigarettes daily.
D. Smoking low-yield cigarettes decreases the harmful cardiovascular effects of cigarette smoking.
E. Smoking low-yield cigarettes is a reasonable alternative to complete smoking cessation for chronic smokers.

ANSWERS

XI-1. **The answer is D.** *(Chap. 366)* Channelopathies, disorders of ion channels that lead to disease, are a growing mechanism to explain a number of neurologic diseases. Most are caused by a mutation in the ion channel gene or by autoimmune alteration of ion channel proteins. Some forms of epilepsy, including benign neonatal familial convulsions and generalized epilepsy with febrile convulsions, are associated with genetic abnormalities of sodium or potassium channels. Familial hemiplegic migraines are associated with genetic abnormalities in sodium and calcium channels. Spinocerebellar ataxia and other ataxias are associated with genetic abnormalities in potassium or calcium channels. Lambert-Eaton syndrome is an example of autoimmune-related abnormalities in calcium channel function. Parkinson's disease is the classic example of neurotransmitter system–mediated disease.

XI-2. **The answer is C.** *(Chap. 366)* Synaptic neurotransmission is the predominant mechanism for neuronal communication. Therefore, it is not surprising that dysfunction with any step in the presynaptic synthesis, vesicular storage, and synaptic cleft release, and receptor binding in the postsynaptic cell may be associated with disease. Neurotransmitters bind to specific receptors that are either ionotropic or metabotropic. Functions related to ionotropic receptors are generally fast (<1 millisecond) and metabotropic receptors are more prolonged. Antibodies to the acetylcholine receptors or motor neuron calcium channels cause myasthenia gravis and Lambert-Eaton syndrome, respectively. Parkinson's syndrome is related to selective cell death in the nigrostriatal dopamine pathway. Stiff-person syndrome is related to antibodies to glutamic acid decarboxylase, the biosynthetic pathway for GABA. Orthostatic tachycardia syndrome is related to mutations in the norepinephrine transporter. Abnormalities with serotonin neurotransmitter function are implicated in mood disorders, migraine pain pathways, and somatic pain pathways.

XI-3 and XI-4. **The answers are D and D, respectively.** *(Chap. 367)* The ability to perform a thorough neurologic examination is an important skill for all internists to master. A careful neurologic examination can localize the site of the lesion and is important in directing further workup. The components of the neurologic examination include mental status, cranial nerves, motor, sensory, gait, and coordination. The motor examination is further characterized by appearance, tone, strength, and reflexes. Pronator drift is a useful tool for determining if upper extremity weakness is present. In this test, an individual is asked to stand with both arms fully extended and parallel to the floor while closing his or her eyes. If the arms flex at the elbows or fingers or there is pronation of the forearm, this is considered a positive test. Other tests of motor strength include tests of maximal effort in a specific muscle or muscle group. Most commonly this type of strength testing is graded from 0 (no movement) to 5 (full power) with varying degrees of weakness noted against resistance. However, many individuals find it more practical to use qualitative grading of strength, such as paralysis, severe weakness, moderate weakness, mild weakness, or full strength.

Babinski sign is a sign of upper motor neuron disease above the level of the S1 vertebra and is characterized by paradoxical extension of the great toe with fanning and extension of the other toes as well. Dysdiadochokinesis refers to the inability to perform rapid alternating movements and is a sign of cerebellar disease. Lhermitte symptom causes electric shock–like sensations in the extremities associated with neck flexion. It has many causes including cervical spondylosis and multiple sclerosis. Romberg sign is performed with an individual standing with feet together and arms at the side. The individual is then asked to close his or her eyes. If the individual begins to sway or fall, this is considered a positive test and is a sign of abnormal proprioception.

XI-5. **The answer is C.** *(Chap. 367)* This patient likely has metastatic disease to the cervical spinal cord. The patient's symptoms are bilateral with sparing of the cranial nerves and normal mental status, localizing the lesion below the level of the brainstem and cerebrum. The patient demonstrates mixed upper and lower motor neuron signs with decreased sphincter tone and a positive Babinski sign, placing the lesion at the level of the spinal cord. As the weakness is involving both the arms and legs, this would indicate a lesion in the lower cervical or upper thoracic spine. Symptoms of abnormalities at the level of the neuromuscular junction include bilateral weakness that can include the face having normal sensation.

XI-6. **The answer is C.** *(Chap. 368)* Appropriate and timely evaluation is needed to determine if a subarachnoid hemorrhage is present as it can be rapidly fatal if undetected. The procedure of choice for initial diagnosis is a CT of the head without IV contrast. On the CT, blood in the subarachnoid space would appear whiter compared to the surrounding brain tissue. The CT of the head is most sensitive when it is performed shortly after the onset of symptoms, but declines over several hours. It can also demonstrate the presence of mass effect and midline shift, factors that increase the severity of the underlying hemorrhage. In the situation where the CT head is negative but clinical suspicion is high, a lumbar puncture can be performed. This may demonstrate increased numbers of red blood cells that do not clear with successive aliquots of cerebrospinal fluid. If the lumbar puncture is performed more than 12 hours after a small subarachnoid hemorrhage, then the red blood cells may begin to decompose, leading to xanthochromia—a yellow to pink coloration of cerebrospinal fluid that can be measured spectrographically. A basic CT of the head with IV contrast is rarely useful in subarachnoid hemorrhage, as the brightness of the contrast material may make it difficult to identify blood in the subarachnoid space. However, a CT angiography that is performed with IV contrast can be useful in identifying the aneurismal vessel leading to the bleeding. Classic angiography is a more direct way to visualize the anatomy of the cranial vasculature and is now often combined with interventional procedures to coiling a bleeding vessel. Transcranial Doppler ultrasound is a test that measures the velocity of blood flow through the cranial vasculature. It is used in some centers following subarachnoid hemorrhage to assess for the development of vasospasm, which can worsen ischemia leading to increased damage to brain tissue following subarachnoid hemorrhage.

XI-7.   **The answer is E.** *(Chap. 368)* Magnetic resonance imaging (MRI) is generated from the interaction between the hydrogen protons in biologic tissues, the magnetic field, and the radiofrequency (Rf) of waves generated by the coil placed next to the body part of interest. The Rf pulses transiently excite the protons of the body with a subsequent return to the equilibrium energy state, a process known as relaxation. During relaxation, the protons release Rf energy creating an echo that is then transformed via Fourier analysis to generate the MR image. The two relaxation rates that influence the signal intensity of the image are T1 and T2. T1 refers to the time in milliseconds that it takes for 63% of protons to return to their baseline state. T2 relaxation is the time for 63% of protons to become dephased owing to interactions among nearby protons. The intensity of the signal is also influenced by the interval between Rf pulses (TR) and the time between the Rf pulse and the signal reception (TE). T1-weighted images are produced by keeping both TR and TE relatively short, while T2-weighted images require long TR and TE times. Fat and subacute hemorrhages have relatively shorted TR and TE times and thus appear more brightly on T1-weighted images. Structures with more water such as cerebrospinal fluid or edema conversely have long T1 and T2 relaxation times, resulting in higher signal intensity on T2-weighted images. T2 images are also more sensitive for detecting demyelination, infarction, or chronic hemorrhage.

   FLAIR stands for fluid-attenuated inversion recovery and is a type of T2-weighted image that suppresses the high-intensity signal of CSF. Because of this, images created by the FLAIR technique are more sensitive to detecting water-containing lesions or edema than the standard spin images.

   MR angiography refers to several different techniques that are useful for assessing vascular structures, but does not provide details of the underlying brain parenchyma.

XI-8.   **The answer is E.** *(Chap. 368)* For many years, MRI imaging was considered the modality of choice for patients with renal insufficiency because it does not lead to acute renal failure. However, gadolinium was recently linked to a rare disorder called nephrogenic systemic fibrosis. This newly described disorder results in widespread fibrosis in skin, skeletal muscle, bone, lungs, pleura, pericardium, myocardium, and many other tissues. Histologically, thickened collagen bundles are seen in the deep dermis of the skin with increased numbers of fibrocytes and elastic fibers. There is no known medical treatment for nephrogenic systemic fibrosis (NSF), although improvement may be seen following kidney transplantation. It has only recently been linked to the receipt of gadolinium-containing contrast agents with a typical onset between 5 and 75 days following administration of the contrast. The incidence of NSF following administration of gadolinium in individuals with a glomerular filtration rate of less than 30 mL/min may be as high as 4% and is thus considered absolutely contraindicated in individuals with severe renal dysfunction.

   Pseudohypocalcemia can occur following administration of gadolinium in individuals with renal dysfunction, but not true hypocalcemia. This occurs because of an interaction of the contrast dye with standard colorimetric assays for serum calcium that are commonly used. If ionized calcium is measured it would be normal, often in the face of very low levels of serum calcium.

   The other reported complications can be seen following administration of iodinated contrast that is used for CT imaging. The most common complication of CT imaging outside of allergic reactions is the development of worsening renal function or acute renal failure. The risk of this can be minimized if the patient is adequately hydrated. Lactic acidosis is a rare but dreaded side effect of iodinated contrast that has been linked to the coadministration of metformin in diabetic patients. Typically a patient is asked to hold metformin for 48 hours before and after a CT scan. The reason for the development of lactic acidosis is actually related to the development of renal insufficiency and a subsequent buildup of lactic acid. In very rare instances, administration of iodinated contrast can unmask hyperthyroidism.

XI-9. **The answer is D.** *(Chap. e45)* While seldom diagnostic, the EEG can often provide clinically useful information in comatose patients. In patients with an altered mental state or some degree of obtundation, the EEG tends to become slower as consciousness is depressed, regardless of the underlying cause. The EEG generally slows in metabolic encephalopathies, and triphasic waves may be present. The findings do not permit differentiation of the underlying metabolic disturbance but help to exclude other encephalopathic processes by indicating the diffuse extent of cerebral dysfunction. As the depth of coma increases, the EEG becomes nonreactive and may show a burst-suppression pattern, with bursts of mixed-frequency activity separated by intervals of relative cerebral inactivity. The EEG is usually normal in patients with locked-in syndrome and helps in distinguishing this disorder from the comatose state with which it is sometimes confused clinically. Epileptiform activity characterized by bursts of abnormal discharges containing spikes or sharp waves may be useful to diagnose and treat nonconvulsive status in a presumed comatose patient. Patients with herpes simplex encephalitis may show a characteristic pattern of focal (often in the temporal regions) or lateralized periodic slow-wave complexes. Periodic lateralizing epileptiform discharges (PLEDs) are commonly found with acute hemispheric pathology such as a hematoma, abscess, or rapidly expanding tumor.

XI-10. **The answer is B.** *(Chap. 369)* The International League against Epilepsy (ILAE) Commission on Classification and Terminology, 2005–2009, has provided an updated approach to the classification of seizures. This system is based on the clinical features of seizures and associated electroencephalographic findings. Seizures are classified as focal or generalized. Focal seizures arise from a neuronal network either discretely localized within one cerebral hemisphere or more broadly distributed but still within the hemisphere. They are frequently associated with a structural lesion. Generalized seizures are thought to arise at some point in the brain but immediately and rapidly engage neuronal networks in both cerebral hemispheres. Focal seizures are subdivided into those with or without dyscognitive features depending on the patient's ability to interact with the environment during an episode. The terms "simple partial seizure" and "complex partial seizure" have been eliminated. Typical absence seizures are characterized by sudden, brief lapses of consciousness without loss of postural control. The seizure typically lasts for only seconds, consciousness returns as suddenly as it was lost, and there is no postictal confusion. Myoclonus is a sudden and brief muscle contraction that may involve one part of the body or the entire body. Although the distinction from other forms of myoclonus (e.g., metabolic, degenerative neurologic disease, anoxic encephalopathy) is imprecise, myoclonic seizures are considered to be true epileptic events since they are caused by cortical dysfunction.

XI-11. **The answer is A.** *(Chap. 369)* Mesial temporal lobe epilepsy is the most common epilepsy syndrome associated with focal seizures with dyscognitive features. Patients are unable to respond to verbal or visual commands during the seizure and they often manifest complex automatisms or complex posturing. An aura is common before the seizures. There is postictal memory loss or disorientation. Patients often have a history of febrile seizures or a family history of seizures. MRI will show hippocampal sclerosis, a small temporal lobe, or enlarged temporal horn. Mesial temporal lobe epilepsy is important to recognize as a distinct syndrome because it tends to be refractory to treatment with anticonvulsants but responds extremely well to surgical intervention. Hypothyroidism, herpes virus infection, diabetes, and tuberous sclerosis are not associated with mesial temporal lobe epilepsy.

XI-12. **The answer is E.** *(Chap. 369)* Focal seizures without dyscognitive features cause motor, sensory, autonomic, or psychic symptoms without an obvious alteration in consciousness. The phenomenon of abnormal motor movements beginning in a restricted area then progressing to involve a larger area is termed *Jacksonian march*. The patient is describing Todd's paralysis, which may take minutes to many hours to return to normal. Although meningitis is a common cause of seizure in young patients, it is unlikely to be the cause in someone who has a known seizure disorder. If his symptoms were to persist beyond many hours, it would be reasonable to investigate a different etiology of his hand weakness with imaging studies. Overt deficits in strength are not compatible with a primary psychiatric disorder. Magnetic resonance angiogram and cerebral angiogram are useful to evaluate for cerebrovascular disorders, but there is no evidence of subarachnoid bleeding or vasculitis.

XI-13. **The answer is C.** *(Chap. 369)* Nuchal rigidity and an elevated white blood cell count are very concerning for meningitis as the etiology for this patient, and lumbar puncture must be performed to rule this out. In addition, acute cocaine intoxication is a plausible reason for this new-onset seizure. Figure XI-13 illustrates the evaluation of

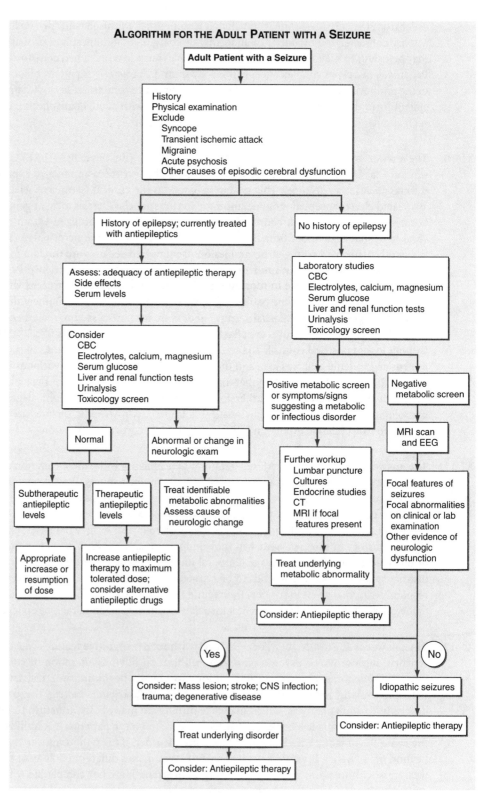

FIGURE XI-13

the adult patient with a seizure. MRI would be indicated if the patient had a negative metabolic and toxicologic screening. Substance abuse counseling, while indicated, is not indicated at this point in his workup since he is postictal. The patient is not having seizures, does not have a known seizure disorder, and has not been treated for the underlying metabolic abnormality, making IV loading with an antiepileptic medication premature at this time.

XI-14. **The answer is B.** *(Chap. 369)* Optimal medical therapy for epilepsy depends on the underlying cause, type of seizure, and patient factors. The goal is to prevent seizures and minimize the side effects of therapy. The minimal effective dose is determined by trial and error. In choosing medical therapies, drug interactions are a key consideration. Certain medications, such as tricyclic antidepressants, may lower the seizure threshold and should be avoided. Patients who respond well to medical therapy and have completely controlled seizures are good candidates for the discontinuation of therapy, with about 70% of children and 60% of adults being able to discontinue therapy eventually. Patient factors that aid in this include complete medical control of seizures for 1–5 years, a normal neurologic examination, a normal EEG, and single seizure type. On the other end of the spectrum, about 20% of these patients are completely refractory to medical therapy and should be considered for surgical therapy. In the best examples, such as mesial temporal sclerosis, resection of the temporal lobe may result in about 70% of these patients becoming seizure-free and an additional 15–25% having a significant reduction in the incidence of seizures. In patients with epilepsy other considerations are critical. Psychosocial sequelae such as depression, anxiety, and behavior problems may occur. Approximately 20% of epileptic patients have depression, with their suicide rate being higher than that of age-matched controls. There is an impact on the ability to drive, perform certain jobs, and function in social situations. Furthermore, there is a two- to threefold increase in mortality for patients with epilepsy compared with age-matched controls. Although most of the increased mortality results from the underlying etiology of epilepsy, a significant number of these patients die from accidents, status epilepticus, and a syndrome known as sudden unexpected death in epileptic patients (SUDEP). A recent meta-analysis demonstrated that treatment of patients with refractory seizures with an antiepileptic drug could reduce the frequency of SUDEP (*Lancet Neurol 2011;10:961*).

XI-15. **The answer is D.** *(Chap. 369)* Adolescence and early adulthood mark the period where idiopathic or genetic epilepsy syndromes become less common and seizures due to acquired central nervous system (CNS) lesions become more common. The most common causes of seizures in the young adults are head trauma, CNS infections, brain tumors, congenital CNS lesions, illicit drug use, or alcohol withdrawal. Fever rarely causes seizure in patients older than 12 years. Amyloid angiopathy and uremia are more common in older adults.

XI-16. **The answer is A.** *(Chap. 369)* Status epilepticus refers to continuous seizures or repetitive, discrete seizures with impaired consciousness in the interictal period. The duration of seizure activity sufficient to meet the definition of status epilepticus has traditionally been specified as 15–30 minutes. Generalized convulsive status epilepticus (GCSE) is typically when seizures last beyond 5 minutes. GCSE is an emergency and must be treated immediately, since cardiorespiratory dysfunction, hyperthermia, and metabolic derangements can develop as a consequence of prolonged seizures, and these can lead to irreversible neuronal injury. Furthermore, CNS injury can occur even when the patient is paralyzed with neuromuscular blockade but continues to have electrographic seizures. The most common causes of GCSE are anticonvulsant withdrawal or noncompliance, metabolic disturbances, drug toxicity, CNS infection, CNS tumors, refractory epilepsy, and head trauma. GCSE is obvious when the patient is having overt convulsions. However, after 30–45 minutes of uninterrupted seizures, the signs may become increasingly subtle. Patients may have mild clonic movements of only the fingers or fine, rapid movements of the eyes. There may be paroxysmal episodes of tachycardia, hypertension, and pupillary dilation. In such cases, the EEG may be the only method of establishing the diagnosis. Thus, if the patient stops having overt seizures yet remains comatose, an EEG should be performed to rule out ongoing status epilepticus. The first steps in the management of a patient in GCSE are to attend to any acute cardiorespiratory problems or hyperthermia, perform a brief medical and neurologic examination, establish venous access, and send samples for laboratory studies to identify metabolic abnormalities. Anticonvulsant therapy should then begin without delay; a treatment approach is shown in Figure XI-16. Carbamazepine is a first-line therapy for focal seizures.

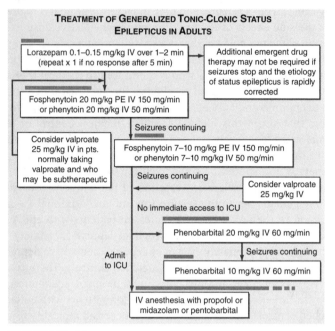

TREATMENT OF GENERALIZED TONIC-CLONIC STATUS EPILEPTICUS IN ADULTS

Lorazepam 0.1–0.15 mg/kg IV over 1–2 min (repeat × 1 if no response after 5 min)

Additional emergent drug therapy may not be required if seizures stop and the etiology of status epilepticus is rapidly corrected

Fosphenytoin 20 mg/kg PE IV 150 mg/min or phenytoin 20 mg/kg IV 50 mg/min

Consider valproate 25 mg/kg IV in pts. normally taking valproate and who may be subtherapeutic

Seizures continuing

Fosphenytoin 7–10 mg/kg PE IV 150 mg/min or phenytoin 7–10 mg/kg IV 50 mg/min

Seizures continuing

Consider valproate 25 mg/kg IV

No immediate access to ICU

Phenobarbital 20 mg/kg IV 60 mg/min

Admit to ICU

Seizures continuing

Phenobarbital 10 mg/kg IV 60 mg/min

IV anesthesia with propofol or midazolam or pentobarbital

FIGURE XI-16

XI-17. **The answer is A.** *(Chap. 370)* Cardioembolism accounts for up to 20% of all ischemic strokes. Stroke caused by heart disease is due to thrombotic material forming on the atrial or ventricular wall or the left heart valves. If the thrombus lyses quickly, only a transient ischemic attack may develop. If the arterial occlusion lasts longer, brain tissue may die and a stroke will occur. Emboli from the heart most often lodge in the middle cerebral artery (MCA), the posterior cerebral artery (PCA), or one of their branches. Atrial fibrillation is the most common cause of cerebral embolism overall. Other significant causes of cardioembolic stroke include myocardial infarction, prosthetic valves, rheumatic heart disease, and dilated cardiomyopathy. Furthermore, paradoxical embolization may occur when an atrial septal defect or a patent foramen ovale exists. This may be detected by bubble-contrast echocardiography. Bacterial endocarditis may cause septic emboli if the vegetation is on the left side of the heart or if there is a paradoxical source.

XI-18. **The answer is D.** *(Chap. 370)* Nonrheumatic atrial fibrillation is the most common cause of cerebral embolism overall. The presumed stroke mechanism is thrombus formation in the fibrillating atrium or atrial appendage. The average annual risk of stroke is around 5%. However, the risk varies with the following factors: age, hypertension, left ventricular function, prior embolism, diabetes, and thyroid function. The risk of stroke can be estimated by calculating the CHADS2 score (see Table XI-18). Patients younger than 60 years of age without structural heart disease or without one of these risk factors have a very low annual risk of cardioembolism of less than 0.5%. Therefore, it is recommended that these patients only take aspirin daily for stroke prevention. Older patients with numerous risk factors may have annual stroke risks of 10–15% and must take a vitamin K antagonist indefinitely. Cardioversion is indicated for symptomatic patients who want an initial opportunity to remain in sinus rhythm. However, studies have shown that there is an increased stroke risk for weeks to months after

TABLE XI-18 Recommendations on Chronic Use of Antithrombotics for Various Cardiac Conditions

Condition	Recommendation
Nonvalvular atrial fibrillation	Calculate CHADS2[a] score
• CHADS2 score 0	Aspirin or no antithrombotic
• CHADS2 score 1	Aspirin or VKA
• CHADS2 score >1	VKA
Rheumatic mitral valve disease	
• With atrial fibrillation, previous embolization, atrial appendage thrombus, or left atrial diameter >55 mm	VKA
• Embolization or appendage clot despite INR 2–3	VKA plus aspirin
Mitral valve prolapse	
• Asymptomatic	No therapy
• With otherwise cryptogenic stroke or TIA	Aspirin
• Atrial fibrillation	VKA
Mitral annular calcification	
• Without atrial fibrillation but systemic embolization, or otherwise cryptogenic stroke or TIA	Aspirin
• Recurrent embolization despite aspirin	VKA
• With atrial fibrillation	VKA
Aortic valve calcification	
• Asymptomatic	No therapy
• Otherwise cryptogenic stroke or TIA	Aspirin
Aortic arch mobile atheroma	
• Otherwise cryptogenic stroke or TIA	Aspirin or VKA
Patent foramen ovale	
• Otherwise cryptogenic ischemic stroke or TIA	Aspirin
• Indication for VKA (deep venous thrombosis or hypercoagulable state)	VKA
Mechanical heart valve	
• Aortic position, bileaflet or Medtronic Hall tilting disk with normal left atrial size and sinus rhythm	VKA INR 2.5, range 2–3
• Mitral position tilting disk or bileaflet valve	VKA INR 3.0, range 2.5–3.5
• Mitral or aortic position, anterior-apical myocardial infarct, or left atrial enlargement	VKA INR 3.0, range 2.5–3.5
• Mitral or aortic position, with atrial fibrillation or hypercoagulable state or low ejection fraction or atherosclerotic vascular disease	Aspirin plus VKA INR 3.0, range 2.5–3.5
• Systemic embolization despite target INR	Add aspirin and/or increase INR: if prior target was 2.5 increase to 3.0, range 2.5–3.5; if prior target was 3.0 increase to 3.5, range 3–4
Bioprosthetic valve	
• No other indication for VKA therapy	Aspirin
Infective endocarditis	Avoid antithrombotic agents
Nonbacterial thrombotic endocarditis	
• With systemic embolization	Full-dose unfractionated heparin or SC LMWH

[a]CHADS2 score is calculated as follows: 1 point for age above 75 years, 1 point for hypertension, 1 point for congestive heart failure, 1 point for diabetes, and 2 points for stroke or TIA; sum of points is the total CHADS2 score.

Abbreviations: Dose of aspirin is 50–325 mg/d; target INR for VKA is 2.5 unless otherwise specified. INR, international normalized ratio; LMWH, low-molecular-weight heparin; TIA, transient ischemic attack; VKA, vitamin K antagonist.

Sources: Modified from DE Singer et al: *Chest* 133:546S, 2008; DN Salem et al: *Chest* 133:593S, 2008.

a successful cardioversion, and these patients must remain on anticoagulation for a long period. Patients who do not respond to cardioversion and do not want catheter ablation have mortality and morbidity with rate control and anticoagulation similar to those of patients who opt for cardioversion. Low-molecular-weight heparin may be used as a bridge to vitamin K–antagonist therapy and may facilitate outpatient anticoagulation in selected patients.

XI-19. **The answer is E.** *(Chap. 370)* Numerous studies have identified key risk factors for ischemic stroke. Old age, family history, diabetes, hypertension, tobacco smoking, and cholesterol are all risk factors for atherosclerosis and therefore stroke. Hypertension is the most significant among these risk factors. All cases of hypertension must be controlled in the setting of stroke prevention. Antiplatelet therapy has been shown to reduce the risk of vascular atherothrombotic events. The overall relative risk reduction of nonfatal stroke is about 25–30% across most large clinical trials. The "true" absolute benefit is dependent on the individual patient's risk; therefore, patients with a low risk for stroke (e.g., younger patients with minimal cardiovascular risk factors) may have a relative risk reduction with antiplatelet therapy but a meaningless "benefit." Numerous studies have shown the benefit of statin therapy in the reduction of stroke risk even in the absence of hypercholesterolemia. Anticoagulation is the treatment of choice to prevent stroke in patients with atrial fibrillation and other potential causes of cardiocerebral emboli. However, data do not support the use of long-term vitamin K antagonists for preventing atherothrombotic stroke for either intracranial or extracranial cerebrovascular disease. The WARSS study found no benefit of warfarin (INR 1.4–2.8) over aspirin 325 mg for secondary prevention of stroke but did find a slightly higher bleeding rate in the warfarin group. A recent European study confirmed this finding. The Warfarin-Aspirin Symptomatic Intracranial Disease (WASID) study demonstrated no benefit of warfarin (INR 2–3) over aspirin in patients with symptomatic intracranial atherosclerosis, and also found higher rates of bleeding complications.

XI-20. **The answer is C.** *(Chap. 370)* Once the diagnosis of stroke is made, a brain imaging study is necessary to determine if the cause of stroke is ischemia or hemorrhage (Figure XI-20). There are no clinical findings that definitively distinguish ischemia from hemorrhage. If the stroke is ischemic, administration of recombinant tissue plasminogen activator (rtPA) or endovascular mechanical thrombectomy may be beneficial in restoring cerebral perfusion. Medical management to reduce the risk of complications becomes the next priority, followed by plans for secondary prevention. For ischemic stroke, several strategies can reduce the risk of subsequent stroke in all patients, while other strategies are effective for patients with specific causes of stroke such as cardiac embolus and carotid atherosclerosis. For hemorrhagic stroke, aneurysmal subarachnoid hemorrhage (SAH) and hypertensive intracranial hemorrhage are two important causes. The National Institute of Neurological Disorders and Stroke (NINDS) recombinant TPA (rtPA) Stroke Study showed a clear benefit for IV rtPA in selected patients with acute stroke. The NINDS study used IV rtPA (0.9 mg/kg to a 90-mg max; 10% as a bolus, then the remainder over 60 minutes) versus placebo in patients with ischemic stroke within 3 hours of onset. Subsequent studies using different dosing and timing ranges have not been as positive. rtPA is being reviewed for approval in the 3- to 4.5-hour window in Europe, but is only approved for 0–3 hours in the United States and Canada. Use of IV rtPA is considered a central component in primary stroke centers as the first treatment proven to improve clinical outcomes in ischemic stroke and is cost-effective and cost saving. Because collateral blood flow within the ischemic brain is blood pressure dependent, there is controversy about whether blood pressure should be lowered acutely. Blood pressure should be lowered if there is malignant hypertension or concomitant myocardial ischemia or if blood pressure is above 185/110 mmHg and thrombolytic therapy is anticipated. When faced with the competing demands of myocardium and brain, lowering the heart rate with a β_1-adrenergic blocker (such as esmolol) can be a first step to decreasing cardiac work and maintaining blood pressure. Endovascular mechanical thrombectomy has recently shown promise as an alternative or adjunctive treatment of acute stroke in patients who are ineligible for, or have contraindications to, thrombolytics or in those who have failed to have vascular recanalization with IV thrombolytics. Studies have

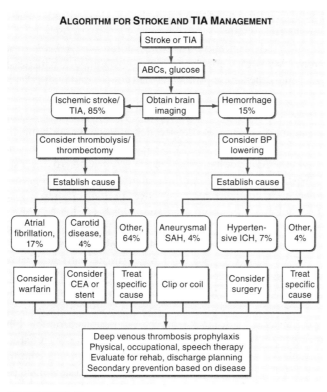

ALGORITHM FOR STROKE AND TIA MANAGEMENT

FIGURE XI-20

shown excellent acute and chronic recanalization rates and the FDA has approved some devices for intracerebral use. Hypothermia is a powerful neuroprotective treatment in patients with cardiac arrest and is neuroprotective in animal models of stroke, but it has not been adequately studied in patients with ischemic stroke.

XI-21. **The answer is B.** (*Chap. 371*) Approximately 10% of all persons over the age of 70 have significant memory loss, and in more than half the cause is Alzheimer's disease (AD). AD can occur in any decade of adulthood, but it is the most common cause of dementia in the elderly. AD most often presents with an insidious onset of memory loss followed by a slowly progressive dementia over several years. Pathologically, atrophy is distributed throughout the medial temporal lobes, as well as lateral and medial parietal lobes and lateral frontal cortex. Microscopically, there are neurofibrillary tangles composed of hyperphosphorylated tau filaments, and accumulation of amyloid in blood vessel walls in the cortex and leptomeninges. The cognitive changes of AD tend to follow a characteristic pattern beginning with memory impairment and spreading to language and visuospatial deficits. Yet approximately 20% of patients with AD present with nonmemory complaints such as word-finding, organizational, or navigational difficulty. In the early stages of the disease, the memory loss may go unrecognized or be ascribed to benign forgetfulness. Slowly the cognitive problems begin to interfere with daily activities, such as keeping track of finances, following instructions on the job, driving, shopping, and housekeeping. Some patients are unaware of these difficulties (*anosognosia*), while others remain acutely attuned to their deficits. Social graces, routine behavior, and superficial conversation may be surprisingly intact. Language becomes impaired—first naming, then comprehension, and finally fluency. In some patients, *aphasia* is an early and prominent feature. Word-finding difficulties and circumlocution may be a problem even when formal testing demonstrates intact naming and fluency. Visuospatial deficits begin to interfere with dressing, eating, or even walking, and patients fail to solve simple puzzles or copy geometric figures. Simple calculations and clock reading become difficult in parallel. Loss of judgment and reasoning is inevitable. Delusions are common and usually simple, with common themes of theft, infidelity, or misidentification. In end-stage AD, patients become rigid, mute, incontinent, and bedridden. Hyperactive tendon reflexes and myoclonic jerks may occur spontaneously or in response to physical or auditory stimulation. Generalized seizures may also occur. Often death results from malnutrition, secondary infections, pulmonary emboli, heart disease, or, most commonly, aspiration. The typical duration of AD is 8–10 years, but the course can range from 1 to 25 years. For unknown reasons, some AD patients show a steady decline in function, while others have prolonged plateaus without major deterioration.

XI-22.   **The answer is D.** *(Chap. 370)* There is currently no robust or curative medical therapy for Alzheimer's disease (AD). The acetylcholinesterase inhibitors donepezil, rivastigmine, and galantamine, as well as the NMDA receptor antagonist memantine are FDA approved for treatment of AD. Double-blind, placebo-controlled crossover studies with these agents have shown improved caregiver ratings of patients' functioning with an apparent decreased rate of decline in cognitive test scores over periods of up to 3 years. The average patient on an anticholinesterase compound maintains his or her MMSE score for close to a year, whereas a placebo-treated patient declines 2–3 points over the same time period. Memantine, used in conjunction with cholinesterase inhibitors or by itself, slows cognitive deterioration and decreases caregiver burden for patients with moderate to severe AD but is not approved for mild AD. Each of these compounds has only modest efficacy for AD. Some studies have suggested a protective effect of estrogen replacement in women. However, a prospective study of a estrogen-progesterone combination increased the prevalence of AD in previously asymptomatic women. A randomized, double-blind, placebo-controlled trial of an extract of *Ginkgo biloba* found modest improvement in cognitive function in subjects with AD and vascular dementia. Unfortunately, a comprehensive 6-year multi-center prevention study using *Ginkgo biloba* found no slowing of progression to dementia in the treated group. Experimental studies are investigating chemical or vaccination strategies to interfere or inhibit amyloid protein deposition. Retrospective studies suggest a beneficial role of statins in the development of dementia. Mild to moderate depression is common in the early stages of AD and may respond to antidepressants or cholinesterase inhibitors. Newer-generation antipsychotics (risperidone, quetiapine, olanzapine) in low doses may benefit neuropsychiatric symptoms. Medications with strong anticholinergic effects should be vigilantly avoided, including prescription and over-the-counter sleep aids (e.g., diphenhydramine) or incontinence therapies (e.g., oxybutynin).

XI-23.   **The answer is D.** *(Chap. 370)* All the choices given in the question are causes of or may be associated with dementia. Binswanger's disease, the cause of which is unknown, often occurs in patients with long-standing hypertension and/or atherosclerosis; it is associated with diffuse subcortical white matter damage and has a subacute insidious course. Alzheimer's disease, the most common cause of dementia, is also slowly progressive and can be confirmed at autopsy by the presence of amyloid plaques and neurofibrillary tangles. Creutzfeldt-Jakob disease, a prion disease, is associated with a rapidly progressive dementia, myoclonus, rigidity, a characteristic EEG pattern, and death within 1–2 years of onset. Vitamin B_{12} deficiency, which often is seen in the setting of chronic alcoholism, most commonly produces a myelopathy that results in loss of vibration and joint position sense, and brisk deep tendon reflexes (dorsal column and lateral corticospinal tract dysfunction). This combination of pathologic abnormalities in the setting of vitamin B_{12} deficiency is also called subacute combined degeneration. Vitamin B_{12} deficiency may also lead to a subcortical type of dementia. Recent studies have demonstrated that elevated levels of MMA, which is a more sensitive measure of vitamin B_{12} deficiency, may increase the risk of cognitive decline in elderly patients. The therapeutic implications of this finding are not yet clear but emphasize the importance of adequate vitamin B_{12} intake. Multi-infarct dementia, as in this case, presents with a history of sudden stepwise declines in function associated with the accumulation of bilateral focal neurologic deficits. Brain imaging demonstrates multiple areas of stroke.

XI-24.   **The answer is D.** *(Chap. 370)* The differential diagnosis of Parkinson's disease is broad, and the disease can be difficult to diagnose, with an estimated misdiagnosis of 10–25% even by experienced physicians. This patient exhibits several atypical features that should alert the physician to search for alternative diagnoses. These include early age of onset, prominent orthostasis, autonomic symptoms of flushing and diaphoresis, and failure to respond to dopaminergic agents. In addition, recurrent urinary tract infections should prompt an evaluation for urinary retention due to autonomic dysfunction in this patient. These symptoms are most consistent with multiple system atrophy with parkinsonian features (MSA-p). The average age of onset is 50 years, and these individuals more frequently present with bilateral, symmetric tremor and more prominent spasticity than those with Parkinson's disease. Orthostasis and autonomic symptoms are typically prominent. On MRI, one would expect to find volume loss and T2-hyperintensity in the area of the putamen, globus pallidus, and white matter. On pathologic examination, α-synuclein–positive inclusions would be seen in the affected areas. Median survival after diagnosis is 6–9 years. Dopaminergic agents are not helpful in the treatment of this disorder and are usually associated with drug-induced dyskinesias of the face and neck, rather than the limbs and trunk. Corticobasal degeneration is a sporadic tauopathy that presents in the sixth to seventh decades. In contrast to Parkinson's disease, this disorder is frequently associated with myoclonic jerks and involuntary purposeful movements of a limb. Its progressive nature leads to spastic paraplegia. Diffuse Lewy body disease has prominent dementia with parkinsonian features. Neuropsychiatric complaints including paranoia, delusions, and personality changes are more common than in Parkinson's disease. Drug-induced Parkinson's disease is not seen with nitrofurantoin, and the patient has no history of illicit drugs such as MTPT, which could cause Parkinson's disease. Finally, this is unlikely to be inadequately treated Parkinson's disease because one would expect at least an initial improvement on dopaminergic agents.

XI-25.   **The answer is C.** *(Chap. 370)* Therapy for Parkinson's disease should be initiated when symptoms interfere with the patient's quality of life. Choice of initial drug therapy is usually with dopamine agonists, levodopa, or MAO inhibitors. The initial choice in most individuals is a dopamine agonist (pramipexole, ropinirole, rotigotine), and monotherapy with dopamine agonists usually controls motor symptoms for several years before levodopa therapy becomes necessary. Over this period, escalating doses are frequently required, and side effects may be limiting. It is thought that dopamine agonists delay the onset of dyskinesias and on-off motor symptoms such as freezing. By 5 years, over half of individuals will require levodopa to control motor symptoms. Levodopa remains the most effective therapy for the motor symptoms of Parkinson's disease, but once levodopa is started, dyskinesias and on-off motor fluctuations become more common. MAO inhibitors (selegiline, rasagiline) work by decreasing the postsynaptic breakdown of dopamine. As monotherapy, these agents have only small effects and are most often used as adjuncts to levodopa. Surgical procedures such as pallidotomy and deep-brain stimulation are reserved for advanced Parkinson's disease with intractable tremor or drug-induced motor fluctuations or dyskinesias. In this setting, deep-brain stimulation can alleviate disabling symptoms.

XI-26.   **The answer is D.** *(Chap. 370)* Restless legs syndrome (RLS) is a neurologic disorder that affects approximately 10% of the adult population, causing significant morbidity in some. It is rare in Asians. The four core symptoms required for diagnosis are as follows: an urge to move the legs, usually caused or accompanied by an unpleasant sensation in the legs; symptoms begin or worsen with rest; partial or complete relief by movement; worsening during the evening or night. Symptoms most commonly begin in the legs, but can spread to or even begin in the upper limbs. In about 80% of patients, RLS is associated with periodic leg movements (PLMs) during sleep and occasionally while awake. These involuntary movements are usually brief, lasting no more than a few seconds, and recur every 5–90 seconds. The restlessness and PLMs are a major cause of sleep disturbance in patients, leading to poor-quality sleep and daytime sleepiness. Primary RLS is genetic, and several loci have been found with an autosomal dominant pattern of inheritance, although penetrance may be variable. The mean age of onset in genetic forms is 27 years, although pediatric cases are recognized. The severity of symptoms is variable. Secondary RLS may be associated with pregnancy or a range of underlying disorders, including anemia, ferritin deficiency, renal failure, and peripheral neuropathy. The pathogenesis probably involves disordered dopamine function, which may be peripheral or central, in association with an abnormality of iron metabolism. Diagnosis is made on clinical grounds but can be supported by polysomnography and the demonstration of PLMs. The neurologic examination is normal. Secondary RLS should be excluded, and ferritin levels, glucose, and renal function should be measured. Most RLS sufferers have mild symptoms that do not require specific treatment. If symptoms are intrusive, low doses of dopamine (pramipexole, ropinirole) may be administered before bedtime. Levodopa can be effective but is frequently associated with augmentation (spread and worsening of restlessness and its appearance earlier in the day) or rebound (reappearance sometimes with worsening of symptoms at a time compatible with the drug's short half-life). Other drugs that can be effective include anticonvulsants, analgesics, and even opiates. Management of secondary RLS should be directed to correcting the underlying disorder.

XI-27. **The answer is E.** *(Chap. 374)* The combination of upper and lower motor neuron findings is highly suggestive of ALS. Indolent presentation is typical and many patients receive alternative diagnoses before defining ALS. There is currently no curative therapy for ALS; therefore, treatable causes of motor nerve dysfunction should be ruled out. Compression of the cervical spinal cord or cervicomedullary junction from tumors in the cervical regions or at the foramen magnum or from cervical spondylosis with osteophytes projecting into the vertebral canal can produce weakness, wasting, and fasciculations in the upper limbs and spasticity in the legs, closely resembling ALS. Absence of pain or of sensory changes, normal bowel and bladder function, normal roentgenographic studies of the spine, and normal cerebrospinal fluid (CSF) all favor ALS. Another important entity in the differential diagnosis of ALS is multifocal motor neuropathy with conduction block (MMCB). In this disorder, remarkably focal blocks in conduction regionally and chronically disrupt lower motor neuron function. Many cases have elevated serum titers of mono- and polyclonal antibodies to ganglioside GM1; it is hypothesized that the antibodies produce selective, focal, paranodal demyelination of motor neurons. MMCB is not typically associated with corticospinal signs. In contrast with ALS, MMCB may respond dramatically to therapy such as IV immunoglobulin or chemotherapy; it is thus imperative that MMCB be excluded when considering a diagnosis of ALS. A diffuse, lower motor axonal neuropathy mimicking ALS sometimes evolves in association with hematopoietic disorders such as lymphoma or multiple myeloma. Lyme disease may also cause an axonal, lower motor neuropathy, although typically with intense proximal limb pain and a CSF pleocytosis.

Other treatable disorders that occasionally mimic ALS are chronic lead poisoning and thyrotoxicosis. Vitamin C deficiency may cause myalgias in addition to fatigue, lethargy, and skin findings, but motor neuron findings are not typical.

XI-28. **The answer is E.** *(Chap. 375)* Postural orthostatic tachycardia syndrome is characterized by symptomatic orthostatic intolerance and either an increase in heart rate to more than 120 beats/min or an increase of 30 beats/min with standing that subsides on sitting or lying down. There is no orthostatic hypotension. Women are affected approximately five times more often than men, and most develop the syndrome between the ages of 15 and 50. Approximately half of affected patients report an antecedent viral infection. Lightheadedness, weakness, and blurred vision combined with symptoms of autonomic over activity (palpitations, tremulousness, nausea) are common. Recurrent, unexplained episodes of dysautonomia and fatigue also occur. The pathogenesis is unclear in most cases; hypovolemia, deconditioning, venous pooling, impaired brainstem regulation, or adrenergic receptor supersensitivity may play a role. Although up to 80% of patients improve, only about 25% eventually resume their usual daily activities (including exercise and sports). Expansion of fluid volume and postural training are initial approaches to treatment. If these approaches are inadequate, then midodrine, fludrocortisone, phenobarbital, beta blockers, or clonidine may provide some benefit. Reconditioning and a sustained exercise program are very important. All of the other listed choices are associated with orthostatic hypotension.

XI-29. **The answer is D.** *(Chap. 375)* Complex regional pain syndrome (CRPS) types I and II are the terms that have replaced reflex sympathetic dystrophy (RSD) or causalgia because of the absence of a proven causative role for the autonomic nervous system. CRPS type I is a regional pain syndrome that usually develops after tissue trauma. Examples of associated trauma include myocardial infarction, minor shoulder or limb injury, and stroke. Allodynia, hyperpathia, and spontaneous pain occur. The symptoms are unrelated to the severity of the initial trauma and are not confined to the distribution of a single peripheral nerve. CRPS type II is a regional pain syndrome that develops after injury to a specific peripheral nerve, usually a major nerve trunk. Spontaneous pain initially develops within the territory of the affected nerve but eventually may spread outside the nerve distribution. Pain is the primary clinical feature of CRPS. Vasomotor dysfunction, sudomotor abnormalities, or focal edema may occur alone or in combination but must be present for diagnosis. Localized sweating and changes in blood flow may produce temperature differences between affected and unaffected limbs. CRPS type I has classically been divided into three clinical phases but is now considered to be more variable. Phase I consists of pain and swelling in the distal extremity occurring within weeks to 3 months after the precipitating event. The pain is diffuse, spontaneous, and either burning, throbbing, or aching in quality. The involved extremity is warm and edematous, and the joints are tender. Increased sweating and hair growth develop. In phase II (3–6 months after onset), thin, shiny, cool skin appears. After an additional 3–6 months (phase III), atrophy of the skin and subcutaneous tissue plus flexion contractures complete the clinical picture. A variety of surgical and medical treatments have been developed for CRPS, with conflicting reports of efficacy. Clinical trials suggest that early mobilization with physical therapy or a brief course of glucocorticoids may be helpful for CRPS type I. Other medical treatments include the use of adrenergic blockers, nonsteroidal anti-inflammatory drugs, calcium channel blockers, phenytoin, opioids, and calcitonin. Stellate ganglion blockade is a commonly used invasive technique that often provides temporary pain relief, but the efficacy of repetitive blocks is uncertain.

XI-30. **The answer is F.** *(Chap. 376)* Trigeminal neuralgia is a clinical diagnosis based entirely on patient history. The disorder is characterized by *paroxysms* of excruciating pain in the lips, gums, cheeks, and chin that resolves over seconds to minutes. It is caused by ectopic action potentials in afferent pain fibers of the fifth cranial nerve, due either to nerve compression or other causes of demyelination. Symptoms are often, but not always, elicited by tactile stimuli on the face, tongue, or lips. An elevated ESR is not part of the clinical syndrome. Elevated ESR is associated with temporal arteritis, a vasculitis associated with jaw claudication, unilateral vision loss, and symptoms of polymyalgia rheumatica. Trigeminal neuralgia is specifically notable for a lack of sensory findings on examination, unless the diagnosis is made in conjunction with another disorder such as a midbrain mass lesion or aneurysm. Deep-seated facial and head pain is more commonly a feature of migraine headache, dental pathology, or sinus disease. First-line therapy is with carbamazepine, not gabapentin. It should be started and increased gradually until pain symptoms subside; 50–75% of patients will respond to this therapy. If treatment is effective, it is continued for 1 month then tapered.

XI-31. **The answer is C.** *(Chap. 376)* Trigeminal neuralgia is a clinical diagnosis based entirely on patient history, and as such should be treated once a patient presents with the virtually pathognomonic complaints of paroxysms of excruciating pain in the lips, gums, cheeks, and chin that resolve over seconds to minutes. Carbamazepine is first-line therapy. Oxcarbazepine likely has equivalent efficacy to carbamazepine with less toxicity. Lamotrigine, orphenytoin, and baclofen are other potential therapeutic options. Surgical approaches, such as radiofrequency thermal rhizotomy, gamma-knife radiosurgery, and microvascular decompression, should be considered only when medical options fail. Steroids have no therapeutic role, as trigeminal neuralgia is not an inflammatory condition. Neuroimaging is not indicated, unless other clinical features or a focal neurologic deficit elicited on history or physical examination suggest another possible diagnosis such as intracranial mass or multiple sclerosis.

XI-32. **The answer is D.** *(Chap. 376)* Brief paroxysms of severe, sharp pains in the face without demonstrable lesions in the jaw, teeth, or sinuses are called tic douloureux, or trigeminal neuralgia. The pain may be brought on by stimuli applied to the face, lips, or tongue or by certain movements of those structures. Aneurysms, neurofibromas, and meningiomas impinging on the fifth cranial nerve at any point during its course typically present with trigeminal neuropathy, which will cause sensory loss on the face, weakness of the jaw muscles, or both; neither symptom is demonstrable in this patient. Amyotrophic lateral sclerosis (ALS) is a motor neuron disease that may present with bulbar motor findings but sensory findings (in the absence of muscle spasms) are uncommon.

XI-33. **The answer is C.** *(Chap. 377)* The MRI shows an infiltrated and collapsed second thoracic vertebral body with posterior displacement and compression of the upper thoracic spinal cord due to metastatic breast cancer. The low-intensity bone marrow signal in panel A of Figure XI-33 signifies replacement by tumor. When a patient presents with possible myelopathy, the first priority is to distinguish between a compressive or noncompressive etiology. The common causes of compressive myelopathy are tumor, epidural abscess or hematoma, herniated disk, or vertebral pathology. Epidural compression due to malignancy or abscess often causes warning signs of neck or back pain, bladder disturbances, and sensory symptoms that precede the development of paralysis. MRI is the optimal diagnostic modality to image the spinal cord. In adults, most neoplasms are epidural in origin, resulting from metastases to the adjacent spinal bones. The propensity of solid tumors to metastasize to the vertebral column probably reflects the high proportion of bone marrow located in the axial skeleton. Almost any malignant tumor can metastasize to the spinal column, with breast, lung, prostate, kidney, lymphoma, and plasma cell dyscrasia occurring particularly frequently. The thoracic spinal column is most commonly involved; exceptions are metastases from prostate and ovarian cancer, which occur disproportionately in the sacral and lumbar vertebrae, probably resulting from spread through Batson's plexus, a network of veins along the anterior epidural space. Retroperitoneal neoplasms (especially lymphomas or sarcomas) enter the spinal canal through the intervertebral foramens and produce radicular pain with signs of root weakness prior to cord compression. Pain is usually the initial symptom of spinal metastasis and characteristically awakens patients at night. A recent onset of persistent back pain, particularly if in the thoracic spine (which is uncommonly involved by spondylosis), should prompt consideration of vertebral metastasis. Infections of the spinal column (osteomyelitis and related disorders) are distinctive in that, unlike tumor, they may cross the disk space to involve the adjacent vertebral body. Management of cord compression includes glucocorticoids to reduce cord edema, local radiotherapy (initiated as early as possible) to the symptomatic lesion, and specific therapy for the underlying tumor type. Spinal epidural abscess presents as a clinical triad of midline dorsal pain, fever, and progressive limb weakness. Risk factors include an impaired immune status (diabetes mellitus, renal failure, alcoholism, malignancy), IV drug abuse, and infections of the skin or other tissues. Two-thirds of epidural infections result from hematogenous spread of bacteria from the skin (furunculosis), soft tissue (pharyngeal or dental abscesses), or deep viscera (bacterial endocarditis). Hemorrhage into the epidural (or subdural) space causes acute focal or radicular pain followed by variable signs of a spinal cord or conus medullaris disorder. Therapeutic anticoagulation, trauma, tumor, or blood dyscrasias are predisposing conditions. Hemorrhage into the substance of the spinal cord is a rare result of trauma, intraparenchymal vascular malformation, vasculitis due to polyarteritis nodosa or systemic lupus erythematosus (SLE), bleeding disorders, or a spinal cord neoplasm. Hematomyelia presents as an acute, painful transverse myelopathy.

XI-34. **The answer is B.** *(Chap. 377)* This patient has a history and examination consistent with a myelopathy. The rapidity of onset and the lack of other antecedent symptoms (e.g., pain) make a noncompressive etiology most likely. An MRI is the initial test of choice and will easily identify a structural lesion such as a neoplasm or subluxation. Noncompressive myelopathies result from five basic causes: spinal cord infarction; systemic disorders such as vasculitis, systemic lupus erythematosus (SLE), and sarcoidosis; infections (particularly viral); demyelinating disease such as multiple sclerosis; and idiopathic. Therefore, serologies for antinuclear antibodies, viral serologies such as HIV and HTLV-I, and lumbar puncture are all indicated. Because the clinical scenario is consistent with a myelopathy, an electromyogram is not indicated.

XI-35. **The answer is A.** *(Chap. 377)* Syringomyelia is a developmental, slowly enlarging cavitary expansion of the cervical cord that produces a progressive myelopathy. Symptoms typically begin in adolescence or early adulthood. They may undergo spontaneous arrest after several years. More than half are associated with Chiari malformations. Acquired cavitations of the spinal cord are referred to as syrinx cavities. They may result from trauma, myelitis, infection, or tumor. The classic presentation is that of a central cord syndrome with sensory loss of pain and temperature sensation, and weakness of the upper extremities. Vibration and position sensation are typically preserved. Muscle wasting in the lower neck, shoulders, arms, and hands with asymmetric or absent reflexes reflects extension of the cavity to the anterior horns. With progression, spasticity and weakness of the lower extremities, and bladder and bowel dysfunction may occur. MRI scans are the diagnostic modality of choice. Surgical therapy is generally unsatisfactory. Syringomyelia associated with Chiari malformations may require extensive decompressions of the posterior fossa. Direct decompression of the cavity is of debatable benefit. Syringomyelia secondary to trauma or infection is treated with decompression and a drainage procedure, with a shunt often inserted that drains into the subarachnoid space. Although relief may occur, recurrence is common.

XI-36. **The answer is A.** *(Chap. 378)* Concussions result from blunt head trauma that causes anterior-posterior movement of the brain within the skull. Transient loss of consciousness is common, as are confusion and amnesia. Many patients do not lose consciousness but feel dazed, stunned, or confused. A brief period of both retrograde and anterograde amnesia is characteristic of concussion and it recedes rapidly in alert patients. Head imaging is typically normal. Postconcussive syndrome is a constellation of symptoms including fatigue, headache, dizziness, and difficulty concentrating that follows a concussion. The patient described fits this diagnosis; strict diagnostic criteria do not exist. Typically patients will improve over a 6- to 12-month period. Patients who were energetic and highly functioning prior to their trauma have an excellent prognosis. Treatment is aimed at reassurance and relieving prominent symptoms. Dizziness can be treated with Phenergan, which acts as a vestibular suppressant. He should avoid contact sports at least until his symptoms resolve.

XI-37. **The answer is D.** *(Chap. 378)* The head CT (Figure XI-37) shows chronic bilateral subdural hematomas of varying age. The collections began as acute hematomas and have become hypodense in comparison to the adjacent brain. Some areas of resolving blood are contained in the more recently formed collection on the left. Acute hematomas (which would be as bright as the resolving blood shown in arrows) become hypodense in comparison with adjacent brain after approximately 2 months. During the isodense phase (2–6 weeks after injury), they may be difficult to discern. Chronic subdural hematoma may present without a history of trauma or injury in 20–30% of patients. Headache is common. Other symptoms may be vague, as in this case, or there may be focal signs including hemiparesis mimicking stroke. Underlying cortical damage may serve as a seizure focus. In relatively asymptomatic patients with small hematomas, observation and serial imaging may be reasonable; however, surgical evacuation is often necessary for large or symptomatic chronic hematomas.

XI-38. **The answer is D.** *(Chap. 378)* Hemorrhages beneath the dural layer (subdural) or between the skull and the dura (epidural) are common sequelae of head trauma. They can be life-threatening, and prompt evaluation and management are imperative. Several clinical features allow these conditions to be distinguished from one another. Acute subdural hematomas typically arise from venous sources, often the bridging veins located immediately under the dura mater. As the brain volume decreases with age, traction on these venous structures increases and even minor head trauma in the elderly can lead to a subdural hematoma. A "lucid interval" of several minutes to hours before coma supervenes is most characteristic of epidural hemorrhage, but it is still uncommon, and epidural hemorrhage is not the only cause of this temporal sequence. Subdural bleeding is typically slower than epidural bleeding due to their different sources. Small subdural bleeds are asymptomatic and often do not require evacuation. Epidural hematomas, on the other hand, can arise quickly and typically represent arterial bleeding. A lacerated middle meningeal artery from an overlying skull fracture often causes these. A rapid increase in intracranial pressure from these bleeds can necessitate arterial ligation or emergent craniotomy. Most patients with epidural bleeding are unconscious when first evaluated; a "lucid interval" can occasionally be seen.

XI-39. **The answer is D.** *(Chap. 379)* Distinguishing CNS toxoplasmosis from primary CNS lymphoma in a patient with HIV infection is often difficult. The standard approach in a neurologically stable patient is to treat the patient for toxoplasmosis for 2–3 weeks then repeat neuroimaging. If the imaging shows clear improvement, continue antibiotics. If there is no response to therapy after 2 weeks, therapy does not need to be continued and a stereotactic brain biopsy is indicated. In this immunocompromised patient who has not responded to treatment for CNS toxoplasmosis, a positive CNS EBV DNA would be diagnostic of CNS lymphoma. Whole-brain radiation therapy is part of the treatment for CNS lymphoma, which is not yet diagnosed in this patient, and should not be instituted empirically. Treatments directed at viral infections of the CNS or CNS lymphomas are not indicated at this time since a diagnosis is still yet to be made. In the absence of a change in neurologic status or evidence of mass effect on CT, there is no indication for dexamethasone. Of note, the incidence of primary CNS lymphoma appears to be increasing in immunocompetent individuals for unclear reasons.

XI-40. **The answer is A.** (*Chap. 379*) Endocrine dysfunction resulting in hypopituitarism frequently follows exposure of the hypothalamus or pituitary gland to therapeutic radiation. Growth hormone is the most sensitive to the damaging effects of WBRT, and thyroid-stimulating hormone is the least sensitive. ACTH, prolactin, and gonadotropins have an intermediate sensitivity. Other complications of radiation therapy to the brain include acute radiation injury manifest by headache, sleepiness, and worsening of preexisting neurologic defects. Early delayed radiation injury occurs within the first 4 months after therapy. It is associated with increased white matter signal on MRI and is steroid responsive. Late delayed radiation injury occurs more than 4 months after therapy, typically 8–24 months. There may be dementia, gait apraxia, focal necrosis (after focal irradiation), or the development of secondary malignancies.

XI-41. **The answer is D.** (*Chap. 379*) The postgadolinium MRI shows multiple meningiomas along the falx and left parietal cortex. Meningiomas derive from the cells that give rise to the arachnoid granulations. They are now the most common primary brain tumor, accounting for approximately 32% of the total, and occur more commonly in women than men. They are usually benign (WHO classification grade 1) and attached to the dura. They rarely invade the brain. Meningiomas are diagnosed with increasing frequency as more people undergo neuroimaging studies for various indications. Their incidence increases with age, and they are more common in patients with a history of cranial irradiation. They are most commonly located over the cerebral convexities, especially adjacent to the sagittal sinus, but can also occur in the skull base and along the dorsum of the spinal cord. Many meningiomas are found incidentally following neuroimaging for unrelated reasons. They can also present with headaches, seizures, or focal neurologic deficits. On imaging studies they have a characteristic appearance usually consisting of a partially calcified, densely enhancing extra-axial tumor arising from the dura. The main differential diagnosis of meningioma is a dural metastasis. Total surgical resection of a meningioma is curative. Low-grade astrocytoma and high-grade astrocytoma (glioblastoma) often infiltrate into adjacent brain and rarely have the clear margins seen in Figure XI-41. Oligodendroma comprise approximately 15% of all gliomas and show calcification in roughly 30% of cases. They have a more benign course and are more responsive than other gliomas to cytotoxic therapy. For low-grade oligodendromas, the median survival is 7–8 years. Brain abscess will have distinctive ring-enhancing features with a capsule, will often have mass effect, and will have evidence of inflammation on MRI scanning.

XI-42. **The answer is D.** (*Chap. 380*) The onset of multiple sclerosis (MS) may be abrupt or insidious. Symptoms may be severe or seem so trivial that a patient may not seek medical attention for months or years. Indeed, at autopsy, approximately 0.1% of individuals who were asymptomatic during life will be found, unexpectedly, to have pathologic evidence of MS. Similarly, in the modern era, an MRI scan obtained for an unrelated reason may show evidence of asymptomatic MS. Symptoms of MS are extremely varied and depend on the location and severity of lesions within the CNS (see Table XI-42). Examination often reveals evidence of neurologic dysfunction, often in asymptomatic locations. For example, a patient may present with symptoms in one leg but signs in both.

TABLE XI-42   **Initial Symptoms of MS**

Symptom	Percentage of Cases	Symptom	Percentage of Cases
Sensory loss	37	Lhermitte's	3
Optic neuritis	36	Pain	3
Weakness	35	Dementia	2
Paresthesias	24	Visual loss	2
Diplopia	15	Facial palsy	1
Ataxia	11	Impotence	1
Vertigo	6	Myokymia	1
Paroxysmal attacks	4	Epilepsy	1
Bladder	4	Falling	1

Source: After WB Matthews et al: *McAlpine's Multiple Sclerosis,* New York, Churchill Livingstone, 1991.

XI-43. **The answer is D.** *(Chap. 380)* The four clinical types of multiple sclerosis (MS) include relapsing/remitting, secondary progressive, primary progressive, and progressive relapsing. Relapsing/remitting MS (RRMS) accounts for 85% of MS cases at onset and is characterized by discrete attacks that generally evolve over days to weeks (rarely over hours). There is often complete recovery over the ensuing weeks to months. However, when ambulation is severely impaired during an attack, approximately half will fail to improve. Between attacks, patients are neurologically stable. Secondary progressive MS (SPMS) always begins as RRMS. At some point, however, the clinical course changes so that the patient experiences a steady deterioration in function unassociated with acute attacks (which may continue or cease during the progressive phase). SPMS produces a greater amount of fixed neurologic disability than RRMS. For a patient with RRMS, the risk of developing SPMS is approximately 2% each year, meaning that the great majority of RRMS ultimately evolves into SPMS. SPMS appears to represent a late stage of the same underlying illness as RRMS. Primary progressive MS (PPMS) accounts for approximately 15% of cases. These patients do not experience attacks but only a steady functional decline from disease onset. Compared to RRMS, the sex distribution is more even, the disease begins later in life (mean age approximately 40 years), and disability develops faster (at least relative to the onset of the first clinical symptom). Despite these differences, PPMS appears to represent the same underlying illness as RRMS. Progressive/relapsing MS (PRMS) overlaps PPMS and SPMS and accounts for about 5% of MS patients. Like patients with PPMS, these patients experience a steady deterioration in their condition from disease onset. However, like SPMS patients, they experience occasional attacks superimposed upon their progressive course. Autoimmune autonomic neuropathy is a distinct clinical syndrome not related to MS. It presents with the subacute development of autonomic disturbances with orthostatic hypotension, enteric neuropathy (gastroparesis, ileus, constipation/diarrhea), and cholinergic failure; the latter consists of loss of sweating, sicca complex, and a tonic pupil. Autoantibodies against the ganglionic ACh receptor (A_3 AChR) are present in the serum of many patients and are now considered to be diagnostic of this syndrome.

XI-44. **The answer is D.** *(Chap. 381)* In a patient with suspected bacterial meningitis empirical therapy should be administered promptly to reduce mortality and morbidity. The decision to obtain an imaging study prior to lumbar puncture (LP) is based on the concern of precipitating herniation in a patient with elevated intracranial pressure or focal CNS lesions. Therefore, patients with the presence of papilledema on physical examination, history of recent head trauma, known or suspected intracranial lesions (immunosuppressed, known malignancy), focal neurologic findings, or depressed level of consciousness should have a head CT or MRI prior to LP. In an immunocompetent patient with no known history of recent head trauma, a normal level of consciousness, and no evidence of papilledema or focal neurologic deficits, it is considered safe to perform LP without prior neuroimaging studies. Kernig's sign is elicited in a supine patient by flexing the thigh and knee. A positive sign occurs when the patient has head/neck pain when passively straightening the knee. The sensitivity and specificity of this sign (also Brudzinski's) for bacterial meningitis are unknown, but they imply meningeal irritation, not an intracranial lesion or elevated intracranial pressure. While cerebrospinal fluid cultures may be impacted by administration of antibiotics prior to LP, stains, antigen tests, and polymerase chain reaction tests will not be affected.

XI-45. **The answer is B.** *(Chap. 381)* The release of bacterial cell wall components after killing by antibiotics may evoke a marked inflammatory cytokine response in the subarachnoid space. This inflammation may lead to increased damage of the blood-brain barrier and central nervous system damage. Glucocorticoids can blunt this response by inhibiting tumor necrosis factor and interleukin-1. They work best if administered before antibiotics. Clinical trials have demonstrated that dexamethasone, 10 mg IV administered 20 minutes *before* antibiotics, reduced unfavorable outcomes, including death. The dexamethasone was continued for 4 days. The benefits were most striking in pneumococcal meningitis. Because this is the most common cause of meningitis in the elderly, empirical coverage should include this intervention as well. The efficacy of dexamethasone therapy in preventing neurologic sequelae is different between high- and low-income countries.

Randomized trials in low-income countries (sub-Saharan Africa, Southeast Asia) failed to show benefit in subgroups of patients. The lack of efficacy of dexamethasone in these trials has been attributed to late presentation to the hospital with more advanced disease, antibiotic pretreatment, malnutrition, infection with HIV, and treatment of patients with probable, but not microbiologically proven, bacterial meningitis. The results of these clinical trials suggest that patients in sub-Saharan Africa and those in low-income countries with negative CSF Gram stain and culture should not be treated with dexamethasone. Empirical antibiotics in this case should include a third-generation cephalosporin, vancomycin, and ampicillin. However, dexamethasone may decrease vancomycin penetration into the CSF, so its use should be considered carefully in cases where the most likely organism requires vancomycin coverage. Acyclovir or valacyclovir may be used as initial empiric treatment in cases of suspected herpes CNS infection. However, in this case the LP is highly suggestive of acute bacterial infection. Intravenous gamma globulin is used as adjunctive therapy in children with known immunoglobulin deficiency who are at risk of viral meningitis/encephalitis.

XI-46. **The answer is D.** *(Chap. 381) Listeria* has become an increasingly important cause of bacterial meningitis in neonates (<1 month of age), pregnant women, individuals more than 60 years old, and immunocompromised individuals. Infection is acquired by eating contaminated foods such as unpasteurized dairy products, coleslaw, milk, soft cheeses, delicatessen meats, and uncooked hot dogs. Ampicillin is the agent most often added to the initial empirical regimen to cover *L. monocytogenes*.

XI-47. **The answer is D.** *(Chap. 382)* Ibuprofen, isoniazid, ciprofloxacin, tolmetin, sulfa-containing medicines, and phenazopyridine have been implicated in drug hypersensitivity leading to meningitis. The cerebrospinal fluid (CSF) will typically show neutrophils, but mononuclear cells or eosinophils are occasionally present. Most causes of chronic (not recurrent) meningitis cause a predominance of mononuclear cells. The differential for chronic meningitis is broad and a diagnosis is often difficult to make. The treating physician needs to consider a diverse array of viral, fungal, bacterial, mycobacterial, helminthic, and protozoal pathogens, both common and exotic, and therefore should obtain a detailed social history and consult an expert in the field. Recurrent meningitis is often due to herpes simplex virus type 2 infection and this should be ruled out, particularly if active genital ulcers develop concurrently. Malignancy, sarcoidosis, and vasculitis are all potential causes, and history, physical examination, and appropriate further testing should dictate the degree to which these possibilities are explored. Medications are often overlooked as a cause of chronic meningitis and should always be carefully considered. When CSF neutrophils predominate after 3 weeks of illness, *Nocardia, Actinomyces, Brucella*, tuberculosis (<10% of cases), and fungal and noninfectious causes of chronic meningitis should be considered.

XI-48. **The answer is E.** *(Chap. 383)* Prions are infectious particles that cause central nervous system degeneration. The human prion diseases described to date include Creutzfeldt-Jacob disease (CJD), kuru, Gerstmann-Sträussler-Scheinker disease, and fatal insomnia. The most common prion disease is sporadic CJD (sCJD), which occurs in a seemingly random pattern in adults in their fifth and sixth decades of life. sCJD accounts for about 85% of cases of CJD and occurs in approximately 1 per 1 million population. Variant CJD (vCJD) results from infection from bovine exposure to tainted beef from cattle with bovine spongiform encephalopathy (BSE). There has been a steady decline of cases of vCJD in Europe over the past decade. Infectious CJD (iCJD) has resulted from injection of tainted human growth hormone, as well as transplant of infected dura mater grafts into humans. Familial CJD (fCJD) is due to germ-line mutations that follow an autosomal dominant inheritance. Kuru is due to infection through ritualistic cannibalism. Gerstmann-Sträussler-Scheinker disease and familial fatal insomnia (FFI) occur as dominantly inherited prion diseases. Sporadic cases of fatal insomnia (sFI) have been described.

XI-49. **The answer is B.** *(Chap. 383)* Startle myoclonus is a worrisome sign but is neither sensitive nor specific for CJD, though it is more worrisome if it occurs during sleep. The constellation of dementia, myoclonus, and periodic electrical bursts in an afebrile

60-year-old patient generally indicates CJD. Clinical abnormalities in CJD are confined to the CNS. Lewy body dementia, Alzheimer's disease, central nervous system infections, and myoclonic epilepsy can all cause myoclonus. Both EEG and MRI can help differentiate CJD from these disorders. The MRI finding of cortical ribboning and intensity in the basal ganglia on fluid-attenuated inversion recovery sequences is characteristic of CJD. EEG is useful if stereotypical periodic bursts every 1–2 seconds are present, but this is seen in only 60% of cases, and other findings may be less specific. Demonstration of specific immunoassays for proteolytic products of disease-causing prion proteins (PrP^{Sc}) at brain biopsy may be necessary to confirm diagnosis in some cases. However, these proteins are not uniformly distributed throughout the brain and false-negative biopsies occur. Both surgeons and pathologists must be warned to use standard precautions under these circumstances. These proteins cannot be measured from cerebrospinal fluid (CSF). CSF in CJD is usually normal except for a minimally elevated protein. Many patients with CJD have elevated CSF stress protein 14-3-3. This test alone is neither sensitive nor specific, as patients with herpes simplex virus encephalitis, multi-infarct dementia, and stroke may have similar elevations.

XI-50. **The answer is A.** (*Chap. 384*) Charcot-Marie-Tooth (CMT) syndrome is the most common type of hereditary neuropathy. CMT is comprised of several similar but genetically distinct conditions with different associated mutations. CMT1 is the most common and is an inherited demyelinating sensorimotor neuropathy. CMT1 affects patients in the first to third decades of life with distal leg weakness, i.e., footdrop. Although patients generally do not complain of sensory symptoms, these can often be elicited on physical examination. Muscle stretch reflexes are unobtainable or reduced throughout and calves are often atrophied, which makes legs appear to have a so-called inverted champagne bottle appearance. Hereditary neuralgic amyotrophy (HNA) is an autosomal dominant disorder characterized by recurrent attacks of pain, weakness, and sensory loss in the distribution of the brachial plexus that often begins in childhood. Hereditary sensory and autonomic neuropathy (HSAN) is a very rare group of hereditary neuropathies in which sensory and autonomic dysfunction predominates over muscle weakness. This would not fit the clinical pattern described here. Guillain-Barré syndrome presents generally acutely with involvement of both proximal and distal weakness and sensory loss. The prolonged symptom period and distribution described here is not typical for Guillain-Barré syndrome. Fabry disease is an X-linked disorder in which men are more commonly affected than women. Patients have angiokeratomas, which are reddish-purple lesions usually found around the umbilicus, scrotum, and inguinal region. Burning pain in the hands and feet often is found in late childhood or early adult life. Patients also have premature atherosclerosis from the underlying mutation in the alpha-galactosidase gene with accumulation of ceramide in nerves and blood vessels.

XI-51. **The answer is F.** (*Chap. 384*) One of the most common side effects of isoniazid treatment is peripheral neuropathy. The elderly, malnourished, and "slow acetylators" are at increased risk for developing the neuropathy. INH inhibits pyridoxal phosphokinase, resulting in pyridoxine (vitamin B$_6$) deficiency and the neuropathy. Prophylactic administration of pyridoxine can prevent the neuropathy from developing. Symptoms are generally dysesthesias and sensory ataxia. Impaired large-fiber sensory modalities are found on examination. Cobalamin (B$_{12}$) is not reduced in this condition and is unaffected by isoniazid. Neurontin and pregabalin may alleviate symptoms but will not reverse the neuropathy. There is no indication that hypothyroidism is present.

XI-52. **The answer is C.** (*Chap. 384*) Diabetes mellitus (DM) is the most common cause of peripheral neuropathy in developed countries and is associated with several different types of polyneuropathy including distal symmetric sensory or sensorimotor polyneuropathy, autonomic neuropathy, diabetic neuropathic cachexia, polyradiculoneuropathies, cranial neuropathies, and other mononeuropathies. Risk factors for the development of neuropathy include long-standing and poorly controlled diabetes and the presence of retinopathy or nephropathy. The patient here appears to have diabetic distal symmetric sensory and sensorimotor polyneuropathy (DSPN), which is the most common form of diabetic neuropathy and presents with sensory loss beginning in the toes and gradually progresses over time up the legs and into the fingers and arms. Symptoms also may include tingling, burning, and deep, aching pains. Nerve biopsy, though rarely indicated, often shows axonal degeneration, endothelial hyperplasia, and occasionally perivascular inflammation. Tight glucose control prevents the development of disease but does not reverse established disease. Diabetic autonomic neuropathy is often seen in combination with DSPN and manifests by abnormal sweating, dysfunctional thermoregulation, dry eyes and mouth, postural hypotension, gastrointestinal abnormalities including gastroparesis, and genitourinary dysfunction.

XI-53.   **The answer is B.** *(Chap. 384)* Peripheral neuropathy is a general term indicating peripheral nerve disorders of any cause. The causes are legion, but peripheral neuropathy can be classified by a number of means: axonal versus demyelinating, mononeuropathy versus polyneuropathy versus mononeuritis multiplex, sensory versus motor, and by the tempo of the onset of symptoms. Mononeuropathy typically results from local compression, trauma, or entrapment of a nerve. Polyneuropathy often results from a more systemic process. The distinction between axonal and demyelinating can often be made only with nerve conduction studies. HIV infection causes a common, distal, symmetric, mainly sensory polyneuropathy. Vitamin B_{12} deficiency typically causes a sensory neuropathy that predominantly involves the dorsal columns. Hypothyroidism and acromegaly may both cause compression and swelling of nerve fibers, resulting first in sensory symptoms and later in disease with motor symptoms. Critical illness polyneuropathy is predominantly motor in presentation. Patients typically present with weakness that can be profound. These patients may recover over the course of weeks to months. The etiology is unknown, but an association may exist with prolonged immobilization, severity of illness, neuromuscular blockade, and corticosteroids.

XI-54.   **The answer is B.** *(Chap. 384)* Carpal tunnel syndrome is caused by the entrapment of the median nerve at the wrist. Symptoms begin with paresthesias in the median nerve distribution. With worsening, atrophy and weakness may develop. This condition is most commonly caused by excessive use of the wrist and situations involving repetitive motion. Most cases are idiopathic other than those related to occupational or environmental associations. Less commonly, systemic disease may result in carpal tunnel syndrome related to nerve compression or infiltrative disease. This may be suspected when bilateral disease is apparent. Tenosynovitis with arthritis, as in the case of rheumatoid arthritis, and thickening of the connective tissue, as in the case of amyloid or acromegaly, may cause carpal tunnel syndrome. Other systemic diseases, such as hypothyroidism and diabetes mellitus, are also possible etiologies. Acute or chronic leukemia is not typically associated with carpal tunnel syndrome.

XI-55.   **The answer is B.** *(Chap. 385)* Guillain-Barré syndrome (GBS) is an acute, severe polyradiculoneuropathy that is autoimmune in nature. GBS manifests as rapidly evolving, areflexic motor paralysis with or without sensory disturbance, usually with ascending paralysis developing over several days. Approximately 70% of GBS cases occur 1–3 weeks after an acute infectious process, usually respiratory or gastrointestinal. Twenty to thirty percent of cases in North America, Europe, and Australia are preceded by infection or reinfection with *Campylobacter jejuni*. Other implicated infections include Epstein-Barr virus, CMV, and *Mycoplasma pneumoniae*. *T. whippelii* is the etiologic agent of Whipple's disease and *B. henselae* is implicated in cat-scratch fever.

XI-56.   **The answer is E.** *(Chap. 386)* Myasthenia gravis (MG) is a neuromuscular disorder characterized by weakness and fatigability of skeletal muscles. The primary defect is a decrease in the number of acetylcholine receptors at the neuromuscular junction secondary to autoimmune antibodies. MG is not rare, affecting at least 1 in 7500 individuals. Women are affected more frequently than men. Women typically present in the second and third decades of life, and men present in the fifth and sixth decades. The key features of MG are weakness and fatigability. Clinical features include weakness of the cranial muscles, particularly the eyelids and extraocular muscles. Diplopia and ptosis are common initial complaints. Weakness in chewing is noticeable after prolonged effort. Speech may be affected secondary to weakness of the palate or tongue. Swallowing may result from weakness of the palate, tongue, or pharynx. In the majority of patients the weakness becomes generalized. The diagnosis is suspected after the appearance of the characteristic symptoms and signs. Edrophonium is an acetylcholinesterase inhibitor that allows ACh to interact repeatedly with the limited number of AChRs, producing improvement in the strength of myasthenic muscles. False-positive tests may occur in patients with other neurologic diseases. Electrodiagnostic testing may show evidence of reduction in the amplitude of the evoked muscle action potentials with repeated stimulation. Testing for the specific antibodies to AChR are diagnostic. In addition to anti-AChR antibodies, antibodies to MuSK have been found in some patients with clinical MG. Antibodies to voltage-gated calcium channels are found in patients with the Lambert-Eaton syndrome.

XI-57.   **The answer is C.** *(Chap. 386)* Except for lumbar puncture, all of the options listed are indicated at this time. Thymic abnormalities are present in 75% of patients with myasthenia gravis. A CT or MRI of the mediastinum may show enlargement or neoplastic changes in the thymus and is recommended upon diagnosis. Hyperthyroidism occurs in 3–8% of patients with myasthenia gravis and may aggravate weakness. Testing for rheumatoid factor and antinuclear antibodies should also be obtained because of the association of myasthenia gravis to other autoimmune diseases. Due to side effects of immunosuppressive therapy, a thorough evaluation should be undertaken to rule out latent or chronic infections such as tuberculosis. Measurements of ventilatory function are valuable as a baseline because of the frequency and seriousness of respiratory impairment in myasthenic patients, and they can be used as an objective measure of response to therapy.

XI-58.   **The answer is E.** *(Chap. 387)* All classes of lipid-lowering agents have been implicated in muscle toxicity including fibrates, HMG-CoA reductase inhibitors, niacin, and ezetimibe. Myalgia, malaise, and muscle tenderness are the most common manifestations, and muscle pain may be exacerbated by exercise. Proximal weakness may be found on examination. In severe cases, rhabdomyolysis and myoglobinuria may occur, though most cases are mild. Concomitant use of statins with fibrates and cyclosporine are more likely to cause adverse muscle reactions. Elevated serum CK is often identified, and muscle weakness is evidenced by myopathic EMG studies and myonecrosis on muscle biopsy. Severe myalgias, muscle weakness, and significant elevations in CK (>3 × upper limit of normal) and myoglobinuria are indications for stopping. After cessation, improvement generally occurs after several weeks.

XI-59.   **The answer is E.** *(Chap. 387)* A number of endocrinologic conditions are associated with myopathy. Both hypo- and hyperthyroidism are associated with proximal muscle weakness. Hypothyroidism is frequently associated with an elevated CK, even with minimal clinical evidence of muscle disease. Thyrotoxic patients may have fasciculations in addition to proximal myopathy, but in contrast to hypothyroid patients, CK is not generally elevated. Hyperparathyroidism is associated with muscle weakness that is generally proximal. Muscle wasting and brisk reflexes are also generally present. Serum CK levels may be normal or slightly elevated. Serum calcium and phosphate levels show no correlation with clinical weakness. Hypoparathyroid patients also often have myopathy due to hypocalcemia. Patients with acromegaly usually have mild proximal weakness without atrophy. The duration of acromegaly, not the serum growth hormone levels, correlate with the degree of myopathy. Diabetes mellitus is a very rare cause of myopathy, generally due to ischemic infarction of muscle and not a primary myopathy. Finally, vitamin D deficiency is associated with muscle weakness, as are glucocorticoid excess states, e.g., Cushing's disease.

XI-60.   **The answer is D.** *(Chap. 387)* There are two recognized clinical forms of myotonic dystrophy, both of which are characterized by autosomal dominant inheritance. Myotonic dystrophy 1 (DM1) is the most common form and the most likely disorder in this patient. Characteristic clinical features of this disorder include a "hatchet-faced" appearance, due to wasting of the facial muscles, and weakness of the neck muscles. In contrast to the muscular dystrophies (Becker and Duchenne), distal limb muscle weakness is more common in DM1. Palatal, pharyngeal, and tongue involvement are also common and produce the dysarthric voice that is frequently heard. The failure of relaxation after a forced hand-grip is characteristic of myotonia. Percussion of the thenar eminence can also elicit myotonia. In most individuals, myotonia is present by age 5, but clinical symptoms of weakness that lead to diagnosis may not be present until adulthood. Cardiac conduction abnormalities and heart failure are also common in myotonic dystrophy. Diagnosis can often be made from clinical features alone in an individual with classic symptoms and a positive family history. An electromyogram would confirm myotonia. Genetic testing for DM1 would show a characteristic trinucleotide repeat on chromosome 19. Genetic anticipation occurs with an increasing number of repeats and worsening clinical disease over successive generations. Myotonic dystrophy 2 (DM2) causes primarily proximal muscle weakness and is also known by the name proximal myotonic myopathy (PROMM). Other features of the disease overlap with DM1. Acid maltase deficiency (glucosidase deficiency, or Pompe's disease) has three recognized forms, only one of which has onset in adulthood. In the adult-onset form, respiratory muscle weakness is prominent and often is the presenting symptom. As stated previously, Becker and Duchenne muscular dystrophies present with primarily proximal muscle weakness and are X-linked recessive disorders. Becker muscular dystrophy presents at a later age than Duchenne muscular dystrophy and has a more prolonged course. Otherwise, their features are similar. Nemaline myopathy is a heterogeneous disorder marked by the threadlike appearance of muscle fibers on biopsy. Nemaline myopathy usually presents in childhood and includes a striking facial appearance similar to that in myotonic dystrophy with a long, narrow face. This disease is inherited in an autosomal dominant fashion.

XI-61. **The answer is B.** *(Chap. 388)* When patients present with proximal muscle weakness and myositis, whether polymyositis, dermatomyositis, or inclusion body myositis, the diagnosis is confirmed by analysis of serum muscle enzymes, EMG findings, and muscle biopsy. The most sensitive serum enzyme is creatinine kinase (CK), which can be elevated as much as 50-fold in active disease. CK levels usually parallel disease activity, but can be normal in some patients with inclusion body myositis or dermatomyositis. CK is always elevated in active polymyositis and thus is considered most sensitive. Other enzymes may be elevated as well including glutamic-oxaloacetic transaminase, glutamate pyruvate transaminase, lactate dehydrogenase, and aldolase.

XI-62. **The answer is B.** *(Chap. 388)* Various autoantibodies against nuclear antigens, e.g., ANAs, and cytoplasmic antigens are found in up to 20% of patients with inflammatory myopathies. The antibodies to cytoplasmic antigens are directed against ribonucleoproteins involved in protein synthesis (antisynthetases) or translational transport (anti–signal-recognition particles). The antibody directed against the histidyl-transfer RNA synthetase, called anti-Jo-1, accounts for 75% of all the antisynthetases and is clinically useful because up to 80% of patients with this autoantibody will have interstitial lung disease. Patients with anti-Jo-1 may also have Raynaud's phenomenon, nonerosive arthritis, and the MHC molecules DR3 and DRw52. Interstitial lung disease associated with anti-Jo-1 is often rapidly progressive and fatal, even if treated aggressively with cyclophosphamide or other immunosuppressants.

XI-63. **The answer is A.** *(Chap. 388)* Dermatomyositis is associated with malignancy in up to 15% of cases, thus age-appropriate cancer screening is indicated when this diagnosis is made. Exhaustive cancer searches are not recommended, however. Dermatomyositis may be associated occasionally with scleroderma and mixed connective tissue disease, but less frequently with systemic lupus erythematosus, rheumatoid arthritis, or Sjögren's syndrome, which are more closely associated with polymyositis or inclusion body myositis (IBM). Viruses may be associated with IBM and polymyositis, but are not proven to be associated with dermatomyositis. Parasites and bacteria such as cestodes and nematodes are associated with polymyositis, but not other forms of inflammatory myopathy. Finally, thyroid-stimulating immunoglobulins are not known to be associated with dermatomyositis.

XI-64. **The answer is A.** *(Chap. 388)* A common mistake in the management of patients with inflammatory myopathy is to "chase the CK" instead of adjusting therapy based on the clinical response. The goal of therapy is to improve strength. If that goal is being achieved, no augmentation of therapy is necessary. In this case, the plan to switch to long-term maintenance with steroid-sparing immunosuppressants should still be pursued. There have been no controlled studies comparing mycophenolate to methotrexate for long-term use in polymyositis, and in the absence of an adverse reaction to mycophenolate, therapy should not be changed. Despite an elevated CK, patients with polymyositis who are responding to therapy do not need a repeat muscle biopsy.

XI-65. **The answer is B.** (*Chap. e47*) The FLAIR MRI shows increased signal bilaterally in the occipital lobes predominantly involving the white matter. This pattern is typical of a hyperperfusion state, in this case secondary to calcineurin-inhibitor toxicity. This clinical-radiographic abnormality was previously described as reversible posterior leukoencephalopathy. However, this characterization is no longer utilized because the syndrome may not be reversible, the territory may not be confined posteriorly, and gray matter may be involved. Hyperperfusion syndrome may be due to a hydrostatic elevation in cerebral capillary pressure or disorders with endothelial dysfunction and capillary leakage. Hydrostatic causes include hypertensive encephalopathy, post–carotid endarterectomy syndrome, (pre)eclampsia, and high-altitude cerebral edema. Endothelial dysfunction causes include calcineurin-inhibitor toxicity, other chemotherapeutic agent toxicity, HELLP syndrome, TTP, SLE, or Wegener's granulomatosis. The diagnosis is clinical and radiographic. CSF findings are nonspecific. In the case of cyclosporine the syndrome may occur with therapeutic serum levels and sporadically after years of treatment. Acoustic neuroma would present on MRI with a discrete mass. The radiologic and clinical appearance is not consistent with pituitary apoplexy. Post–liver transplant patients are at risk of acute (streptococcal) and chronic (tuberculous) meningitis, but the clinical and radiologic findings in this case would not be typical.

XI-66. **The answer is B.** (*Chap. e47*) Acute neurologic events, such as encephalopathy or stroke (often related to intraoperative hypotension or embolism), are common after open heart surgery or coronary artery bypass graft (CABG). Additionally, a chronic syndrome of cognitive impairment is now increasingly recognized after surgery. Small or microemboli during surgery are thought to be the etiology of a hyper- or hypoactive confusional state in the postoperative period. A smaller burden of microemboli may be responsible for the more subtle post–cardiac surgery syndrome characterized by confusion and depressive symptoms as described in this case. Cardiac surgery may also unmask the early manifestations of vascular dementia or Alzheimer's disease. Off-pump CABG patients have a shorter length of hospital stay and fewer perioperative complications. Recent studies do not confirm the hypothesis that off-pump surgery results in less cognitive impairment than on-pump surgery. Ongoing studies are testing the efficacy of microfilters to capture emboli and reduce CNS complications. Given the temporal relation to CABG surgery and the lack of temporal variability, multiple sclerosis is not likely in this case. Similarly, in the absence of meningitis or encephalitis signs or symptoms, streptococcal or West Nile virus disease is unlikely. vCJD is associated with ingestion of prion-contaminated product. It is characterized by rapidly developing delirium and dementia, often associated with myoclonic jerks.

XI-67. **The answer is E.** (*Chap. e47*) The peroneal nerve winds around the head of the fibula below the lateral aspect of the knee. This superficial location makes it vulnerable to trauma. Poorly applied leg braces, fibular fracture, tight-fitting stockings, or casts may cause peroneal nerve injury and neuropathy. Patients may present with footdrop (dorsiflexion defect) with weakness of foot eversion. Intact foot inversion at the ankle distinguishes peroneal nerve injury from L5 radiculopathy, which involves the muscles innervated by the tibial nerve. Sensory loss due to peroneal nerve injury involves the lateral aspect of the leg below the knee and the dorsum of the foot. Cauda equina syndrome is caused by compression of the spinal nerve roots of the lumbar plexus usually due to tumor, trauma, or spinal stenosis. It typically presents with weakness of the muscles innervated by the involved nerves, incontinence, and decreased anal sphincter tone. Cauda equina syndrome is usually a medical emergency to avoid permanent functional loss. The femoral nerve branches into anterior and posterior portions in the leg. Injury of the anterior branches may lead to sensory findings in the thigh and muscular findings in the sartorius and the quadriceps. L4 radiculopathy causes symptoms in the anterior thigh and knee extensors (including the patellar reflex).

XI-68.   **The answer is A.** *(Chap. 389)* Chronic fatigue syndrome (CFS) is a disorder characterized by persistent and unexplained fatigue resulting in severe impairment in daily functioning. Besides intense fatigue, most patients with CFS report concomitant symptoms such as pain, cognitive dysfunction, and unrefreshing sleep. Additional symptoms can include headache, sore throat, tender lymph nodes, muscle aches, joint aches, feverishness, difficulty sleeping, psychiatric problems, allergies, and abdominal cramps. Criteria for the diagnosis of CFS have been developed by the U.S. Centers for Disease Control and Prevention (see Table XI-68). CFS is seen worldwide, with adult prevalence rates varying between 0.2% and 0.4%. In the United States, the prevalence is higher in women, members of minority groups (African and Native Americans), and individuals with lower levels of education and occupational status. Approximately 75% of all CFS patients are women. The mean age of onset is between 29 and 35 years. It is probable that many patients go undiagnosed and/or do not seek help.

TABLE XI-68   **Diagnostic Criteria for Chronic Fatigue Syndrome**

Characterized by Persistent or Relapsing Unexplained Chronic Fatigue

Fatigue lasts for at least 6 months.

Fatigue is of new or definite onset.

Fatigue is not the result of an organic disease or of continuing exertion.

Fatigue is not alleviated by rest.

Fatigue results in a substantial reduction in previous occupational, educational, social, and personal activities.

Four or more of the following symptoms are concurrently present for 6 months:

Impaired memory or concentration, sore throat, tender cervical or axillary lymph nodes, muscle pain, pain in several joints, new headaches, unrefreshing sleep, or malaise after exertion.

Exclusion Criteria

Medical condition explaining fatigue

Major depressive disorder (psychotic features) or bipolar disorder

Schizophrenia, dementia, or delusional disorder

Anorexia nervosa, bulimia nervosa

Alcohol or substance abuse

Severe obesity (BMI >40)

XI-69.   **The answer is B.** *(Chap. 389)* Cognitive behavioral therapy (CBT) and graded exercise therapy (GET) have been found to be the only beneficial interventions in chronic fatigue syndrome (CFS). CBT is a psychotherapeutic approach directed at changing condition-related cognitions and behaviors. CBT for CFS aims at changing a patient's perpetuating factors by exploiting various techniques and components. The intervention, which typically consists of 12–14 sessions spread over 6 months, helps CFS patients gain control over their symptoms. GET is based on the model of deconditioning and exercise intolerance and usually involves a home exercise program that continues for 3–5 months. Walking or cycling is systematically increased, with set target heart rates. Evidence that deconditioning is the basis for symptoms in CFS is lacking, however. The primary component of CBT and GET that results in a reduction in fatigue is a change in the patient's perception of fatigue and focus on symptoms. CBT is generally the more complex treatment, which might explain why CBT studies tend to yield better improvement rates than GET trials. Not all patients benefit from CBT or GET. Predictors of poor outcome are somatic comorbidity, current disability claims, and severe pain. CBT offered in an early stage of the illness reduces the burden of CFS for the patient as well as society in terms of decreased medical and disability-related costs. Full recovery from untreated CFS is rare: the median annual recovery rate is 5% (range 0–31%) and the improvement rate 39% (range 8–63%). Major depressive disorder, bipolar disorder, eating disorder, and schizophrenia are exclusion criteria for the diagnosis of chronic fatigue syndrome.

XI-70. **The answer is D.** *(Chap. 391)* This patient is experiencing her first episode of a panic attack and does not meet the criteria for panic disorder. In this situation, no specific treatment is required. The patient should be reassured in a manner that is empathetic and supportive that she does not have any evidence of a serious medical disorder. Panic attacks are common, with about 1–3% of the population experiencing at least one panic attack. Panic attacks begin abruptly, most commonly without an immediate precipitating cause, and peak in severity over 10 minutes. The symptoms usually subside spontaneously over the course of an hour. Diagnostic criteria for a panic attack include a minimum of four of the following criteria: palpitations or racing heart, sweating, trembling, shortness of breath, feeling of choking, chest pain, nausea or GI distress, dizziness, derealization, fear of losing control, fear of dying, paresthesias, or chills/hot flushes. If a patient subsequently develops panic disorder, a variety of treatment options can be pursued. Panic disorder is marked by at least 1 month of recurrent panic attacks associated with excessive worry about or change in behavior as a result of the attacks. The goals of therapy for panic attacks are to decrease the frequency of attacks and the severity of symptoms during the attack. Antidepressant medications are the cornerstone of therapy with selective serotonin reuptake inhibitors being the most frequently used class of medication. The dose of medication for panic disorder is typically lower than the antidepressant dose. For fluoxetine, this would be 5–10 mg daily. As these medications take 2–6 weeks to become effective, they are often combined with benzodiazepines to be used on an as-needed basis for immediate relief of attacks. Alprazolam and clonazepam are common agents used for panic disorder, although alprazolam may have more associated dependence with the need for escalating doses of medications. In combination with pharmacologic therapy, psychotherapy and education are also useful for the treatment of panic disorder. The therapy often includes breathing techniques, cognitive behavioral therapy, and even homework assignments.

XI-71. **The answer is A.** *(Chap. 391)* There are increasing numbers of antidepressant medications available in a variety of classes. Selective serotonin reuptake inhibitors (SSRIs) are the most commonly used antidepressant drugs. This class of medications includes fluoxetine, sertraline, paroxetine, fluvoxamine, citalopram, and escitalopram. These medications are taken once daily and have side effects including sexual dysfunction, headache, and insomnia. Tricyclic antidepressants were commonly used in past decades for the treatment of depression. However, overdoses can be lethal, and anticholinergic side effects including dry mouth, constipation, and urinary retention can limit the dose. Medications in the tricyclic class of antidepressants include amitriptyline, nortriptyline, imipramine, desipramine, doxepin, and clomipramine. Mixed norepinephrine/serotonin reuptake inhibitors and receptor blockers are a newer class of medications. These medications are increasing in use as they are quite effective and do not have the same frequency of sexual dysfunction. Medications in this class include venlafaxine, desvenlafaxine, duloxetine, and mirtazapine. Monoamine oxidase inhibitors were once a common antidepressant class of medication, but these medications are now only rare used. There is a wide range of drug and food interactions that can lead to hypertensive crises. Examples of medication in this class include phenelzine, tranylcypromine, and isocarboxazid. A final class of antidepressants is called simply mixed action drugs and includes trazodone, bupropion, and nefazodone.

XI-72. **The answer is E.** *(Chap. 391)* Post-traumatic stress disorder (PTSD) was only added as a discrete disorder in 1980. The diagnostic criteria for PTSD are long and require that an individual experiences an event where there was an actual or perceived threat of death or serious injury and that the individual's reaction included intense fear or helplessness. Following the event, the individual continues to re-experience the event and avoids stimuli associated with the trauma. In association with this, there is also often a generalized withdrawal and decrease in responsiveness. At the same time, the patient exhibits an increase in arousal that is often exhibited by insomnia, irritability, hypervigilance, and difficulty concentrating. Treatment of PTSD is almost always multifactorial, including both pharmacotherapy and psychotherapy. It is not uncommon for an individual with PTSD to develop a dependence on drugs or alcohol as an attempt to control the symptoms, and any substance abuse issues need to be treated simultaneously as well. This patient's treatment would include avoidance of alcohol and intensive substance abuse treatment as needed. Treatment with antidepressant medications can decrease anxiety and avoidance behaviors. Trazodone is often given at night for its sedating properties. Psychotherapeutic strategies include cognitive behavioral therapy to overcome avoidance behaviors as well.

XI-73. **The answer is B.** *(Chap. 391)* Fifteen percent of the population will experience at least one episode of major depression over the course of a lifetime, and most episodes of major depression are treated by primary care practitioners. Treatment can be any of a number of medications across a variety of classes. Despite the popularity of newer antidepressants, there is no evidence that these medications are more efficacious than older drugs like tricyclic antidepressants. Indeed, 60–70% of patients will respond to any drug chosen if given in a sufficient dose for 6–8 weeks. Once a patient has been on treatment for about 2 months, the response should be evaluated, and if there has been an insufficient response, a dosage increase should be considered. In this patient, a dosage increase yielded control of depressive symptoms at 4 months. Once control of symptoms has been achieved, the drug should be continued for an additional 6–9 months to prevent relapse. If a patient experiences any additional episodes of major depression, he or she will likely require indefinite maintenance treatment.

XI-74. **The answer is A.** *(Chap. 392)* Alcohol is primarily absorbed through the proximal small intestine, but small to moderate amounts can also be absorbed in the mouth, esophagus, stomach, and large intestines. Several factors can increase the rate of absorption. One factor that increases absorption is rapid gastric emptying, which can be induced by concurrent consumption of carbonated beverages. Another factor that increases absorption from the gut to the blood is the ingestion of alcohol in the absence of other calorie sources such as proteins, fat, or carbohydrates. A final factor that can increase absorption is to drink alcohol that is diluted to a modest concentration (~20% or less). At high alcohol concentrations absorption is decreased, although high blood levels may be achieved because the amount of alcohol ingested is high.

XI-75. **The answer is C.** *(Chap. 392)* Alcohol has effects on many neurotransmitters in the brain. The predominant effect of alcohol lies in its ability to cause the release of γ-aminobutyric acid (GABA) and acts primarily at the $GABA_A$ receptors. GABA is the primary inhibitory neurotransmitter in the brain and is associated with the sedative effects of alcohol. Many other drugs affect the GABA system including benzodiazepines, nonbenzodiazepine sleep aids such as zolpidem, anticonvulsants, and muscle relaxants. The euphoric effects of alcohol consumption are related to increases in dopamine, which is common to all pleasurable activities. The effects on dopamine are thought to be important in alcohol craving and relapse. In addition, alcohol alters opioid receptors and can lead to a release of beta endorphins during acute ingestion. In addition to these effects, alcohol also inhibits postsynaptic N-methyl-D-aspartate excitatory glutamate receptors. Glutamate is the primary excitatory neurotransmitter of the brain, and its inhibition further contributes to the sedative effects of alcohol. Additional important effects on neurotransmitters include increased serotonin activity and decreased nicotinic acetylcholine receptors.

XI-76. **The answer is D.** *(Chap. 392)* The acute effects of any drug depend on many factors including amount consumed and absorbed, presence of other drugs, and past experience with the drug. In an individual who is naïve to alcohol, drug levels as low as 0.02 g/dL can lead to a decrease in inhibitions and a slight feeling of intoxication. In the United States, "legal" intoxication occurs at a blood alcohol level of 0.08 g/dL in most states. At this level, decreases in cognitive and motor abilities are seen. Once an alcohol level of 0.20 g/dL is achieved, an individual is obviously impaired with slurred speech, poor judgment, and impaired coordination. Light coma and depression of respiratory rate, blood pressure, and pulse occur at levels of around 0.30 g/dL, and death is likely to occur at levels of 0.40 g/dL. However, in individuals who drink heavily, tolerance begins to develop to alcohol. After a period of 1–2 weeks of daily alcohol consumption, liver metabolism of alcohol increases by as much as 30%, but disappears quite quickly with abstinence. Cellular or pharmacodynamic tolerance also occurs and refers to the neurochemical changes that allow an individual to maintain more normal physiologic functioning despite the presence of alcohol.

XI-77. **The answer is C.** *(Chap. 392)* Alcohol abuse is defined as repetitive problems in any one of four life areas that can be attributed to alcohol. The four life areas that can be affected by alcohol include social, interpersonal, legal, or occupational. In addition, an individual who repetitively engages in hazardous behaviors while under the influence of alcohol would be considered to suffer from alcohol abuse. However, this is to be differentiated from alcohol dependence. Alcohol dependence is defined in the DSM-IV as repeated alcohol-related difficulties in three of seven life areas and includes the development of tolerance and dependence. If tolerance or dependence is present, this predicts a more severe clinical course, and the presence of alcohol dependence decreases overall life span by about a decade. Only about 50% of individuals with alcohol abuse will continue to experience similar alcohol-related problems 3–5 years later, and only 10% will go on to develop alcohol dependence. The lifetime risk of alcohol dependence in most Western countries is about 10–15% in men and 5–8% in women. However, there may be higher rates in Ireland, France, and Scandinavian countries. In addition, native cultures appear to be especially susceptible to problems with alcohol dependence. This has been seen in Native Americans, Maoris, and the aboriginal tribes of Australia.

About 60% of the risk for alcohol use disorders is attributed to genetic influences. Children of alcoholics do have a higher risk of alcohol abuse and dependence; however, this risk is about 4 times higher, not 10. Identical twins also exhibit a higher risk of concurrent alcohol abuse and dependence when compared to fraternal twins. The genetic factors that appear to be most strongly linked to alcohol use disorders include genes that are linked to impulsivity, schizophrenia, and bipolar disorder. In addition, genes that affect alcohol metabolism or sensitivity to alcohol also contribute to the genetics of alcoholism. A mutation in aldehyde dehydrogenase that is more common in individuals of Asian descent results in intense flushing when alcohol is consumed and confers a decreased risk of alcohol dependence. Conversely, genetic variants that lead to a low sensitivity to alcohol increase the risk of subsequent alcohol abuse and dependence, as higher and higher doses of alcohol are required to achieve the same effects.

XI-78. **The answer is B.** *(Chap. 392)* Individuals with alcohol dependence are susceptible to alcohol withdrawal when alcohol intake is stopped abruptly. The individual in this case scenario is likely alcohol dependent given his large amount of alcohol intake on a daily basis. Symptoms of alcohol withdrawal can range from mild tremulousness to hallucinations, seizures, or the development of delirium tremens. Other clinical features of alcohol withdrawal include anxiety, insomnia, and autonomic nervous system overactivity manifested as tachycardia, tachypnea, elevated blood pressure, and fever. This patient exhibits symptoms of the more severe delirium tremens, with mental confusion, agitation, and fluctuating levels of consciousness. While minor symptoms of alcohol withdrawal may begin as soon as 5–10 hours after cessation of alcohol intake, the symptoms do not peak for 48–72 hours, putting this patient in the appropriate time frame for alcohol withdrawal.

The best approach for the alcohol-dependent patient who abruptly stops all alcohol intake is to take a prophylactic approach and screen early for symptoms of alcohol withdrawal. Tools such as the Revised Clinical Institute for Withdrawal Assessment for Alcohol (CIWA-Ar) may help clinicians and nurses screen for the early development of symptoms and allow intervention before symptoms escalate. In this setting, most experts recommend the use of oral long-acting benzodiazepines such as chlordiazepoxide or diazepam beginning on the first day. However, in this case, the patient received no such treatment and is now experiencing severe alcohol withdrawal and delirium tremens. Intravenous medications that have a rapid onset of action and can be titrated for more aggressive symptom management are often employed in this setting. Thus, the use of IV lorazepam or diazepam is preferred in this patient. Following an initial bolus, repeated doses can be used in short intervals until the patient is calm but arousable. In some instances a continuous infusion may be required, although bolus dosing is preferred. In the most severe cases, propofol or barbiturates may be required, although the patient would most likely need to be intubated for airway protection with use of these medications.

The other options listed are not appropriate for initial management of this patient. Intravenous fluids and thiamine had been administered since hospital admission. Administration of glucose-containing fluids without thiamine in the alcohol-dependent patient can precipitate Wernicke's encephalopathy, which would present with ophthalmoparesis, ataxia, and encephalopathy. Given the patient's fever, an infectious etiology can be considered, and it would be appropriate to perform blood cultures in this patient. However, given the clear symptoms of alcohol withdrawal and lack of necrotizing pancreatitis on CT abdomen, empiric treatment with antibiotics is not required. Likewise, without focal neurologic findings, a head CT would be a low-yield diagnostic procedure that would be difficult to perform in the patient's current agitated condition and would only delay appropriate therapy. Finally, restraints are best avoided if the patient's safety can be ensured through the appropriate use of benzodiazepines, as restraints are only likely to make the patient's agitation worse and may lead to iatrogenic harm. Haloperidol may have some sedative effect on the patient, but could lead to torsades de pointe arrhythmia as this patient is at risk for electrolyte deficiencies from his alcoholism and pancreatitis.

XI-79. **The answer is D.** *(Chap. 392)* In individuals recovering from alcoholism several medications may have a modest benefit in increasing abstinence rates. The two medications with the best risk-benefit ratio are acamprosate and naltrexone. Acamprosate inhibits NMDA receptors, decreasing symptoms of prolonged alcohol withdrawal. Naltrexone is an opioid antagonist than can be administered orally or as a monthly injection. It is thought to act by decreasing activity in the dopamine-rich ventral tegmental area of the brainstem and subsequently decreasing the pleasurable feelings associated with alcohol consumption. There is some research to suggest that the use of these medications in combination may be more effective than either one alone. Disulfiram is an aldehyde dehydrogenase inhibitor that has been used for many years in the treatment of alcoholism. However, it is no longer a commonly used drug due to its many side effects and risks associated with treatment. The primary mechanism by which it acts is to create negative effects of vomiting and autonomic nervous system hyperactivity when alcohol is consumed concurrently with use of the medication. As it inhibits an enzyme that is part of the normal metabolism of alcohol, it allows the buildup of acetaldehyde, which creates these symptoms. Because of the autonomic side effects, it is contraindicated in individuals with hypertension, a history of stroke, heart disease, or diabetes mellitus.

XI-80. **The answer is E.** *(Chap. 393)* Prescription drug abuse has increased dramatically among all age groups and is strikingly common in teenagers. Since 2007, prescription opiates have passed marijuana as the most common illicit drugs that adolescents initially abuse. This has occurred at the same time as rates of prescription narcotic abuse have increased across all age groups. The annual prevalence of heroin abuse is approximately 0.14% of the population. In contrast, this prevalence is only one-third the rate of prescription opiate abuse. Among prescription narcotics, oxycodone is the single most commonly abused drug. Other common prescription narcotics that are abused include morphine and hydrocodone. Among health care professionals, meperidine and fentanyl are more frequently abused.

XI-81. **The answer is B.** *(Chap. 393)* Tolerance and withdrawal begin within 6–8 weeks of chronic daily opioid use. Tolerance develops not because of increased metabolism, but through a change in the pharmacodynamics of the drugs, requiring increasing doses to achieve the euphoric effects and prevent withdrawal. With the abrupt cessation of narcotics, acute withdrawal symptoms begin within 8–10 hours after the last dose. While the symptoms of narcotic withdrawal are noxious, they are not life threatening, as is the case with benzodiazepine or barbiturate withdrawal. The primary symptoms of opiate withdrawal are related to over activity of the autonomic nervous system. This manifests as increased lacrimation, rhinorrhea, and sweating. In addition, patients frequently will have diffuse piloerection (chill bumps), giving rise to the term "cold turkey." As withdrawal symptoms progress, patients appear restless with myalgias, nausea, vomiting, and diarrhea. Hypertension, hyperthermia, and tachypnea can occur as well. Hypotension is not a symptom of opioid withdrawal. A patient with known infection and new-onset hypotension should be evaluated for systemic infection, not withdrawal.

XI-82. **The answer is E.** *(Chap. 393)* The patient is presenting with an acute overdose of an unknown quantity of extended-release opioid medications taken with alcohol. When evaluating and treating a patient with an intention overdose, the first priority is to stabilize the patient's condition. The patient was appropriately given the opiate antagonist naloxone by emergency responders as the patient was near-apneic. In addition, the patient was also appropriately intubated and stabilized for transport to the hospital. In the emergency room, however, the patient remained hypotensive and unresponsive. At this point, the next step in stabilizing the patient is to support the blood pressure with bolus fluid resuscitation, and if the patient fails to respond, IV vasopressors would be required. Given his ongoing unresponsive state and the expected long duration of effect with a sustained-release preparation, it is appropriate to initiate a continuous infusion of naloxone. After a bolus dose, the expected onset of action is 1–2 minutes, but the duration of effect is only a few hours. Some care must be taken when giving naloxone as one only wants to reverse the respiratory and cardiovascular depression associated with the overdose. Particularly in chronic drug abusers, high doses of naloxone can precipitate the distressing symptoms of narcotic withdrawal. When long-acting preparations of opioids are taken, activated charcoal and gastric lavage are appropriate considerations to decrease the absorption of any undigested pills. While the patient is being stabilized from a cardiovascular and respiratory standpoint, it is important that the clinician consider if any other concurrent ingestion may have occurred that would affect the patient's outcome. As the patient is unable to provide any history and the overdose was not witnessed, one must not focus solely on the opioids. The appropriate approach is to perform a comprehensive toxicology evaluation that should include a urine drug screen, blood alcohol level, and acetaminophen levels, at a minimum. One could also consider sending for levels of aspirin or tricyclic antidepressants.

XI-83. **The answer is C.** *(Chap. 394)* Marijuana is the most commonly used illegal drug in the United States with over 6% of all individuals reporting current usage in 2009 (http://www.whitehousedrugpolicy.gov/publications/pdf/nsduh.pdf, accessed July 25, 2011). In part, the prevalence of marijuana use is related to the widespread belief that marijuana is thought to have few negative health effects. Acutely, marijuana causes a sense of relaxation and mild euphoria, not unlike that of alcohol intoxication. In addition, impaired judgment, cognition, and psychomotor performance are seen. Occasionally, acute intoxication can lead to negative emotional responses as well. A consensus about the chronic effects of marijuana usage is not clearly defined. Traditionally, marijuana usage has been linked with an "amotivational syndrome." While it is true that chronic users of marijuana may lose interest in day-to-day activities and spend more time using the drug, this is certainly not specific for marijuana uses, and a specific "amotivational syndrome" is not defined with chronic marijuana use. Other symptoms that have been attributed to chronic marijuana use that lack good evidence for causation include depression and maturational dysfunction. In individuals with a history of schizophrenia, however, chronic marijuana use has been associated with an increased risk of psychotic symptoms.

The physical effects of chronic marijuana use are also not clearly known. Acutely, marijuana causes increased heart rate, but tolerance for this effect occurs rapidly. Acute ingestion can also precipitate angina. The chronic effects on lung function are not known, as tobacco products are frequent confounders. Acute decreases in vital capacity and diffusion capacity are seen, but whether this translates into an increased risk of emphysema has not yet been determined. Most studies have not found an association with emphysema. A variety of other adverse physical effects have been described but not confirmed in a systematic fashion. This includes reports of low testosterone levels, decreased sperm count, impaired fetal growth, and chromosomal abnormalities.

Contrary to popular belief, chronic use of marijuana is associated with the development of tolerance as well as a withdrawal syndrome. Signs of physical tolerance include tolerance to the development of tachycardia and conjunctival injection. The psychological tolerance that develops is more prominent and predictable. This occurs rapidly, with individuals often seeking more potent compounds or smoking the drug more frequently. With cessation of marijuana use, a withdrawal syndrome can be demonstrated with irritability, anorexia, and sleep disturbance.

XI-84. The answer is E. *(Chap. 395)* Approximately 400,000 individuals die yearly in the United States as a result of cigarette smoking, accounting for about 20% of all deaths. While heart disease, lung cancer, and chronic obstructive pulmonary disease are most commonly connected with tobacco-related deaths, multiple cancers have also been associated with cigarette smoking. Of all cancers, cancers of the lung, oropharynx, and larynx have the strongest associations. The relative risk of lung cancer in current male cigarette smokers is as high as 23.3. However, the relative risk of lung cancer is only 12.7 among current female smokers. Other cancers that have been associated with cigarette smoking include esophageal, bladder, kidney, pancreatic, stomach, cervical, and acute myeloid leukemia. Postmenopausal breast cancer is not associated with current cigarette use, although there may be a link with premenopausal breast cancer that has not yet been fully determined.

XI-85. The answer is B. *(Chap. 395)* Smoking cessation is vitally important in promoting health and preventing adverse outcomes related to cigarette use. However, nicotine is a remarkably addictive substance, and most smokers require several attempts at smoking cessation prior to success. It is estimated that 33% of current smokers attempt to quit each year, with 90% of unassisted attempts at smoking cessation resulting in failure. Even with the appropriate support and best medical treatments available, sustained quit rates of 20–30% are typical. Short counseling sessions by a physician alone do increase quit rates. Therefore, questions about current tobacco use and prior quit attempts should be part of every office visit. Even when patients do not express the desire to stop smoking, they should be encouraged to consider the potential benefits of smoking cessation. As part of counseling, the physician should negotiate a quit date with the patient, typically 2 or 3 weeks after the appointment, and follow-up phone calls may be helpful. However, most often counseling should be combined with pharmacologic interventions to improve quit rates. A variety of options are available, and the most commonly used treatments are nicotine replacement therapy, bupropion, and varenicline. In this patient with a history of depression that is inadequately treated, combined therapy with bupropion and nicotine replacement would have the greatest likelihood of success. Bupropion is an antidepressant medication that has been studied for smoking cessation in randomized clinical trials. Pretreatment with bupropion for 1–2 weeks prior to the quit date increases success. Concomitant use of nicotine replacement therapy can be administered in a variety of forms including patches, gum, lozenges, and nasal or oral inhalers. Some programs advocate combining patches with a more rapidly acting nicotine product that can alleviate acute cravings for nicotine. Varenicline is a recently introduced medication that acts as a partial agonist at the nicotinic acetylcholine receptor. Concomitant nicotine administration is not felt to be helpful. Use of varenicline in this patient is contraindicated given the patient's history of untreated depression. Varenicline has been associated with severe psychiatric symptoms, and there are reports of suicide that have been related to its use.

XI-86. The answer is D. *(Chap. 395)* Cigarette smoking is associated with early mortality from a variety of causes including cardiovascular, respiratory, cerebrovascular, and oncologic. It is also associated with increased complications during pregnancy (premature rupture of membranes, placenta previa, abruption placenta), delay in healing of peptic ulcers, osteoporosis, cataracts, macular degeneration, cholecystitis in women, and impotence in men. Children born to smoking mothers are more likely to have preterm delivery, higher perinatal mortality, higher rates of infant respiratory distress, and higher rates of sudden infant death. Moreover, 400,000 individuals die prematurely each year in the United States from cigarette use, representing 1 out of every 5 deaths.

XI-87. The answer is B. *(Chap. 395)* Smokers regulate their blood levels of nicotine by adjusting the frequency and intensity of their tobacco use. Smokers can compensate for the lower levels of nicotine in low-yield cigarettes by smoking more cigarettes or by adjusting their smoking technique with a deeper inhalation and breath hold. Therefore, smoking low-yield cigarettes is not a reasonable alternative to smoking cessation. Moreover, there is no difference in the harmful physical effects of smoking or in the potential for drug interactions. Finally, although not definitively proven, there is some thought that the rise in adenocarcinoma of the lung over the past 50 years is associated with introduction of the low-tar cigarette and the resultant change in smoking behavior associated with this.

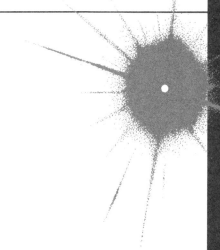

QUESTIONS

DIRECTIONS: Choose the **one best** response to each question.

XII-1. A 34-year-old woman seeks evaluation for a skin lesion. On examination, the lesion is present on the extensor surface of the right elbow. It measures 2.4 cm in diameter and is raised, with a flat top and distinct edge. Overlying the lesion is an excess accumulation of stratum cornea. Further examination reveals several smaller lesions also located on extensor surfaces. Which term best characterizes the primary lesion for which the patient is seeking evaluation?

A. Macule with lichenification
B. Patch with a scale
C. Plaque with a crust
D. Plaque with a scale
E. Tumor

XII-2. What term is used in dermatology to describe a coin-shaped lesion?

A. Herpetiform
B. Lichenoid
C. Morbilliform
D. Nummular
E. Polycyclic

XII-3. A 5-year-old boy is brought in by his mother complaining of approximately 6 months of itching and scaling of the skin inside the elbows (see Figure XII-3). The area gets red occasionally and improves with over-the-counter topical steroid creams. There is no fever, chills, night sweats, or red streaks ascending the arm. The family has a pet cat and lives in a clean apartment. All of the following statements concerning this child are true EXCEPT:

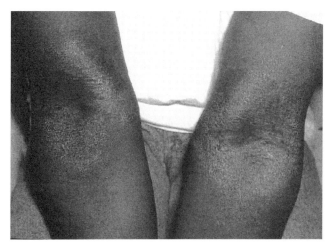

FIGURE XII-3 (see Color Atlas) *(Courtesy of Robert Swerlick, MD; with permission.)*

A. Both of his parents likely have a history of atopic dermatitis.
B. He likely has a history of asthma or atopic rhinitis.
C. His serum IgE levels are elevated.
D. He has a greater than 70% chance of spontaneous resolution.
E. His lesions will likely respond to topical tacrolimus.

XII-4. A 63-year-old woman has a 5-year history of psoriasis involving her elbows that has been controlled with topical glucocorticoids and a vitamin D analogue. However, in the past 9–12 months she has developed worsening and new lesions involving her knees, gluteal regions, and scalp. She is increasingly uncomfortable and has noted swelling of her digits with pain and stiffness. She is up to date on all cancer screening and has no sign of systemic infection. Her physical examination is only notable for the psoriatic plaques that are red and scaling, and swollen, tender DIPs on both hands. All of the following therapies are indicated for worsening widespread systemic psoriatic disease EXCEPT:

A. Alefacept
B. Cyclosporine
C. Infliximab
D. Methotrexate
E. Prednisone

XII-5. A 67-year-old man presents with complaints of diffuse rash with blistering. The lesions began as pruritic plaques distributed on the trunk and abdomen. Lesions are now appearing on the flexor surfaces of the arms. Some of the lesions have developed into tense blisters that rupture. As the lesions have healed, no scarring is present. A photo of the patient's rash is shown in Figure XII-5. What would be the expected finding on biopsy of the lesion?

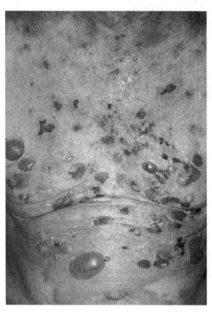

FIGURE XII-5 (see Color Atlas) *(Courtesy of the Yale Resident's Slide Collection; with permission.)*

A. Cell surface deposition of IgG on keratinocytes
B. Cell surface deposition of IgG and C3 on keratinocytes
C. Granular deposits of IgA in dermal papillae
D. Linear band deposition of IgA in the epidermal basement membrane zone
E. Linear band deposition of IgG and/or C3 in the epidermal basement membrane zone

XII-6. A 24-year-old woman seeks evaluation for a rash that is present diffusely on her back, buttocks, elbows, and knees. The rash began abruptly and the patient is complaining of severe pruritus and burning associated with the rash. A biopsy of the rash demonstrates neutrophilic dermatitis within the dermal papillae, and immunofluorescence highlights granular deposition of IgA in the papillary dermis and along the epidermal basement membrane zone. What treatment do you recommend for this patient?

A. Dapsone 100 mg daily
B. Gluten-free diet
C. Prednisone 40 mg daily
D. A and B
E. All of the above

XII-7. A patient presents to you for evaluation of ear lesions worsening over the last 6–9 months. Each lesion began as a red papule with a thick adherent scale (see Figure XII-7). Since that time, they have progressed to the current pictured lesions with variable coloration, raised borders, and scars. There has been no improvement with use of topical glucocorticoids, which the patient borrowed from a friend. What is the best course of action for this patient at this time?

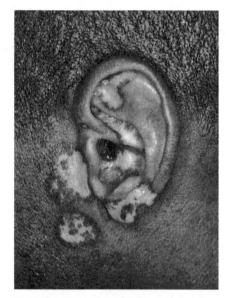

FIGURE XII-7 (see Color Atlas)

A. Aminoquinoline antimalarials
B. Azathioprine
C. Systemic glucocorticoids
D. Vitamin E ointment
E. Wide surgical excision with regional lymph node dissection

XII-8. A 55-year-old man presents with fever and a blistering skin rash that has developed after taking allopurinol for gout. The patient also is complaining of a sore throat and painful watery eyes. On examination, the patient is found to have blisters developing over a targetoid lesion with oral mucosal involvement. The estimated body surface area that is currently affected is 33%. Which of the following statements regarding this patient's diagnosis and treatment are TRUE?

A. Immediate treatment with intravenous immunoglobulin will decrease the extent of the disease and improve mortality.
B. Long-term treatment with glucocorticoids is required to prevent relapse of the disease.
C. The expected mortality rate from this syndrome is about 30%.
D. The most common drug to cause this syndrome is penicillin.
E. Younger individuals have a higher mortality than older individuals with this syndrome.

XII-9. A 32-year-old man receives amoxicillin/clavulanate for presumed bacterial sinusitis. One week later he presents with a diffuse itchy rash (see Figure XII-9). His mucous membranes are normal. Which of the following is the most likely diagnosis?

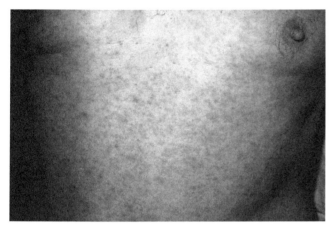

FIGURE XII-9 (see Color Atlas)

A. Morbilliform drug eruption
B. Pemphigus vulgaris
C. Stevens-Johnson syndrome
D. Toxic shock syndrome
E. Urticaria

XII-10. A 22-year-old woman comes to your office concerned about sun exposure. She brings a few sunblock creams into your office and wants to know which one is best for preventing wrinkling and blotchiness. She is less concerned about sunburn because she is trying to get a better tan. Blocking which ultraviolet rays will achieve her desired result?

A. UV-A
B. UV-B
C. Both UV-A and UV-B equally
D. Neither UV-A nor UV-B

XII-11. A 45-year-old patient with HIV/AIDS presents to the emergency department. He complains of a rash that has been slowly spreading up his right arm and is now evident on his chest and back. The rash consists of small nodules that have a reddish-blue appearance. Some of them are ulcerated, but there is minimal fluctuance or drainage. He is unsure when these began. He notes no foreign travel or unusual exposures. He is homeless and unemployed, but occasionally gets work as a day laborer doing landscaping and digging. A culture of a skin lesion grows a *Mycobacterium* in 5 days. Which of the following is the most likely organism?

A. *M. abscessus*
B. *M. avium*
C. *M. kansasii*
D. *M. marinum*
E. *M. ulcerans*

XII-12. A 22-year-old man presents to the emergency department complaining of generalized malaise and rash. The patient has a history of illicit drug use with intranasal heroin and cocaine. He admits to engaging in unprotected sexual intercourse with men in exchange for drugs. He was negative for the HIV virus 8 weeks previously. He has a prior history of syphilis and gonorrhea that were treated appropriately 2 years previously. Following treatment, his rapid plasma reagin test fell to a titer of 1:8 from a high of 1:128 after 12 months. On physical examination, the patient has normal vital signs without fever. He is well developed and has no wasting. Diffuse lymphadenopathy measuring up to 2.5 cm is palpable in the cervical, axillary, and femoral areas. Genital examination shows no ulcerations or lesions. The rash is shown in Figure XII-12. Which test is most likely to yield the appropriate diagnosis in this patient?

A. Fluorescent treponemal antibody test
B. HIV antibody
C. HIV viral load
D. Rapid plasma reagin test
E. Venereal Disease Research Laboratory test

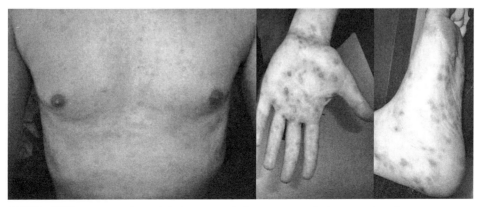

FIGURE XII-12 (see Color Atlas) *(Courtesy of Jill McKenzie and Christina Marra.)*

XII-13. While on a medical mission to the Ivory Coast, you are asked to see a 17-year-old boy with a large skin lesion on his forearm (see Figure XII-13). The lesion began as a small bump about 3 weeks ago and has grown to the size of a raspberry. He has tender axillary adenopathy on the ipsilateral side but no other physical findings. His siblings report similar lesions that healed after about 6 months. Which of the following is the most appropriate therapy?

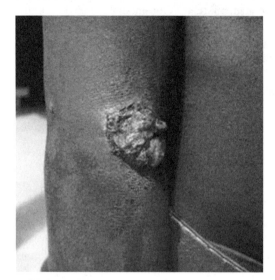

FIGURE XII-13 (see Color Atlas)

A. Albendazole
B. Ivermectin
C. Penicillin
D. Praziquantel
E. Vancomycin

XII-14. Infection by what organism causes the rash shown in Figure XII-14?

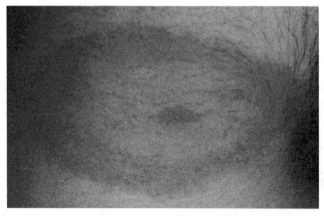

FIGURE XII-14 (see Color Atlas) *(Courtesy of Vijay K. Sikand, MD; with permission.)*

A. *Anaplasma phagocytophilum*
B. *Bartonella henselae*
C. *Borrelia burgdorferi*
D. *Ehrlichia chaffeensis*
E. *Rickettsia rickettsii*

XII-15. A 36-year-old man with HIV/AIDS (CD4+ lymphocyte count = 112/μL) develops a scaly, waxy, yellowish, patchy, crusty, pruritic rash on and around his nose. The rest of his skin examination is normal. Which of the following is the most likely diagnosis?

A. Molluscum contagiosum
B. Kaposi's sarcoma
C. Psoriasis
D. Reactivation herpes zoster
E. Seborrheic dermatitis

XII-16. A 34-year-old man seeks the advice of his primary care physician because of an asymptomatic rash on his chest. There are coalescing light-brown to salmon-colored macules present on the chest. A scraping of the lesions is viewed after a wet preparation with 10% potassium hydroxide solution. There are both hyphal and spore forms present, giving the slide an appearance of "spaghetti and meatballs." In addition, the lesions fluoresce to a yellow-green appearance under a Wood's lamp. Tinea versicolor is diagnosed. Which of the following microorganisms is responsible for this skin infection?

A. *Fusarium solani*
B. *Malassezia furfur*
C. *Penicillium marneffei*
D. *Sporothrix schenckii*
E. *Trichophyton rubrum*

XII-17. A 19-year-old college freshman comes to the clinic complaining of blistering skin lesions on the back of his hands and arms that are painful. He's noticed these occasionally during his childhood, and they were often precipitated by sunlight and healed with scarring. He now notices that since starting college they are more frequent, and often occur after drunken parties. His hands and forearms have numerous hypopigmented scars that he says are from previous episodes. The skin over the back of his hands appears thick and coarse. Otherwise his review of systems and physical examination is normal. The lesions on his hands are shown in Figure XII-17. Which of the following tests will most likely yield the correct diagnosis?

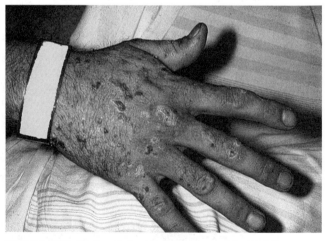

FIGURE XII-17 *(see Color Atlas) (Courtesy of Dr. Karl E. Anderson; with permission.)*

A.   ANA
B.   Anti-SCL-70
C.   Plasma cortisol
D.   Plasma porphyrin
E.   Urine porphobilinogen

XII-18. A 22-year-old male comes to the clinic reporting severe penile itching and new skin lesions. His last sexual encounter was unprotected sex 3 weeks prior with a new female partner in her bed. He has not seen her since. Over the last 3 days he's noticed new lesions on his penis and scrotum. The lesions are extremely pruritic, particularly at night and after a shower. His physical examination is shown in Figure XII-18. Which of the following is the best therapy?

A.   Ceftriaxone plus azithromycin
B.   Metronidazole
C.   Penicillin G
D.   Permethrin
E.   Vancomycin

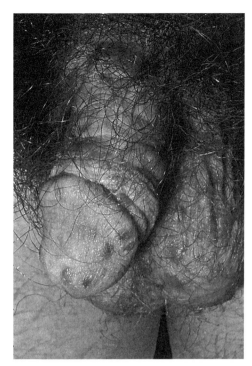

FIGURE XII-18 (see Color Atlas)

ANSWERS

XII-1. **The answer is D.** *(Chap. 51)* Rashes and skin lesions are the most common reasons for visits to primary care physicians. Accurately characterizing a skin lesion is important for determining the underlying cause of the disease. Four basic features that are important when describing a skin lesion are the distribution, types of primary and secondary lesions, shape, and arrangement of lesions. The primary description of a skin lesion takes into account size, whether the lesion is raised or flat, and whether the lesion is fluid filled. Raised lesions can be papules, nodules, tumors, or plaques. A plaque is a raised lesion with a flat top that measures more than 1 cm in diameter. The edges may be distinct or gradually blend in with the surrounding skin. Papules, nodules, and tumors are similar raised solid lesions of the skin. These lesions differ only by size, with papules being smaller than 0.5 cm, nodules measuring 0.5–5.0 cm, and tumors measuring more than 5 cm. Macules and patches are not raised and also differ only by size, with macules being less than 2 cm and patches being greater than 2 cm. Vesicles are small (<0.5 cm) fluid-filled lesions, and pustules are vesicles containing leukocytes. Larger fluid-filled lesions are called bullae. A secondary description of a skin lesion takes into account features of the lesion. An excess accumulation of stratum corneum on a skin lesion is called a scale. Thus, this patient would be characterized as having a plaque with a scale. Other secondary descriptors include lichenification, which refers to a distinctive thickening of the skin that accentuates skinfold markings, and crusting, which refers to dried body fluids. In addition, the lesion may have erosions, ulceration, excoriation, atrophy, or scarring.

XII-2. **The answer is D.** *(Chap. 51)* Characteristic terms are used in dermatology to describe a skin lesion. Nummular lesions are coin shaped and are closely related to annular lesions, which are ring shaped. A polycyclic eruption consists of a configuration of skin lesions that coalesce to form a ring or incomplete rings. Herpetiform lesions are grouped in a fashion that is seen in herpes simplex virus infection, whereas morbilliform lesions are generalized macules or papules that are similar to those seen in a measles eruption. Lichenoid rashes are violaceous lesions that resemble those seen in lichen planus.

XII-3. **The answer is D.** *(Chap. 52)* These lesions are typical examples of childhood atopic dermatitis, the cutaneous expression of the atopic state. Over 75% of patients present by 5 years of age, and a similar proportion has concomitant asthma and/or allergic rhinitis. There is a strong genetic predisposition. Over 80% of children whose parents both have atopic dermatitis will have similar skin findings; the prevalence is approximately 50% when one parent is affected. In addition to the antecubital fossae, the face, neck, and other extensor surfaces are commonly affected. The typical course involves exacerbations and remissions. In the adult form, the disease is often localized lichen simplex chronicus or hand eczema. Treatment of atopic dermatitis involves adequate moisturizing, topical anti-inflammatories, and avoidance of secondary bacterial infection. Topical tacrolimus and pimecrolimus are approved as therapy. They do not cause some of the complications of topical corticosteroids, but recent reports have raised the concern of a potentially increased risk of lymphoma. Children with atopic dermatitis may have spontaneous resolution, but about 40% of children with symptoms will have dermatitis as adults. Interestingly, for unknown reasons the worldwide prevalence of atopic dermatitis is increasing.

XII-4. **The answer is E.** *(Chap. 52)* All patients with psoriasis should be advised to avoid excessive drying of the skin and maintain hydration. Secondary bacterial infection should be suspected with local worsening and treated appropriately. Topical glucocorticoids often cause skin atrophy and lose effectiveness over time. Topical vitamin D analogues and retinoids have effectively replaced topical coal tar, salicylic acid, and anthralin as local adjunctive therapies. UV-A (with psoralen) and/or UV-B light is an effective therapy for widespread psoriasis in many cases. These therapies may be associated with an increased risk of skin cancer, particularly in patients who are immunocompromised. Methotrexate is often effective in patients with psoriatic arthritis (up to 30% of patients with psoriasis). Cyclosporine and other modulators of T-cell mediated immunity are effective in psoriasis. Alefacept is an intramuscular biologic that is anti-CD2 and is indicated in psoriasis. It may cause lymphopenia, increased risk of infection, or secondary malignancy. Infliximab, etanercept, and adalimumab are anti-TNF biologics indicated for use in psoriasis arthritis (etanercept is indicated for psoriasis). They are associated with an increased risk of serious systemic infection, neurologic events (progressive multifocal leukoencephalopathy), and hypersensitivity reactions. Oral glucocorticoids should not be used for the treatment of psoriasis due to the potential for developing life-threatening pustular psoriasis when the therapy is discontinued.

XII-5. **The answer is E.** *(Chap. 54)* Bullous pemphigoid is an autoimmune skin disease associated with the development of tense vesicles and bullae on erythematous bases. The disease is more common in elderly individuals and typically begins as urticarial plaques that are located on the lower abdomen, groin, and flexor surfaces of the extremities. These lesions often evolve to tense bullae on erythematous or normal-appearing skin. Oral mucosal lesions can occur, and pruritus is variable from none to severe. The blisters often rupture with secondary erosions and crusting. Without secondary trauma, these lesions will heal without scarring. Biopsy of early lesions shows subepidermal blisters with a variable inflammatory infiltrate. Lesions on an erythematous base demonstrate eosinophilic infiltrates, whereas lesions on normal skin have minimal perivascular infiltrate only. Direct immunofluorescence shows linear deposits of IgG and C3 along the epidermal basement membranes. In about 70% of individuals, autoantibodies can be found that bind to the epidermal basement membrane. The disease tends to be chronic with relapses and remissions over a period of months to years. The treatment of choice is systemic glucocorticoids at doses of prednisone equivalent to 0.75–1 mg/kg daily.

XII-6. **The answer is D.** *(Chap. 54)* Dermatitis herpetiformis (DH) is an immunologic skin disorder characterized by severe pruritus with skin lesions symmetrically distributed along the extensor surfaces, buttocks, back, scalp, and posterior neck. The lesions of DH may be papular, papulovesicular, or urticarial plaques. Because of the severity of the associated pruritus, many patients do not exhibit the primary skin lesions but have excoriations and crusted papules. Burning and stinging are also frequently reported along with the pruritus, and these symptoms are present prior to the manifestation of skin lesions. Almost all patients have an associated gluten-sensitive enteropathy, although it may be clinically unrecognized on presentation. Pathologically, the lesions demonstrate a neutrophilic inflammatory infiltrate in the dermal papillae. On immunofluorescence, granular deposits of IgA are found in the papillary dermis and along the epidermal basement membrane. The primary treatment of DH is dapsone at doses of 50–200 mg daily with most patients reporting remarkable improvement within 24–48 hours. At doses greater than 100 mg daily, one must pay close attention to side effects as methemoglobinemia and hemolysis frequently occur. In addition to dapsone, gluten-free diets are recommended. However, many months of the diet are required to achieve a clinical benefit and are not recommended as the sole treatment. Corticosteroids are not used in the treatment of DH.

XII-7.   **The answer is A.** *(Chap. 54)* The patient has discoid lupus erythematosus (DLE) or chronic cutaneous lupus erythematosus. It is characterized by discrete lesions most often on the face, scalp, or ears. The lesions are usually erythematous papules or plaques with a thick scale that occludes hair follicles. The lesions persist for years and grow slowly. Less than 10% of patients with DLE meet the criteria for systemic lupus erythematosus (SLE), although skin lesions are common in patients with SLE. Chronically, the lesions evolve to look similar to the one pictured. Treatment consists of topical or intralesional glucocorticoids. If that is ineffective, systemic therapy with an aminoquinoline antimalarial may be indicated. Systemic glucocorticoids or immunosuppressives are not indicated for localized disease. Although malignant melanoma may take on myriad appearances, the location, progress, and description of this lesion is more suggestive of discoid lupus; therefore, surgical excision and lymph node dissection are not indicated at this time. Vitamin E ointment has no proven role in the treatment of DLE.

XII-8.   **The answer is C.** *(Chap. 55)* Stevens-Johnson syndrome (SJS) and toxic epidermal necrolysis (TEN) are the most dreaded drug reactions and are characterized by diffuse blistering and epidermal necrosis with skin detachment. In both syndromes, the lesions typically begin with blisters developing over target lesions with mucosal involvement. In SJS, the amount of skin detachment is between 10% and 30% with the more severe TEN associated with skin detachment of more than 30%. Mortality is directly related to the amount of skin detachment with a mortality of about 10% in SJS and 30% in TEN. Other risk factors for mortality in SJS/TEN include older age and intestinal or pulmonary involvement. The most common drugs to cause SJS/TEN are sulfonamides, allopurinol, nevirapine, lamotrigine, aromatic anticonvulsants, and the oxicam nonsteroidal anti-inflammatory drugs (NSAIDs). There is no evidence that any therapy changes outcomes in SJS or TEN. Clearly, immediate cessation of the offending agent is necessary. Supportive therapy to prevent secondary infections is important. In many instances, these patients are treated in burn wards. Systemic corticosteroids may be useful for the short-term treatment of SJS/TEN, but these drugs increase long-term complications and have a higher associated mortality. Early data suggested that intravenous immunoglobulin (IVIG) may be helpful, but more recent studies have not shown benefit. Future studies are required to determine the role of IVIG in the treatment of SJS/TEN.

XII-9.   **The answer is A.** *(Chap. 55)* Morbilliform drug eruptions are the most common drug reactions. They typically begin on the trunk and consist of symmetric macules and papules that may become confluent. Moderate to severe pruritus is common. In contrast to Stevens-Johnson syndrome and toxic shock syndrome, involvement of the mucous membranes is uncommon. The principal differential diagnosis is viral exanthem, particularly in children. The rash usually develops within 1 week of initiation of therapy and resolves with discontinuation within 2 weeks. The most common drugs that cause morbilliform eruptions include penicillin derivatives, allopurinol, sulfonamides, and nonsteroidal anti-inflammatories. Urticaria consists of superficial well-defined wheals that are pruritic. Penicillins may cause IgE-mediated urticaria. Pemphigus is an autoimmune bullous disease of the skin and mucous membranes that is rarely associated with drugs such as penicillin.

XII-10.   **The answer is A.** *(Chap. 56)* The UV spectrum reaching the earth is arbitrarily divided into two major segments: UV-A and UV-B. The outermost epidermal layer, the stratum corneum, is a major absorber of UV-B, and less than 10% of incident UV-B wavelengths penetrate through the epidermis to the dermis. In contrast, UV-A readily penetrates to the dermis. Photons in the UV-B are 1000-fold more efficient than photons in the UV-A in evoking the sunburn response. UV-B is primarily responsible for the sunburn response and for vitamin D photochemistry. UV-A is important in the pathogenesis of photoaging in human skin.

XII-11. The answer is A. *(Chap. 167)* Nontuberculous mycobacteria (NTM) were originally classified into "fast-growers" and "slow-growers" based on the length of time they took to grow in culture. Although more sophisticated tests have been developed, this classification scheme is still used and is of some benefit to the clinician. Fast-growing NTM include *M. abscessus, M. fortuitum,* and *M. chelonae.* They will typically take 7 days or less to grow on standard media, allowing relatively fast identification and drug-resistance testing. Slow-growing NTM include *M. avium, M. marinum, M. ulcerans,* and *M. kansasii.* They often require special growth media and therefore a high pretest suspicion. The patient described likely has a cutaneous infection from one of the "fast-growing" NTM, which could be diagnosed with tissue biopsy, Gram stain, and culture.

XII-12. The answer is D. *(Chap. 169)* This vignette presents a patient with symptoms consistent with secondary syphilis. The causative organism of syphilis is *Treponema pallidum,* and it can penetrate normal skin to disseminate via the bloodstream long before the appearance of the typical skin lesion of primary syphilis. This lesion appears at the initial site of inoculation only after a period of 4–6 weeks. It will heal spontaneously, and symptoms of secondary syphilis begin approximately 6–8 weeks after it heals. However, as much as 15% of individuals will have evidence of healing chancres at the time of the manifestation of secondary syphilis. The primary manifestations of secondary syphilis are a generalized rash with generalized lymphadenopathy. The skin rash of secondary syphilis is most commonly macular or maculopapular and nonpuritic with a pink color. The rash begins on the trunk and upper extremities and classically progresses to involve the palms and soles. Ten percent of individuals with secondary syphilis also exhibit condylomata lata, which are papular lesions that develop in intertriginous areas. It is notable that the skin lesions of secondary syphilis do harbor bacteria and are infectious. A variety of constitutional symptoms can be present in secondary syphilis including malaise, fever, weight loss, sore throat, and headache.

Diagnosis of secondary syphilis in this patient with a prior diagnosis of syphilis is best accomplished by means of nontreponemal antibody testing. There are two common nontreponemal antibody tests: the rapid plasma reagin (RPR) test and the Venereal Disease Research Laboratory (VDRL) test. This patient's prior syphilis infection was diagnosed and treated based on a positive RPR, which demonstrated the appropriate fourfold decrease in titers after appropriate therapy. As VDRL titers do not directly correspond to RPR titers, it is recommended that sequential testing be performed via the same nontreponemal test. In this case, that would be the RPR, as the VDRL would be difficult to interpret in the absence of previous titers. The fluorescent treponemal antibody test (FTA-Abs) is a specific treponemal antibody test. It does cross-react in the presence of other treponemal infections such as yaws or pinta. More importantly in this case, it remains positive after treatment of prior infection and lacks the ability to differentiate between new and past infections.

Primary HIV infection is certainly a concern in this patient given his risk factors. It can present similarly with a fever, rash, malaise, and generalized lymphadenopathy. The rash of primary HIV infection is also a maculopapular disseminated rash, but it is much less likely to affect the palms and soles. Acute HIV infection would be best diagnosed by obtaining an HIV viral load and would be reasonable to consider as additional testing in this patient, but would not yield the appropriate diagnosis. Given his recent negative antibody testing, the HIV antibody test would not likely be positive in the setting of recent infection.

XII-13. The answer is C. *(Chap. 170)* The lesion shown is typical of primary yaws skin infection caused by the endemic treponeme *T. pallidum* subsp. *Pertenue.* Yaws remains a health problem in parts of West Africa (including Ivory Coast and Ghana), Central Africa Republic, rural Congo, Indonesia, Papua New Guinea, Haiti, and parts of South America. India has not had a reported new case since 2003. As in syphilis, endemic treponemal infections typically have primary, secondary, and late stages. Yaws (also known as pian, framboesia, or bouba) is characterized by a primary raspberry-like lesion at the site of inoculation. Early skin lesions are infectious by contact and may persist for months.

Cutaneous relapses are common, and late disease affects approximately 10% of patients with destructive skin, bone, and joint lesions. Primary infection is often associated with regional lymphadenopathy. Late yaws is characterized by gummas of the bones and skin. Destruction of the nose, maxilla, palate, and pharynx similar to leprosy and leishmaniasis may occur. Darkfield examination is diagnostic, and because of cross-reactivity the same serologic tests used for syphilis are positive. Therapy of yaws is based on treatment of syphilis because there are no controlled treatment trials of yaws. Penicillin, doxycycline, and tetracycline are thought to be effective therapies. Albendazole, ivermectin, and praziquantel are used for a variety of worm infections.

XII-14. **The answer is C.** *(Chap. 174)* The picture shows the characteristic rash of erythema migrans, the defining lesion of Lyme disease caused by *Borrelia burgdorferi*. Erythema migrans appears at the site of the tick bite within 3–32 days following the initial bite. It typically begins as a red macule or papule and expands slowly to form an annular lesion. As the lesion gets larger, the classic targetoid appearance develops with a bright red outer ring as well as ongoing erythema at the central lesion with clearing in between. The most common sites of erythema migrans are the classic locations of tick bites, including the groin, axilla, and thigh. The presence of this lesion in an endemic area for Lyme disease is an indication for treatment and does not require serologic confirmation.

   Anaplasma phagocytophilum is the causative organism of human granulocytic anaplasmosis. This rickettsial disease is also transmitted through a tick bite and is prevalent in the upper Midwest, New England, parts of the Mid-Atlantic, and northern California. Rash occurs in about 6% of cases, although no specific rash is identified. The most common manifestations are fevers, malaise, and myalgia. *Bartonella henselae* (option B) is the organism responsible for cat-scratch fever, which can present with mild erythema near the site of the injury and markedly enlarged lymph nodes. *Ehrlichia chaffeensis* is another rickettsial organism that is transmitted by the bite of a tick and is common in the southeast, northeast, Texas, and California. Human monocytic ehrlichiosis is the disease causes by the organism and presents with nonspecific symptoms of fever, malaise, and myalgia. Rash is also not common in ehrlichiosis. *Rickettsia rickettsii* is the rickettsial organism responsible for Rocky Mountain spotted fever (RMSF). About 90% of individuals with RMSF have a rash during the course of the illness. The rash most commonly presents with diffuse macules beginning on the wrists and ankles, and spreading to the trunk.

XII-15. **The answer is E.** *(Chap. 189)* Dermatologic problems occur in more than 90% of patients with HIV infection. Seborrheic dermatitis is perhaps the most common rash in HIV-infected patients, affecting up to 50% of patients. The prevalence increases with falling CD4+ T-cell count. The rash involves the scalp and the face, appearing as described in the question. Therapy is standard topical treatment, although often a topical antifungal is added because of concomitant infection with *Pityrosporum*. Herpes zoster reactivation is painful and dermatomal, with progression of papules to vesicles to small pustules and then crusting. Molluscum contagiosum typically appears as one or many small pearly umbilicated asymptomatic papules occurring anywhere on the body. They can be a significant cosmetic issue in patients with AIDS. Psoriasis is not more common in patients with HIV infection but may be more severe and generalized. It would be uncommon to involve the face only. Kaposi's sarcoma is due to coinfection with HHV-8 in patients with HIV/AIDS. It typically presents as more than one red/purple nodular painless lesion anywhere on the body.

XII-16. **The answer is B.** *(Chap. 206)* Tinea versicolor is the most common superficial skin infection. It is caused by lipophilic yeasts of the genus *Malassezia*, most commonly *M. furfur*. In tropical areas, the prevalence of tinea versicolor is 40–60%, whereas in temperate areas it is about 1%. In general, most individuals seek evaluation for cosmetic reasons as the lesions in tinea versicolor are asymptomatic or only mildly pruritic. The lesions typically appear as patches of pink or coppery-brown skin, but the areas may be hypopigmented in dark-skinned individuals. Diagnosis can be made by demonstrating the organism on potassium hydroxide preparation where a typical "spaghetti and meatballs" appearance may be seen. This is due to the presence of both spore forms and hyphal forms within the skin. Under long-wave UV-A light (Wood's lamp), the affected areas fluoresce to yellow-green. The organism is sensitive to a variety of antifungals. Selenium sulfide shampoo, topical azoles, terbinafine, and ciclopirox have all been used with success. A 2-week treatment regimen typically shows good results, but the infection typically recurs within 2 years of initial treatment. *Fusarium solani* is an environmental fungus that usually causes infection in immunocompromised hosts. It can cause keratitis, onychomycosis, pneumonia, and hematogenous dissemination. *Sporothrix schenckii* is the usual etiologic agent of sporotrichosis. *Penicillium marneffei* is endemic in Vietnam, Thailand, and other southeast Asian countries. It causes a clinical syndrome similar to disseminated histoplasmosis. *Trichophyton rubrum* is a dermatophyte that causes ringworm.

XII-17. **The answer is D.** *(Chap. 358)* This patient has porphyria cutanea tarda (PCT). The major clinical feature of PCT is scarring skin lesions predominantly affecting the back of the hands that also may involve the forearms, face, legs, and feet. The lesions start as blisters that rupture and crust over, leaving scarring. Chronically, the areas most involved can develop thickened skin similar to systemic sclerosis. PCT is the most common porphyria; it usually occurs sporadically, but there is also a familial form. It is due to a deficiency of hepatic URO-decarboxylase, which must have more than 20% activity for symptoms. Excess hepatic iron is involved in the pathogenesis, and phlebotomy aiming for a low normal ferritin is a component of treatment. Precipitating factors should be avoided. Episodes are typically provoked by alcohol intake or sun exposure. Plasma porphyrins should be measured in patients suspected of PCT. Urinary ALA may be slightly increased, but urinary porphobilinogen is normal. Urine porphobilinogen is elevated during attacks of acute intermittent porphyria. ANA is utilized in the diagnosis of SLE, which may present with photosensitivity. Anti-SCL-70 is used to diagnose systemic sclerosis, which may also present with thick skin.

XII-18. **The answer is D.** *(Chap. 397)* Scabies, the human itch mite, remains a common problem due to its high degree of infectivity and ability to cause symptoms. It is a common reason for seeking attention from dermatologists and is thought to affect over 300 million people worldwide. Transfer is facilitated by intimate contact, and outbreaks may occur in nursing homes, mental institutions, and hospitals. The itching and rash associated with scabies derive from a sensitization reaction directed against the excreta that the mite deposits in its burrow. An initial infestation remains asymptomatic for up to 6 weeks, and a reinfestation produces a hypersensitivity reaction without delay. Intense itching worsens at night and after a hot shower. Typical burrows may be difficult to find because they are few in number and may be obscured by excoriations. Burrows appear as dark wavy lines in the epidermis and measure up to 15 mm. Lesions occur most frequently on the volar wrists, between the fingers, on the elbows, and on the penis. Small papules and vesicles, often accompanied by eczematous plaques, pustules, or nodules, are distributed symmetrically in those sites and in skinfolds under the breasts and around the navel, axillae, belt line, buttocks, upper thighs, and scrotum. Except in infants, the face, scalp, neck, palms, and soles are spared. Burrows should be sought and unroofed with a sterile needle or scalpel blade, and the scrapings should be examined microscopically for the mite, its eggs, and its fecal pellets. Permethrin cream is effective therapy. Ivermectin has not been approved by the U.S. Food and Drug Administration (FDA) for use against any form of scabies, but a single oral dose effectively treats scabies in otherwise healthy persons. Ceftriaxone plus azithromycin is recommended treatment for suspected gonorrhea and chlamydia infection, and metronidazole for trichomonas in women. The lesions shown in Figure XII-18 are not consistent with the single painless chancre of syphilis that is treated with penicillin G.

COLOR ATLAS

Monocular Prechiasmal Field Defects:

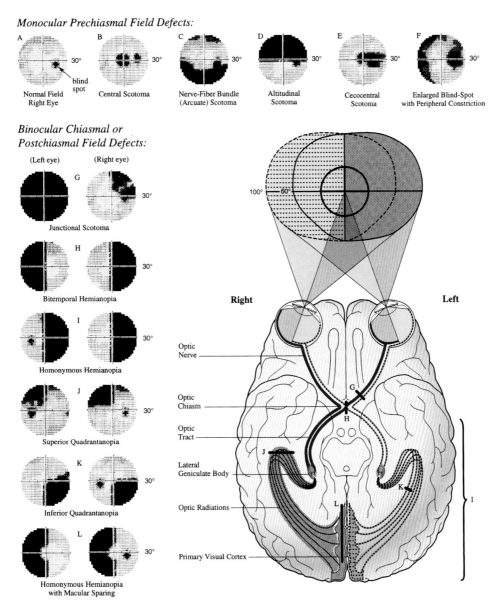

A — Normal Field Right Eye · 30° · blind spot

B — Central Scotoma · 30°

C — Nerve-Fiber Bundle (Arcuate) Scotoma · 30°

D — Altitudinal Scotoma · 30°

E — Cecocentral Scotoma · 30°

F — Enlarged Blind-Spot with Peripheral Constriction · 30°

Binocular Chiasmal or Postchiasmal Field Defects:

(Left eye) (Right eye)

G — Junctional Scotoma · 30°

H — Bitemporal Hemianopia · 30°

I — Homonymous Hemianopia · 30°

J — Superior Quadrantanopia · 30°

K — Inferior Quadrantanopia · 30°

L — Homonymous Hemianopia with Macular Sparing · 30°

100° · 60° · 30°

Right

Left

Optic Nerve

Optic Chiasm

Optic Tract

Lateral Geniculate Body

Optic Radiations

Primary Visual Cortex

FIGURE I-94

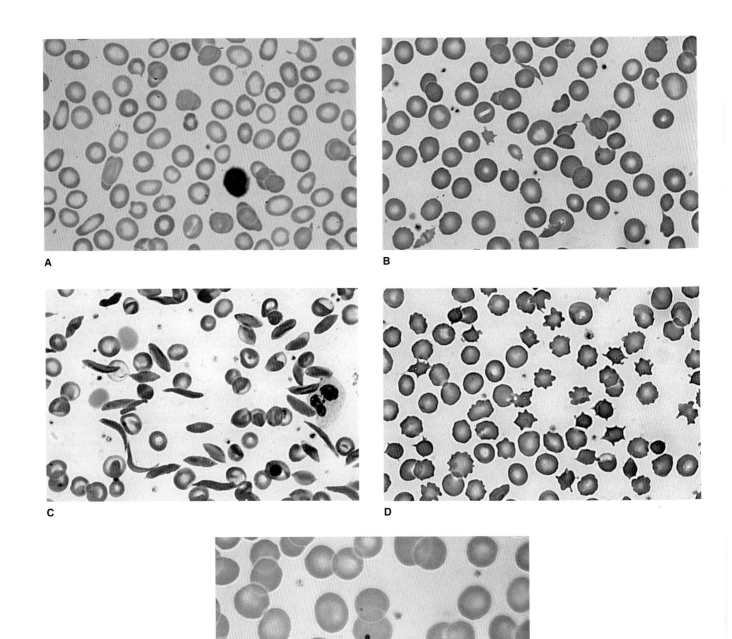

A

B

C

D

E

FIGURE III-1 A-E

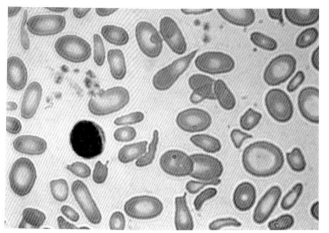

FIGURE III-2

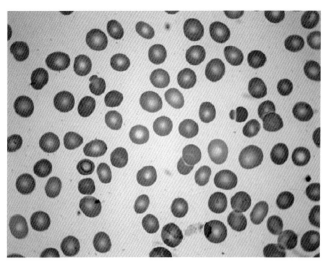

FIGURE III-67

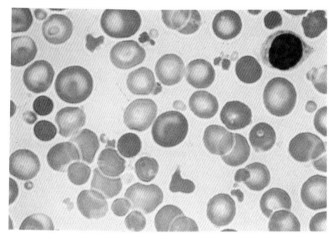

FIGURE III-4

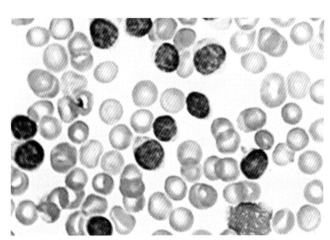

FIGURE III-89

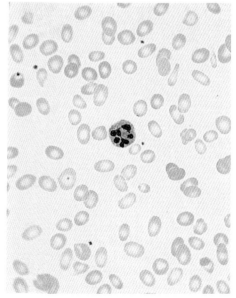

FIGURE III-64

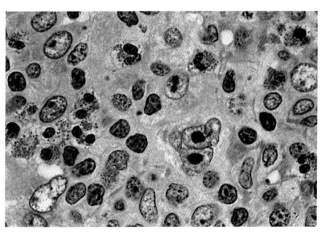

FIGURE III-91

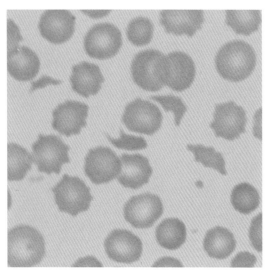

FIGURE III-99

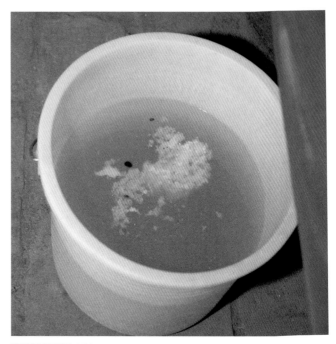

FIGURE IV-100

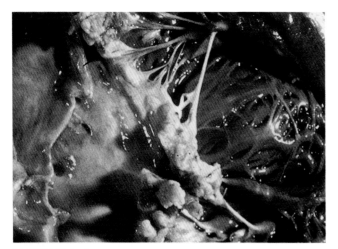

FIGURE IV-13

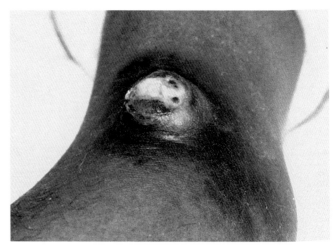

FIGURE IV-104

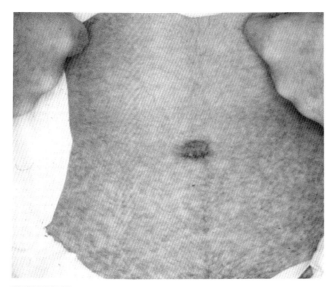

FIGURE IV-143

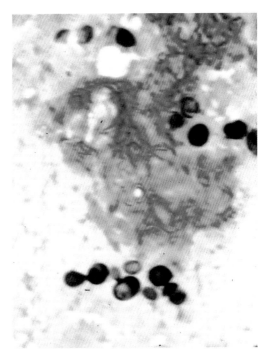

FIGURE IV-188

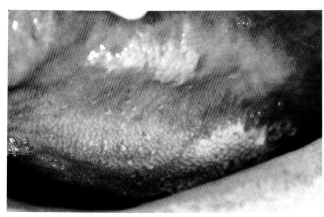

FIGURE IV-173

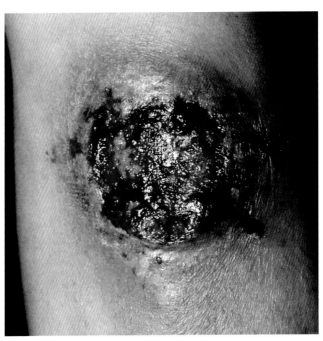

FIGURE IV-194 *(Used with permission from Elizabeth M. Spiers, MD.)*

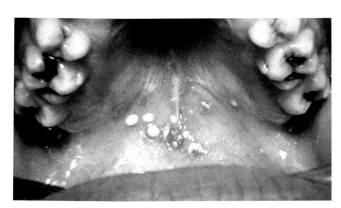

FIGURE IV-179

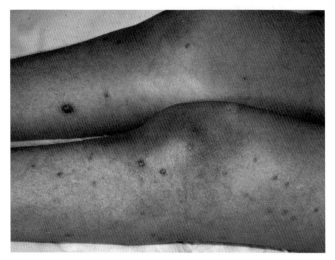

FIGURE IV-198

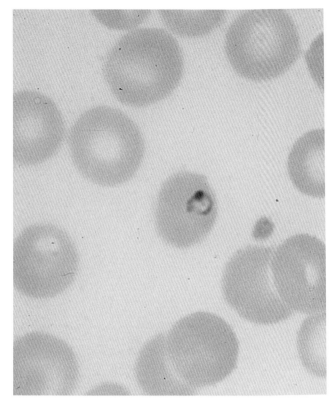

FIGURE IV-219

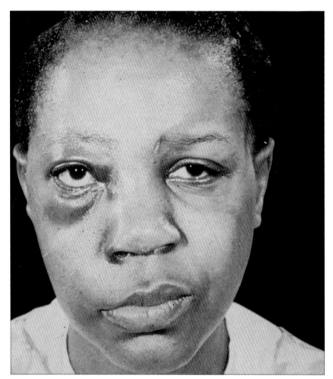

FIGURE IV-210

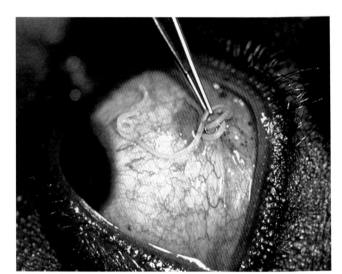

FIGURE IV-245

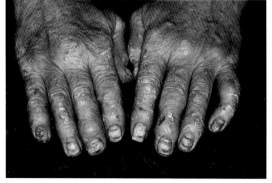

FIGURE IX-40

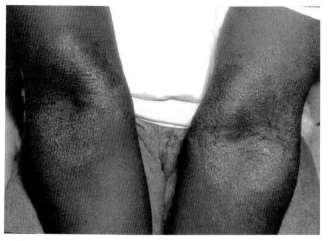

FIGURE XII-3 (Courtesy of Robert Swerlick, MD; with permission.)

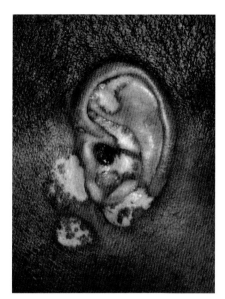

FIGURE XII-7

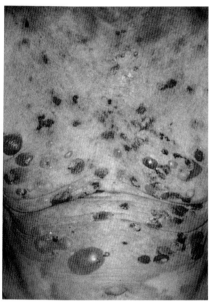

FIGURE XII-5 (Courtesy of the Yale Resident's Slide Collection; with permission.)

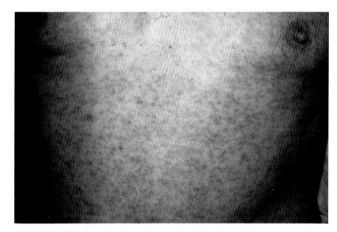

FIGURE XII-9

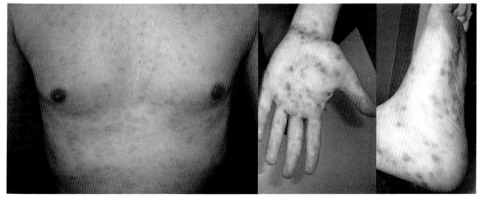

FIGURE XII-12 (Courtesy of Jill McKenzie and Christina Marra.)

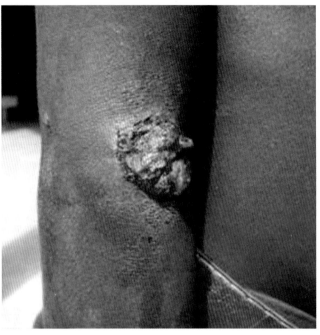

FIGURE XII-13

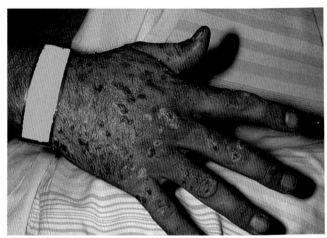

FIGURE XII-17 (*Courtesy of Dr. Karl E. Anderson; with permission.*)

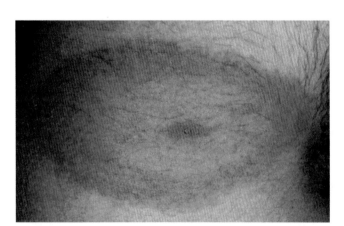

FIGURE XII-14 (*Courtesy of Vijay K. Sikand, MD; with permission.*)

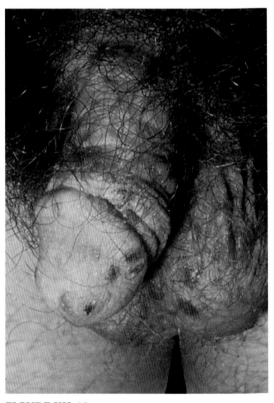

FIGURE XII-18

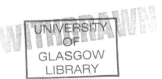